Jianne Lien

Scott-Brown's Otolaryngology
Fifth edition

Paediatric Otolaryngology

Scott-Brown's Otolaryngology

Fifth edition

General Editor

Alan G. Kerr FRCS

Consultant Otolaryngologist, Royal Victoria Hospital, Belfast and Belfast City Hospital;
Formerly Professor of Otorhinolaryngology, The Queen's University, Belfast

Advisory Editor

John Groves FRCS

Consultant Otolaryngologist, Royal Free Hospital, London

Other volumes

1 **Basic Sciences** *edited by* David Wright

2 **Adult Audiology** *edited by* Dafydd Stephens

3 **Otology** *edited by* John B. Booth

4 **Rhinology** *edited by* Ian S. Mackay and T. R. Bull

5 **Laryngology** *edited by* P. M. Stell

Paediatric Otolaryngology

Editor

John N. G. Evans MB, BS, DLO, FRCS

Consultant Ear, Nose and Throat Surgeon, The Hospitals for Sick Children, Great Ormond Street, and St Thomas's Hospital, London

Butterworths

London   Boston   Durban   Singapore   Sydney   Toronto   Wellington

First edition, 1952
Second edition, 1965
   Reprinted, 1967, 1968
Third edition, 1971
   Reprinted, 1977
Fourth edition, 1979
   Reprinted 1984
Fifth edition, 1987

Butterworth International Edition, 1987

ISBN-0-407-00518-8   ISBN-0-407-00521-8
ISBN-0-407-00522-6   ISBN-0-407-00523-4
ISBN-0-407-00524-2   ISBN-0-407-00525-0
ISBN-0-407-00517-X (set of six volumes)

© **Butterworth & Co. (Publishers) Ltd, 1987**

British Library Cataloguing in Publication Data

Scott-Brown, Walter Graham
    Scott-Brown's otolaryngology.—5th ed.
    1. Otolaryngology
    I. Title   II. Kerr, A. G.   III. Groves, John,
    1925-   IV. Scott-Brown, Walter Graham.
    Scott-Brown's diseases of the ear, nose and throat
    617'.57   RF46

    ISBN 0-407-00511-0   ISBN 0-407-00512-9
    ISBN 0-407-00513-7   ISBN 0-407-00514-5
    ISBN 0-407-00515-3   ISBN 0-407-00516-1
    ISBN 0-407-00510-2 (set of six volumes)

Library of Congress Cataloging-in-Publication Data
Paediatric otolaryngology.

    (Scott-Brown's otolaryngology; v. 6)
    Includes bibliographies and indexes.
    1. Paediatric otolaryngology.   I. Evans, John N. G.
II. Series.   [DNLM: 1. Otorhinolaryngologic Diseases—in infancy
and childhood. WV 100 S4313 v. 6]   RF20.S37   vol. 6
617'.51 s   87-15105   [RF47.C4]   [618.92'09751]
ISBN 0-407-00516-1

Photoset by Butterworths Litho Preparation Department
Printed and bound in Great Britain by Butler and Tanner, Frome, Somerset

Historical introduction

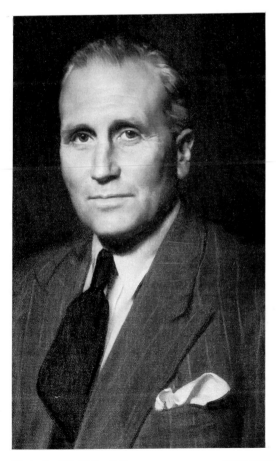

Portrait of W. G. Scott-Brown, CVO, MD, FRCS (1897–1987)

About 36 years ago Bill Scott-Brown suffered a major coronary infarct and being strictly ordered to 'rest' for six months set himself to create, as Editor (not author, because that would have been too strenuous, he thought) this work of his own inspiration. In 1952 I was among the first generation of FRCS candidates for whom it was the Bible. We all revered 'Negus' for the nose and throat (some of us still do) but Scott-Brown, in two volumes as it then was, provided the first post-war text for otolaryngology across the board. SB (as he was known) was probably the only person to be at all surprised by the success of his achievement, and to find himself in due course under notice from Butterworth's to prepare a second edition. It was at this stage that he recruited John Ballantyne and myself and the second, third and fourth editions were produced by the two of us under his friendly eye. For the third edition we succumbed to the inevitable by expanding two fat volumes into four (slightly) thinner ones, only to find that the fourth edition in its turn required four fat ones.

Throughout this 20 year period John Ballantyne and I derived constant satisfaction and pleasure from the ongoing association with so many willing friends and contributors past and present. We thank them warmly.

We know that the ENT fraternity world-wide has pleasure in the knowledge that SB continued in his retirement still to take satisfaction from the perpetuation of his work. The sad news of his death came just as this new edition went to press. Those who knew him will perhaps see in this Fifth Edition, and the 35th year of his book, a memorial to his achievement.

John Groves
Advisory Editor

Introduction

When I was first invited to edit the Fifth Edition of *Scott-Brown's Otolaryngology*, I thought I was aware of the enormity of the task and my own limitations. As time progressed, I realized that I had misjudged both.

This work has represented the mainstream of British otolaryngological thinking for over thirty years. However, the increase in the breadth and depth of our specialty is such that only a gifted few can be conversant with all aspects of it. Hence, I realized that I could not undertake the task without help. I have been most fortunate in having such a distinguished group of volume editors, all of whom are already well-known in British otolaryngology, and all of whom have beeen delightful and stimulating colleagues in this work. It has been a joy to work with them.

Modern otolaryngology has widened in recent decades, and procedures are now being performed that are no longer covered by the term 'ear, nose and throat surgery'. This work attempts to embrace all the areas that so-called ear, nose and throat surgeons are covering at the present time, and hence the change of the title to *Scott-Brown's Otolaryngology*.

For the new edition *Scott-Brown* has grown from four to six volumes. An entirely new volume has been introduced in recognition of the subspecialty of paediatric otolaryngology and the amount of material in audiological medicine is now great enough to justify its separation from the Ear volume. Although these are now specialties in their own rights, they are also, and will continue to be beyond the lifetime of this edition, part of the routine practice of most British otolaryngologists. To enable these new volumes to stand alone, a certain amount of overlap with other volumes has been necessary.

In any multi-author and multi-volume production, overlap is always necessary if each chapter is to be developed freely, and if there is to be easy reference to subjects dealt with in more than one volume. Consequently, I ask for the reader's indulgence in those sections where overlap has been planned and deliberate. Where it has occurred as a result of my ineptitude, I apologize.

The editorial team have been very pleased at the response of those invited to contribute, although, unfortunately, a few leading members of our specialty were unable to accept the invitation. However, by and large, those asked were both cooperative and energetic in their responses, and have given freely of themselves in their contributions. I have been most impressed by the spirit of goodwill among the otolaryngologists in this country, and I am grateful to them.

In the production of this edition, I have seen myself as custodian of a great British institution. I have always been aware of the privilege and responsibility of my position, and am grateful for the advice I have received from many senior and not so senior members of our specialty. I am particularly indebted to the Advisory Editor, John Groves, and to his former editorial colleague, John Ballantyne. My respect and admiration for these colleagues has risen, not simply because of the invaluable help they have given so freely in this edition, but because I now realise the enormity of their accomplishment and their contribution to British otolaryngology in editing the last three editions.

I also wish to express my thanks to those in Belfast who have helped with, or suffered because of, the Fifth Edition. Some have done both, and without their backing and encouragement this work would not have been possible. It would be invidious to try to name everyone. Various secretaries have been of enormous help, and without this I could not have produced this edition. My consultant colleagues have advised and encouraged me, and my junior colleagues have given very practical advice in their down-to-earth comments and invaluable help with proof-reading. My family have been both encouraging and remarkably tolerant of the long hours required to edit such a work as this.

The staff at Butterworths were helpful and encouraging throughout. Initially, Peter Richardson set the wheels in motion. He was followed as publisher by Charles Fry, who was assisted by Anne Smith and Jane Bryant. The sub-editors have been Anne Powell and Jane Sugarman. The general spirit of pleasant cooperation and tolerance has been delightful.

I am sufficiently optimistic to believe that there will be a Sixth Edition. I do not know who will be editing it. However, if the reader has any constructive comments or criticisms, I should be pleased to have them … in writing! I can not guarantee to acknowledge these, but I promise that, if I am the editor, I shall give them due consideration, and, if not, I shall make them available to my successor.

Alan G. Kerr

Preface

This is the first comprehensive textbook on Paediatric Otolaryngology to be published in the British Isles since T. G. Wilson's *Diseases of the Ear, Nose and Throat in Children*. The fact that Paediatric Otolaryngology now merits a complete volume in a standard otolaryngology text is a fitting tribute to the established importance of this branch of the specialty. It gives me great pleasure to acknowledge the magnitude of Bob Pracy's contribution to this achievment. I was delighted therefore that he agreed to write the introduction to this volume and that he was persuaded to write the chapter on congenital anomalies of the ear. I am most grateful for his friendship, guidance and wise counsel during an extremely happy and rewarding association at The Hospitals for Sick Children.

I would like also to thank my colleagues and the nursing staff at Great Ormond Street for their help and guidance, and Martin Bailey for his support and help in preparing manuscripts. I am greatly indebted to Ted Battersby whose unrivalled ability to anaesthetize very sick babies with precarious airways has helped immeasurably in the development of techniques for the correction of airway disorders in infants. I would like also to thank my old chief Sir Geoffrey Bateman who stimulated my interest in laryngeal and tracheal stenosis during my training at St Thomas's Hospital. It was he who first suggested using a 'swiss-roll' of silastic sheeting as an internal splint for laryngotracheal stenosis.

It is with gratitude that I acknowledge all the contributors, who have given unstintingly of their time and expertise and without whom a book of this wide-ranging complexity would be impossible to assemble. My grateful thanks go also to the publishers for their forbearance and especially to Alan Kerr for his indefatigable patience and unfailing politeness at all times.

To Mrs Sara Wood my secretary I owe a particular debt since without her help and organizational skills this book would not have been published. Above all I would like to acknowledge the unfailing support of my wife and family during the preparation of this volume.

John Evans
London 1987

'The child first and always'

Contributors to this volume

David A. Adams, BSc, MSc, FRCS (Ed)
Senior Lecturer, Department of Otolaryngology,
The Queen's University, Belfast

C. M. Bailey, BSc, FRCS
Consultant Otolaryngologist, The Hospitals for
Sick Children, Great Ormond Street and The
Royal National Throat, Nose and Ear Hospital,
London

Edward F. Battersby, MB, ChB, DA, FFARCS
Consultant Anaesthetist, The Hospitals for Sick
Children, Great Ormond Street, London

Sue Bellman, MA, MB, BChir (Cantab), FRCSI, DLO
Consultant Audiological Physician, The Hospitals
for Sick Children, Great Ormond Street, London

Denzil N. Brooks, PhD
Regional Audiology Unit, Withington Hospital,
Manchester

Michael J. Cinnamond, FRCS (Ed)
Professor and Head of Department, Department
of Otorhinolaryngology, The Queen's University,
Belfast

Charles B. Croft, FRCS, FRCS (Ed)
Consultant Surgeon, The Royal National Throat,
Nose and Ear Hospital, London

Robert Dinwiddie, MB, FRCP, DCH
Consultant Paediatrician, The Hospitals for Sick
Children, Great Ormond Street, London

Adrian Brendan Drake-Lee, MB, ChB, FRCS
Consultant ENT Surgeon, Queen Elizabeth
Hospital, Birmingham; Honorary Senior Lecturer,
The Institute of Laryngology and Otology,
London

P. D. M. Ellis, MA, FRCS
Consultant ENT Surgeon, Addenbrooke's
Hospital, Cambridge

John N. G. Evans, MB, BS, DLO, FRCS (Eng)
Consultant Ear, Nose and Throat Surgeon, The
Hospitals for Sick Children, Great Ormond Street
and St. Thomas's Hospital, London

George Robert Fraser, MD (Camb), PhD, DSc (Lond),
FRCP (C)
Consultant in Genetics, Imperial Cancer Research
Fund; Honorary Consultant in Medical Genetics,
Oxfordshire Health Authority; Honorary Visiting
Geneticist, St Bartholomew's Hospital, London

Andrew P. Freeland, MB, BS, FRCS
Consultant Otolaryngologist, Radcliffe Infirmary,
Oxford; Clinical Lecturer, University of Oxford

John Hibbert, MA, ChM, FRCS
Consultant ENT Surgeon, Guy's Hospital, London

Martyn L. Hyde, PhD
Research Fellow, Mount Sinai Hospital, Toronto;
Associate Professor of Otolaryngology, University
of Toronto

David R. James, FRCS(Ed), FDSRCS(Eng)
Consultant Oral and Maxillofacial Surgeon, Centre
for Craniofacial Anomalies, The Hospitals for Sick
Children, Great Ormond Street, and University
College Hospital, London

Douglas S. McManamny, MB, BS, FRACS
Plastic and Reconstructive Surgeon, 29 Royal
Parade, Parkville, Victoria; Associate Plastic
Surgeon, Royal Children's Hospital, Melbourne

A. Richard Maw, MB, BS, MS, FRCS
Consultant Otolaryngologist, Bristol Royal
Infirmary and The Royal Hospital for Sick
Children, Bristol; Clinical Lecturer and Head of
the Department of Otolaryngology, University of
Bristol

Ronald W. Pigott, BA, MB, FRCS, FRCS(I)
Consultant Plastic Surgeon, South Western
Regional Health Authority, Frenchay Hospital,
Bristol

Peter D. Phelps, MD (Lond), FRCS, FRCR, DMRD
Consultant Radiologist, Walsgrave Hospital,
Coventry; Honorary Consultant, Royal National
Throat, Nose and Ear Hospital, London

D. A. Plint, BDS (Rand), FDSRCS, DOrth(Eng)
Consultant Dental Surgeon in Orthodontics and
Children's Dentistry, The Hospitals for Sick
Children, Great Ormond Street, London;
Consultant Orthodontist, University College
Hospital Dental School, London; Late Consultant,
Royal Dental Hospital, London

P. N. Plowman, MA, MD, MRCP, FRCP
Consultant, Department of Oncology, The
Hospitals for Sick Children, Great Ormond Street;
Department of Radiotherapy, St Bartholomew's
Hospital, London

Robert Pracy, MB, BS (Lond), FRCS (Eng), FRCSI (Hon),
MPhil (Lond)
Formerly Dean, The Institute of Laryngology and
Otology, Consultant Surgeon, The Hospitals for
Sick Children, Great Ormond Street; Consultant
Surgeon, The Royal National Throat and Ear
Hospital, London

Jon Pritchard, FRCP
Consultant and Senior Lecturer, Hospital for Sick
Children and Institute of Child Health, London;
Honorary Consultant in Paediatric Oncology, St
Bartholomew's Hospital, Oxford, and Oxford
Regional Health Authority

Joselen Ransome, MB, BS, FRCS
Honorary Consultant in Otolaryngology, Charing
Cross Hospital; Consultant Emeritus in
Otolaryngology, St Mary Abbot's and St Stephen's
Hospitals, London

J. H. Rogers, MA, BM, BCh, FRCS, DLO
Consultant Ear, Nose and Throat Surgeon, Royal
Liverpool Hospital, and Royal Liverpool
Children's Hospital, Alder Hey

Lewis Rosenbloom, MB, ChB, FRCP (Lond), DCH(Eng)
Consultant Paediatric Neurologist, Royal
Liverpool Children's Hospital, Alder Hey,
Liverpool

Debbie Sell, LCST, MCST
Speech Therapy Department, The Hospitals for
Sick Children, Great Ormond Street, London

O. H. Shaheen, MS, FRCS
Consultant Otolaryngologist, Guy's Hospital and
Royal National Throat, Nose and Ear Hospital,
London

Susan Snashall, MB, BS (Lond)
Consultant Audiological Physician, Royal Surrey
County Hospital, Guildford

Lewis Spitz, PhD, FRCS
Nuffield Professor of Paediatric Surgery, Institute
of Child Health, University of London; Consultant
Paediatric Surgeon, The Hospitals for Sick
Children, Great Ormond Street, London

M. Stuart Strong, MD, FRCS (Eng)
Associate Chief of Staff for Ambulatory Care,
Bedford VA Medical Center

Gillian M. Tym, SRN, RSCN
Sister in Charge, Tracheostomy Unit, The
Hospitals for Sick Children, Great Ormond Street,
London

Contents

Colour plates in this volume

1

Introduction

Robert Pracy

Why have a volume devoted to the otorhinolaryngological problems of children? The reason is that, over the past 25 years, otorhinolaryngologists all over the world have come to appreciate that children have special problems and, more important, that children do not react to disease in the same way as adults.

History

The first attempts to stimulate a special interest in the otorhinolaryngological problems of children occurred in Poland in the 1930s. The pioneer in the field was Professor Jan Danielowicz of Warsaw. Many children were referred to him with strictures of the oesophagus and he rapidly came to appreciate that they did not react, and that they should not be managed, in the same way as adults. After the Second World War Poland became one of the countries of the Soviet bloc and the spread of interest in this discipline to the West was delayed. When the immediate post-war crisis was over and doctors began to travel again between the East and West contacts were made. Professor Gatti Mancini of Brescia, Italy, worked hard to build up the speciality in Europe. North America followed suit and made rapid progress in the field aided by the establishment of professorial chairs in the speciality. In the UK interest has been slow to develop but has now reached the point where it is recognized that there are conditions which are better managed by those with a special interest in the problems of children. In the larger cities centres are developing where children with the rarer problems of paediatric otolaryngology can be both investigated and managed.

Development versus maturity

The majority of hospital patients are adults. This is because, on the whole, childhood is a period of health rather than a period susceptible to disease. In early life the commonest cause of death is malignant disease, including the embryomata and the malignant blood disorders. Between the ages of 3 and 15 years the commonest cause of death is an accident. Thus the average doctor has very little appreciation of the processes of maturation which are so vital to an understanding of paediatrics. It is of fundamental importance to realize that the child is not just 'a small adult' anatomically, physiologically or immunologically. The rates of growth in the different 'systems' vary with age (*Figure 1.1*).

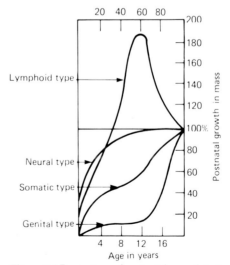

Figure 1.1 Percentage of postnatal growth in time (taken from Minckler (1971) *Pathobiology*, with permission)

1

Obviously during the first year of life there is immense activity in both the peripheral and central nervous systems. Normal progress in the achievement of muscular control and the acquisition of knowledge about the environment by the use of sight and sound are essential for any child to be able to lead a 'normal' existence. The acquisition of skills through the medium of the nervous system is the yardstick that the family use to predict the child's future. However, in order that the nervous system should be permitted to develop most advantageously the other less glamorous support systems of oxygen transport and waste disposal, the gastrointestinal system and the immunological system must be developed too. Happily, at the time of writing, breast-feeding is fashionable once again and this means that there is a period of passive immunity conferred from the mother's milk. It also means that there is less possibility of the early development of infantile atopic disease which can cause so much distress. In susceptible children atopy is eleven times more common in those fed upon artificial milk than among the breast-fed.

The development of immune competence is just as important for the child as the more spectacular feats of the central nervous system. Once passive immunity is lost the child has to acquire immunity by exposure to disease. It is desirable that this immunity should be acquired gradually by exposure to the less serious infections first of all. However, it is of paramount importance that any possibility of infection should be avoided in the first weeks of life. It is for this reason that children who are born in hospital should be discharged as early as possible after delivery so that they are not exposed to those 'antibiotic-resistant' infections which are endemic in hospital. The complete lack of immune competence in the early days of life will lead almost inevitably to a fatal outcome.

The otolaryngologist expects to see more children in his practice than specialists in disciplines other than paediatrics because the natural development of the young child involves the transfer of respiratory infection from one child to another. Inevitably the symptoms and signs of infection, particularly in a first child cause parental anxiety and lead them to seek medical advice. When, as is sometimes the case, these infections are frequent and debilitating it is possible that the primary care doctor will refer the child, asking whether surgery is indicated. However, the ablation, or the attempted ablation, of lymphoid tissue in Waldeyer's ring should always be looked upon as the last resort. Even though the outcome is seldom fatal the effect on the child's immune system may be to produce recurring morbidity with a marked tendency to the development of atopy. A great deal of unnecessary and potentially harmful surgery can be avoided by explaining to the parents exactly what is happening to their child, emphasizing that this is a necessary part of the normal process of development and that surgery should be resorted to only when it is clear that the general development is being hindered as a result of repeated respiratory infections.

The approach

The surgeon whose advice is sought for a child has to ask himself initially, 'is this part of the normal process of development?' or, 'how far has development advanced in this particular child?' Having satisfied himself as to the answers to these questions he must ask himself, 'what will happen to the child's development if I decide upon active surgical treatment?' and then again, 'what will *not* happen to the patient's development if I operate?' In many cases the answer will be clear. For example there is little time to be lost in cases of acute respiratory obstruction and almost unlimited time available when faced with a unilateral aplasia of the ear with good hearing on the other side. However, he must take endless pains to 'carry' the parents with him all the way. Immense technical skill is of no avail if the parents do not understand what is proposed for their child and they can undoubtedly communicate their anxiety to the patient. It is equally important to have an excellent rapport with the patient and time is not wasted if every effort is made to communicate with the child without condescension. Children do not appreciate being 'talked down to' and if approached in a compassionate and kindly manner make excellent patients. They do not like being hurt any more than adults; but they are prepared to suffer some discomfort if they understand that this may be necessary to make them better.

Since approximately one-third of all outpatients attending departments of otolaryngology are children, it is highly desirable that only those who enjoy working with children and who can therefore develop a good rapport with them should consider training in the speciality. Experience in paediatrics is clearly desirable for the trainee surgeon; experience in paediatric nursing should be mandatory for those responsible for the inpatient care. Although there are physicians specializing in paediatric audiology in many centres in the country, it is necessary also for the paediatric otolaryngologist to have the expertise to make a first assessment of the hearing capability, because many of the first referrals are to the surgeon rather than to the audiological physician.

What type of work should be referred to the special centre? Special centres have personnel expert in dealing with both acute and chronic respiratory obstruction. Nursing in the early stages of treatment calls for experts who are trained to detect those signs which indicate that the airway is compromised and that active measures are called for, such as the cleaning of a tracheostomy tube or suction of the tracheobronchial tree. Endoscopy, requiring the use of special small laryngoscopes and bronchoscopes may be required and it is preferable that such investigations are carried out by those surgeons and anaesthetists trained in the procedure. Special centres accumulate experience in the management of the congenital abnormalities of the ear and the nose in addition to those of the laryngotracheobronchial tree, and it is desirable that patients with such disorders should be referred to the special centre. The surgeon working in such a centre will also be called upon by his paediatrician colleagues for advice about those children with syndromes containing otorhinolaryngological signs.

The surgeon working in a mixed adult/paediatric department must be able to manage the spectrum of the normal child's problems and must therefore be conversant with the essential differences in the response to disease, to inflammation and to repair, for such knowledge affects the advice which is tendered and the timing of possible surgery.

Advances in knowledge of how the immature human being reacts to disease has accumulated rapidly over the past 25 years. Advances in technology of both optics and electronics have extended the possibilities both for investigation and surgical management. The pharmacological chemists have produced a bewildering array of preparations which are said to satisfy the needs in management for many of the intractable conditions of former years.

However, there is much work still to be done in research in paediatric otolaryngology before such technology can be exploited to the full. Although a vast amount of work has been undertaken on the processes by which the child's immune system is gradually changed to the adult pattern, there is still a great deal to be discovered about which children are liable to have abnormal patterns of immunity and how such children can be expected to react when exposed to particular allergens.

Antibiotics are still used, particularly in primary care, with too little thought as to possible sequelae and the development of sensitivity. Knowledge of the effects of deafness in childhood has been gathered over 65 years and, happily in this field, thanks to the work of educationalists such as Sir Alexander Ewing, the UK was among the countries who pioneered research. However, with the access to antibiotics the acute infections of previous generations of young children have been aborted but less florid deafness, in the form of secretory otitis media – the so-called 'glue ear' – has produced a serious problem in education. On the whole, the approach to the management of these conditions has been empirical. Drainage tubes for secretory otitis media can certainly offset the problems of deafness, only to leave the problem of tympanosclerosis in its wake. There is therefore an urgent need for systematic research into all phases of development in this field in order to temper the judgement and to improve prognosis and management. Money is never found easily for such projects but a small amount of money spent now could reduce morbidity in the next generation and cut the costs of looking after the sick child.

Reference

MINCKLER, J. (1971) Disturbances in growth. In *Pathobiology: An Introduction*, edited by J. Minckler, H. B. Anstall and T. M. Minckler, pp. 117–126. St Louis: C. V. Mosby Company

2

Radiology of the ear, nose and throat

P. D. Phelps

The principles of technique which apply to imaging in adults apply equally to the demonstration of head and neck lesions in infants and children. Optimum spatial and density resolution with lowest possible level of patient irradiation and freedom from movement artefacts must be achieved. Limitation of radiation dose is particularly important in this age group, and minimal patient movement is hard to obtain. Consequently, many of the more sophisticated modes of imaging such as xerography, conventional tomography and computerized tomography (CT) are used less in the younger age group and most imaging assessments rely on plain films. However, the role of CT continues to increase and, with scan times of a few seconds possible on the latest machines, these examinations can now usually be performed without sedation.

Sedation and anaesthesia in paediatric radiology

A completely immobile patient is necessary for most imaging, especially when there are long radiographic exposure times. This may be difficult to achieve in young patients, especially those who are hyperactive, mentally retarded or disturbed; Hutton (1981) has described a regimen of sedation and anaesthesia for children undergoing tomography and electrocochleography. He recommends ketamine anaesthesia for children under 3 years of age, and conventional inhalation anaesthesia for those above this age.

Upper respiratory tract

Air within the structures of the upper respiratory tract provides a natural contrast medium for the accurate delineation and evaluation of the adjacent soft tissues of the neck. Most of these assessments are made on the lateral neck film obtained during inspiration with the neck partially extended. Additional views can be employed as the need arises, and radiology can often provide information as to the specific cause of airway obstruction and to its site. Well-coned frontal and lateral films are obtained; inspiratory and expiratory films may be needed in each projection to reveal the abnormality fully.

The prevertebral soft tissues and the airway in general are extremely pliable in infants, and with expiration and flexion of the neck a wide variety of distortions and bizarre appearances can result; these are discussed in Chapter 30. High kilovoltage techniques with special filters in the X-ray beam can give detailed radiographs of the upper airway for reduced radiation dose (Joseph *et al.*, 1976). Such techniques can usually obviate the need for xerography. Although xerography can give an enhanced demonstration of the air–soft tissue interface (*Figure 2.1*), the radiation dose is higher, and in the opinion of the author little further information is obtained.

Inflammatory disease of the pharynx, larynx and epiglottis are common causes of upper respiratory obstruction and potentially very serious. Radiological examination is rarely necessary to demonstrate these conditions directly but is needed to exclude pulmonary disease. A soft tissue lateral view of the neck may show soft tissue swelling of the larynx, and can reveal the extent of a retropharyngeal abscess (*see Figure 24.1*).

Conventional tomography is particularly useful in the frontal projection for showing subglottic stenosis and webs (*Figure 2.2*). It can be combined with CT to assess congenital abnormalities such as

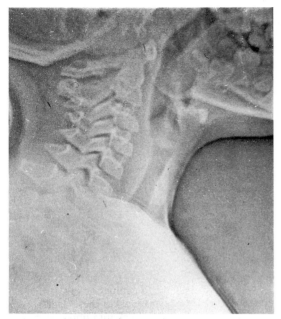

Figure 2.1 Lateral neck xerogram in a child. Note the high position of the larynx

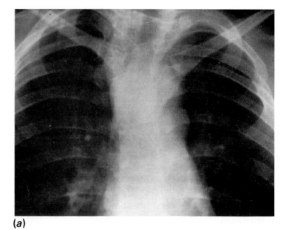

(a)

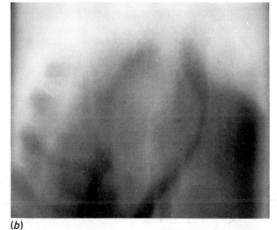

(b)

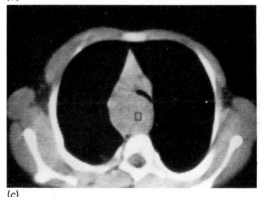

(c)

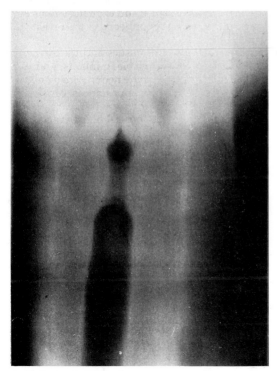

Figure 2.2 Frontal linear tomogram of the larynx showing subglottic stenosis. Note the vocal cords in full adduction

Figure 2.3 A child with stridor, due to a mediastinal tracheal duplication cyst. (a) Chest radiograph shows an ill-defined midline soft tissue mass and a vertebral anomaly at the same level. The presence of such a congenital osseous abnormality suggests that the soft tissue lesion may also be of congenital origin; (b) lateral tomogram shows the cyst indenting and narrowing the trachea from behind; (c) axial CT shows the round cyst at the level of the right main bronchus which is slightly compressed. Attenuation values in the area depicted by the square confirmed a cyst

vascular rings or developmental cysts which cause stridor by distortion of the trachea at a lower level (*Figure 2.3*).

Face and sinuses

The sinuses are present in the infant and can become infected. At birth small antra and ethmoid sinuses can be demonstrated radiologically. The frontal and sphenoid sinuses develop later. The lateral view does not present any problem, but proper positioning is essential to show infant sinuses. The most important plain film sinus view in the adult is the occipitomental with the baseline at 45° to the plane of the film (*see* Volume 4). In the older child this angle must be decreased to about 28° or the projection will be too steep for proper evaluation of the maxillary antra. In the infant the angle must be even less so that the view is almost a posteroanterior view (Hayden and Swischuk, 1984). Radiographically the findings of sinusitis vary according to age but, as in the adult, loss of the normal radiolucency usually indicates disease. As well as the loss of normal aeration, more specific features such as mucosal thickening and fluid levels may be recognized (*Figure 2.4*). Mucocoeles from obstruction of the sinus ostium are rare in children, and are best demonstrated by sectional imaging (*Figure 2.5*).

Choanal atresia

Choanal atresia is the commonest congenital abnormality of the nose, but cannot be demons-

trated by plain film views. Although CT would probably now be the investigation of choice in the first instance, a very satisfactory demonstration of the site of obstruction can be made by instilling an oily contrast medium into the nasal cavity and obtaining films in the lateral and base projections (*Figure 2.6*).

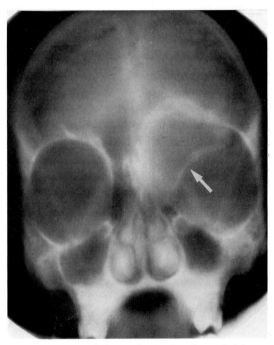

Figure 2.5 Expansile lesion depressing the roof of the orbit (arrow). Hypocycloidal coronal section tomogram

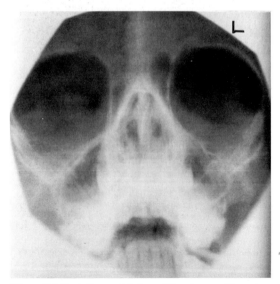

Figure 2.4 Occipitomental view of the sinuses. There is mucosal thickening in the left antrum. The frontal sinuses are unformed

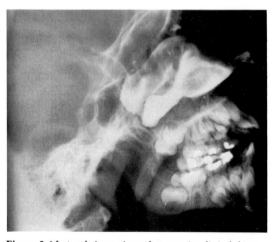

Figure 2.6 Lateral sinus view after pouring lipiodol into the obstructed nasal cavity in a case of unilateral choanal atresia. The soft tissue obstruction is not shown although the site is clearly apparent

Developmental mass lesions

Developmental mass lesions affecting the upper respiratory tract include meningoencephalocoeles and arachnoid or dermoid cysts. Encephalocoeles occur in the midline in the nasofrontal and nasoethmoidal regions (*Figure 2.7*). Although they

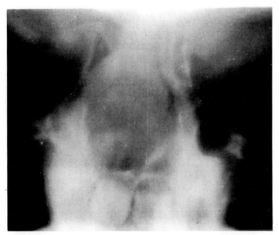

Figure 2.7 Coronal section tomogram showing a pear-shaped mass in the nasal cavity. A nasoethmoidal encephalocoele

may be demonstrated by conventional imaging techniques, CT scanning is the investigation of choice. This is particularly so for the much rarer lateral protrusions through the base of the skull. They may present as masses in the infratemporal fossa which subsequently expand and bulge into the aerodigestive tract (*Figure 2.8*). Dehiscences in the skull base occur with neurofibromatosis and defects in the back of the orbit may result in proptosis (*Figure 2.9*).

Juvenile nasopharyngeal angiofibroma

Although the pathogenesis of so-called juvenile nasopharyngeal angiofibroma is uncertain and it occurs in an older age group, this vascular tumour also appears to be of developmental origin. Lloyd and Phelps (1986) in a recent study of 30 cases have shown that angiofibroma takes origin at the sphenopalatine foramen. It enlarges the foramen and erodes bone locally: at the base of the medial pterygoid plate, the floor of the sphenoid sinus and the posterior wall of the maxillary antrum. Further extension leads to invasion of the infratemporal fossa, orbit and middle cranial fossa (*Figure 2.10*). Severe bleeding may accompany biopsy and for this reason most surgeons are

reluctant to undertake biopsy of a nasopharyngeal mass in an adolescent male patient, and prefer to rely upon clinical and radiological features to decide whether the mass is likely to be an angiofibroma or a non-vascular lesion such as an antrochoanal polyp. Traditionally this involved angiography to show the characteristic vascular blush, supported by the 'antral sign' or indentation of the posterior wall of the maxillary antrum shown on lateral plain films or tomography.

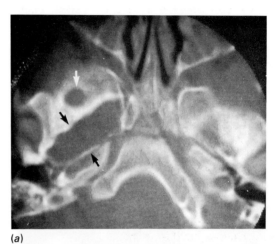

(*a*)

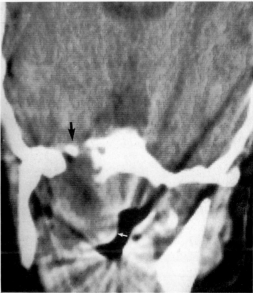

(*b*)

Figure 2.8 (*a*) Axial, (*b*) coronal CT scans showing a large meningocoele protruding through a grossly widened sphenopetrosal suture (black arrows) and bulging into the nasopharynx (small white arrow). Note the enlargement of the ipsilateral foramen ovale and the low attenuation within the mass

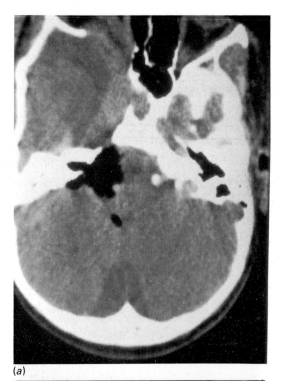

(a)

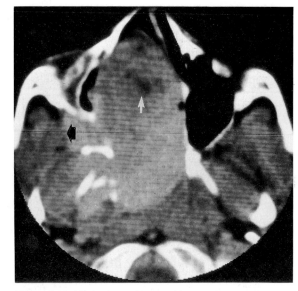

Figure 2.10 A large juvenile angiofibroma fills the nasal cavity and extends through the pterygomaxillary fissure into the infratemporal fossa (black arrow). The white arrow indicates an area of necrosis. Axial enhanced CT section

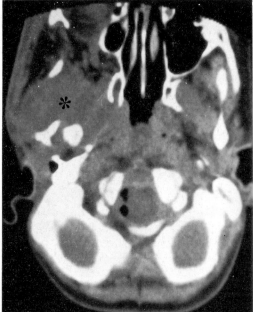

(b)

Figure 2.9 (*a*) Axial CT section on a patient with neurofibromatosis and deficient floor of the middle cranial fossa and back of the orbit. The patient was deaf, and the air meatogram examination was performed to exclude an acoustic neuroma. (*b*) The encephalocoele (asterisk) appears as a soft tissue mass in the infratemporal fossa

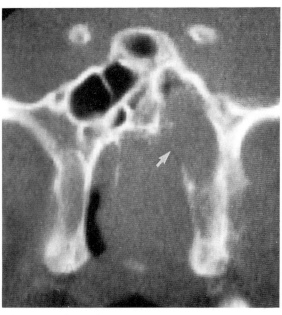

Figure 2.11 Coronal CT section at the level of the choana. A juvenile angiofibroma has eroded the base of the medial pterygoid plate (arrow) and extended into the sphenoid sinus

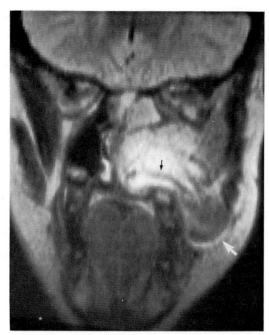

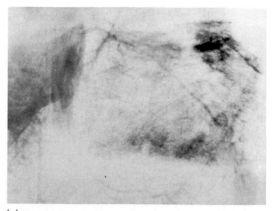

(a)

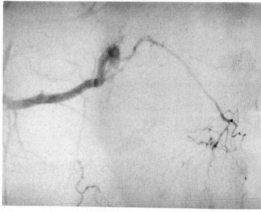

(b)

Figure 2.12 Coronal MR section showing an angiofibroma which has extended into the soft tissues of the cheek (white arrow). The black arrow points to a large vessel on the surface of the tumour. Demonstration of these vessels by MR can be diagnostic. (From Lloyd and Phelps, 1986, *Clinical Otolaryngology,* with permission)

Figure 2.13 External carotid angiogram with subtraction, to show the blood supply to a large juvenile angiofibroma (*a*) before and (*b*) after therapeutic embolization. (Courtesy of Dr Brian Kendall, The National Hospital, London)

However, the antral sign is not specific for angiofibromata. It can occur with any slow-growing mass in the infratemporal fossa (*see* Volume 5, *Figure 2.17*) and was only positive in 81% of the author's patients with angiofibroma.

A more reliable sign is erosion of the base of the medial pterygoid plate, associated with enlargement of the sphenopalatine foramen which was demonstrated in 100% of 28 patients examined by conventional or computerized tomography (*Figure 2.11*). Once the diagnosis is established then the role of the radiologist is to define the limits of the tumour prior to surgery since this may influence the surgical approach. Three-plane magnetic resonance tomography is the method of choice (*Figure 2.12*). It best demonstrates the extent of the tumour, it uses non-ionizing radiation, and it will show the vascular nature of the angiofibroma and confirm the diagnosis. Angiography need only be performed if embolization is deemed necessary prior to surgery (*Figure 2.13*).

The natural history of angiofibroma, treated or untreated, is highly variable. It has long been known that there is a tendency to involute with age, and these clinical observations have been supported by histological evidence that individual tumours show an increase in fibrous elements with time. However, at least partly because of the difficulty of assessment of the area of origin, and because of the reluctance of clinicians to intervene in the absence of symptoms, there seems to be no firm evidence in the literature that spontaneous involution of untreated lesions occurs (Chandler *et al.*, 1984). Recently, complete regression of a small tumour that persisted after surgical removal of the original mass has been described (Stansbie and Phelps, 1986). Involution of this tumour was fully documented by serial CT scans over a period of 4 years (*Figure 2.14*).

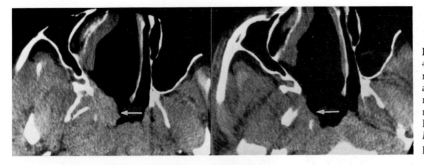

Figure 2.14 Axial CT sections 4 years apart, showing regression of a small angiofibroma which had reappeared after surgical removal. (From Stansbie and Phelps, 1986, *Journal of Laryngology and Otology*, with permission)

Lesions of the jaws

Congenital deformities of the face and jaws usually present to plastic surgeons or to oral surgeons and orthodontists because of bite problems. The two most important of the first arch syndromes are:

(1) hemifacial microsomia in which there is under-development of one half of the face (*Figure 2.15*). In the 20% of cases where the deformity is bilateral there is always dissymmetry between the two sides
(2) mandibulofacial dysostosis or the Treacher Collins syndrome, where there is characteristic bilateral and symmetrical hypoplasia of jaw and ear structures. The pathogenesis of both conditions has been discussed by Poswillo (1974).

Underdevelopment of the ascending ramus and condyle of the mandible appears to be the hallmark of hemifacial microsomia, and these abnormalities can be well shown by lateral and frontal radiographs and especially by orthopanto-mography (*Figure 2.16*). It has long been recognized that this hypoplasia affects not only bony structures but also the soft tissues, and in

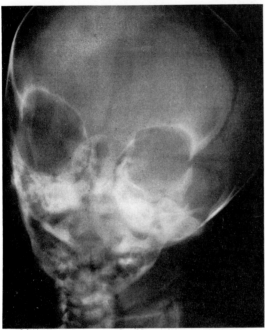

Figure 2.15 Underdevelopment of one half of the face, including the orbit, in a child with oculo-auricular-vertebral dysplasia

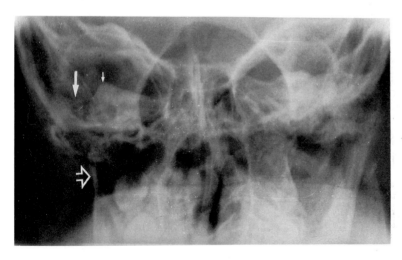

Figure 2.16 Another case of oculo-auricular-vertebral dysplasia. The Towne's view shows a large foramen magnum which was associated with an occipital meningocoele. The open arrow points to the hypoplastic mandibular ramus; the small arrow points to the arcuate eminence; the large arrow to the depressed tegmen, so typical of hemifacial microsomia

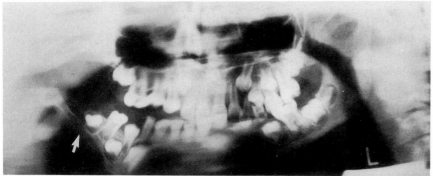

(a)

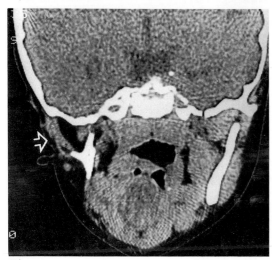

(b)

Figure 2.17 Hemifacial microsomia.
(a) Orthopantomograph showing gross underdevelopment of part of the body of the mandible on the right (arrow); (b) coronal CT section shows the hypoplastic musculature and can be compared to the normal muscles shown on the left. The open arrow points to temporalis, which inserts into a horizontal shelf of bone, presumably representing a deformed coronoid process

particular the muscles and the parotid gland. Only recently has the use of CT scanning enabled this soft tissue hypoplasia to be adequately demonstrated (*Figure 2.17*). Characteristically there is most underdevelopment of the masseter muscle and the parotid gland, a feature often apparent on clinical examination, although the pterygoid muscles are also commonly affected.

Symmetrical hypoplasia of jaws and muscles is a feature of the Treacher Collins syndrome but this is more uniform and less pronounced than in hemifacial microsomia and the salivary glands are not affected. Antegonal notching of the body of the mandible is a feature of the condition (*Figure 2.18*), and crowding of teeth causes orthodontic problems.

Fibrous dysplasia

Tumours and tumour-like lesions of the jaws are uncommon in children, and fibro-osseous abnormalities such as fibrous dysplasia predominate (*Figure 2.19*). They cause a painless and slowly developing expansion of the jaws and may have characteristic appearances on plain films or CT, but are more often cystic with non-specific features, although a well corticated margin confirms the benign nature of the lesion. A giant cell reparative granuloma of the upper alveolus is shown in Volume 4 (*Figure 2.30*).

Rare malignant neoplasms cause extensive ragged destruction of the jaws. Sometimes calci-

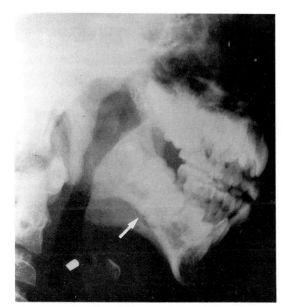

Figure 2.18 Treacher Collins syndrome. Antegonal notching of the body of the mandible

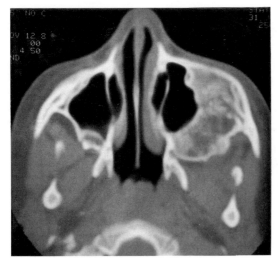

Figure 2.19 Fibrous dysplasia of the maxilla in a 4-year-old child. This axial CT scan shows the lesion to be of the mixed type, with islands of bone in a largely fibrous bed

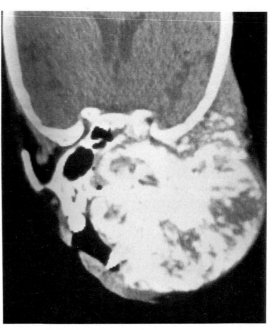

Figure 2.20 Coronal CT scan showing a massive osteogenic sarcoma arising from the maxilla

fication or even new bone formation within the tumour may be diagnostic, especially in osteogenic sarcoma (*Figure 2.20*).

Bone marrow tumours

Bone marrow tumours in children not infrequently involve the mandible. Leukaemia, lymphoma and metastatic neuroblastoma can produce mottled destruction of the mandible and destruction or disruption of the teeth. Lytic destructive lesions are a common feature of histiocytosis and the mandible is often involved (*Figure 2.21*).

The petrous temporal bone

The middle and inner ears are fully developed at birth, but the temporomandibular joint and mastoid process are not. Postnatal changes in the temporal bone consist of growth and pneumatization of the mastoid process and alteration in the shape of the tympanic ring. Prior to full ossification of the petrous pyramid, the dense bone of the labyrinthine capsule can be clearly identified on plain mastoid views, enabling gross developmen-

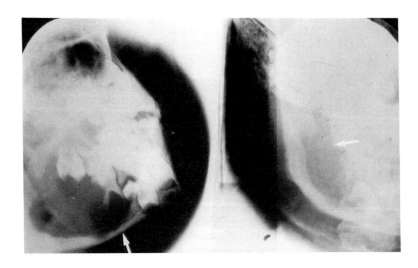

Figure 2.21 Large lytic lesion of the mandible with the 'floating teeth' sign so typical of histiocytosis

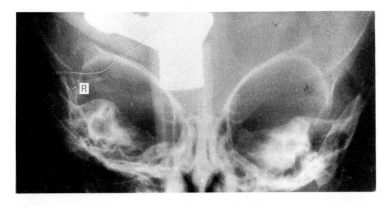

Figure 2.22 Perorbital view. Normal appearances on the left. On the right there is no labyrinth, but just a primitive otocyst with endolymphatic appendage

tal abnormalities to be identified without the need for sectional imaging (*Figure 2.22*). In the middle ear the ossicles can be shown and, in the neonate, even marrow spaces (*Figure 2.23*).

Congenital ear deformities

Many congenital abnormalities of the hearing organ do not involve bony structures and therefore cannot be shown by radiological methods. Nevertheless, structural abnormalities of the inner, middle and external ear can be shown in considerable detail by tomographic techniques. Unfortunately, affected children are usually referred between the ages of 2 and 4 years, when the deafness is first confirmed, and sedation or a general anaesthetic is required for the examination. If, after careful consideration, it is felt that the results of the investigation would be unlikely to affect patient management it may be reasonable to defer the examination until the child can cooperate. In the neonatal period a few tomographic sections can usually be obtained for those relevant

external deformities or syndromes in which temporal bone abnormalites are a feature. These syndromes with recognized structural abnormalities of the temporal bone are reviewed in Chapter 4 of *Radiology of the Ear* (Phelps and Lloyd, 1983).

The purpose of the radiological examination is first to demonstrate any bony abnormality of the inner ear, and particularly of the cochlea. This is complementary to the audiological assessment and ideally electrophysiological studies (either auditory brainstem response or electrocochleography) should be undertaken at the same time. Deformities associated with an actual or potential cerebrospinal fluid fistula may be demonstrated.

Congenital abnormalities of the middle and external ears are shown much more often than deformities of the inner ear, although combined deformities occur in about 20% of cases. The study of the outer ear relates to the prospects for surgical intervention to improve the sound conducting mechanisms and is mandatory before any exploration of congenital atresia. Surgery is now, however, rarely performed for unilateral lesions, but in bilateral atresias the radiological examination is crucial to indicate the best side for exploration.

Sectional imaging with a profound knowledge of normal and abnormal temporal bone anatomy on the part of the observer is required. For bony abnormalities of the inner ears, conventional tomography is just as good as CT, but for the middle ear and external meatus, thin section, high resolution CT with its ability to demonstrate both bone and soft tissue abnormalities is essential before any surgical exploration; particularly for the all-important assessment of the presence, state and size of the middle ear cavity.

Inner ear deformities

Congenital malformations of the bony labyrinth, internal auditory meatus and vestibular aqueduct, which vary widely in severity from minor anomalies with normal cochlear function to severe

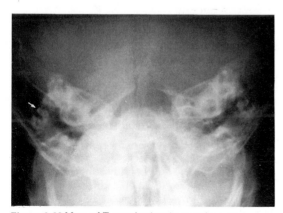

Figure 2.23 Normal Towne's view in an infant. The arrow points to the bodies of malleus and incus and marrow spaces can be identified

deformities which preclude any level of hearing whatever, may be suggested by audiological assessment. Traditionally two eponyms are enshrined in accounts of congenital deafness and so need to be defined:

(1) Michel defect (Michel, 1863) – complete lack of development of any inner ear structures
(2) Mondini defect (Mondini, 1791) – a cochlea with one and a half turns and the apical coil replaced by a distal sac. Although the subject of Mondini's dissection had been completely deaf, the normal basal turn of the true Mondini defect means that some hearing is possible. Mondini's case also had very dilated vestibular aqueducts (Phelps, 1986).

Line drawings of some examples of labyrinthine deformities are shown in *Figure 2.24*. A primitive sac with one or more appendages (*Figures 2.22* and *2.24*) is commoner than a Michel deformity.

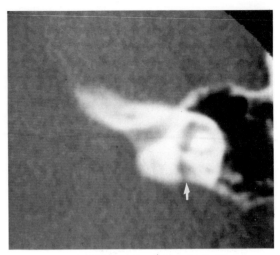

Figure 2.25 Axial CT scan showing a widely dilated vestibular aqueduct in a child with progressive sensorineural deafness. Note the normal vestibule and lateral semicircular canal ('signet ring' sign, *see* Volume 3, Chapter 2)

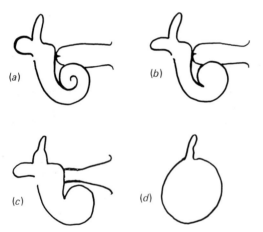

(a)   (b)

(c)   (d)

Figure 2.24 Line drawings of some important abnormalities of the inner ear, based on coronal section imaging. (*a*) Solitary dysplastic semicircular canal; (*b*) Mondini deformity with a deficient bony spiral in the cochlea; (*c*) dilated dysplastic labyrinth with tapering internal auditory meatus; (*d*) primitive otocyst

The semicircular canals may be missing or dilated in varying degree, but the commonest inner ear anomaly, namely a solitary dilated dysplasic lateral semicircular canal (*Figure 2.24*) is often associated with normal cochlear function. Dilatation of the vestibular aqueduct often accompanies minor abnormalities of the bony cochlea and vestibule and congenital hearing loss (*Figure 2.25*) (Valvassori, 1983). The deafness may be fluctuant and/or progressive giving rise to speculation that endolymphatic hydrops is also a feature.

Anomalies of the internal auditory meatus include the bulbous type which is usually of no significance; unusual direction which is the result of skull base aberrations; and very narrow or double internal auditory meatus which usually indicate severe or total deafness (Phelps and Lloyd, 1983).

Inner ear lesions associated with cerebrospinal fluid fistula

Congenital cerebrospinal fluid fistula into the middle ear cavity is a rare but potentially fatal condition which is frequently misdiagnosed. When the fistula occurs spontaneously it usually presents in the first 5 or 10 years of life as:

(1) cerebrospinal fluid rhinorrhoea if the eardrum is intact. Cerebrospinal fluid passes down the eustachian tube causing a nasal discharge
(2) cerebrospinal fluid otorrhoea if there is a perforation in the eardrum, or if myringotomy has been performed for presumed serous otitis media
(3) Attacks of meningitis which are usually recurrent. At times meningitis is the sole presenting manifestation of a cerebrospinal fluid fistula.

Deafness is usually severe or complete, but it is difficult to diagnose and assess, especially in a young child. It is frequently unrecognized if unilateral. The conductive and sensorineural components of the deafness are also hard to define.

Spontaneous cerebrospinal fluid fistulae from the subarachnoid space into the middle ear cavity

may be classified as perilabyrinthine or translabyrinthine. The very rare perilabyrinthine group,
through bony defects close to but not involving
the labyrinth, usually have normal hearing initially. The commoner translabyrinthine group is
nearly always associated with anacusis, severe

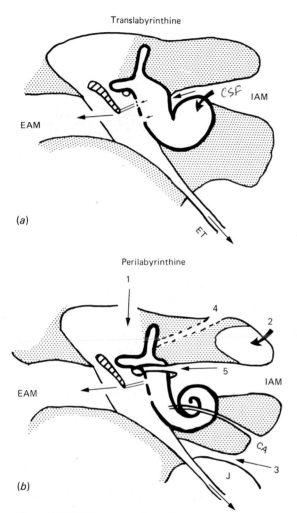

(a)

(b)

Figure 2.26 (*a*) Diagram to show the commonest inner
ear anomaly associated with cerebrospinal fluid fistula.
Note the wide communication between vestibule and
cochlear sac. This diagram is based on coronal section
tomograms. (*b*) Diagram based on coronal section
tomograms to show the various routes of
perilabyrinthine fistulae around a labyrinth of normal
configuration: (1) through the tegmen tympani;
(2) through large apical air cells; (3) via Hyrtl's fissure;
(4) via petromastoid canal (not a proven route); (5) via
the facial nerve canal. EAM = external auditory meatus;
IAM = internal auditory meatus; ET = eustachian tube;
CA = cochlear aqueduct; J = jugular fossa. (From
Phelps, P. D., 1986. *Clinical Otolaryngology,* with
permission)

labyrinthine dysplasia and a route via the internal
auditory meatus. The labyrinthine deformity is
more severe than the type classically described by
Mondini, and evidence of a dilated cochlear
aqueduct in these cases is also unconvincing.

The perilabyrinthine and translabyrinthine
routes (*Figure 2.26*) are discussed in a recent paper
by Phelps (1986). The most important route is via
an abnormally shaped internal auditory meatus
that usually tapers at its lateral end (*Figures 2.24*
and *2.27*). The cochlea is an amorphous sac which
lacks a modiolus or central bony spiral. The
cochlear sac may be bigger or smaller than a
normal cochlea. No proper basal turn can be
recognized as in a true Mondini deformity, and
there is a wide communication between the
cochlear sac and the vestibule which is itself
abnormal and enlarged, especially in the horizontal plane. The semicircular canals may be dilated to
a varying degree, especially the lateral.

The labyrinthine malformation is often accompanied by a defective stapes – usually a hole in the
footplate – and the exit route of cerebrospinal fluid
into the middle ear is via the oval or, less
commonly, the round window. It should be
stressed that the fistula is usually spontaneous or
the result of a minor head injury.

Congenital fixation of the stapes footplate is
likely to be associated with a profuse perilymph or
cerebrospinal fluid leak following stapedectomy.
The surgical results of stapedectomy for congenital
stapedial fixation are not very satisfactory, but
there is little radiological evidence of structural
abnormalities of the labyrinth in these 'gushers'.

The management of cerebrospinal fluid fistulae
into the middle ear depends on a high degree of
clinical suspicion. Perilabyrinthine fistulae are
extremely rare and usually associated with normal
hearing. Bone defects around the labyrinth may be
shown by sophisticated bone imaging, but tracer
cerebrospinal fluid contrast studies may be necessary to confirm the aural route. The commoner
translabyrinthine type is almost always associated
with labyrinthine dysplasia. Sensorineural deafness or two unexplained attacks of meningitis
make a polytomographic or CT study of the
temporal bones mandatory.

Middle ear deformities

Radiology of congenital deformities of the middle
and external ear relates almost exclusively to the
prospects of improvement of conductive deafness
by surgical intervention. The size and shape of the
middle ear cavity is the most important assessment to be made, especially where there is atresia
of the external auditory meatus.

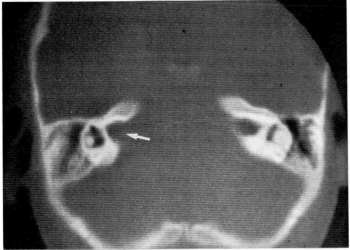

(a)

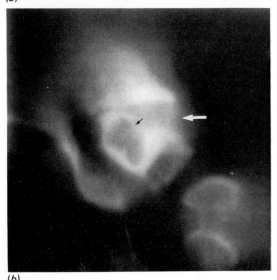

(b)

Figure 2.27 (*a*) Axial CT scan in a child with a spontaneous cerebrospinal fluid fistula through the labyrinth. The arrow points to the wide tapering internal auditory meatus. (*b*) Axial pyramidal tomogram shows the large dysplastic cochlea with wide communication from the internal auditory meatus (small arrow)

In the majority of unilateral atresias with associated deformity of the pinna but no other congenital abnormality, there is a normally formed mastoid with good pneumatization and the middle ear cavity is of relatively normal shape. Even in the most severe deformities there is rarely complete absence of the middle ear and usually at least a slit-like hypotympanum can be shown lateral to the basal turn of the cochlea. The middle ear cavity may be reduced in size by encroachment of the atretic plate laterally, by a high jugular bulb

inferiorly or by descent of the tegmen superiorly. In craniofacial microsomia and mandibulofacial dysostosis, the attic and antrum are typically absent or slit-like, being replaced in varying degrees by solid bone or by descent of the tegmen (*Figure 2.28*).

If the middle ear cavity is air containing, its shape and contents are relatively easy to assess. Frequently, however, the middle ear in congenital abnormalities contains undifferentiated mesenchyme, a thick glue-like substance which is radiologically indistinguishable from soft tissue or retained mucus. Thin bony septa may divide the middle ear cavity into two or more compartments.

Facial nerve

The next most important structure from a surgical point of view is the facial nerve. The nerve is very rarely absent, although it might be hypoplastic. The main problem is aberration in the course of the nerve.

In early embryonic life, the developing seventh cranial nerve lies anterior to the otocyst, so if development is arrested at this stage, a tract for the facial nerve is found anterior to a primitive otic sac. If development is arrested at a later stage, after the cochlea has formed to some extent, then the first part of the facial nerve is found in its usual situation above and lateral to the cochlea. The facial nerve is, therefore, relatively unaffected by developmental abnormalities of the labyrinth, and aberrations of the first part of the facial nerve canal are most unusual.

The course of the second and third parts is, however, dependent on normal development of the branchial arches, the facial nerve being the nerve of the second arch. During its development

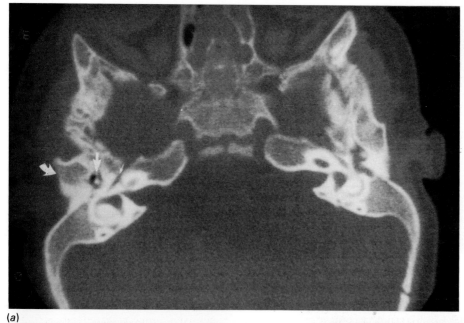

(a)

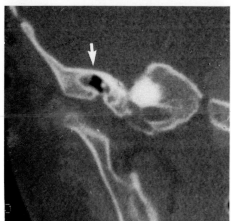

(b)

(c)

Figure 2.28 Severe congenital deformity of the middle and external ears in a case of Treacher Collins syndrome. The inner ears are normal. (*a*) Axial section at the level of the lateral semicircular canals. On both sides the antrum is replaced by solid bone. On the right a very small air-containing attic encloses a diminutive ossicle (large arrow). The curved arrow indicates the uncannulated tympanic bone and the small arrow the second part of the facial nerve canal, which is in relatively normal position; (*b*) coronal section anteriorly shows the small attic; (*c*) more posterior coronal section through the vestibule shows the short descending facial canal. (Courtesy of Dr E. A. Burrows)

and migration, the facial nerve curves behind the branchial cartilage to reach the anterior aspect of the same cartilage. At the same time, part of the cartilage adheres to the otic capsule to form the fallopian canal. If, during development, the external pharyngeal groove of the first branchial arch is active and atresia is due only to mal-

development of the tympanic ring, then the second and third parts of the facial canal follow a relatively normal course (*Figure 2.29*). In major atresias, when the external pharyngeal groove is not active, then development of malformations is much worse. The temporomandibular joint may abut directly onto the mastoid process.

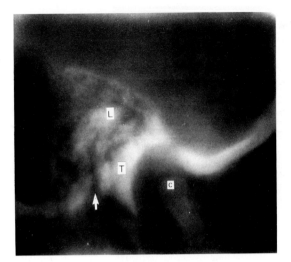

Figure 2.29 Lateral tomogram of congenital atresia with well-pneumatized mastoid. T = the uncannulated tympanic bone, L= lateral semicircular canal, c = condyle of the mandible. The arrow points to the descending facial canal, which is in normal position

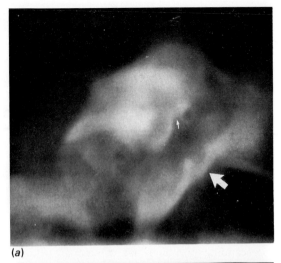

(*a*)

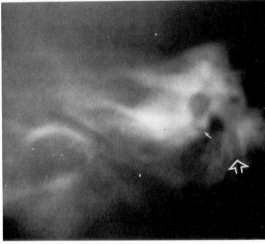

(*b*)

Figure 2.30 Congenital bony atresia with a normal sized air-containing middle ear cavity. (*a*) Semiaxial section shows the oval window (small arrow) obscured by an overhanging fallopian canal. This feature would make it difficult or impossible to insert any form of strut during attempts at reconstructive surgery. (*b*) Coronal section slightly more posterior at the level of the short descending facial canal (open arrow). The small arrow points to the round window niche. Note the absence of the normal pyramidal eminence, suggesting that there is dehiscence of the facial nerve at the second genu

The greater the deformity the more marked is the tendency for the facial nerve to follow a more direct route out into the soft tissues of the face. Exposed facial nerves in the middle ear cavity are the most common abnormalities recorded at surgery for congenital malformations. Usually the fallopian canal is dehiscent but the descending segment may also be exposed, and overhang of the facial ridge with absence of the second genu is a usual finding in the Treacher Collins syndrome making access to the oval window difficult for the surgeon. A short vertical segment of the facial canal and high stylomastoid foramen mean that the nerve turns forwards into the cheek in a high position (*Figure 2.30*).

In the preoperative radiological assessment the descending facial canal and its relationship to other structures must be demonstrated, preferably in both coronal and lateral sections (*Figure 2.31*). Axial CT sections will show the descending canal in cross-section and identification is less certain. Grossly displaced nerves that cross the middle ear cavity are more difficult to identify even by CT, but two useful signs of aberrant pathways through the middle ear cavity are:

(1) an exit foramen through the floor of the middle ear cavity or lateral atretic plate may be identified
(2) absence, at the back of the middle ear cavity, of the pyramidal eminence which normally contains the stapedius muscle and tendon (*see* Volume 3, Chapter 2).

The pyramid was identified in only two of the cases noted at operation to have anomalies of the facial canal in the middle ear and, in these, the dehiscence was in the second part. Absence of the pyramid is, therefore, good presumptive evidence of an exposed facial nerve. Bifurcation of the

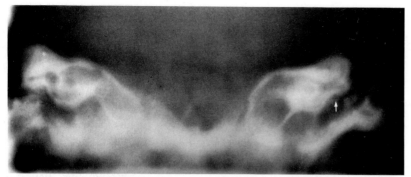

Figure 2.31 Coronal section tomogram at vestibule level in bilateral atresia. On both sides the ossicles were abnormal. The arrow on the left points to the second part of the facial nerve canal. Note that on the other side the fallopian canal is double. This is most unusual, and not nearly so common as bifurcation of the descending facial canal

descending portion is far commoner with congenital malformations than in normal patients (*Figure 2.31*).

Ossicles

A normal ossicular chain is rarely found where there is atresia of the external ear, but complete absence of the ossicles is also unusual. In most cases at least some vestige of the ossicular chain is evident. The ossicles are often thicker and heavier than normal (*Figure 2.32*) or, less frequently, thin and spidery. They may be fixed to the walls of the middle ear cavity by bosses of bone but the more usual deformity discovered at surgery is a fusion of the bodies of malleus and incus. The ankylosis varies in degree and may be bony or fibrous. The radiological recognition of this ossicular union is difficult but is, in any case, not of great practical importance and an irregular lump of bone in the

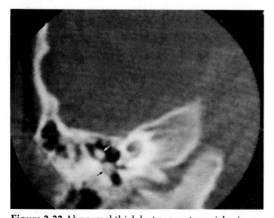

Figure 2.32 Abnormal thick but separate ossicles in an air-containing middle ear behind a pneumatized atretic plate. This axial CT section was made at the level of the round window niche

middle ear cavity usually represents an ossicular mass.

Because of the partial or complete replacement of the tympanic membrane by a bony plate, the handle of the malleus is not surprisingly that part of the chain which is most often abnormal and most easily recognized on the tomograms. If the handle is absent the 'molar tooth' appearance of the ossicles will no longer be evident in the lateral projection and a triangular appearance of the ossicular mass will be seen. Often, the handle of the malleus is bent towards the atretic plate to which it may be fixed and this gives the typical L-shaped appearance to the ossicular mass. A slit-like attic so typical of Treacher Collins syndrome or an overhanging facial ridge may obstruct the free movement of the ossicular chain.

External auditory meatus

In congenital deformities of the external ear, the external auditory meatus may be narrow, short, completely or partially atretic or it may run in an abnormal direction. It often slopes up towards the middle ear and in such cases it may be curved in two planes, becoming more horizontal at its medial end. The obstruction in atresia may be due to soft tissue or bone but usually both are involved. The tympanic bone may be hyperplastic (rarely), deformed or absent.

The so-called atretic plate may therefore be composed partly of a deformed tympanic bone (*Figure 2.33*) and partly of downwards and forward extension of squamous temporal and mastoid bones, in which case it may be pneumatized.

A diagrammatic representation of some of the congenital structural abnormalities of the middle and external ears as shown by coronal section imaging is given in *Figure 2.34*.

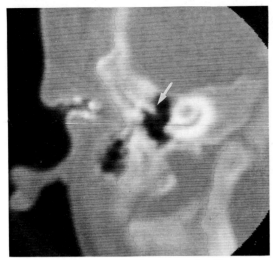

Figure 2.33 A short blind ending external auditory meatus containing droplets of oily contrast medium. The abnormal malleus (arrow) is attached to the deformed tympanic bone. An axial CT section showing a mixture of bony and soft tissue atresia

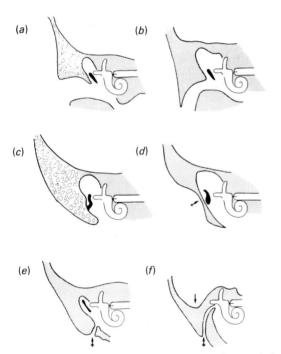

Figure 2.34 A diagrammatic representation of congenital deformities of middle and external ears based on coronal section tomograms. (*a*) Normal appearances; (*b*)–(*f*) various types of atretic plate, reduced middle ear cavity, ossicular deformity and anterior facial nerve ↦.
↦ = thin atretic plate, → = depression of the tegmen.
(From Phelps, P. D., Lloyd, G. A. S. and Sheldon P. W. E., 1977. *British Journal of Radiology*, with permission)

Syndromes

It is not intended to discuss the radiological features of syndromic ear deformities except for the two commonest and most important.

Hemifacial microsomia

The ear lesions are usually bizarre and severe. The pinna is often represented by a small tag. Meatal atresia and middle ear abnormalities are almost constant findings and there may be gross descent of the tegmen to, or even below, the level of the lateral semicircular canal (*see Figure 2.34b*). Occasionally, some degree of hyperplasia of external ear structures, particularly the tympanic bone, occurs but the mastoid is hypoplastic and unpneumatized. The middle ear cavity is usually small, being encroached upon by the low tegmen and thick atretic plate. The ossicles in such cases are absent or hypoplastic and malformed (*Figure 2.35*). Three of the author's patients had an ossicular mass displaced laterally, far from the oval window. This anomaly is only seen in cases of facial microsomia. The condition is not exclusively unilateral and often involves the bones of the skull base. Though bilateral, there is always considerable dissymmetry between the two sides. This dissymmetry distinguishes the syndrome from Treacher Collins syndrome, with which it has often been confused in the past. There is no hereditary factor in craniofacial microsomia. It is the most common of the otocraniofacial syndromes (Phelps, Lloyd and Poswillo, 1983).

Treacher Collins syndrome

The middle ear abnormalities in Treacher Collins syndrome are symmetrical and characteristic, although they may vary in severity (Phelps, Poswillo and Lloyd, 1981). The mastoid is unpneumatized and the attic and antrum are often reduced to slit-like proportions (*Figure 2.36*). Atresia of the external auditory meatus is a less constant feature and in 50% of patients the meatus may be patent, although it tends to be curved, running upwards in its lateral part. Ossicular abnormalities are common and, in nearly all the operated ears in the author's series, the facial nerve followed a more direct path with opening out of the bends. It usually appeared at surgery as an overhanging facial ridge.

Bone dysplasias

Deafness is a common childhood feature of rare congenital generalized bony dysplasias. Only a brief account of the radiological features of

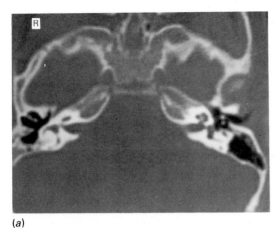

(a)

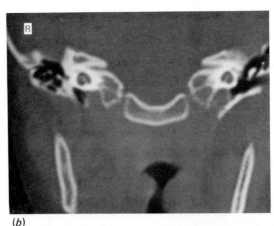

(b)

Figure 2.35 Hemifacial microsomia. (a) Axial, (b) coronal sections. Normal appearances on the left. On the right there is some depression of the tegmen and thin bony atresia, but there is a large air-containing middle ear cavity. Note, however, that the small hypoplastic ossicles lie medial and lateral instead of anterior and posterior as on the normal side

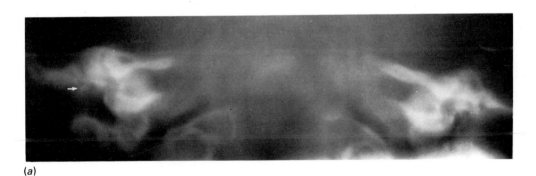

(a)

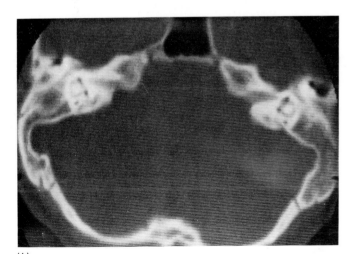

(b)

Figure 2.36 Treacher Collins syndrome. (a) Coronal section tomogram showing normal external auditory meatus and relatively normal lower middle ear cavities. There are, however, virtually no attics present and some hypoplastic ossicles (arrow). (b) Axial CT section at the level of the lateral semicircular canals showing solid bone replacing the antrum on each side. Note the typical symmetry of these lesions

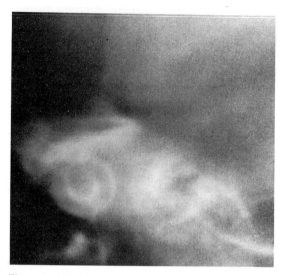

Figure 2.37 Demineralization of bone surrounding the cochlea in a case of osteogenesis imperfecta, shown on this coronal tomogram

osteogenesis imperfecta and of the dysplasias with increased bone density is given here. For more extensive descriptions other works need to be consulted (Booth, 1982; Phelps and Lloyd 1983).

Deafness in osteogenesis imperfecta tarda may be conductive, sensorineural or mixed. The radiological appearances consist of demineralization in the labyrinthine capsule indistinguishable from otospongiosis but, in contrast to otospongiosis which only affects the capsule, dehiscent ossification occurs in other sites in the petrous pyramid (*Figure 2.37*).

The osteopetroses are a group of uncommon genetic disorders that are characterized by increased skeletal density and abnormalities of bone modelling. Common to all of these disorders, is a proclivity for involvement of the calvarium and skull base. An associated constellation of neurotological symptoms may result, presumably secondary to bony encroachment on the cranial foramina. Sectional imaging of the petrous temporal bones shows generalized sclerosis and narrowing

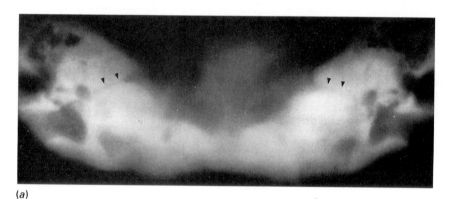

(a)

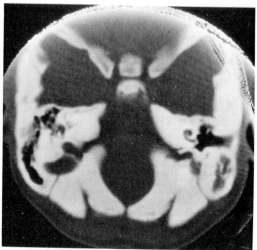

(b)

Figure 2.38 (*a*) Coronal section tomogram, (*b*) axial CT showing very dense sclerotic bone and a very narrow internal auditory meatus, although the labyrinth is normal. In spite of the gross narrowing of the internal auditory meatus, this 13-year-old child at the moment has normal hearing

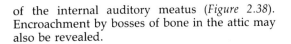

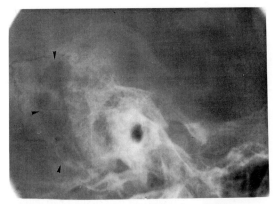

Figure 2.39 Acute otitis media. Plain lateral view showing mastoid cell wall breakdown (coalescent mastoiditis)

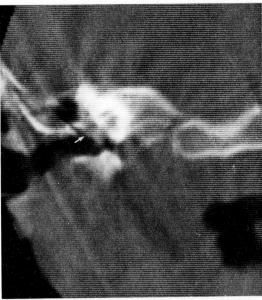

(a)

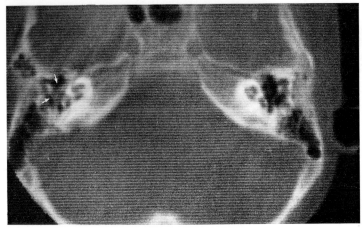

(b)

of the internal auditory meatus (*Figure 2.38*). Encroachment by bosses of bone in the attic may also be revealed.

Otitis media

Radiology has little part to play in conditions such as otitis media, which is essentially a clinical diagnosis. Loss of aeration of the middle ear cleft and mastoid may suggest infection, but cell wall breakdown (coalescent mastoiditis) and abscess formation in mastoiditis are hard to demonstrate on plain films, and are better shown by CT (*Figure 2.39*).

Cholesteatoma in children

Cholesteatoma in childhood is less common than in adults but is a more aggressive and dangerous disease and shows some special features. Often, large cholesteatomata are associated with small perforations of the eardrum and well pneumatized mastoids (Jahnke, 1982). The cholesteatomata in the author's patients appeared to be primary attic lesions and are considered to be 'acquired' even when the eardrum was intact. There was usually no bone erosion seen upon radiological examination.

While not wishing to discuss the aetiology of cholesteatoma, it does seem that a high proportion of childhood cholesteatomata affecting the middle ear have a congenital origin with an intact, unscarred eardrum and no bone erosion (*Figure 2.40*). Characteristically they are localized in the mesotympanum and later extend to the attic. Any discussion of congenital childhood cholesteatoma is complicated by two phenomena which are difficult to explain:

Figure 2.40 Congenital cholesteatoma. (*a*) Coronal; (*b*) axial CT sections of the middle ear cavity. This 6-year-old child was found to have a small cholesteatoma, presumably of congenital origin, confined to the mesotympanum (arrows), behind an intact eardrum. Note the normal outer attic wall or spur, and the air in the attic

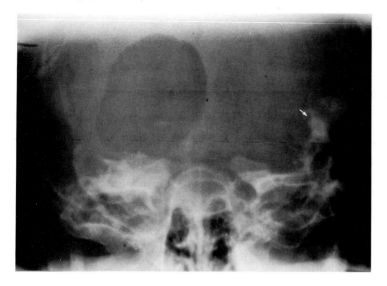

Figure 2.41 Gross disruption of the base of the skull by Hand-Schüller-Christian disease. Only a part of the labyrinth remains on the left (arrow). More typical of this condition is the punched out erosion in the skull vault. Plain Towne's view

(1) Cholesteatoma of the base of the skull not affecting the middle ear cavity, and therefore undoubtedly of congenital origin, is predominantly a disease of later life. These lesions from presumed squamous cell rests are therefore considered in Volume 3, Chapter 2

(2) The external auditory meatus develops by recannulation of a solid plug of ectodermal cells of the first branchial arch. This process begins at the medial end, with the membrane separating the primitive meatus from the tubotympanic recess developing into the eardrum. Failure of recannulation will result in congenital atresia of the external auditory meatus, potentially with the epidermis trapped medial to the atretic plate. This situation would seem to have all the potential for development of a cholesteatoma, especially if, as is often found at operation, there is a vestigial eardrum present.

Congenital atresia of the external auditory meatus is not rare but, surprisingly, cholesteatoma beyond the atresia is most unusual. Phelps, Lloyd and Sheldon (1977) found only four cases of cholesteatoma or retained squamous desquamation in 270 congenital deformities of the middle and external ear. Of these four cases, two were due to stenosis of the external auditory meatus and two were true soft-tissue atresias. Unfortunately, because the cholesteatoma is radiologically indistinguishable from soft tissue, these could not have been diagnosed even in retrospect. Other authorities have had similar experience with cholesteatoma, in association with congenital ear malformations. It is probable, that in such cases lack of a stimulus, such as infection, means that any squamous cell rests remain dormant.

Neoplasms

Occasionally tumours such as rhabdomyosarcoma or tumour-like conditions such as Hand-Schüller-Christian disease (histiocytosis X) may affect the temporal bone or mastoid (*Figure 2.41*). Massive destruction of bone is the usual feature.

References

BOOTH, J. B. (1982) Medical management of sensorineural hearing loss. *Journal of Laryngology and Otology*, **96**, 673–684

CHANDLER, J. R., GOULDING, G. R., MOSKOWITZ, L. and QUENCER, R. M. (1984) Nasopharyngeal angiofibromas, staging and management. *Annals of Otology, Rhinology and Laryngology*, **93**, 322–329

HAYDEN, E. K. and SWISCHUK, L. E. (1984) Editors. Head and neck imaging. In *Head and Neck Imaging*, **15**, p. 686. St Louis: C. V. Mosby Co.

HUTTON, J. N. T. (1981) Sedation and anaesthesia in audiological medicine. In *Audiology and Audiological Medicine*, edited by H. A. Beagley, ch. 34, pp. 809–815. Oxford: Oxford University Press

JAHNKE, V. (1982) Clinical, pathological and therapeutic aspects of cholesteatoma in children. In *Cholesteatoma and Mastoid Surgery*, edited by J. Sade, p. 25. Amsterdam: Kugler Publications

JOSEPH, P. M., BERDON, W. E., BAKER, D. H., SLOVIS, T. L. and HALLER, J. O. (1976) Upper airway obstruction in infants and small children. *Radiology*, **121**, 143–148

LLOYD, G. A. S. and PHELPS, P. D. (1986) Juvenile angiofibroma: imaging by magnetic resonance, CT and conventional techniques. *Clinical Otolaryngology*, (in press)

MICHEL (1863) Memoire sur les anomalies congenitals de l'oreille interne. *Gazette Medicale de Strasbourg*, **4**, 55–58

MONDINI, C. (1791) Anatomica surdi nati section. Bononiensi scientarium et artium instituto atque academia commentarii. *Bononiae*, **VII**, 419–428

PHELPS, P. D. (1986) Congenital cerebrospinal fluid fistulae of the petrous temporal bone. *Clinical Otolaryngology*, **11**, 79–92

PHELPS, P. D. and LLOYD, G. A. S. (1983) Syndromes with congenital hearing loss. In *Radiology of the Ear*, p. 121. Oxford: Blackwell Scientific Publications

PHELPS, P. D., LLOYD, G. A. S. and POSWILLO, D. E. (1983) The ear deformities in craniofacial microsomia and oculo-auriculo-vertebral dysplasia. *Journal of Laryngology and Otology*, **97**, 995–1005

PHELPS, P. D., LLOYD, G. A. S. and SHELDON, P. W. E. (1977) Congenital deformity of the middle and external ear. *British Journal of Radiology*, **50**, 714–727

PHELPS, P. D., POSWILLO, D. and LLOYD, G. A. S. (1981) The ear deformities in mandibulofacial dysostosis (Treacher Collins syndrome). *Clinical Otolaryngology*, **6**, 15–18

POSWILLO, D. (1974) Otomandibular deformity: pathogenesis as a guide to reconstruction. *Journal of Maxillofacial Surgery*, **2**, 64–72

STANSBIE, J. M. and PHELPS, P. D. (1986) Involution of juvenile nasopharyngeal angiofibroma (a case report). *Journal of Laryngology and Otology*, **100**, 599–603

VALVASSORI, G. E. (1983) The large vestibular aqueduct and associated anomalies of the inner ear. *Otolaryngolic Clinics of North America*, **16**, 95–101

3

The genetics of deafness

G. R. Fraser

Definition

Except where expressly stated otherwise, deafness should be taken to be synonymous within the context of this chapter with profound hearing impairment in childhood. In general, this may be taken to connote bilateral hearing loss of sufficient severity and of sufficiently early onset to necessitate special or supplementary educational measures for the learning of speech. It should be noted that such hearing loss is not necessarily congenital. Indeed, it is virtually impossible to distinguish between deafness which is congenital and that which is of rapid onset in the first few weeks or months of life.

This definition may be justified both on pragmatic and on biological grounds. The inability to acquire speech by normal methods of education because of hearing loss represents a useful way of identifying that group of children with the conditions which form the subject matter of this chapter and which give rise, in the majority of cases, to this type and degree of hearing loss. About one in 1000 children suffer from severe educational handicap to this extent as a result of deafness and, of these, approximately one-half owe their handicap primarily to hereditary causes. In the other half, the hearing impairment is due primarily to acquired causes.

Mendelian inheritance and deafness

Autosomal recessive deafness

This is the most common type of Mendelian inheritance of deafness. The autosomes are the 22 pairs of chromosomes which are not sex chromosomes (X, Y). Autosomal recessive deafness is biologically heterogeneous and may be determined by genes at many different sites, or loci, on these chromosomes. In the simplest case, the gene concerned with hearing exists in alternative forms, a normal and an abnormal, which are known as alleles.

In the vast majority of cases, the normally hearing parents of a child with autosomal recessive deafness are both carriers of an abnormal allele at the same locus. They are said to be heterozygous in that they possess two different alleles at the locus in question, one abnormal and the other normal. The presence of the normal allele ensures that they themselves do not suffer from hearing loss. In such a family, each parent has a 50% chance of transmitting the chromosome carrying the abnormal allele to each child. Thus, there is a 25% chance that any child will inherit two abnormal alleles without any compensating normal allele and, as a consequence, be deaf. Such a child is said to be homozygous for the abnormal allele.

Autosomal recessive deafness, therefore, generally occurs within a single sibship and usually is not transmitted from a deaf parent to a child. Because of the tendency of the deaf to marry similarly affected individuals, exceptions to this rule occur in that some unions involve two persons with the same type of autosomal recessive deafness. In such a case, all the offspring will be deaf since they cannot inherit a normal allele from either parent and, like their parents, will be homozygous for the abnormal allele. This is a very rare situation because there are so many different causes of profound childhood deafness that each cause individually is of low frequency in the deaf population. Even when the two parents suffer from autosomal recessive deafness which is determined at different gene loci, the offspring will hear normally in that they will inherit a normal as well as an abnormal allele at each locus and will be doubly heterozygous.

A person with autosomal recessive deafness may occasionally marry a heterozygote at that locus who hears normally, or who may be deaf due to an entirely distinct cause. In such a case, each child will inherit the abnormal allele from the first parent and have a 50% chance of inheriting the same abnormal allele from the other parent. The chance of deafness occurring in a homozygous abnormal child of such a union is therefore 50%. This type of family also occurs very uncommonly since the abnormal alleles concerned are individually very rare and the frequency in the population of heterozygotes for even the most common of them is not substantially more than 1%.

A characteristic finding relating to autosomal recessive inheritance of rare conditions such as deafness, is an increased frequency of consanguineous marriages, usually involving first cousins, among the parents of affected children, as compared with the general population. This happens because the alleles concerned are rare and, therefore, a relative of a heterozygote is far more likely to carry the same abnormal allele, inherited from a common ancestor, than is an unrelated marriage partner.

Because the chance of any child of a marriage between heterozygotes being deaf is only 25% and because of the small family size which is now the rule in economically advanced countries, autosomal recessive deafness most frequently occurs in a single individual who represents an isolated case within the sibship and within the family. It is very important to make every effort to identify the cause of the deafness in such an isolated case since, if autosomal recessive inheritance is operative, a risk of 25% exists for recurrence in subsequent offspring. Occasionally this will be revealed by the fact that the parents are related. More often, clinical findings associated with the deafness will serve to identify a syndrome known to be inherited in an autosomal recessive manner.

The Pendred syndrome (deafness with goitre)

Perhaps the most common autosomal recessive syndrome involving deafness, in European populations at least, is that first described by Pendred in 1896 as an association of deaf-mutism with goitre. Deaf-mutism is of course no longer used as a term to describe this group of children since it has been realized that the difficulty in learning speech is secondary to the hearing impairment.

Brain (1927) first invoked the hypothesis of autosomal recessive inheritance in this syndrome. Furthermore, he clearly foresaw the later discoveries by Morgans and Trotter (1958), that the goitre in this condition is due to an inborn error of thyroid hormone synthesis, and he showed great perspicacity in suggesting that it represented only one of several such errors which could exist. Morgans and Trotter (1958) showed that this defect consists of a partial block in the enzymatic step involving the incorporation of inorganic iodide into organic form in the thyroid gland. Compensatory hyperplasia of the thyroid gland, often leading to a large goitre, may overcome the deficiency in thyroid hormone synthesis and affected individuals often remain euthyroid throughout life. In the past, surgical removal of the goitre often led to hypothyroidism. This unsatisfactory treatment has been superseded by the administration of exogenous thyroid hormone immediately after diagnosis, which maintains euthyroid status even without compensatory hyperplasia of the gland and, indeed, may lead to a regression in size of a gland which is already hyperplastic. Such treatment has no effect on the hearing impairment.

A specific test of thyroid function can be employed to make an unequivocal diagnosis of the Pendred syndrome in a deaf child with thyroid enlargement. The test is too complex to be used as a routine screening procedure among deaf children without clinical enlargement of the gland, who may be presymptomatic cases of the Pendred syndrome. The test depends on the phenomenon that inorganic iodide contained in the thyroid gland is expelled by perchlorate or thiocyanate. Thus, if a dose of such a compound is given to an affected individual one hour after administration of radioactive iodide, there is a marked fall in counting rate over the thyroid. In normal individuals, all the radioactive iodide trapped by the gland is converted instantaneously into organic form and no such fall occurs.

The audiogram of cases of the Pendred syndrome characteristically shows complete sensorineural loss of hearing in the high frequencies, often with an island of residual hearing being retained in the low frequencies. This pattern is found in many types of autosomal recessive deafness, but the correspondence between the aetiology of hearing loss and audiometric patterns is in general not close and exceptions to this rule occur frequently in cases of the Pendred syndrome, as in other types of autosomal recessive deafness. There is no firm evidence as to whether progression of the hearing loss occurs in the Pendred syndrome.

The Usher syndrome (deafness with retinitis pigmentosa)

The Usher syndrome is one of the more common types of deafness in European populations, although it is less common than the Pendred syndrome. In 1858, only a few years after the discovery of the ophthalmoscope had made the detection of this syndrome possible, the famous German ophthalmologist, Albrecht von Graefe, briefly mentioned in a paper on retinitis pigmentosa that a cousin of his, Alfred Graefe, while assisting him in his Berlin clinic, had seen a sibship of five children in which three deaf brothers had the condition.

Liebreich (1861) systematically surveyed the deaf population of Berlin for retinitis pigmentosa and found that the association was more common among the Jewish deaf. Other early surveys of deaf populations were conducted by Adler (1876), Lee (1883) and Hammerschlag (1907). The last of these authors conducted a survey of deaf individuals in Vienna and confirmed the findings of Liebreich (1861), that the association with retinitis pigmentosa was more common among deaf persons who were Jewish.

In general, the different types of autosomal recessive deafness may vary greatly in frequency between population groups. These variations are associated with the fact that marriages do not occur at random within the human population and the choice of marriage partner may be constrained by religious, ethnic, social, or geographical factors. Because of these deviations from random mating (panmixia), abnormal alleles and the autosomal recessive conditions to which they give rise may reach high frequencies in certain groups. These are known as mating isolates because marriages often occur within the group (inbreeding). The Jews of Central Europe may have constituted one such isolate in which the allele for the Usher syndrome reached a high frequency. Another such isolate has been described more recently. In the Acadian population of Louisiana consisting of 57 000 individuals, 44 cases of the Usher syndrome were identified (Kloepfer, Laguaite and McLaurin, 1966). This figure for the prevalence of the condition is far higher than any reported from other populations, and it must be assumed that one or more of the restricted number of founders of this isolated and inbred population carried the abnormal allele on arrival from the original home of the Acadians on the Eastern seaboard of Canada. Subsequently, as population numbers grew in their new home, the condition reached its present high prevalence. This is known as a founder effect.

It was actually more than half a century after the findings of von Graefe (1858) and Liebreich (1861) in Berlin that Usher (1914), in studying the incidence of deafness in a series of cases of retinitis pigmentosa referred to his ophthalmological clinic in London, noted the existence of the syndrome which now carries his name. This eponym is probably best reserved for the autosomal recessive association of retinitis pigmentosa with profound childhood deafness, although the existence of genetical subtypes comprising milder deafness of later onset, and even a distinct mode of inheritance, has been postulated on inadequate grounds.

Typically, the sensorineural hearing loss in the Usher syndrome shows the same audiometric configuration as that in the Pendred syndrome, the high tones being more severely involved than the low, although many exceptions occur to this rule. Marked disturbances of vestibular function are commonly found.

Subjective and objective signs of retinal involvement usually do not appear until late childhood, or even adult life, unlike the deafness which is of very early onset and is usually diagnosed before the age of 3 years. Contraction of the visual fields (tunnel vision) and night blindness may precede objective evidence of retinitis pigmentosa as determined by ophthalmoscopy; when they occur, the ophthalmoscopic lesions are characteristically peripheral in distribution. It is probable that more sensitive electrodiagnostic tests, such as the electroretinogram (ERG) and the electro-oculogram (EOG), would reveal abnormalities at a much earlier age, perhaps even at birth.

Cataracts are a common complication in later life and, in combination with progressive retinal degeneration, may lead to virtual blindness. Nevertheless, the prognosis for vision is not always poor since cataracts may never form and the retinal degeneration may remain stationary indefinitely. Thus, in some cases, Usher's syndrome may first be diagnosed in middle age, or even later, by routine ophthalmoscopy without the patient being aware of undue visual difficulties.

The Jervell and Lange-Nielsen syndrome (deafness with electrocardiographic abnormalities)

Bizarre abnormalities of the electrocardiogram are associated with deafness in this condition which is less common than the syndromes of Usher and Pendred. The QT interval is markedly prolonged due to lengthening of the ST segment and the T wave, with normal appearance and duration of the QRS complex. The large T waves may be upright, biphasic, or inverted. A disorder of the later stages of cardiac repolarization is probably the underlying cause of these very unusual anomalies. It gives rise to a susceptibility to episodes of ventricular fibrillation which are manifested as recurrent fainting attacks (being, in fact, attacks of cardiac syncope) beginning in early infancy. Any one of these attacks is potentially fatal and sudden death is a component of this autosomal recessive syndrome.

In view of the dramatic nature of this condition, it is perhaps surprising that its recognition and delineation had to await the published description of Jervell and Lange-Nielsen (1957). These authors described a family in Norway in which four of six sibs were deaf. From early childhood all four had been subject to fainting attacks during which three had died at the ages of 4, 5 and 9 years. Of course, the recognition of the syndrome was not possible before the discovery of the electrocardiograph and, in addition, sudden death in childhood has been more common than it is now and, therefore, attracted less interest. In addition, the taking of an electrocardiogram may not form part of the routine investigation of recurrent fainting attacks which tend to be ascribed to neurological or even psychological causes. It was only because Jervell and Lange-Nielsen showed unusual perspicacity in obtaining ECGs from their patients that they were able to characterize the syndrome which now bears their name. There are, in fact, several suggestive accounts in the earlier literature of sudden death in deaf children which may well represent this condition, the first being reported by Meissner in 1856, long before the discovery of the electrocardiograph.

In the past, a substantial proportion of individuals with this syndrome died before reaching adolescence. A process of gradual adaptation to the disorder of cardiac conduction occurs so that, once adolescence is reached, the frequency of the fainting attacks is much diminished and the danger of sudden death recedes. The prognosis in childhood has improved greatly with modern treatment with drugs, and with the use of the implantable automatic defibrillator.

The hearing loss is characteristically similar to that seen in the syndromes of Pendred and Usher with complete loss of hearing in the high tones and some retention in the low.

Other autosomal recessive syndromes including deafness

There are only three autosomal recessive syndromes currently identified (those of Pendred, of Usher, and of Jervell and Lange-Nielsen) which are at all common among deaf persons. Other autosomal recessive syndromes involving deafness are much less frequent, and even their status as distinct entities is in doubt in many cases. The reason for these uncertainties is simple. Autosomal recessive deafness, as a whole, is a relatively common condition and it is not surprising, therefore, that, among the many thousands of persons with this handicap who have been studied, some should fortuitously be affected with other genetically-determined traits.

It is pertinent to consider at this stage the criteria on which the definition of the associations of deafness with goitre, with retinitis pigmentosa, and with ECG abnormalities as autosomal recessive syndromes is based. In each case, many families have been described in which multiple sibs suffer from the association in question. In these families, persons do not have deafness without the associated abnormality and vice versa. Even though no concrete knowledge exists concerning the biochemical mechanisms through which the abnormal alleles in question exert their pleiotropic effects (that is effects on different organ systems), it would be stretching coincidence too far to suppose that deafness and the associated abnormality were present in the same persons fortuitously in all cases. An alternative hypothesis to that of pleiotropism of abnormal alleles in the homozygous state at a single locus is that closely linked loci are responsible for the deafness and the associated abnormality. Experimental breeding techniques are not, of course, available in man and, therefore, such a theory cannot be formally invalidated but, in the light of current knowledge concerning gene action, the hypothesis of pleiotropism provides a far more likely explanation.

The number of such syndromes involving deafness which have been tentatively defined is very large and little would be gained by deriving a listing from various compilations which are available (Fraser 1976; Konigsmark and Gorlin, 1976; McKusick, 1986). It should be noted that in many of these syndromes the hearing loss is rarely or never profound in childhood. Instead of such a listing, one syndrome will be mentioned since it illustrates some basic principles concerning the genetics of deafness. This is the multiple malformation syndrome, sometimes known as the cryptophthalmos syndrome after one of its most striking component features.

The cryptophthalmos syndrome; modes of gene action and deafness

Cryptophthalmos means hidden eye and, in a fully expressed case, the eyelids are fused and the ocular globe is represented only by some disorganized remnants. This cardinal feature illustrates the principle of variability of expressivity of the abnormal allele in this condition. The extent of the eye involvement is variable and sometimes the eyelids and ocular globe may be virtually normal, giving rise to the paradox that the cryptophthalmos syndrome may exist without the presence of cryptophthalmos. In such a case, the diagnosis must be made by identifying some of the large number of other malformations, affecting virtually all organ systems, which may occur in this condition. Not only its presence, but also the degree to which each of these malformations is expressed is variable, giving rise to an almost infinite range of clinical manifestations, or phenotypes. The involvement of the auditory apparatus in this condition is as variable as that of any other organ system. Deafness, when it occurs, may be profound and is associated with malformations of the middle ear ossicles. Thus, it is conductive rather than sensorineural; this is true of only a small minority of cases of genetically-determined profound deafness in childhood.

It is perhaps surprising that only one of all these malformations is potentially lethal – renal dysplasia. Thus, stillbirths or neonatal deaths are seen in a substantial proportion of cases of the cryptophthalmos syndrome and are associated with renal aplasia, an extreme degree of this malformation. The cryptophthalmos syndrome may therefore be regarded as a semi-lethal genetic condition, one of a number of autosomal recessive multiple malformation syndromes with a limited potential for survival. Of course, semi-lethal abnormal alleles do not necessarily cause multiple malformations. The syndrome of Jervell and Lange-Nielsen, described above, may also be regarded as being the result of such an allele.

It is reasonable to assume that biochemical defects are involved in the causation of the syndrome of Jervell and Lange-Nielsen and of the syndromes of Pendred and of Usher, even though nothing is known of the nature of such defects, which may be presumed to be caused by the absence of normal alleles at the gene loci in question. However, by analogy with other autosomal recessive conditions such as galactosaemia, phenylketonuria and sickle-cell anaemia, which also comprise constellations of widely disparate clinical manifestations, it seems likely that point mutations in the chromosomal DNA have led to amino acid substitutions in an essential protein whose deranged function gives rise to deafness and its accompanying manifestations in these three syndromes.

It should be noted that, at a time when the nature of these biochemical defects will be elucidated, which may be far in the future, much will be learnt about the mechanisms of normal and abnormal hearing, cardiac conduction, thyroid hormone synthesis, and retinal function. Such discoveries will also have profound implications with respect to the treatment of deafness. In this context, it has been noted above that it is not known whether these abnormal alleles exert their full effect on the auditory apparatus in fetal life, or soon after birth. In the mouse, where detailed histological studies of the auditory apparatus are possible, both types of abnormal alleles are known. If the main brunt of the damage is in fact postnatal, this would be encouraging for prospects of prevention of deafness on the model of the dietary treatment of phenylketonuria; in this autosomal recessive condition damage to the brain occurs after birth unless a phenylalanine-free diet is provided.

In the case of the cryptophthalmos syndrome such a 'simple' biochemical explanation seems unlikely. Perhaps a whole region of the chromosome rather than a single DNA base pair is involved. Such a chromosomal lesion must be presumed to be beyond the present resolving power of cytogenetical techniques but this need not always be the case. Lesions of this type in a particular chromosomal region may well be variable in extent, giving rise to the wide clinical diversity which has been observed in the cryptophthalmos syndrome and which occurs mainly between, rather than within, families, as is to be expected on the basis of such a hypothesis. Thus, although variable between families, the particular genetic constitution, or genotype, within a family will be associated with a particular pair of small abnormal allelic chromosomal regions which will be constantly present in affected members of the same family.

Clinically undifferentiated (non-syndromal) autosomal recessive deafness

Despite the large number of syndromes mentioned above, the great majority of cases of deafness caused by autosomal recessive inheritance are clinically undifferentiated – the deafness does not form part of a recognizable syndrome in which it is associated with visible malformation or in which other organs and body systems are involved. There are undoubtedly several gene loci at which autosomal recessive non-syndromal deafness may be determined. Thus, it has been mentioned above that marriages between individuals both of whom have an unequivocal family history indicative of such a condition (consanguineous parents or affected siblings) most often give rise to offspring who are hearing. This suggests that these offspring are doubly heterozygous at the two gene loci at which the deafness of their parents is caused. Only in rare families are all the offspring deaf suggesting that the same locus is involved.

Another line of evidence suggesting that there are multiple gene loci involved is the consanguinity rate among the parents of children with non-syndromal autosomal recessive deafness. The rarer an autosomal recessive condition, the higher is the rate of consanguinity among the parents because the chance of an unrelated marriage partner carrying the same abnormal allele decreases with its frequency. The consanguinity rate among the parents of children with autosomal recessive non-syndromal deafness is higher than would be expected if this were a single condition, suggesting that it is made up of a number of component entities.

It is very difficult from these types of evidence to make an estimate of the number of gene loci which may be involved in the causation of non-syndromal autosomal recessive deafness. Fraser (1976) has suggested that there may be two or three relatively common types with a prevalence in the population of the UK similar to that of the Pendred syndrome, two or three moderately common types with a prevalence similar to that of the Usher syndrome, and up to 12 rarer types of which the syndrome of Jervell and Lange-Nielsen is an example.

Autosomal dominant deafness

Mendelian dominant inheritance of deafness occurs when a single abnormal allele is sufficient to cause the condition, even in the presence of a normal allele of the same locus on the paired chromosome. Thus, affected individuals are heterozygous at the locus in question and they pass the abnormal allele on to one-half of their offspring. Not all of these offspring are profoundly and bilaterally deaf, however, since the abnormal allele does not give rise to its full potential adverse effect in every individual who carries it. Thus, the deafness may vary from profound to mild, and may be unilateral rather than bilateral. This is known as variable expressivity of the abnormal allele. Some individuals may escape the effects of the abnormal allele altogether and enjoy normal hearing. This is known as reduced penetrance.

Autosomal dominant deafness, like the recessive variety, is extremely heterogeneous and distinct abnormal alleles at many different loci may be involved. The degrees of expressivity and penetrance of these abnormal alleles vary widely and, as a result, some families will show the classical pattern of Mendelian autosomal dominant inheritance with full expressivity and penetrance through several generations. In such families, on average, one-half of the offspring of affected individuals manifest profound bilateral deafness.

The Waardenburg syndrome

Of all the syndromes of which deafness is a component, this is the best known because of the striking anomalies of pigmentation which occur in association with hearing impairment. Heterochromia of the irides may be present and is often very striking, one eye showing a deep blue pigmentation and the other a deep brown. It may be partial rather than total with segments of two different colours in one or both eyes. In addition, there may be partial hypopigmentation of skin, eyebrows, ocular fundi, and hair (white forelock). Even if the irides are not heterochromic, they may often show an unusual blue colour, associated with hypopigmentation and hypoplasia of the stroma. Other features include overgrowth of the eyebrows leading to confluence, a broad and prominent root of the nose and a peculiar configuration of the eyelids associated with lateral displacement of the medial canthi (telecanthus or dystopia canthi medialis lateroversa).

There are many indications in the earlier literature of the existence of such a syndrome, but it was Waardenburg, in 1951, who first clearly delineated all the clinical features of this autosomal dominant condition which now bears his name as an eponym. Many families have since been reported coming from all ethnic groups (the condition is one of the causes of the rare appearance of blue eyes in non-white individuals). It has become clear, as Waardenburg (1951) had suggested, that there is genetic heterogeneity even within this very specific association of hearing impairment with pigmentary anomalies, in that at least two distinct clinical forms, or phenotypes, are to be found. The main distinguishing feature between these two forms is the presence or absence of lateral displacement of the medial canthi. Within a single family, only one form occurs in affected individuals, suggesting that different alleles, and possibly even different gene loci, are involved.

Variable expressivity and reduced penetrance of these abnormal alleles are commonly found in the Waardenburg syndrome and may affect each clinical manifestation independently. Thus, some individuals may escape the effect on hearing of the abnormal allele altogether (reduced penetrance) or may be unilaterally or mildly deaf, but still show clearly that they are transmitting the allele responsible because of the presence of pigmentary anomalies. When the deafness is bilateral and profound, it is often similar to that seen in autosomal recessive deafness with only a residual island of hearing being preserved in the low tones. When the hearing loss is more moderate, the audiogram often shows a flatter pattern; there is even sometimes an improvement in the high tones.

The Treacher Collins syndrome

The Treacher Collins syndrome (mandibulofacial dysostosis) (Collins, 1900) is a well-known but rare cause of profound deafness. The complete syndrome consists of abnormalities of the outer, the middle, and occasionally the inner ears, associated with antimongoloid palpebral fissures, colobomas of the lower eyelids, hypoplasia of the malar bone and mandible, macrostomia, high palate and malformed teeth, blind fistulae between the angles of the mouth and the ears, and abnormal implantation of the facial hair. These deformities may occur in any combination and with varying degrees of severity; they may be unilateral. The deafness is usually conductive since involvement of the inner ear is unusual, and it is only rarely bilateral and profound. The condition is autosomal dominant, but is often difficult to trace through several generations because of variable expressivity and reduced penetrance of the abnormal allele concerned. Furthermore, a substantial proportion of cases described seem to be due to fresh mutations; that is to say that the abnormal allele first appeared in the germ cell derived from one or other of the parents who are not themselves affected since they do not carry the abnormal allele in their somatic cells.

Other autosomal dominant syndromes including deafness

As in the case of autosomal recessive deafness, there are many of these syndromes and descriptions may be found in the compilations mentioned above. The Alport syndrome of sensorineural deafness with nephritis is very well known but virtually never leads to profound hearing impairment in childhood, the deafness typically being initially mild with an onset in late childhood or adolescence and with subsequent progression.

Clinically undifferentiated (non-syndromal) autosomal dominant deafness

As in the case of autosomal recessive non-syndromal deafness, there is likely to be genetical heterogeneity in the autosomal dominant variety. This is strongly suggested by the variability of audiometric pattern and degree of hearing loss, the variation being more marked between than within families, suggesting that different alleles may be at the origin of such variation. This is also true of the familial patterns of variable expressivity, reflected in unilateral involvement, and failure of penetrance, reflected in the presence of family members who have normal hearing but who have transmitted the abnormal allele.

As in autosomal recessive non-syndromal deafness, cases of the autosomal dominant variety are often isolated in one family. This may be because they represent fresh mutations, or it may occur because the allele has not been recognized to be present in other family members because of variable expressivity or reduced penetrance.

X-linked deafness

In 1836, at the very beginning of serious scientific inquiry concerning the subject of the causation of deafness, Kramer wrote as follows in discussing hereditary predisposition:

'Most frequently the parents of deaf-dumb children hear perfectly well; in this respect nature often observes the most strange and inexplicable laws of formation, for the determination of which we have no data. In place of many similar instances, I may merely detail one which comes under my notice every day. A man and his wife, of the name of Hartnuss, of Berlin, both of them healthy and having no predisposition to any disease of the ear in their family on either side, have five daughters and six sons; the latter were all born deaf-dumb, whilst the daughters, without exception, hear perfectly well. The mother of these eleven children is not aware of any circumstances that distinguish her pregnancies from each other, though the children are so remarkably differently endowed.'

It seems very likely that this family represents X-linked deafness, but because such patterns characteristic of X-linked inheritance (occurrence in males with transmission by unaffected females) have only rarely been reported, deafness of this type is probably very uncommon. References are to be found in Fraser (1976) where some additional pedigrees are presented. It is there pointed out that sibships containing two or more deaf brothers without deaf sisters were observed in a survey of the population of the British Isles with greater frequency than is to be expected, suggesting that some owe their deafness to X-linked rather than autosomal recessive inheritance.

X-linked syndromes including deafness

A strikingly large pedigree described in Israel by Ziprkowski *et al.* (1962) and by Margolis (1962) showed an association of deafness with pigmentary anomalies reminiscent of the Waardenburg syndrome. In this family, however, the association was clearly inherited in an X-linked recessive, as opposed to an autosomal dominant manner.

While most X-linked deafness is sensorineural, Nance *et al.* (1971), in a careful study of a family in which profound deafness was segregating in a pattern consistent with X-linked inheritance, showed that the hearing loss in six affected males was of a mixed type with both conductive and perceptive components. Furthermore, at operation in one case, a fixation of the footplate of the stapes was found. In addition, operation was complicated by a profuse flow of perilymphatic fluid thought to be under increased pressure as a result of an abnormal patency of the cochlear aqueduct.

A spectrum of Mendelian causation

It has been shown that deafness inherited in a Mendelian manner is very heterogeneous. It is extremely difficult to establish a balance sheet of causes, especially since these may vary substantially between populations. Furthermore, the methods available for establishing such a balance sheet are very limited since virtually nothing is known of the mode of action of the genes involved and only very partial clinical differentiation is possible.

Fraser (1976) in a study of the causation of deafness in the British Isles concluded that about one-half of all cases were determined in a Mendelian manner. This would give a population prevalence for Mendelian deafness in childhood of about 1 in 2000. Of these cases, about 66% were determined in an autosomal recessive manner, 31% in an autosomal dominant, and 3% in an X-linked recessive manner. Of the autosomal recessive cases, the syndromes of Pendred, Usher and Jervell and Lange-Nielsen accounted for 17, 9 and 2% respectively while, of the autosomal dominant cases, syndromes involving associated disorders of pigmentation such as that of Waardenburg accounted for 20%. These can only be regarded as very rough guidelines but, taking into account the large number of rarer syndromes, and the fact that the majority of cases of Mendelian deafness are non-syndromal and may be determined at many different loci, these figures are indicative of the considerable genetical heterogeneity underlying what is biologically a homogeneous handicap.

Congenital malformations and deafness

The Treacher Collins syndrome has been mentioned as an autosomal dominant congenital malformation syndrome which may include deafness as one of its components and the cryptophthalmos syndrome as an autosomal recessive one. Many other such syndromes, both dominant and recessive, have been described. A substantial proportion of cases in which deafness occurs as part of a congenital malformation syndrome are not determined in a simple Mendelian manner, but must be assumed to be caused by the synergistic interaction of multiple genes modified by environmental factors. An example of this group of conditions may well be the Wildervanck (1960) syndrome which combines hearing loss, associated with malformations of the outer, middle and/or internal ear, with Klippel-Feil anomaly of the spine. Although the malformation itself seems to occur with equal frequency in the two sexes, its association with impaired hearing occurs much more often in girls, in a ratio of 10 or more to one boy. The reason for this is not clear but a predilection for one or other sex is a characteristic feature of congenital malformations as a whole, although it is usually less pronounced.

Presumably, this phenomenon is due to the fact that one sex has a lower threshold of resistance to the combination of genetic and environmental factors determining a particular defect of embryogenesis. Since embryogenesis takes a substantially different course in the two sexes, such variations in resistance would not be surprising. The Wildervanck syndrome in fact accounts for 2% of deafness among girls.

The genetic component contributing to acquired forms of deafness

As much as one-half of cases of profound deafness in childhood are due primarily to acquired causes but the contributory hereditary component should not be forgotten. Thus, susceptibility to the teratogenic effects of the rubella virus is to some extent dependent on the genotypes of both mother and fetus. Deafness connected with perinatal mishaps is also due in part to genetic factors which may include those associated with low birthweight and those which determine the nature and extent of susceptibility to ototoxic drugs. Meningitis is a common cause of deafness acquired in early childhood. Again, genetic factors intervene in determining susceptibility both to the infecting organism and to ototoxic drugs used in treatment. Such genetic determinants in primarily acquired deafness are not easy to define but they are, nonetheless, of considerable importance.

References

ADLER, H. (1876) Beobachtungen und Bemerkungen über das Sehen der Taubstummen. *Klinische Monatsblätter für Augenheilkunde*, **14**, 65–96

BRAIN, W. R. (1927) Heredity in simple goitre. *Quarterly Journal of Medicine*, **20**, 303–319

COLLINS, E. T. (1900) Congenital abnormalities. 8. Case with symmetrical congenital notches in the outer part of each lower lid and defective development of the malar bones. *Transactions of the Ophthalmological Society of the United Kingdom*, **20**, 190–192

FRASER, G. R. (1976) *The Causes of Profound Deafness in Childhood: A study of 3535 Individuals with Severe Hearing Loss Present at Birth or of Childhood Onset*. Baltimore and London: The Johns Hopkins University Press

HAMMERSCHLAG, V. (1907) Zur Kenntnis der hereditär-degenerativen Taubstummheit. V. Über pathologische Augenbefunde bei Taubstummen und ihre differential-diagnostische Bedeutung. *Zeitschrift für Ohrenheilkunde*, **54**, 18–36

JERVELL, A. and LANGE-NIELSEN, F. (1957) Congenital deaf-mutism, functional heart disease with prolongation of Q-T interval and sudden death. *American Heart Journal*, **54**, 59–68

KLOEPFER, H. W., LAGUAITE, J. K. and McLAURIN, J. W. (1966) The hereditary syndrome of congenital deafness and retinitis pigmentosa. *The Laryngoscope*, **76**, 850–862

KONIGSMARK, B. W. and GORLIN, R. S. (1976) *Genetic and Metabolic Deafness*. Philadelphia: Saunders

KRAMER, W. (1836) *Die Erkenntniss und Heilung der Ohrenkrankheiten*. Berlin: Nicolai. Bennett, J. R. (1837) Translated as *Diseases of the Ear*. London: Longman

LEE, C. G. (1883) Notes on the ophthalmic conditions of deaf-mutes. *British Medical Journal*, **2**, 1184–1185

LIEBREICH, R. (1861) Abkunft aus Ehen unter Blutsverwandten als Grund von Retinitis pigmentosa. *Deutsche Klinik*, **13**, 53–55

McKUSICK, V. A. (1986) *Mendelian Inheritance in Man: Catalogs of Autosomal Dominant, Autosomal Recessive, and X-linked Phenotypes*, 7th edn. Baltimore and London: The Johns Hopkins University Press

MARGOLIS, E. (1962) A new hereditary syndrome – sex-linked deaf-mutism associated with total albinism. *Acta Genetica et Statistica Medica*, **12**, 12–19

MEISSNER, F. L. (1856) *Taubstummheit und Taubstummenbildung*. Leipzig and Heidelberg: Winter

MORGANS, M. E. and TROTTER, W. R. (1958) Association of congenital deafness with goitre; the nature of the thyroid defect. *The Lancet*, **1**, 607–609

NANCE, W. E., SETLEFF, R. C., McLEOD, A., SWEENEY, A., COOPER, C. and McCONNELL, F. E. (1971) X-linked mixed deafness with congenital fixation of the stapedial footplate and perilymphatic gusher. *Birth Defects: Original Article Series*, **7**, 64–69

PENDRED, V. (1896) Deaf-mutism and goitre. *The Lancet*, **2**, 532

USHER, C. H. (1914) On the inheritance of retinitis pigmentosa, with notes of cases. *Royal London Ophthalmic Hospital Reports*, **19**, 130–236

VON GRAEFE, A. (1858) Vereinzelte Beobachtungen und Bemerkungen. 6. Exzeptionelles Verhalten des Gesichtsfeldes bei Pigmentenartung der Netzhaut. *Albrecht von Graefes Archiv für Ophthalmologie*, **4**, 250–253

WAARDENBURG, P. J. (1951) A new syndrome combining developmental anomalies of the eyelids, eyebrows and nose root with pigmentary defects of the iris and head hair and with congenital deafness. *American Journal of Human Genetics*, **3**, 195–253

WILDERVANCK, L. S. (1960) Een cervico-oculo-acusticus syndroom. *Nederlands Tijdschrift voor Geneeskunde*, **104**, 2600–2605

ZIPRKOWSKI, L., KRAKOWSKI, A., ADAM, A., COSTEFF, H. and SADE, J. (1962) Partial albinism and deafmutism due to a recessive sex-linked gene. *Archives of Dermatology*, **86**, 530–539

4

The causes of deafness

David A. Adams

It is often difficult to identify accurately the cause of deafness in a child because exposure to a known pathogen, such as rubella, does not necessarily imply responsibility for the deafness. Nevertheless, the clinician must not be deterred from making a thorough search for the cause. Fraser (1976) pointed out that this search is not of purely academic interest, but does have considerable practical implications. Parents naturally want to know the cause of deafness in their child and often this is one of the first questions they ask. Awareness of the causes of deafness helps to identify high risk groups and is therefore useful in assisting early detection. It also assists in the planning of programmes for prevention or reduction in the size of the problem.

Classification

A good history, examination and full audiological investigation will usually permit classification of the deafness, whether *conductive, sensorineural mixed* or *non-organic*.

Confusion may occur when attempts are made to classify deafness according to whether it is congenital or acquired. In this chapter the following form is used.

Congenital disorders causing or predisposing to deafness

(1) Genetic, with anatomical abnormalities of external or middle ear
  (a) deafness present at birth
  (b) hearing probably normal at birth, deafness begins in childhood

(2) Non-genetic, due to disease affecting the developing embryo or fetus
(3) Other congenital disorders predisposing to development of deafness during childhood

Perinatal causes of deafness

Acquired disorders causing deafness

Conductive deafness

Table 4.1 summarizes the conditions in which the hearing loss is mainly conductive. Many other syndromes present with external and middle ear

Table 4.1 Causes of conductive deafness

(1) Congenital disorders
(a) Genetic, with abnormality of external or middle ear
  (i) Deafness present at birth
    Down's syndrome
    Crouzon's disease
    Marfan's syndrome
    Treacher Collins syndrome
    Pierre Robin syndrome
    achondroplasia
    Duane syndrome
    Apert's syndrome
    otopalatodigital syndrome
  (ii) Deafness appearing in childhood
    osteogenesis imperfecta
    otosclerosis
(b) Congenital disorders predisposing to secretory otitis media or infection (*see Table 4.2*)
(c) Miscellaneous disorders (*see Table 4.3*)

(2) Acquired disorders (see Table 4.4)

deformity although the hearing loss is usually mixed or predominantly sensorineural. These are discussed later.

Congenital disorders causing conductive deafness

Down's syndrome (trisomy 21)

Down's syndrome is a common disorder occurring in 1 in 600 of all live births. The incidence has been estimated at 1 in 1000 births in mothers under the age of 25 years and 1 in 100 births in mothers aged 40 or older. The affected individual usually has an extra number 21 chromosome. The characteristic facies makes the disorder easily recognizable.

Children with Down's syndrome present multiple problems to the otologist. Cunningham and McArthur (1981) estimated that as many as 50% of Down's syndrome children with hearing loss passed the normal childhood screening tests as carried out by local authorities. Maurizi *et al.* (1985) concluded that middle ear pathology is more common than might be expected on a purely clinical basis and that objective tests including evoked response audiometry are essential for reliable evaluation. The present author has found this technique to be of limited value if there is only a slight conductive loss, since it is often difficult to determine if there is a response present at near normal threshold levels.

These children are very susceptible to repeated upper respiratory tract infections, including sinusitis and otitis media, both infected and secretory (with effusion). In one series, 60% of children with Down's syndrome, examined during the summer months, were found to have secretory otitis media (Schwartz and Schwartz, 1978). Down's syndrome is associated with narrow external auditory canals, making it difficult to insert ventilation tubes.

In addition, there may be ossicular chain abnormalities, usually of the stapes. Balkany *et al.* (1979) found that 40% of a group of Down's syndrome children had a conductive deafness not due to infection or secretory otitis media. Exploratory surgery in 17 of these children revealed congenital ossicular malformations or destruction probably as a consequence of previous chronic infection.

There may also be an underlying sensorineural deafness, a short cochlea being the commonest reported finding.

It is therefore important to re-assess hearing thresholds after insertion of ventilation tubes as residual hearing loss is a major additional handicap in these children (Cunningham and McArthur, 1981).

Crouzon's disease (craniofacial dysostosis)

As with most of the hereditary causes of conductive deafness this is inherited as an autosomal dominant trait. Affected children have hypoplasia of the mandible and maxilla with a parrot-beak nose. There is usually skull deformity (craniostenosis) and exophthalmos.

Associated with the syndrome may be stenosis or atresia of the external auditory canal. The tympanic membrane may be absent and the malleus fused to the bony wall of the epitympanum. Other features include a deformed stapes, often fused to the promontory, and a narrow round window niche. A conductive hearing loss is present in one-third of children with Crouzon's disease.

Marfan's syndrome

This is inherited as an autosomal dominant trait. Affected children are tall, often with scoliosis and have long fingers and toes. Other features include hypotonic muscles, a tendency for lens dislocation and cardiac problems, especially aortic aneurysm. Deafness is a rare finding (Konigsmark and Gorlin, 1976).

Treacher Collins syndrome (mandibulofacial dysostosis)

The features of this autosomal dominant trait are confined to the head. The commonest feature of the syndrome is hypoplasia of the malar bones and maxilla. There is an antimongoloid slant to the palpebral fissures. The mandible is usually hypoplastic.

There may be deformities of the pinna, usually microtia, with stenosis or atresia of the external auditory canal. The tympanic membrane may be replaced by a bony plate. The ossicular chain can have a variety of malformations and, in some cases, the middle ear cleft is absent. Tensor tympani and stapedius muscles are often absent. Inner ear abnormalities, if present, would appear to be confined to the vestibular labyrinth (Schuknecht, 1974).

McKenzie (1958) proposed that the basic defect in Treacher Collins syndrome is a temporary deficiency in the blood supply to those structures which develop from the first arch cartilage.

In spite of their appearance the distribution of intelligence in these children would appear to be similar to that in the normal population (Fisch, 1981).

Pierre Robin syndrome

This is considered to be an autosomal dominant trait, although, in some cases, it may be due to intrauterine disease during the first trimester. The features of this syndrome include cleft palate, hypoplasia of the mandible, glossoptosis, congenital dislocation of the hip and club foot. There may be mental retardation associated with either microcephaly or hydrocephalus.

The external ears may be cup-shaped and appear to be low set because of the hypoplastic mandible (*Figure 4.1*). The middle ear cleft may be

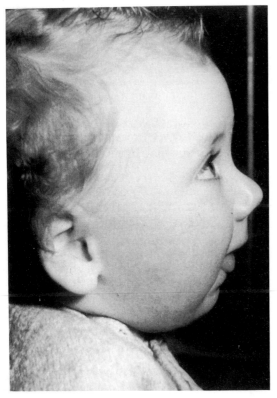

Figure 4.1 Pierre Robin syndrome

absent, or there may be thickening of the stapes footplate and crura. Inner ear deformities include abnormal communications between the middle and apical turns of the cochlea, a poorly developed modiolus or a narrow internal auditory canal.

The audiogram shows a conductive deafness, but in cases with inner ear abnormalities the hearing loss is mixed.

Achondroplasia (dwarfism)

Although this is inherited as an autosomal dominant trait, about three-quarters of cases may be due to fresh mutation. The incidence rises with increasing parental age.

The main effects are on the skeletal system. There is slow growth of cartilage and delayed endochondral ossification. The result is stunted growth, with disproportionately short limbs and a large head with prominent forehead and depressed nasal bridge.

In the middle ear, the ossicles may be fused to the bony margins of the middle ear cleft. The cochlea may be deformed. The hearing loss, if present, is usually conductive as a result of the middle ear abnormality and also of a predisposition to secretory otitis media.

Duane syndrome (cervical oculoacoustic dysplasia)

The affected children with this autosomal dominant syndrome have a very short neck, congenital paralysis of the sixth cranial nerve, and enophthalmos with conductive deafness.

Abnormalities of the external ear include microtia and atresia of the external auditory canal. In the middle ear, the ossicles may be fused and not connected to the oval window. The oval window may be closed by a membrane. Some children have a mixed hearing loss.

Apert's syndrome (acrocephalosyndactyly)

This is occasionally inherited as an autosomal dominant trait, although most of the cases are thought to be the result of fresh mutation with a high mutation rate related to advancing parental age. These children have a high, tower skull and flat forehead (acrocephaly). There is maxillary hypoplasia with a high-arched cleft palate and saddle nose. The fingers and toes are fused (syndactyly).

The audiogram shows a flat conductive loss of varying degrees. Surgical exploration has demonstrated congenital fixation of the stapes footplate.

Otopalatodigital syndrome

This X-linked trait is characterized by bossing of the frontal and occipital bones. There is hypertelorism, hypoplasia of the mandible and cleft palate. The fingers are short and clubbed. Most cases show mild mental retardation.

The pinnae are low set and small. There is a conductive deafness due to abnormalities of the ossicular chain.

Osteogenesis imperfecta

The association of fragile bones, blue sclerae and conductive deafness is known as the syndrome of van de Hoeve and de Kleyn. Not all children with osteogenesis imperfecta have blue sclerae and not all have deafness. There would appear to be two distinct forms of the disorder: osteogenesis imperfecta congenita (autosomal recessive) and osteogenesis imperfecta tarda (autosomal dominant).

The basic defect of osteogenesis imperfecta seems to be that collagen does not mature properly, giving a faulty framework for the hydroxyapatite crystals deposited during ossification.

The congenital form is usually lethal, often *in utero*, with skull fractures being the commonest cause of death. In osteogenesis imperfecta tarda the deafness may begin soon after puberty. Morrison (1979) reported a series in which the onset of deafness started as early as 6 years and as late as 51 years, with a peak in the third decade. The deafness is conductive initially, although some cases develop a mixed loss. Schuknecht (1974) summarized the findings of several authors, noting that the disease was characterized by the presence of new soft vascular bone in the region of the oval window, resembling that found in otosclerosis. Bergstrom (1977) reported deformity of the stapes.

It has been argued that otosclerosis is a localized form of osteogenesis imperfecta as they share many common features. Shea and Postma (1982), however, reported that the results of surgery in a group of patients with osteogenesis imperfecta were not as good as those obtained in otosclerotic ears. This, with the earlier age of onset of deafness in osteogenesis imperfecta, would suggest that the two conditions are at least clinically distinct.

Otosclerosis

This is a disease of uncertain aetiology. In many cases it is inherited as an autosomal dominant trait with variable penetrance (Sando, Suehiro and Wood, 1983).

Deafness does not usually begin until puberty and is, on average, later than that in osteogenesis imperfecta. Cawthorne (1955) reported that 70% of patients with clinical otosclerosis first noticed their hearing loss between the ages of 11 and 30 years. In another large series of 610 patients, in whom the deafness began before 18 years of age, the average age of onset of deafness was surprisingly low at 11.5 years (Robinson, 1983). One-half of the patients in this series had a family history of otosclerosis.

There is general agreement that the deafness in children is conductive, with normal or good inner ear function. The results of stapedectomy in children are good, but it should be remembered that middle ear infection is common in this age group. The additional risk to the cochlea which

this might present may be avoided by fitting a hearing aid until the child is older.

Congenital disorders predisposing to secretory otitis media or infection
(*Table 4.2*)

Cystic fibrosis (mucoviscidosis)

Cystic fibrosis is the commonest autosomal recessive disease in the UK, occurring in approximately 1 in 2000 births. The precise nature of the defect is unknown. It affects both mucus and non-mucus secreting glands. The nasal airway, sinus ostia, eustachian tube and middle ear are blocked by viscid mucus. There is also involvement of the salivary glands, bile duct and intestine with fat malabsorption and impaired digestion.

Table 4.2 Congenital disorders predisposing to secretory otitis media or infection

Cystic fibrosis
Immotile cilia syndrome
Cleft palate
Immune deficiency disease

Children with this disease are susceptible to secretory otitis media and middle ear infection. In addition, these children are often treated with potentially ototoxic antibiotics in high dosage and are therefore also at risk of developing a sensorineural deafness.

The diagnosis is established by the finding of an increased concentration of sodium in the sweat to above 60 mmol/l.

Immotile cilia syndrome

In this rare disease there is impairment of the normal ciliary mechanism of respiratory tract mucosa. The clinical spectrum of disease varies from children with a chronic cough to the sinusitis, bronchiectasis and situs inversus of Kartagener's syndrome. These children are very susceptible to secretory otitis media. The diagnosis is confirmed by electron microscopy of biopsies of upper respiratory tract mucosa.

Cleft palate

The incidence of cleft lip-palate is 1 in 500–750 live births (Rood and Stool, 1981). Otitis media, especially the secretory type is common. Paradise, Bluestone and Felder (1969) found that virtually all children with cleft palates under the age of 20 months had otitis media which was usually secretory in nature.

Two factors may be responsible for this. First, regurgitation of irritant food and fluids around the eustachian tube orifice will cause oedema and obstruction. Second, there is usually some degree of eustachian tube dysfunction associated with failure of the tube to open properly on swallowing. There is no midline anchorage in the unrepaired cleft palate and this prevents the tensor palati muscle exerting sufficient force on the eustachian tube orifice to open it.

Rood and Stool (1981) found that the incidence of secretory otitis media reduced after palatal repair and also with advancing age. Repair of the cleft palate does not, however, always solve the eustachian tube problem. Scarring may inhibit movement of the tensor palati. Furthermore, infracture of the pterygoid hamulus is sometimes used to relieve tension on the palatal repair. This in itself disturbs the functional opening of the eustachian tube.

Immune deficiency disease

Disorders of the immune system predispose to infection of various body systems, including the middle ear.

Miscellaneous congenital causes of conductive deafness (*Table 4.3*)

Isolated malformations of the external and middle ears

These, and their management, are discussed in Chapter 5.

Table 4.3 Congenital disorders with conductive deafness – miscellaneous conditions

Isolated malformations
Congenital cholesteatoma
Rhabdomyosarcoma
Fibrous dysplasia
Goldenhar's syndrome

Congenital cholesteatoma

True congenital (primary) cholesteatoma may be due to an epithelial rest left behind as the otic cyst sinks in from the surface of the developing embryo. More recently, Aimi (1983) postulated that most congenital cholesteatomata occurred near the tympanic isthmus of the middle ear, at the junction of first and second branchial arches. This would suggest that the origin of the cholesteatoma was related to migration of external canal ectoderm into the middle ear at an early stage of development, perhaps because of the failure of the inhibitory function of the tympanic ring.

Derlacki and Clemis (1965) outlined three criteria for diagnosis:

(1) development behind an intact tympanic membrane
(2) no history of ear infections
(3) the lesion must arise from inclusion of squamous epithelium during embryonic development.

It must not be forgotten, however, that cholesteatoma, limited to the middle ear and mastoid behind an intact tympanic membrane, may be due to epidermal ingrowth followed by healing of a perforation of the tympanic membrane (Schuknecht, 1974).

Congenital cholesteatoma may be classified according to the site of origin (Schuknecht, 1974):

(1) petrous apex
(2) middle ear and mastoid
(3) external auditory canal.

The lesion behaves in the same way as acquired cholesteatoma, with enlargement of the cyst and bony erosion. The spectrum of symptoms ranges from conductive deafness to facial paralysis and the intracranial complications of the disease. In some cases the hearing may be normal because sound is conducted from the tympanic membrane through the cyst to the stapes footplate.

McDonald, Cody and Ryan (1984) reported a series of 21 patients considered to have congenital cholesteatoma. This group represented 2% of all the cholesteatomata considered by the authors, suggesting that congenital cholesteatoma may not be as rare as previously supposed. Conductive deafness was the commonest presenting symptom in 18 patients and in 13 of those the tympanic membrane was described as opaque, white or had a cyst visible through it. The disease was confined to the middle ear and mastoid in 20 patients, in the other patient there was extension to the petrous apex.

Rhabdomyosarcoma

Rhabdomyosarcoma, although rare, is the commonest type of malignant neoplasm arising in the soft tissues of the head and neck in children (Chasin, 1984).

The tumour probably originates from a primitive skeletal muscle cell (the myoblast) or from a mesenchymal stem cell. Those related to the ear present with a friable mass in the external auditory canal. There is discharge, bleeding, conductive deafness and occasionally facial paralysis.

The prognosis is poor, although treatment with a combination of radiotherapy, chemotherapy and surgery may give some benefit.

Fibrous dysplasia of bone

A comprehensive review of this disorder was provided by Nager, Kennedy and Kopstein (1982). It is a disease of unknown aetiology. There are two types – monostotic and polyostotic. In monostotic disease a single bone is involved with the skull or face being the site in about 10% of cases. If the lesion involves the temporal bone, it may present as a slowly progressive, hard, painless swelling in the mastoid or squamous portion. Temporal bone disease usually becomes evident during childhood with progressive conductive deafness, increase in size or change in shape of the temporal bone, and progressive obliteration of the external auditory canal (Nager and Holliday, 1984).

Polyostotic fibrous dysplasia, if associated with café-au-lait spots and precocious sexual development, is known as McCune Albright syndrome. In polyostotic disease, both temporal bones may be affected.

The radiological features vary with the amount of fibrosis and calcification, with areas of radiotranslucency adjacent to areas of increased bony density.

The complications include exposure of dura, predisposition to acquired cholesteatoma and cranial nerve involvement.

Hereditary fibrous dysplasia is very rare. Adams and Kerr (1983) described a unique family, many members of which have polyostotic fibrous dysplasia of bone. In this family the disorder would appear to be inherited as an autosomal dominant trait with variable penetrance. Deafness is an early symptom in affected children and is purely conductive. The tympanogram shows a very high compliance in most cases. The hearing loss is progressive and eventually becomes mixed. Seven of the patients have had exploratory middle ear surgery with the commonest finding being the replacement of the long process of the incus by fibrous tissue. There is at present considerable debate as to the nature of the disease in this family. The histology has some features in keeping with a diagnosis of Paget's disease, although the clinical and biochemical findings are quite different.

Goldenhar's syndrome (oculoauriculovertebral dysplasia)

The aetiology of this condition is unknown, although it is probably not hereditary. Lesions of the eye include a cleft upper lid, dermoids and defects of the extraocular muscles. There may be auricular appendages, microtia and atresia of the external auditory canal (*Figure 4.2*). There is often unilateral hypoplasia of the mandible with hemivertebrae and club foot.

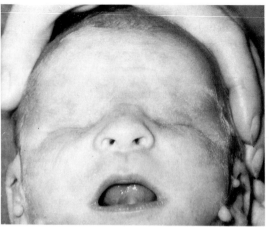

Figure 4.2 Goldenhar's syndrome

Approximately 50% of cases have a conductive deafness due to the external ear abnormalities.

Acquired disorders causing conductive deafness

The conditions acquired during childhood which cause hearing loss are summarized in *Table 4.4*. Otitis media, whether suppurative or secretory, is the commonest cause of deafness in childhood. These disorders are discussed in Chapters 13 and 12 respectively.

Table 4.4 Acquired causes of conductive deafness

Inflammation
  otitis externa
  acute (suppurative) otitis media
  chronic (suppurative) otitis media
  acute secretory otitis media
  chronic secretory otitis media
Trauma
Foreign body
Wax

Otitis externa

In children, acute (infected) otitis externa and eczematous otitis externa are the commonest forms of this disorder.

Swimming in chlorinated pools predisposes to the condition. The irritation of the skin of the external canal makes the child scratch and the subsequent trauma allows the skin to become infected.

Some children develop an allergy to acrylic or silicone earmoulds. This can be successfully overcome by using non-allergic moulds made from vulcanite, although these are expensive.

Conductive deafness is not a feature of otitis externa unless the external canal is blocked by debris or oedematous skin.

Trauma

Conductive deafness can be caused by direct or indirect trauma to the ear. Direct trauma is from a foreign body perforating the tympanic membrane or a longitudinal fracture of the petrous temporal bone.

Many parents are obsessed with the need to remove wax manually from a child's ear using cotton buds. The child's head may jerk during this manoeuvre and the object may be driven through the tympanic membrane. There may be damage to the ossicular chain and on occasions to the cochlea. Perforation of the tympanic membrane also occurs during clumsy attempts to syringe an ear.

Head injuries, as the result of accidents involving traffic or falls at home, are common in the young. The child's skull is more deformable than that of an adult and will often dent without fracture (Pond fracture). The sutures have not united and fissure fractures may persist as separated sutures. As in adults, fractures of the temporal bone are classified relative to the axis of the petrous portion. Longitudinal fractures are commonest (80% of cases) and are associated with a blow to the side of the head. The fracture line usually spares the cochlea and the deafness tends to be conductive in nature but may be sensorineural or mixed. There is often bleeding from the ear if the skin of the external canal is lacerated and the tympanic membrane torn. In other cases there may be a haemotympanum or cerebrospinal fluid behind an intact tympanic membrane. The ossicular chain may be damaged by dislocation or fracture.

The hearing loss in a child may not be noticed until some time after the injury. The child may be unconscious, or admitted to a paediatric unit and not complain of deafness. The ear must not be cleaned or syringed to obtain a better look at the tympanic membrane since this might introduce infection.

Radiology is difficult in the young as they tend to be restless and uncooperative. In some cases, fractures of the temporal bone are not visible on X-ray.

Most cases will settle spontaneously with healing of the perforation and the hearing will return to normal assuming there is no damage to the ossicular chain or cochlea. Cholesteatoma, as a result of entrapment of squamous cells in the fracture line is a rare complication (Freeman, 1983).

Indirect trauma occurs as the result of a slap on the ear, an explosion or to barotrauma. Children are more likely than adults to have eustachian tube dysfunction and may experience problems when flying, usually during descent.

Foreign body

Children often present with a foreign body in the external auditory canal and in many cases it is an incidental finding.

Foreign bodies may be of two types: those which are hygroscopic (peas, beans, paper) and those which are not (beads, gravel). A foreign body will only cause deafness if it completely occludes the ear canal or is pushed through the tympanic membrane during attempts to remove it.

Most are easily removed by syringing, although this must be avoided if the foreign body is hygroscopic. If the object is in the outer one-third of the ear canal it can often be removed using a hooked probe. This is not always easy since children are much more likely to move about with subsequent risk of damage to the tympanic membrane. It is best to try once only and if unsuccessful to arrange removal of the foreign body under general anaesthesia.

Wax

The ear's self-cleansing mechanism will usually keep the external ear free of wax. The use of cotton buds may cause impaction of wax deep in the external canal.

Children who use hearing aids often have excessive wax in the ear canal. This must be removed on each visit to the clinic as it may block the earmould. In a profoundly deaf child, with high-powered aids, accumulation of wax in the ear canal can cause feedback and limit the useful output of the aid.

Sensorineural deafness

Sensorineural deafness in children may result from the various known congenital or acquired disorders summarized in *Table 4.5*. In published series the incidence of deafness with cause unknown may be as high as 50%.

Four patterns of pathological abnormality of the cochlea have been described in patients with sensorineural deafness.

Michel dysplasia is the most severe, with total absence of the labyrinth, perhaps as a result of failure of the otic vesicle to separate from the neural ridge.

Mondini dysplasia affects the cochlea and semicircular canals. The cochlear duct is reduced to the basal coil only. The organ of Corti may be absent

Table 4.5 Causes of sensorineural deafness

(1) Congenital disorders
(a) Genetic
    (i) Deafness present at birth
        deafness alone
        syndromes associated with deafness
    (ii) Deafness appearing in childhood
        deafness alone
        syndromes associated with deafness
(b) Non-genetic, due to intrauterine disease
    infections
    ototoxic drugs
    metabolic disorders

(2) Perinatal disorders (see Table 4.6)

(3) Acquired disorders (see Table 4.7)

or reduced to a mound of undifferentiated cells. This type of dysplasia is seen in the Klippel-Feil and Pendred's syndromes. It may be visible on polytomography. Alexander (1904) described this dysplasia in association with auditory nerve involvement.

In *Bing-Siebenmann dysplasia*, the bony labyrinth is normal with underdevelopment of the membranous part.

Scheibe (cochleosaccular) dysplasia is the least severe and is thought to be present in about 70% of cases of congenital deafness. The stria vascularis has alternating areas of aplasia and hyperplasia. The organ of Corti is rudimentary and the hair cells sparse or absent. The saccule is collapsed. The utricle and semicircular canals are normal. It has been identified in Waardenburg's, Usher's and Refsum's syndromes and also in rubella deafness.

Genetic disorders with deafness present at birth

A fuller discussion of the genetics of deafness is given in Chapter 3. Holmes (1977) described hereditary deafness, *without any other abnormality*, which could be any combination of the following:

(1) inherited as a dominant, recessive or X-linked trait
(2) slight or profound
(3) affecting low, middle or high frequencies
(4) present at birth, or developing during childhood
(5) progressive or stable.

Klippel-Feil syndrome (brevicollis)

The aetiology of this condition is uncertain, although some cases would appear to be the result of an autosomal recessive trait. It is much commoner in females than males.

The external ear may have microtia with preauricular appendages and atresia of the external auditory canal. Middle ear manifestations include deformity of the incudostapedial joint or stapes and fusion of the short process of incus to the floor of the attic. The cochlea is short and there may be distortion of the internal auditory meatus. Most have a sensorineural loss, although it may be mixed.

Turner's syndrome (gonadal aplasia)

These patients have an abnormal genetic constitution, with an XO pattern. It is present in 1 in 5000 live births. The external ears are low set, with large lobes. The mastoid air cell system is poorly developed and there may be abnormalities of the stapes. There is some debate as to whether or not the disorder is associated with sensorineural deafness, although cases have been reported. Anderson *et al.* (1969) stated that, in their series, 64% of patients had a sensorineural deafness with a bilaterally symmetrical loss in the mid-frequency range. A conductive or mixed loss, was present in 22%; perhaps, in some cases, as a consequence of repeated attacks of otitis media.

Fanconi's syndrome

This autosomal recessive condition presents with congenital anaemia, skin pigmentation, skeletal deformities and mental retardation. The hearing loss appears to affect the high frequencies first, and is slowly progressive.

Pili torti

In this autosomal recessive disease dry, brittle hair is associated with sensorineural deafness.

Usher's syndrome

Inherited as an autosomal recessive trait, this is an association of retinitis pigmentosa with progressive sensorineural deafness. These children may also have vertigo and epilepsy.

Pendred's syndrome

This is inherited as an autosomal recessive trait. A congenital defect in thyroxine synthesis eventually causes goitre, which usually becomes obvious between the ages of 5 and 10 years. The sensorineural deafness is severe to profound, is said to be present at birth, and is certainly present by 6 months. This condition may not be diagnosed in the first child until 8–10 years of age when the goitre appears. The diagnosis will then be made much earlier in subsequent siblings.

Congenital hypothyroidism (cretinism)

The cause of the hearing loss in this condition is different from that in Pendred's syndrome (Fisch, 1981). The detection of partial deafness, sensorineural or mixed, is often made difficult by associated mental or physical abnormalities. Objective assessment is usually necessary. Fisch pointed out that this cause of deafness might be prevented by effective screening of neonates for hypothyroidism.

Waardenburg's syndrome

This is an autosomal dominant trait. Of those affected, 20% have a white forelock, 45% have irides of different colours or have different colours in one iris (heterochromia iridis) and 90–95% have lateral displacement of the medial canthi. This, not the white forelock, is the most common finding and gives a wide appearance to the bridge of the nose. The hearing loss may be moderate or profound, unilateral or bilateral. If the hearing loss is partial it may affect the low rather than the high frequencies.

Jervell and Lange-Nielsen syndrome

One-half of affected children with this autosomal recessive disorder, die before the age of 20 years. The deafness is bilateral and severe to profound. It is associated with abnormalities of the electrocardiograph, in particular a prolongation of the Q-T interval.

Genetic disorders with deafness developing after birth

Various authors have reported examples of hereditary sensorineural deafness with no other abnormality, in which the hearing appears to be normal at birth with a gradual onset of deafness, which may progress, occurring during childhood (Konigsmark and Gorlin, 1976; Holmes, 1977; Creamers, 1979).

Alport's syndrome

There is debate as to the aetiology of this disorder. The renal lesion may be inherited as a partially X-linked dominant trait (Fisch, 1981). Children present with haematuria and albuminuria within the first decade. Males are much more seriously affected than females and often die before 30 years of age.

In approximately 50% of patients a high frequency sensorineural deafness begins around the age of 10 years. This loss usually progresses to become severe. Ruben (1985) suggested that a renal lesion must be excluded in all adolescents with a newly found, progressive sensorineural deafness.

Renal tubular acidosis

This is a rare autosomal recessive disorder with only 23 cases reported in the world literature (Takanobu *et al.*, 1984). The present author has seen one child, thought to be the first in Ireland. The child's deafness was first noticed at 3 years of age and was found at that time to be a flat, moderate to severe sensorineural deafness. His most recent audiogram shows a profound loss, worse for the high frequencies.

Refsum's disease

Retinitis pigmentosa with peripheral neuropathy and cerebellar ataxia are the features of this autosomal recessive disorder. Sensorineural deafness usually starts between the ages of 10 and 20 years and is asymmetrical in some cases.

Cogan's syndrome

The aetiology of this is unknown, although it has been suggested that it is an autoimmune disease and, as such, is a localized manifestation of polyarteritis nodosa (Stephens, Luxon and Hinchcliffe, 1982). There is non-syphilitic interstitial keratitis with sensorineural deafness and vertigo. It usually first manifests in adolescence with sudden onset of vertigo, tinnitus and rapidly progressive deafness. Treatment with high doses of steroids may halt the deterioration in hearing.

Norrie's syndrome

In this X-linked recessive disorder there is progressive blindness with, in some cases, mental retardation. Progressive sensorineural deafness is present in about one-third of patients.

Non-genetic disorders: deafness due to intrauterine disease

These conditions, sometimes referred to as the embryopathies, are common and often preventable causes of congenital sensorineural deafness. The best known of these are the maternal infections which may be transmitted to the fetus across the placenta, through the cervix or at the time of birth.

Rubella

This is the commonest identifiable cause of congenital sensorineural deafness in children (Martin, 1982). Deafness occurs in about one-third of rubella children. Affected children may also have microcephaly with mental retardation, eye lesions including cataracts and retinitis, abnormalities of the cardiovascular system and lower limb deformities.

There is a mistaken belief that deafness only occurs if infection is within the first trimester. Hardy (1973) pointed out that infection with rubella at any stage in the pregnancy can cause deafness: infection at 0–8 weeks – 86% of children born with deafness, 9–12 weeks – 85%, 13–20 weeks – 53%, 21–35 weeks – 20%.

The virus enters the mother either through the nose or mouth and is transmitted through the placenta to the fetus. The maternal infection may be subclinical in about 40% of cases. Deafness is sometimes the only abnormality.

There is seasonal variation in the incidence of rubella (Martin, 1982). The numbers of children with rubella deafness born in December and January are much greater than those born in the summer months (*Figure 4.3*). This is not due to a

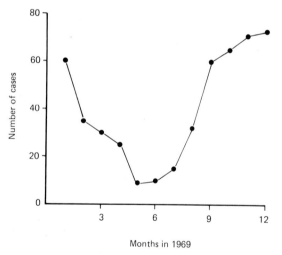

Figure 4.3 Distribution by month of birth for all cases of perceptive deafness due to rubella (EEC 469 cases). (From Martin, J. A. M., 1982, *Audiology*, **21**, by courtesy of the author and publisher)

seasonal variation in birth rate. It would appear that children conceived in March and April are more at risk of rubella than at any other time of year.

Hemenway, Sando and McChesney (1969) described the abnormal findings in the ear. There may be abnormalities of the stapes or cartilaginous fixation of the stapes footplate. The child's middle ear may contain fetal mesenchyme. The cochlea and saccule have Scheibe-type dysplasia.

The sensorineural hearing loss is usually severe to profound. If moderate it may progress to a severe loss (Fraser, 1976). Fisch (1981) described the typical hearing loss as flat, affecting all frequencies more or less evenly, although it may be trough-shaped with a maximum loss for the middle frequencies. The hearing loss is often asymmetrical and may even be unilateral. Occasionally, the deafness is of the mixed type. Some children may have normal peripheral hearing with central auditory imperception.

The diagnosis of rubella is often made on clinical grounds. It is possible to culture the virus from throat swabs or samples of stool or urine up to the age of 6 months. Persistence of IgG antibody after the disappearance of maternal IgG indicates congenital infection. Rubella specific IgM is present in the infected child for about the first 6 months after birth.

Martin (1982) pointed out that eradication of rubella would abolish one-fifth of all congenital sensorineural deafness. The policy in the UK at present is to offer vaccination to all girls between 10 and 14 years of age and also to screen all women at antenatal clinics. There are several problems with this policy. For it to be successful in abolishing congenital rubella there would have to be almost a 100% uptake in the target population. This is known not to be the case. In addition, the vaccine would need to be 100% effective (Begg and Noah, 1985). At present no check is made on girls after vaccination. Around 40% of babies damaged by rubella are first born. Antenatal screening for rubella is therefore too late since the fetus may already be infected (Kudesia *et al.*, 1985). These authors advocated a change in policy with testing before and after vaccination to ensure a primary response. This technique would also distinguish women who were protected by the vaccine from those with antibodies to the natural virus.

Cytomegalovirus

There is controversy as to the importance of cytomegalovirus in the aetiology of congenital sensorineural deafness. Fraser (1976) thought that it was a relatively minor cause of hearing loss. More recently, several authors have suggested that the importance of cytomegalovirus as a cause of congenital deafness has been underestimated. Bergstrom (1977) stated that 10 times as many children were born with cytomegalovirus infection as with rubella. Pappas (1983), in a review of children with subclinical infection, found that cytomegalovirus is the most common viral agent causing sensorineural deafness in children. It may well be that many cases of congenital sensorineural deafness in the 'cause unknown' group are due to cytomegalovirus.

There are two clinical types of the infection. The *systemic* infection (10% of patients) is obvious at birth or in the neonatal period. This has a much worse prognosis with the child often being severely handicapped. Children with *focal infection* (90% of patients) appear to be normal at birth and, in other words, have subclinical disease.

Pappas (1983) summarized the pathological findings. Cells with intranuclear inclusion bodies were found in Reissner's membrane and the stria vascularis. Immunofluorescent techniques demonstrated viral antigens among the inner ear cells including the organ of Corti and neurons of the spiral ganglion. Cytomegalovirus infection can cause destruction of both cochlear and labyrinthine structures.

The hearing loss is usually severe to profound and bilateral, but may, in a few cases, be unilateral (Saigal *et al.*, 1982; Pappas, 1983).

If the disorder is suspected at birth the virus can be cultured from urine samples. This is only useful during the first few weeks of life. Serological tests which show either a rising *titre* of IgG antibody or the presence of cytomegalovirus-specific IgM will confirm the diagnosis.

Toxoplasmosis

The causative organism of this infection is *Toxoplasma gondii*. The disease is much less common than either rubella or cytomegalovirus infection. The condition is usually subclinical at birth but may eventually manifest itself with progressive blindness because of chorioretinitis. Some children present with hepatosplenomegaly and jaundice. In some, cerebral calcification may result in epilepsy or hydrocephalus.

Kelemen (1958) reported the pathological findings in two children. Both had calcium deposits in the stria vascularis and spiral ligament.

The diagnosis may be made by injecting material from a lymph node or cerebrospinal fluid into mice and examining the brain for calcification 4–6 weeks later. The Sabin-Feldman dye test and the indirect fluorescent antibody test will confirm the presence of infection. Radiology of the skull can be useful if there is focal calcification of the brain.

Congenital syphilis

Deafness caused by congenital syphilis may begin in childhood, although in most cases the onset occurs between the ages of 25–35 years (Karmody and Schuknecht, 1966). In early onset disease the infection is severe and often fatal. The ear symptoms are overshadowed by systemic disease. In the later onset or tardive form, deafness with vertigo and tinnitus may be presenting symptoms. There may be profound unilateral deafness.

In the middle ear there may be thickening of the malleus with fusion of the malleus head and incus. There is osteitis of the temporal bone with mononuclear leucocytic infiltration. Obliterative endarteritis and hydrops are found, resulting in degeneration of the cochlear and vestibular end organs.

Herpes simplex

Congenital deafness has also been attributed to infection with herpes simplex virus, although specific reports are not available (Veltri *et al.*, 1981). These authors demonstrated, histopathologically, infection of the labyrinthine sensory cells.

Ototoxic drugs

The effect of these drugs on the fetal cochlea is discussed in the section dealing with acquired causes of deafness.

Irradiation

Irradiation can cause deafness in adults. It is sometimes quoted as a potential cause of congenital sensorineural deafness. The present author cannot find any reports in the literature in which this relationship has been established.

Ultrasound

Pye, Knight and Arnett (1984) described cochlear hair cell damage in guinea pigs due to ultrasound of 12.5 kHz. Ultrasonic scanning, using frequencies of 3.5 or 5 MHz, is a commonly employed technique in obstetric practice. At present, there is no evidence that this is harmful to the fetal ear.

Maternal diabetes

Fraser (1976) stated that the role of maternal diabetes as a cause of congenital deafness had not been established. Gratz, Pollack and Zimmerman (1981) described the radiological findings in two children of unrelated, insulin-dependent mothers. In each case there was hypoplasia of the internal auditory meatus. The cochlea, vestibule and semicircular canals were radiologically normal.

Perinatal disorders causing sensorineural deafness

Perinatal mortality has decreased dramatically over the last two decades. This may mean that more children survive with handicaps such as deafness. The main risk factors in the perinatal period are summarized in *Table 4.6*.

Table 4.6 Perinatal causes of sensorineural deafness

Hypoxia
Hyperbilirubinaemia
Preterm delivery and low birthweight

Hypoxia

Hall (1964) described the otopathological findings in neonatal asphyxia, including a decrease in cell numbers in the cochlear nuclei. The cochlea appeared histologically normal. A review of the literature would suggest that perinatal asphyxia only rarely causes a hearing loss. D'Souza *et al.* (1981) found a sensorineural hearing loss in one child from a group of 26 with a history of severe perinatal asphyxia. Significantly, one-third of these children had speech and language defects. Karjalainen *et al.* (1982) examined the hearing in 20 known cases of severe placental insufficiency and intrauterine hypoxia. There was no evidence of sensorineural deafness in any of these children.

Hyperbilirubinaemia

The best known cause of this condition is Rhesus disease, although it may also be found with other blood group incompatibilities, hereditary spherocytosis and liver immaturity. The incidence of deafness caused by hyperbilirubinaemia has fallen, presumably as a result of increased awareness of the problem and the availability of exchange transfusions.

Uziel, Marot and Pujol (1983) used hyperbilirubinaemia in the Gunn rat as an experimental model of this condition. Functional and morphological studies showed no cochlear abnormality, although evoked response audiometry suggested the presence of a defect in the brainstem auditory pathways of these rats. Schuknecht (1974), on the other hand, believed the lesion to be in the cochlea in man.

Hyperbilirubinaemia may cause kernicterus (bilirubin encephalopathy). In this condition, 20–40% of affected children have sensorineural deafness. The hearing loss is bilateral and predominantly high frequency in type.

Low birthweight and preterm children

Preterm delivery (before the end of the thirty-seventh week) and low birthweight (weighing less than 2500 g) are usually concomitant conditions and are therefore best considered together.

These infants have a higher incidence of hearing loss than normal (Fraser, 1976; Abramovich *et al.*, 1979; Minoli and Moro, 1985). There are several reasons for this. They are more likely to have suffered episodes of hypoxia or acidosis. In addition, these children have immature metabolic functions and kernicterus can result from smaller increases in serum bilirubin levels than in mature neonates. There is also the possibility that the deafness and low birthweight are concomitantly caused by the same factor, for example rubella.

In the immediate postnatal period these children spend a variable amount of time in intensive care units in noisy incubators. This is discussed later in this chapter. They are very prone to life-threatening infections and are given antibiotics which are potentially ototoxic.

Some experimental animals seem to have a 'critical period' during which structural and functional development of hearing occurs (Uziel, 1985). Deafness is likely to result from exposure to noxious agents at different times during this critical period. There is no evidence at present that there is a similar critical period in humans.

In summary, it is often difficult to ascertain the causative agent in these children because of the number of potential risk factors. It is possible that these factors exert a synergistic effect on the auditory system.

Acquired disorders causing sensorineural deafness

These conditions are summarized in *Table 4.7*. Extension of middle ear infection to cause cochlear damage is discussed in Chapter 14.

Various different viral agents, in addition to those already discussed, have been identified as

Table 4.7 Acquired conditions causing sensorineural deafness

Infections
    complication of otitis media
    viral labyrinthitis
Immunization
Autoimmune deafness
Meningitis
Ototoxic drugs
Trauma
Metabolic disease
Neoplastic disease

pathogenic in the ear. These include mumps, measles, herpes simplex, herpes varicella-zoster and influenza viruses.

Davis (1982) provided the first experimental evidence for viraemic spread to the ear and it seems likely that this is the common route by which the viruses reach the auditory system. Labyrinthitis may also be caused by extension of infection from the meninges.

Mumps

The deafness in mumps is usually of sudden onset, occurring within the first week of infection, although its recognition may be delayed. In some cases the deafness may follow subclinical infection. The loss may affect the high frequencies only but, more commonly, is profound. It is usually unilateral, but may on occasions affect both ears.

Measles

Schuknecht (1974) reported the incidence of deafness with measles as the suspected cause to be about 4–10% of populations of deaf children. The hearing loss tends to be bilateral and moderate to severe.

The pathological findings include degeneration of the organ of Corti, spiral ganglion and vestibular sensory cells.

Reye's syndrome

This acute, and sometimes fatal, illness usually starts during recovery from a viral illness especially influenza and varicella. More recently it has been linked to the use of aspirin in children. Clinically the child's condition deteriorates with vomiting, lethargy or irritability. In severe cases cerebral oedema will progress to coma and death. Rarey *et al.* (1983) described the pathological features in a 2-month old child with Reye's syndrome. The inner hair cells of the organ of Corti were damaged more severely than the outer cells with various degrees of degeneration of non-sensory epithelial cells lining the cochlear duct. Similar lesions were found in the vestibular end organs.

The present author is not aware of any published reports of auditory function in children who have recovered from Reye's syndrome; those seen in Belfast to the present have normal hearing.

Immunization

Tetanus immunization and antitoxin are known to cause peripheral neuropathies in some patients. In a review of the literature Mair and Elverland (1977) identified nine cases in which deafness occurred 2–10 days after tetanus immunization or tetanus antitoxin. These authors pointed out that it is extremely difficult to be certain that the two events are related, although in the absence of other aetiological factors a cause–effect relationship may be assumed. The present author has seen one child in which triple vaccination was followed within 2 days by a 'flu-like illness and severe bilateral sensorineural loss.

There are no reports in the literature of deafness after diphtheria or polio immunization.

Autoimmune sensorineural hearing loss

Immunological destruction of the auditory and vestibular systems is a recognized feature of many diseases (Stephens, Luxon and Hinchcliffe, 1982; Brookes, 1985; Naclerio, 1985).

Damage may be caused in several ways. Immune complexes lodge in the microcirculation of the ear causing obstruction and hypoxia in the distal tissues. Complement fixation may cause a vasculitis with subsequent inflammatory response. It is also possible that there is an inappropriate direct immune reaction against cells derived from the neural crest.

Brookes and Newland (1986) presented eight cases, one a child of 11 years, with deafness and evidence of circulating immune complexes. Plasma exchange, thought to remove the immune complexes, was of marginal benefit in restoring hearing in about one-half of the cases, although in some, relief was only temporary.

Meningitis

The most frequent cause of acquired deafness in childhood is meningitis (Martin, 1982). Rahko *et al.* (1984) presented the audiological and vestibular findings in 219 cases. These authors considered that deafness was due to labyrinthitis following spread of infection through the cochlear aqueduct, internal acoustic meatus or endolymphatic duct. It would appear, in some cases, that either the onset or detection of deafness may be delayed for up to 6 months after the illness.

About 10% of children with meningitis will develop some degree of hearing loss. In some children the initial hearing loss in bacterial meningitis will recover within 6 months (Munoz *et al.*, 1983).

Haemophilus influenzae is responsible for about 45% of cases of bacterial meningitis, especially in children aged 2 months to 4 years. Nylen and Rosenhall (1979) published a series of 97 children treated for this illness. Fifteen had moderate to severe sensorineural deafness, in six of these the loss was unilateral. In many other children there were minor abnormalities on audiometric testing.

Neisseria meningitidis causes 15–25% of bacterial meningitis. It is probably the most dangerous with respect to hearing loss, causing about 50% of all deafness from meningitis (Rahko *et al.*, 1984).

Streptococcus pneumoniae is estimated to cause about 20–25% of cases of meningitis. It is often accompanied by acute otitis media (Schuknecht, 1974).

Streptococcal and staphylococcal meningitis are much less common than the above. Tuberculous meningitis is associated with a high incidence of hearing loss and other neurological deficits.

Nadol (1978) considered the findings in 304 patients thought to have viral meningitis. The causative virus was identified in only one-sixth of the group and included mumps, measles, herpes simplex and varicella-zoster viruses. None of these patients had a sensorineural hearing loss.

Ototoxic drugs

The potential ototoxicity of many drugs is well recognized, the two most important groups being the 'loop' diuretics and the aminoglycoside antibiotics. A comprehensive summary of the pharmacology of these drugs and pathological lesions produced was provided by Harper (1982).

Animal research has demonstrated that aminoglycosides will cause intrauterine cochlear damage (Uziel, 1985). There also appears to be interspecies and interstrain variability. In humans, there are surprisingly few reports of deafness due to the administration of aminoglycosides either during pregnancy or childhood (Abramovich *et al.*, 1979; Crifo *et al.*, 1980). It would appear that neonates and older children have reduced risks from the ototoxic effects of these drugs. Children with cystic fibrosis often receive prolonged treatment with high doses of these drugs. Crifo *et al.* (1980) found only one such child, in a group of 30, with a bilateral slight high frequency loss assumed to be due to gentamicin.

Similar findings were reported in 53 children with cystic fibrosis who were given tobramycin. Only one developed a transient high frequency loss (Thomsen and Friis, 1979).

Erythromycin is commonly used in children with a history of penicillin allergy. Schweitzer and Olson (1984) presented a case report in which pharmacological doses were used. The patient developed a hearing loss 5 days after erythromycin was first given. On stopping the drug the hearing improved, although the high frequency loss persisted. A survey of the literature revealed a further 32 cases with a reversible high frequency loss.

This apparent decrease in ototoxicity in children must not be allowed to induce a feeling of complacency. Bernard (1981) demonstrated alterations in the brainstem evoked potentials of preterm babies due to conventional doses of aminoglycosides. As with adults, the serum peak and trough levels must be carefully monitored, especially in children with renal disease.

Trauma

The effects of trauma on the cochlea are fully discussed in Volumes 2 and 3.

A blow to the head, sufficient to render a child unconscious can cause cochlear concussion with a fracture of the temporal bone (Schuknecht, 1974). Transverse fractures of the petrous temporal bone are associated with damage to the cochlea or auditory nerve. In children, the deafness may not be noticed for some time after the injury. Rupture of the round or oval window may be caused by sudden violent exercise and is predisposed to by anatomical abnormalities (Pashley, 1982). Surgical trauma, even after minor procedures such as myringotomy may damage the cochlea.

The effects of noise exposure on the adult ear are well known. Most women continue to work for the first few months of their pregnancy. Mothers' abdominal and uterine walls will provide protection from noise. Szmeja *et al.* (1979) found that, when the mother was exposed to 100 dB noise, there was a change in fetal heart rhythm and also fetal movements. These may reflect distress. The effects of excessive environmental noise on the ears of the fetus are unknown.

Many neonates spend their first few days or weeks of life in incubators in constant noise levels of 60–80 dB. Added to this is the 5–25 dB generated by other life-support equipment such as ventilators, humidifiers and monitors. Medical and nursing staff will often stimulate apnoeic babies by striking the side of the incubator. This can cause impulse signals up to 140 dB SPL (Bess, Peek and Chapman, 1979).

Animal experiments have demonstrated outer hair cell loss in neonatal guinea pigs and rats exposed to noise (Douek *et al.*, 1976; Uziel, 1985). In human neonates, however, the noise levels currently found in incubators do not seem to cause a hearing loss (Schulte and Stennert, 1978; Abramovich *et al.*, 1979).

Children and adolescents live in a self-induced noisy environment. Portable stereo radiocassette players with headphones can generate noise intensity levels potentially hazardous to human ears (Catalano and Levin, 1985). Much has been written about the potential dangers of rock concert music and there are many reports of temporary threshold shifts in both musicians and the audience. Ruben (1985) pointed out that an adolescent with a seemingly insignificant high frequency loss may become severely handicapped in middle age due to the additive effects of industrial noise exposure and other causes of sensorineural deafness.

Menière's disease

This is extremely rare in children and presents a similar clinical picture to that found in adults.

Metabolic disease

Disorders of the microcirculation are common in diabetes mellitus and it is quoted as a cause of deafness. Seiger *et al.* (1983), in a survey of the literature, found conflicting views. One explanation of this was the heterogenicity of the different groups studied. These authors presented the findings in a group of 51 insulin-dependent diabetic children. None had evidence of deafness. This may have been due to many factors including short duration of the illness and lack of sensitivity in the auditory tests used.

Neoplastic disease

Acoustic neuroma (schwannoma) may be present at birth, but only become clinically obvious in later life. There are very few reported cases of acoustic neuroma in children.

Leukaemia may affect the temporal bone in two ways (Schuknecht, 1974). Leukaemic infiltrates may be found in middle ear mucosa and perilymph spaces. Haemorrhage may cause sudden deafness, usually with dizziness.

Sudden deafness

Children rarely complain of sudden loss of hearing. Tieri *et al.* (1984) suggested the following as possible causes:

(1) infection – mumps, measles, meningitis, varicella
(2) trauma – concussion, fractures of temporal bone, perilymph fistula
(3) idiopathic – the mechanism may be vascular with spasm, thrombosis, embolism or haemorrhage causing cell anoxia and death.

Mixed deafness

The conditions which cause a mixed deafness are summarized in *Table 4.8*. Otosclerosis in children is usually associated with conductive deafness only.

Earpits-deafness syndrome

Slack and Phelps (1985) presented a description of four families and a review of the literature. The

Table 4.8 Causes of mixed deafness

(1) Congenital abnormalities, deafness present at birth
    earpits-deafness syndrome
(2) Congenital abnormalities, deafness occurring in childhood
    osteopetrosis (Albers-Schönberg disease)
    histiocytosis X
    mucopolysaccharidosis
(3) Acquired disease
    infection

condition is characterized by unilateral or bilateral auricular deformities in 75% of cases. These are preauricular pits or appendages with unilateral or bilateral branchial fistulae or cysts in 50% of affected children. The ossicular chain may be abnormal and there is distortion of the basal turn of the cochlea. Two of the patients in this series had ossiculoplasties with no improvement in hearing. This confirmed the findings of other otologists dealing with this condition.

Osteopetrosis (Albers-Schönberg disease)

This may be inherited in a dominant form (benign) or as a recessive trait (clinically malignant). There is abnormal bone growth with failure of reabsorption of calcified cartilage and persistence of primitive bone. The bony labyrinths and ossicles consist of dense calcified cartilage. The mastoid is usually not pneumatized. These patients present to otologists with mixed deafness and recurrent facial nerve palsy.

Histiocytosis X (Langerhans cell histiocytosis)

The three forms of this disease, eosinophilic granuloma, Hand-Schüller-Christian disease and Letterer-Siwe disease, are probably different expressions of the same basic disorder.

Eosinophilic granuloma is the mildest form. There is localized skeletal destruction which, if present in the temporal bones, is manifest by swelling over the mastoid process with otorrhoea and granulations in the external auditory canal. There is a mixed hearing loss and occasionally facial paralysis.

Hand-Schüller-Christian disease often presents with a triad of symptoms: diabetes insipidus, exophthalmos and osteolytic lesions of the cranium. Temporal bone involvement produces a similar clinical picture to that in eosinophilic granuloma.

The most severe form of histiocytosis X is found in Letterer-Siwe disease. This is usually fatal.

A review of histiocytosis X was provided by De-Marino *et al.* (1985). There is proliferation of abnormal histiocytes. The ear manifestations in children may mimic those of chronic otitis media with mastoiditis, but are resistant to the usual treatments. The diagnosis is made by histological examination of a biopsy, taking care to obtain a sample of tissue deep to surface granulations. Treatment uses a combination of surgery, radiotherapy and chemotherapy.

Mucopolysaccharidoses

The best known of these are Hurler's (type 1) and Hunter's (type 2) syndromes. There is abnormal metabolism of intracellular high molecular weight carbohydrates. Most of the mucopolysaccharidoses are autosomal recessive traits except for Hunter's syndrome which is X-linked.

Fisch (1981) noted that all affected children examined by him had a hearing loss. In many of the children the hearing loss was conductive, although it was sometimes superimposed on a moderate high frequency sensorineural deafness to give a mixed loss. Schuknecht (1974) indicated that deafness is not always present in these children but, if present, is of the mixed type.

Schachern, Shea and Paparella (1984) presented the findings from the temporal bones of three patients with Hurler's syndrome. They included otitis media, residual mesenchyme in the round window niche, partial occlusion of the middle ear and basophilic concretions in the stria vascularis. Other reports note the absence of the incudostapedial joint and obliteration of both oval and round windows with fibrous tissue invading the otic capsule.

Infection

This is the commonest cause of mixed deafness in children and is discussed elsewhere.

Non-organic deafness (psychogenic deafness)

There are three types of this condition.

Functional (hysterical) deafness

This is apparent deafness in the absence of a pathological process affecting the auditory pathway. The deafness is a product of the subconscious. It is estimated that functional deafness is responsible for about 5% of all audiological clinic attendances. It would appear to be very uncommon under the age of 5 years.

It may be a reaction to stress, especially if the child is not doing well at school and the parents' expectations are unrealistically high. In some cases

it is a means of identifying with another member of the family who has a hearing problem.

The deafness may be moderate to severe with evidence of other psychological disturbances such as mutism, tremors, aggressive or withdrawn behaviour. The child's voice is usually unaltered with no deterioration in the quality of speech. These children often give different serial audiograms with better speech discrimination scores than would be expected from the pure-tone readings. Clinically the child's hearing is usually much better than the audiogram would suggest. This group must be differentiated from those children who seem to have difficulty in understanding what is involved in pure-tone audiometry.

Malingering

In this type there is intention on the part of the child to deceive. This is rare in children as most are not sophisticated enough to maintain the pretence for long and there is rarely the motivation for financial gain as sometimes seen in adults.

Organic deafness with psychogenic overlay

Children with true ear disease occasionally appear to be much deafer than can be explained by the pathology.

In all three types of non-organic deafness, objective tests, including evoked response audiometry, will reveal the true hearing thresholds.

These children present difficult management problems. It is important to stress to parents the need to avoid accusing the child of feigning a hearing loss. Attempts should be made to look for areas of conflict at home or school. This will often mean referral to a child psychologist or psychiatrist. These children must not be issued with hearing aids for fear of reinforcing their 'deafness'.

Conclusions

This chapter attempts to cover the major causes of deafness in children. The space given to each is not a reflection of its importance or prevalence.

Table 4.9 Different prevalence rates of deafness between various studies

Causes	Percentage of cases
Genetic	24–39
Embryopathies (mainly rubella)	6–24
Perinatal	6–23
Unknown	25–45

Taylor (1979) discussed the reasons for the differences in prevalence rates betwen various studies (*Table 4.9*). In retrospective studies serological data are not available, access to accurate hospital records is not always possible and sample groups differ. True comparisons are therefore difficult to make.

A more recent multicentre study of EEC children with a hearing loss of 50 dB or worse was reported by Martin (1982). In this study rubella was responsible for 20% of deafness in children in the UK. Deafness was identified as having a genetic basis in about 12% of cases, caused by perinatal anoxia or jaundice in 10% and in 40% of cases the cause was unknown.

The large size of the 'cause unknown' group is a feature of all reported series. Much discussion has ensued as to possible aetiologies in this group. At present, it is generally assumed that most of these are the result of recessive genes or to gene mutations. Many of the others are caused by undiagnosed intrauterine infection or to the effects of other unrecognized cochlear pathogens. Barr (1982) underlined the marked interspecies differences in response to thalidomide. This suggests an interaction between genetic factors and exogenous pathogens in the causation of deafness. It would seem that a genetically deficient auditory pathway is more susceptible to external agents. A better understanding of the processes causing deafness, together with appropriate and early investigation of the deaf child, should reduce the size of the 'cause unknown' group.

References

ABRAMOVICH, S. J., GREGORY, S., SLEMINK, M. and STEWART, A. (1979) Hearing loss in very low birth weight infants treated with neonatal intensive care. *Archives of Disease in Childhood*, **54**, 421–426

ADAMS, D. A. and KERR, A. G. (1983) Fibrous dysplasia of the ear – the multiple registrar syndrome. *Proceedings of the Irish Otolaryngological Society*, edited by J. E. T. Byrne, pp. 28–29

AIMI, K. (1983) Role of the tympanic ring in the pathogenesis of congenital cholesteatoma. *The Laryngoscope*, **93**, 1140–1146

ALEXANDER, G. (1904) Zur Pathologie und pathologischen Anatomie der kongenitalen Taubheit. *Archiv für klinische und experimentelle Ohren-, Nasen- und Kehlkopfheilkunde*, **61**, 183–219

ANDERSON, H., FILIPSSON, R., FLUUR, E., KOCH, B., LINDSTEN, J. and WEDENBERG, E. (1969) Hearing impairment in Turner's syndrome. *Acta Oto-Laryngologica Supplementum*, **247**, 1–26

BALKANY, T. J., MISCHKE, R. E., DOWNS, M. P. and JAFEK, O. W. (1979) Ossicular abnormalities in Down's syndrome. *Otolaryngology and Head and Neck Surgery*, **87**, 372–384

BARR, B. (1982) Teratogenic hearing loss. *Audiology*, **21**, 111–127

BEGG, N. T. and NOAH, N. D. (1985) Immunisation targets in Europe and Britain. *British Medical Journal*, **291**, 1370–1371

BERGSTROM, L. (1977) Osteogenesis imperfecta. Otologic and maxillofacial aspects. *The Laryngoscope*, **87** (suppl. 6) 1–42

BERNARD, P. A. (1981) Freedom from ototoxicity in aminoglycoside treated neonates: a mistaken notion. *The Laryngoscope*, **91**, 1985–1994

BESS, F. H., PEEK, B. E. and CHAPMAN, J. J. (1979) Further observations on noise levels in infant incubators. *Pediatrics*, **63**, 100–106

BROOKES, G. B. (1985) Immune complex associated deafness. *Journal of the Royal Society of Medicine*, **78**, 47–55

BROOKES, G. B. and NEWLAND, A. C. (1986) Plasma exchange in the treatment of immune complex associated sensorineural deafness. *Journal of Laryngology and Otology*, **100**, 25–33

CATALANO, P. J. and LEVIN, S. M. (1985) Noise induced hearing loss and portable radios with headphones. *International Journal of Paediatric Otorhinolaryngology*, **9**, 59–67

CAWTHORNE, T. (1955) Otosclerosis. *Journal of Laryngology and Otology*, **69**, 437–456

CHASIN, W. D. (1984) Rhabdomyosarcoma of the temporal bone. *Annals of Otology, Rhinology and Laryngology*, **93**, (Suppl. 112), 71–73

CREAMERS, C. W. R. J. (1979) Autosomal recessive, non-syndromal progressive sensorineural deafness in childhood: a separate clinical and genetic entity. *International Journal of Paediatric Otorhinolaryngology*, **1**, 193–199

CRIFO, S., ANTONELLI, M., GAGLIARDI, M., LUCARELLI, N. and MARCOLINI, P. (1980) Ototoxicity aminoglycoside antibiotics in long-term treatment for cystic fibrosis. *International Journal of Paediatric Otorhinolaryngology*, **2**, 251–253

CUNNINGHAM, C. C. and McARTHUR, K. (1981) Hearing loss and treatment in young Down's syndrome children. *Child: Care, Health and Development*, **7**, 357–374

DAVIS, L. E. (1982) Experimental viral infections of the inner ear. III. Viraemic spread of reovirus to hamster eighth nerve ganglion cells. *Annals of Otology, Rhinology and Laryngology*, **91**, 90–93

DeMARINO, D. P., DUTCHER, P. O. Jr., PARKINS, C. W. and HENGERER, A. S. (1985) Histiocytosis-X: otologic presentations. *International Journal of Paediatric Otorhinolaryngology*, **10**, 91–100

DERLACKI, E. and CLEMIS, J. (1965) Congenital cholesteatoma of the middle ear and mastoid. *Annals of Otology, Rhinology and Laryngology*, **74**, 706–727

DOUEK, E., DODSON, H. C., BANNISTER, L. H., ASHCROFT, P. and HUMPHRIES, K. N. (1976) Effects of incubator noise on the cochlea of the newborn. *The Lancet*, **2**, 1110–1113

D'SOUZA, S., McCARTNEY, E., NOLAN, M. and TAYLOR, I. G. (1981) Hearing, speech and language in survivors of severe perinatal asphyxia. *Archives of Disease in Childhood*, **56**, 245–252

FISCH, L. (1981) Syndromes associated with hearing loss. In *Audiology and Audiological Medicine*, Volume II, edited by H. A. Beagley, pp. 595–639. Oxford: Oxford University Press

FRASER, G. R. (1976) *The Causes of Profound Deafness in Childhood*. London: Baillière Tindall

FREEMAN, J. (1983) Temporal bone fractures and cholesteatoma. *Annals of Otology, Rhinology and Laryngology*, **92**, 558–560

GRATZ, E. S., POLLACK, M. A. and ZIMMERMAN, R. D. (1981) Congenital facial palsy and ipsilateral deafness: association with maternal diabetes mellitus. *International Journal of Paediatric Otorhinolaryngology*, **3**, 335–341

HALL, J. G. (1964) The cochlea and cochlear nuclei in neonatal asphyxia. *Acta Oto-Laryngologica Supplementum*, **194**, 1–93

HARDY, J. B. (1973) Foetal consequences of maternal viral infections in pregnancy. *Archives of Otolaryngology*, **98**, 218–227

HARPER, E. S. (1982) The pharmacology of ototoxic drugs. *British Journal of Audiology*, **16**, 81–93

HEMENWAY, W., SANDO, I. and McCHESNEY, D. (1969) Temporal bone pathology following maternal rubella. *Archiv für klinische und experimentelle Ohren-, Nasen-, Kehlkopfheilkunde*, **193**, 287–300

HOLMES, L. B. (1977) Medical genetics. In *Hearing Loss in Children*, edited by B. F. Jaffe, pp. 253–265. Baltimore: University Park Press

KARMODY, C. S. and SCHUKNECHT, H. F. (1966) Deafness in congenital syphilis. *Archives of Otolaryngology*, **83**, 18–27

KARJALAINEN, S., KARJA, J., SUONIO, S. and YLISKOSKI, M. (1982) Intrauterine hypoxia as a cause of hearing impairment in children. *International Journal of Paediatric Otorhinolaryngology*, **4**, 233–243

KELEMEN, G. (1958) Toxoplasmosis and congenital deafness. *Archives of Otolaryngology*, **68**, 547–561

KONIGSMARK, B. W. and GORLIN, R. J. (1976) *Genetic and Metabolic Deafness*. Philadelphia: W. B. Saunders

KUDESIA, G., ROBINSON, E. T., WILSON, W. D. *et al.* (1985) Rubella: immunity and vaccination in schoolgirls. *British Medical Journal*, **290**, 1406–1408

McDONALD, T. J., CODY, D. T. R. and RYAN, R. E. Jr. (1984) Congenital cholesteatoma of the ear. *Annals of Otology, Rhinology and Laryngology*, **93**, 637–640

McKENZIE, J. (1958) The first arch syndrome. *Archives of Disease in Childhood*, **33**, 477–486

MAIR, I. W. S. and ELVERLAND, H. H. (1977) Sudden deafness and vaccination. *Journal of Laryngology and Otology*, **91**, 323–329

MARTIN, J. A. M. (1982) Aetiological factors relating to childhood deafness in the European Community. *Audiology*, **21**, 149–158

MAURIZI, M., OTTAVIANI, F., PALUDETTI, G. and LUNGAROTTI, S. (1985) Audiological findings in Down's children. *International Journal of Paediatric Otorhinolaryngology*, **9**, 227–232

MINOLI, I. and MORO, G. (1985) Constraints of intensive care units and follow-up studies. *Acta Oto-Laryngologica Supplementum*, **421**, 62–67

MORRISON, A. W. (1979) Diseases of the otic capsule – II. Other diseases. In *Scott-Brown's Diseases of the Ear, Nose and Throat*, 4th edn, edited by J. Ballantyne and J. Groves, Vol. 2, pp. 465–496. London: Butterworths

MUNOZ, O., BENITEZ-DIAZ, L., MARTINEZ, M. C. and GUISCAFRE, H. (1983) Hearing loss after *Haemophilus influenzae* meningitis. Follow-up study with auditory brainstem potentials. *Annals of Otology, Rhinology and Laryngology*, **92**, 272–275

NACLERIO, R. (1985) Recent advances in immunology with reference to otolaryngology. *Otolaryngologic Clinics of North America*, **18**, 821–832

NADOL, J. B. (1978) Hearing loss as a sequela of meningitis. *The Laryngoscope*, **88**, 739–750

NAGER, G. T. and HOLLIDAY, M. J. (1984) Fibrous dysplasia of the temporal bone. Update with case reports. *Annals of Otology, Rhinology and Laryngology*, **93**, 630–633

NAGER, G. T., KENNEDY, D. W. and KOPSTEIN, E. (1982) Fibrous dysplasia. A review of the disease and its manifestations in the temporal bone. *Annals of Otology, Rhinology and Laryngology*, **91**, (suppl. 92) 1–52

NYLEN, O. and ROSENHALL, V. (1979) *Haemophilus influenzae* meningitis and hearing. *International Journal of Paediatric Otorhinolaryngology*, **1**, 97–101

PAPPAS, D. G. (1983) Hearing impairments and vestibular abnormalities among children with subclinical cytomegalovirus. *Annals of Otology, Rhinology and Laryngology*, **92**, 552–557

PARADISE, J. L., BLUESTONE, C. D. and FELDER, H. (1969) The universality of otitis media in 50 infants with cleft palate. *Pediatrics*, **44**, 35–42

PASHLEY, N. R. T. (1982) Simultaneous round and oval window fistulae in a child. *Annals of Otology, Rhinology and Laryngology*, **91**, 332–335

PYE, A., KNIGHT, J. J. and ARNETT, J. M. (1984) Sensory hair cell damage from high frequency noise exposure. *British Journal of Audiology*, **18**, 231–236

RAHKO, T., BAER, M., VIROLAINEN, E. and KARMA, P. (1984) Audiological and vestibular findings in 219 cases of meningitis. *Archives of Otorhinolaryngology*, **240**, 15–20

RAREY, K. E., DAVIS, J. A., DAVIS, L. E. and HAWKINS, J. E. Jr. (1983) Inner ear pathology associated with Reye's syndrome. *International Journal of Paediatric Otorhinolaryngology*, **6**, 255–263

ROBINSON, M. (1983) Juvenile otosclerosis – a 20-year study. *Annals of Otology, Rhinology and Laryngology*, **92**, 561–565

ROOD, S. R. and STOOL, S. E. (1981) Current concepts of aetiology, diagnosis and management of cleft palate related otopathologic disease. *Otolaryngologic Clinics of North America*, **14**, 865–884

RUBEN, R. J. (1985) Otorhinolaryngologic disorders of adolescents: a review. *International Journal of Paediatric Otorhinolaryngology*, **9**, 1–30

SAIGAL, S., LUNYK, O., LARKE, R. P. B. and CHERNESKY, M. A. (1982) Outcome in children with congenital cytomegalovirus infection: a longitudinal follow-up study. *American Journal of Diseases of Children*, **136**, 896–901

SANDO, I., SUEHIRO, S. and WOOD, R. P. (1983) Congenital anomalies of the external and middle ear. In *Paediatric Otolaryngology*, edited by C. D. Bluestone and S. E. Stool, pp. 309–346. Philadelphia: W. B. Saunders

SCHACHERN, P. A., SHEA, D. A. and PAPARELLA, M. M. (1984) Mucopolysaccharidosis I-H (Hurler's syndrome) and human temporal bone histopathology. *Annals of Otology, Rhinology and Laryngology*, **93**, 65–69

SCHUKNECHT, H. F. (1974) *Pathology of the Ear*. Cambridge: Harvard University Press

SCHULTE, F. J. and STENNERT, E. (1978) Hearing defects in pre-term infants. *Archives of Disease in Childhood*, **53**, 269–270

SCHWARTZ, D. M. and SCHWARTZ, R. M. (1978) Acoustic impedance and otoscopic findings in young children with Down's syndrome. *Archives of Otolaryngology*, **104**, 652–656

SCHWEITZER, V. G. and OLSON, N. R. (1984) Ototoxic effect of erythromycin therapy. *Archives of Otolaryngology*, **110**, 258–260

SEIGER, A., WHITE, N. H., SKINNER, M. W. and SPECTOR, G. J. (1983) Auditory function in children with diabetes mellitus. *Annals of Otology, Rhinology and Laryngology*, **92**, 237–241

SHEA, J. J. and POSTMA, D. S. (1982) Findings and long-term surgical results in the hearing loss of osteogenesis imperfecta. *Archives of Otolaryngology*, **108**, 467–470

SLACK, R. W. T. and PHELPS, P. D. (1985) Familial mixed deafness with branchial arch defects (earpits-deafness syndrome). *Clinical Otolaryngology*, **10**, 271–277

SMEJA, Z., SLOMKO, Z., SIKORSKI, K. and SOWINSKI, H. (1979) The risk of hearing impairment in children from mothers exposed to noise during pregnancy. *International Journal of Paediatric Otorhinolaryngology*, **1**, 221–229

STEPHENS, S. D. G., LUXON, L. and HINCHCLIFFE, R. (1982) Immunological disorders and auditory lesions. *Audiology*, **21**, 128–148

TAKANOBU, A., YAMAMOTO, J., MATSUDA, I., TANIGUCHI, N. and NAGAI, B. (1984) Siblings with renal tubular acidosis and nerve deafness. The first family in Japan. *Human Genetics*, **66**, 282–285

TAYLOR, I. G. (1979) The deaf child. In *Scott-Brown's Diseases of the Ear, Nose and Throat*, 4th edn, edited by J. Ballantyne and J. Groves, Vol. 2, pp. 499–532. London: Butterworths

THOMSEN, J. and FRIIS, B. (1979) High dose tobramycin treatment of children with cystic fibrosis. Bacteriological effect and clinical ototoxicity. *International Journal of Paediatric Otorhinolaryngology*, **1**, 33–40

TIERI, L., MASI, R., MARSELLA, P. and PINELLI, V. (1984) Sudden deafness in children. *International Journal of Paediatric Otorhinolaryngology*, **7**, 257–264

UZIEL, A. (1985) Non-genetic factors affecting hearing development. *Acta Oto-Laryngologica Supplementum*, **421**, 57–61

UZIEL, A., MAROT, M. and PUJOL, R. (1983) The Gunn rat: an experimental model for central deafness. *Acta Oto-Laryngologica Supplementum*, **95**, 651–656

VELTRI, R. W., WILSON, W. R., SPRINKLE, P. M., RODMAN, S. M. and KAVESH, D. A. (1981) The implication of virus in idiopathic sudden hearing loss: primary infection or reactivation of latent virus. *Otolaryngology and Head and Neck Surgery*, **89**, 137–141

5

Congenital anomalies of the ear

Robert Pracy

Congenital anatomical anomalies of the ear are rare. It is difficult to assess acurately the incidence of anomalies per thousand live births because some are not associated with a gross anatomical deformity of the external ear. Since the majority appear to be unilateral, it is probable that there are people who go through life with a unilateral congenital conductive deafness which is never detected.

Furthermore, as there is a great variation in the incidence between the rarer syndromes and the commoner abnormalities, there would appear to be little value in suggesting an overall incidence. However, it is considered that the incidence over all possible causes is in the region of 1:60 000 live births. Broadly speaking anomalies may arise on their own, or in association with other abnormalities which may result from exposure of the mother to drugs during the first trimester of pregnancy or to genetic irregularity. Where the abnormality occurs in association with other obvious defects the dysplasia may be part of a syndrome. Some of these syndromes will be considered below and the dysplasia may be unilateral or bilateral. For a more comprehensive list of all syndromes which may be associated with congenital conductive deafness the appropriate chapter should be consulted.

The purpose of this chapter is to describe the management of congenital abnormalities of the ear as they present, without confusing the reader with lists of very rare syndromes. However, where the anomaly presents as part of a syndrome it is of cardinal importance to take into account the complete picture before offering elaborate surgical procedures. Indeed, as with congenital abnormalities in other sites, it is very desirable to have the patient examined by a developmental paediatrician for other possible abnormalities before pro-

ceeding with investigation. A brief recapitulation of the essential developmental and pathological anatomy will be given here (Bowden, 1977). A fuller account of the normal anatomy will be found in Volume 1.

Developmental anatomy

Anatomically the ear consists of three distinct parts, the external, middle and inner ear. Each develops as a separate entity and will be considered separately.

The external ear

This may be divided into two subdivisions, the pinna and the external auditory meatus.

The pinna develops around the first branchial cleft. By the time the pinna begins to appear, the cleft is represented by a pit and this becomes surrounded anteriorly by three small hillocks derived from the tissue of the first branchial arch and posteriorly by three hillocks derived from the tissue of the second branchial arch. The anterior hillocks form the tragus, the crus of the helix and the helix. The posterior hillocks form the antihelix, the antitragus and the lobule. The concavity of the concha is derived from the wall of the branchial pit. Initially the developing pinna lies ventromedially but as development proceeds it moves in a dorsolateral direction. By the twentieth week of intrauterine life the hillocks have fused forming the adult appearance, but of course much smaller than the final size. After birth the pinna continues to enlarge and the development cannot be considered as complete before the twelfth year.

The pinna consists of fibroelastic cartilage covered on either surface by skin, bound down firmly laterally with fibrous strands and loosely medially by connective tissue.

The external auditory canal also consists of two parts. The outer one-third is cartilaginous and the medial two-thirds are bony. By the fourth or fifth week of intrauterine life the branchial pit is in contact with the first pharyngeal diverticulum and the tympanic membrane will be formed at this point of contact. However, the stimulus for the formation of the tympanic membrane comes from the handle of the malleus and if this is abnormal no membrane will appear. By the eighth week a solid cord of epithelium extends from the primitive external auditory meatus to the tympanic membrane in its lower portion. This cord is called the meatal plate and canalization of the plate takes place during the twenty-first week of intrauterine life. Bone forms in membrane round this tube and eventually becomes the external osseus meatus. Anteroinferiorly the ossification is incomplete at birth but is completed by the end of the first year. At birth the tympanic membrane lies posterosuperiorly and is horizontal.

The middle ear

This consists of the tympanic membrane, the tympanic cavity, ossicles, muscles, nerves and blood vessels communicating with the nasopharynx by the eustachian tube. The middle ear develops from the first branchial pouch which springs from the epipharynx. It is separated from the external ear by the tympanic membrane and from the inner ear by the bone of the otic capsule.

The tympanic membrane consists of two parts, the pars flaccida and the pars tensa which lies inferiorly. Histologically there are three layers in the pars tensa. A middle fibrous layer is divided into a lateral portion in which the fibres run in a radial direction and a medial portion in which the fibres run in a generally circular pattern. The lateral surface is covered by squamous epithelium which is continuous with the epithelium lining the external auditory meatus. The medial covering is by mucosa of the middle ear. The pars flaccida consists of two layers, an outer epithelial layer and an inner mucosal layer. The membrane is lodged in the tympanic ring which is formed from four centres in the medial end of the bone forming the tympanic plate. It is incomplete superiorly. The handle of the malleus is embedded in the layers of the tympanic membrane.

The eustachian tube extends from the epipharynx to the tubotympanic recess and appears at about the third week of intrauterine life. In the infant it passes more or less horizontally and laterally from the epipharynx to the middle ear. In childhood the development of the skull and nasopharynx results in an inclination of about 45° passing upwards and posteriorly and laterally from the nasopharyngeal orifice. The tube has two portions, a medial cartilaginous part which tapers to a narrow diameter as it passes laterally; this represents two-thirds of the length of the tube. The lateral one-third is bony beginning medially at the isthmus and widening as it passes laterally to the middle ear. The tube is lined with respiratory epithelium which is continuous with that lining the nasal cavity. It is rich in goblet cells particularly at the medial end.

The middle ear proper consists of three parts, the epitympanum, the mesotympanum and the hypotympanum. The floor and roof of the mesotympanum form the roof and floor of the hypotympanum and epitympanum. This is merely an anatomical boundary and is represented by no structure. Essentially the three parts of the cavity lie in that area bounded above by the tegmen tympani, below by the plate of bone over the jugular bulb, medially by the bone of the otic capsule, laterally by the tympanic membrane, posteriorly by the fallopian canal and the facial recess, and anteriorly it merges with the opening of the eustachian tube.

The middle ear contains the three ossicles, intratympanic muscles, nerves and blood vessels. *The ossicles* are derived from cartilage from the dorsal ends of the first two branchial cartilages. The cartilage of the first arch is called Meckel's cartilage and that of the second Reichert's cartilage. There has been considerable discussion as to the extent to which each contributes to individual ossicles. The current consensus appears to be that the handle of the malleus, the long process of the incus and the stapes, except for the medial layer of the footplate, are derived from Reichert's cartilage and the head and neck of the malleus and short process of the incus from Meckel's cartilage. Development of the cartilage begins at the eighth week of intrauterine life and is complete by 16–18 weeks. Ossification begins at 16 weeks and is complete by 32 weeks. The ossicles are suspended in the middle ear by ligaments and surrounded by four mucosal pouches described by Proctor (1964).

The tympanic antrum appears at the twenty-second week of intrauterine life as a posterolateral extension of the epitympanum. At birth it is about 7 mm in diameter. Pneumatization of the mastoid process begins late in fetal life and continues through childhood until the adult state is attained at between 10 and 12 years. The degree of pneumatization varies from ear to ear but total absence of pneumatization should be looked upon as pathological.

The inner ear

The inner ear comprises a membranous labyrinth housed in a bony capsule (the otic capsule) which is part of the petrous bone. At birth the inner ear has already attained adult size.

The membranous labyrinth appears at the third week of intrauterine life as thickenings on the side of the rhombencephalon known as the otic placodes. During the fourth week each placode invaginates giving rise initially to an otic pit and later an otocyst. Subsequently the otocyst divides into a dorsal and a ventral portion. The dorsal portion forms the utricle, semicircular canals and endolymphatic duct and the ventral portion, the saccule and the cochlea. Development is complete by the sixth fetal month.

Pathological anatomy

The normal anatomy may be distorted in either the external, middle or inner ear or, indeed, in all three in the same patient.

Abnormalities of the external ear

The commonest abnormality is an accessory skin tag which may result from incomplete fusion of the tubercles which coalesce to form the pinna. The whole pinna may be smaller on the affected side. The meatus may be stenosed or totally atretic and occasionally the tympanic membrane may be normal but obscured from view by an otherwise uncanalized meatus. When there is a total atresia, a thick wedge of dense bone lies between the mastoid process and the ascending ramus of the mandible in the position normally taken up by the external meatus. In such cases the epitympanum lies superior to the atresia.

Abnormalities of the middle ear

The tympanic membrane may be absent and replaced by a solid bony plate. The whole conformation of the middle ear cleft may be distorted being narrower in some diameters and wider in others. The angle of presentation of the lateral semicircular canals may be altered. The handle of the malleus may be absent or turned through a right angle to face anteriorly where it is ankylosed with the anterior meatal wall (*Figure 5.1*).

The malleus and incus may be fused to form one ossicle of considerable mass in which the contribution from malleus or incus is impossible to analyse. The incus may not articulate with the

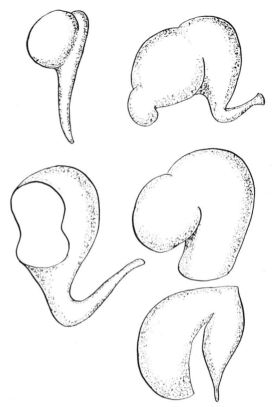

Figure 5.1 Abnormalities of the malleus and incus. Five types are illustrated. The malleus and incus must be considered together because they are frequently found to be fused into one large ossicular mass which may or may not articulate with the stapes

stapes or the long process may be considerably shorter than normal and the connection is established by a fibrous strand. There are many possible types of stapes abnormality. Broadly they may be divided into two categories:

(1) The superstructure may be missing or the crura may be replaced by a solid column of bone (*Figure 5.2a*). It is then said to be monopodal. Frequently the single crus bends forward from the oval window region and points towards the eustachian tube opening (*Figure 5.2b*).

(2) The stapes footplate may be abnormal. The normal footplate is formed from two origins. The lateral portion is derived from the second branchial arch and the medial from the bone of the otic capsule. The inner lamina can remain attached to the otic capsule and give rise to congenital stapes footplate fixation (Steele 1969) (*Figure 5.3*). On other occasions there may be a hole in the centre of the footplate perhaps covered with a fine membrane.

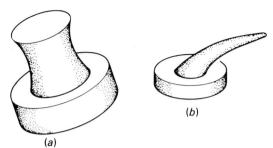

(a)

(b)

Figure 5.2 Abnormalities of the stapes superstructure. Two varieties are illustrated: (*a*) the crura are replaced with a single stout column of bone; (*b*) a single crus tapers as it passes anteriorly. There is no articulation with the other ossicles

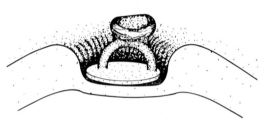

Figure 5.3 Abnormality of the stapes footplate. The inner lamina remains fused with the wall of the labyrinth

In addition to the bony deformities there are commonly abnormalities in the course of the facial nerve and the blood vessels. The normal covering of the bone of the fallopian canal may be missing and the nerve may prolapse over the oval window. Frequently the descending portion is found in what appears to be the posterior border of the tympanic membrane in those cases where a membrane is present. The descending portion of the nerve may curve backwards sharply as it begins its descent and it then approaches the lateral sinus. On occasion the descending portion of the nerve may be found in two strands which diverge as the nerve travels caudally. Where there is a substantial atretic plate of bone in place of a meatus, the nerve may pass forwards at the level of the neck of the malleus to disappear from the middle ear in the region of the temporo-mandibular joint (*Figure 5.4*). Access to the middle ear cleft may be made more difficult by overhanging dura with large veins on its inferior surface. The stapedial artery may be larger than normal and interfere with instrumentation in the oval window region.

Abnormalities of the inner ear

Sometimes the development of the cochlea is grossly abnormal. Such a child may well be born severely deaf but may appear to have relatively good bone conduction and may be considered to

be suffering from congenital conductive deafness. However, surgery in these cases frequently results in a dead ear and on occasion to a perilymph 'gusher'. When the cochlea is found on radiology to consist of a single large cavity with no sign of the normal cochlear turns this is termed the Mondini deformity. It is not amenable to treatment.

The problem

The surgeon must plan with great care the investigation of the patient, the counselling of the parents and the timing of any surgery proposed. His objective should be to have the surgery completed and any hearing aid which may be required, fitted in time for the explosion in language development which occurs normally soon after the age of 2 years. In this way the really important time for language development can be exploited most advantageously. In addition, the child will have little memory of his period of hospitalization. Anatomically there is no reason why this should not be done. The middle ear is almost of adult size at birth and, unless the cleft is greatly distorted by the abnormality, it should be possible to provide a skin-lined cavity with some form of artificial tympanic membrane linked to the ossicular conducting mechanism.

A great deal has been written about how this may be achieved and the fact that there are many opinions as to how it should be done indicates that no perfect solution to the problem has yet been found. The method described below has been

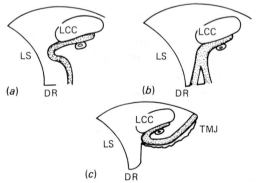

Figure 5.4 Some of the common variations in the course of the facial nerve. (*a*) Unusual degree of posterior extension before the turn from horizontal to vertical portions; (*b*) bifurcation of descending portion; (*c*) absence of descending portion. The nerve passes laterally and then anteriorly to leave the temporal bone in the region of the temporomandibular joint. LCC = Lateral semicircular canal; LS = lateral sinus; DR = digastric ridge; TMJ = region of temporomandibular joint

evolved over the past 25 years and in the author's hands has proved to give reasonably reliable results which can be kept in a stable condition throughout the period of childhood upper respiratory tract inflammations. As in the case of the normal child, otitis media may occur but, if it is treated promptly, there is no reason why there should be any sequelae. After the age of 12 years one can expect to have a dry stable cavity which will require the same occasional inspection and cleaning as every mastoid cavity.

Clinical presentation of types of dysplasia

(1) *There may be no abnormality of the pinna or the outer part of the external auditory meatus.* The tympanic membrane may be present and may appear to be normal or the meatus may be stenosed or not patent in the medial portion.

(2) *Absence of one or each external auditory meatus with no other obvious abnormality.* This is the commonest presentation. The pinna on the affected side is rarely normal but the degree of abnormality may vary from being slightly smaller than normal through presentation as a crumpled skin tag to complete absence. There will be no palpable space between the rudimentary mastoid process and the ascending ramus of the mandible (*Figure 5.5*). Gill (1969) has provided a useful 'rule of thumb' in stating that the greater the degree of abnormality of the pinna the more complex the abnormality of the middle ear will prove to be.

(3) *Absence of one or each pinna with an associated facial weakness on the homolateral side.* The presentation is thus much the same as described above in (2). However, the facial weakness indicates that the nerve to the second branchial arch is involved and it is

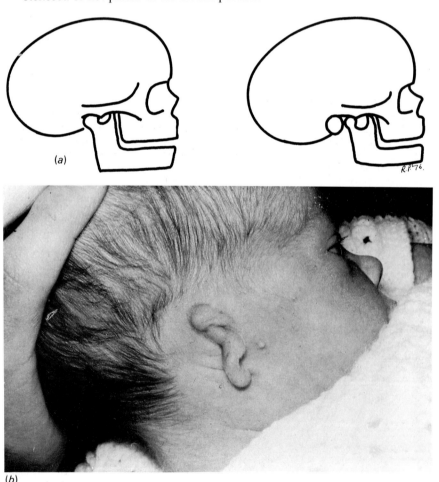

(a)

(b)

Figure 5.5 (*a*) The relationship between the ascending ramus of the mandible and the mastoid process. The absence of the meatus means that there is no intervening space. (*b*) A case of unilateral microtia with meatal atresia

therefore possible that exploration of these cases will expose an abnormal stapes or even absence of the stapes. This was the condition found quite commonly in those children whose mothers had taken thalidomide in the first trimester of pregnancy and in some cases was associated with abnormalities of the inner ear. On the whole the hearing results in these children were poor and in the author's series all required the use of a hearing aid.

(4) *Absence of the pinna on one or each side associated with other signs indicating a congenital abnormality of other first branchial arch structures.* The most common form of this presentation is the Treacher Collins' syndrome (*Figure 5.6*). In

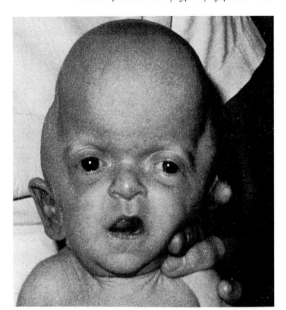

Figure 5.7 Crouzon's syndrome may or may not be associated with meatal atresia, cardiac abnormality and choanal atresia. The bones of the vault fuse early. The characteristic features are the high crown, exophthalmos and shortened external nose

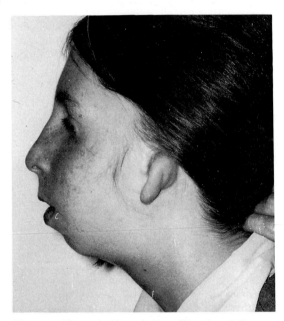

Figure 5.6 The typical lateral view of Treacher Collins syndrome. Observe the underdevelopment of the mandible and zygoma, the antimongoloid slant to the palpebral fissure and the low placement of the pinna

such cases it is likely that there will be dysplasia of the lower jaw, flattening of the zygomatic arch and 'antimongoloid' slant to the palpebral fissure. The pinna will lie at a lower level on the side of the head than in a normal child (Wright, Phelps and Fraser, 1977).

(5) *Dysplasia of the ear may be part of a more obvious syndrome* such as Crouzon's syndrome in which there are other facial and structural abnormalities of the head which will draw attention to the obvious difference between the patient and the normal baby (*Figure 5.7*).

(6) *Dysplasia of the ear may be one of multiple abnormalities of the head and other organs present-*

ing no recognizable features of any syndrome (*Figure 5.8*). In such cases the abnormality of the ear, disabling though it undoubtedly is, must be considered to take a second place to the other more serious disabilities. Surgery should not be offered.

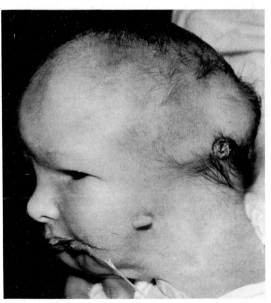

Figure 5.8 Multiple abnormalities of the head and neck. Meatal atresia is only one facet of the total disability

The assessment of the patient and counselling of the parents

The parents of every child born with an obvious structural abnormality, particularly one which cannot be hidden, are going to be very concerned. The baby is therefore likely to be brought for advice at a very early age. Naturally the worried parent is going to expect to be told how his or her child is going to be affected physiologically as a result of the anatomical abnormality. It cannot be emphasized too strongly that until there is objective evidence of some cochlear function, it is unwise to discuss the prognosis of the particular patient. However, it is equally important that the whole picture of the patient with bilateral atresia should be discussed with the parents if their child presents in this way. If the preliminary examination indicates that the atresia is merely one facet of a syndrome or of multiple disabilities then the first step should be to seek the advice of the developmental paediatrician in order to get some idea of the prognosis for the future pattern of life.

If the condition is unilateral, once the cochlear function on the healthy side has been verified as being normal the parents should be reassured and

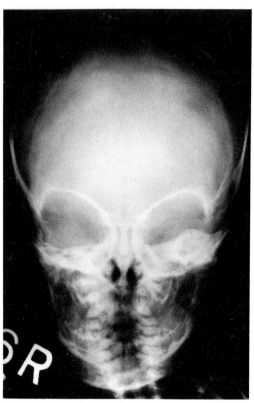

Figure 5.9 The transorbital view of the cochlea. The cochlea is present on the left side only

every effort made to postpone surgery on the atretic side until the child is old enough to make up his own mind about surgery. If the condition is bilateral, a bone conductor hearing aid should be fitted immediately in order to bring ambient sound to the child at the earliest possible moment. It then becomes necessary to carry out a radiological examination to confirm that a cochlea is present on each side. A 'transorbital' view (*Figure 5.9*) is the best way to obtain this information as only one exposure is required and, if the cochlea is present on both sides, it will be necessary at a later stage to ask for hypocycloidal polytomography in order to have detailed information about the anatomy of the inner ear on both sides. If the cochlea is present on one side only this represents an *absolute contraindication* to all attempts to construct an artifical sound pathway because of the possibility of producing a dead ear as the result of surgery.

If the patient is found to have a cochlea on each side it is necessary to wait until about the age of 4 months in order to be able to verify that there is a cochlear reserve. (It is not always easy to verify that it is equal on the two sides.) Once this has been established the whole plan for the future managment of the child can be discussed with the parents. Hypocycloidal polytomography is best left until shortly before it is proposed to operate. It is usually possible to obtain better films with less risk to the patient and the anatomic findings can then be discussed with the radiologist (*see* Chapter 2).

No possible service can be done for either the patient or the parent by offering optimistic prognoses for hearing or for the ultimate 'natural' appearance of the pinna. Experience shows that the hearing results are poor in the majority of cases, stenosis of the new meatus is common and the final appearance of the pinna bears little resemblance to the norm. The first step towards forming a satisfactory relationship with the family is to be quite open about what is 'on offer'. The promise of relatively little will of course be disappointing to the parents, but this is infinitely better for both the surgeon and the family than the inevitable frustrations and misunderstandings which are bound to follow from an unwarranted optimism on the part of the surgeon. Furthermore, the better the rapport with the parents the more chance of their cooperation if the course of management has to be modified.

The practice of offering to create only a meatus without making a definitive link with the ossicular chain has much to commend it. This has been the author's practice for many years, with an offer to combine this procedure with an ossicular link if it can be accomplished relatively easily without danger to important structures such as the facial nerve. The modern hearing aid is small and can be fitted fairly satisfactorily to the new meatus and will almost certainly provide more satisfactory hearing than a surgical linkage. In about 5% of cases it is possible to achieve a good hearing result which will not require the provision of a hearing aid. Experience shows that what the child wants more than anything is to have an 'earhole' like other children. This requirement can be met in a high percentage of cases.

Operations on both ears

There can be no justification in operating on both ears in early childhood. The object of the operation is to provide an effective meatus to which, if necessary a hearing aid may be fitted. The possibility of providing stereophonic hearing by operations on both sides is so remote that it cannot be weighed in the balance against the additional trauma to the patient and the family. The difficulty is that a very successful result achieved on one side is very likely to result in extreme pressure from the parents for the other side to be treated immediately. This should be resisted because a good result on both sides proves to be a very rare occurrence.

Surgery for conductive deafness without meatal atresia

The approach of choice for this condition is by the tympanotomy route. The actual reconstructive procedure employed will naturally depend upon the underlying pathology and may vary from stapedectomy procedures to the establishment of a functioning ossicular chain by the use of a prosthesis, wire or a bone graft. Surgery should not be attempted until the meatus is large enough to accommodate the instruments required and, at the same time, to provide an adequate view of the operative field down the microscope. Generally this is not earlier than 4 years of age. Experience shows that it is often helpful to use a small endaural incision to allow better access. Extreme caution should be adopted in turning the tympanomeatal flap forward because of the possibility of damage to an exposed facial nerve which, as has been described above, may lie in the free border of the membrane or in the immediate vicinity. If, in attempting to free a fixed footplate, a perilymph 'gusher' occurs the leak should be controlled with a plug of fat or muscle kept in position with a strut or short piston attached to the incus; the original objective of ossicular reconstruction should be abandoned.

Surgery when there is atresia of the external ear

The complications of procedures designed to correct meatal atresia are infection of the cavity with resulting death of the skin graft, leading to granulation tissue formation and subsequent stenosis or closure. Poor hearing may result either from failure to anchor the new tympanic membrane to the ossicular chain, which then moves laterally, or a dead ear following drilling on an intact and mobile ossicular chain. As in the tympanotomy procedure described above, there is always a risk of damage to the facial nerve. Earlier operations for this condition were of the 'open' type (Ombredanne, 1947; Livingstone, 1959, 1965), in which a bony meatus was shaped by drilling and then lined by a Tiersch graft fashioned in the form of a tube which was then splinted by packing. Once the packing had been removed the site became prone to infection as a result of investigation by the patient's fingers. If the operation was delayed until a more cooperative patient had developed, the objective of attaining a stable meatus in time for the language explosion was lost (Colman, 1974).

For this reason a two-stage operation was developed which could be carried out in the second year of life. The principle behind the operation was to create a closed skin-lined cavity not accessible to the introduction of infection from outside which could be converted into a meatus after an interval of 3 or 4 months, by which time the graft both of the tympanic membrane and of the meatal wall would have had time to 'bed down'. Initially the attachment of the new meatus to the pinna was left until the child was older, but now that the fashion is to wear the hair longer, the second stage can be combined with a Z-plasty of the pinna rudiment, with or without rotation, and this provides a satisfactory result without the need

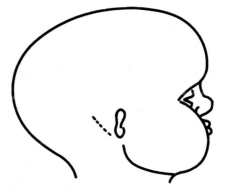

Figure 5.10 The incision for the first operation. It is straight and passes upwards and backwards from the base of the mastoid process

for multiple procedures. The first stage of the operation is carried out once the child is clean and dry at about 14–16 months and the second stage at 18–20 months. Many paediatricians feel that this is early for toilet training to be complete but experience of over 70 cases shows that adequate training can be achieved with full parental cooperation.

A fuller description of the operation will be found elsewhere (Pracy, 1977) but the broad steps will be given here. The incision should be planned with the Z-plasty in mind. It should be straight and angled at 45° to the vertical (*Figure 5.10*). It extends from the lower border of the mastoid process to the lower border of the temporalis muscle.

Once the soft tissues have been retracted and the bone uncovered the mastoid antrum is exposed. It should be appreciated that this will lie apparently more posteriorly because the mastoid process in these cases lies against the ascending ramus of the mandible. Once the antrum has been defined, the opening should be enlarged superiorly as far as the middle fossa dura, posteriorly as far as the lateral sinus and anteriorly just below the tegmen tympani until the upper portion of the ossicular mass is exposed (*Figure 5.11*).

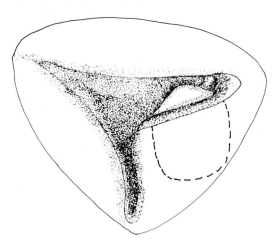

Figure 5.11 The antrum has been identified and, working forwards from the antrum, the superior aspect of the ossicular mass has been uncovered. The broken line indicates the area of hard atretic bone which remains to be removed

It is then possible to remove the atretic plate from above working from the epitympanum without danger to the facial nerve. The drilling should proceed with caution as the region of the neck of the malleus is approached, since it is in this area that the facial nerve can turn forwards horizontally. If the ossicular chain is fixed the

malleus and incus should be disarticulated from the stapes in order to avoid damage to the cochlea by noise or vibration. Once an adequate view of the medial wall of the middle ear has been obtained the drilling can be directed to forming a suitable bed for the tympanic membrane graft. When this has been done a decision should be made about the use of the ossicles removed to provide a rounded columella which can be shaped to fit over the stapes (*Figure 5.12*).

The middle ear region is now completed by the positioning of a graft made from temporalis fascia, taking care to ensure that it lines at least the medial one-third of the newly defined anterior meatal wall (*Figure 5.13*).

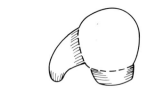
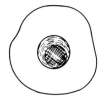

Figure 5.12 Fashioning of the ossicles to produce a 'boss columella'. It is important to drill a cavity on the medial surface which will fit easily on to the head of the stapes

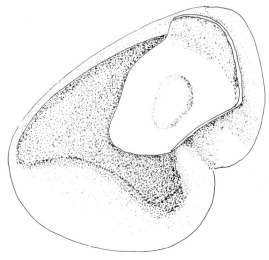

Figure 5.13 Placing of the fascial graft; particular care is taken to 'lead' it up the anterior meatal wall

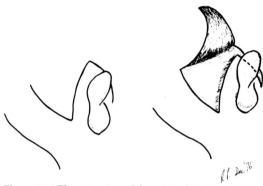

Figure 5.14 The extension of the original incision for the fashioning of the meatus at the second operation

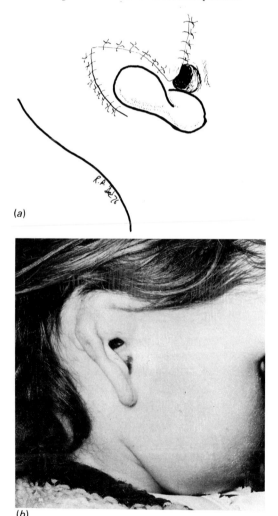

(a)

(b)

Figure 5.15 (*a*) The Z-plasty is now completed and the skin of the external ear sutured to the well-bedded Tiersch graft used to line the cavity at the original operation. (*b*) The postoperative appearances in a typical case of bilateral atresia

The remainder of the cavity is lined with a Tiersch graft taken from the inner side of the homolateral thigh and supported by a sterile non-absorbable plastic sponge. The final piece of skin is turned so that the outer surface faces inwards on to the sponge. The wound is closed in layers without drainage.

In the second stage of the procedure the incision is reopened and extended into a Z-plasty (*Figure 5.14*). The cyst formed deliberately by the first operation is opened and will be found to be lined by healthy skin. There will be enough skin to suture that inside the cavity to the external skin and, by the use of the Z-plasty, the opening can be brought out anterior to and above the pinna remnant (*Figure 5.15*). The cavity should be lightly packed for a further 14 days and subsequently treated like a mastoid cavity.

Results

Results have to be judged from the surgical standpoint and from the degree to which it has been possible to offset the pathological anatomy. A recent review of 20 cases, treated by two surgeons by the method described, and reported to a meeting of the Section of Otology of the Royal Society of Medicine (Pracy, 1987), offers a good illustration of what may be expected. Twenty parents were circulated and only 10 replied. One mother was totally dissatisfied. Her child was not suitable for surgery and therefore did not perform well at school as she had virtually no cochlear reserve and did not find a hearing aid of much use. All of the remaining parents who replied said that the advice that they had been given at counselling was accurate. The children were being educated in normal schools. In some the language development was retarded, but all performed normally from an educational point of view. Only one child did not need to use a hearing aid. Due to complications discussed above some had required a second meatoplasty but all had manageable cavities.

References

BOWDEN, R. E. M. (1977) Development of the middle and external ear in man. *Proceedings of the Royal Society of Medicine*, **70**, 823–826

COLMAN, B. H. (1974) Congenital atresia – the otological problem. *Proceedings of the Royal Society of Medicine*, **67**, 1203–1204

GILL, N. W. (1969) Congenital atresia of the ear. *Journal of Laryngology and Otology*, **83**, 551–587

LIVINGSTONE, G. H. (1959) Sound conduction in congenital deformities of the external ear. *Journal of Laryngology and Otology*, **73**, 231–241

LIVINGSTONE, G. H. (1965) Congenital ear abnormalities due to thalidomide. *Proceedings of the Royal Society of Medicine*, **58**, 493–497

OMBREDANNE, M. (1947) Surgery for deafness: fenestration in cases of congenital atresia of the external auditory canal. *Oto-rhino-laryngologie internationale*, **31**, 229–236

PRACY, R. (1977) Surgery for conductive deafness. *Proceedings of the Royal Society of Medicine*, **70**, 823–826

PRACY, R. (1987) Results of management of twenty cases of congenital aplasia. Presented at the Royal Society Medicine June 1985. *International Journal of Paediatric Otolaryngology* (in press)

PROCTOR, B. (1964) Development of middle ear spaces and their surgical significance. *Journal of Laryngology and Otology*, **78**, 631–648

STEELE, B. C. (1969) Congenital fixation of the stapes footplate. *Acta Oto-Laryngologica Supplementum*, **245**

WRIGHT, J. L. W., PHELPS, P. D. and FRASER, I. (1977) Anatomical findings in congenital conductive deafness. *Proceedings of the Royal Society of Medicine*, **70**, 816–821

6

Testing and screening of hearing

Sue Bellman

When testing the hearing of young children different methods may be used from those employed for an older child or adult, but the information that is being sought is similar. The aim is to identify as accurately as possible the threshold of hearing at a range of frequencies in both ears and to identify the nature and cause of any hearing impairment that may be present. As the main effect of hearing loss in young children is on their verbal communication skills, the tests of threshold are supplemented as early as possible by tests of speech discrimination. Screening tests, whatever their nature, are designed to identify two groups of children, those with normal hearing and those who fail the screen and need definitive testing as above. If a hearing loss is identified by testing, the child will then need further investigation and following this may undergo corrective surgery or may enter a rehabilitative programme. These topics are covered elsewhere, but it is important to recognize that testing is only one aspect of the assessment of the child with a hearing problem.

Development of response to sound

The behavioural response to sound matures with the child's development in the same way as other skills. Before a tester can start to assess the hearing of children, it is essential to have a good working knowledge of how these responses develop in a normal child. It is also necessary to understand the normal development of the child in other fields, as the hearing responses and communication skills have to be related to the child's overall level of maturation.

Neonatal responses

In the period after birth a baby responds to loud sounds by a form of startling reflex. This reaction includes the aural-palpebral reflex, which is the most consistent response to sound, a change in heart rate and pattern of respiration, a backward head jerk and an increase in general body activity (the Moro reflex). These responses are not elicited by quiet sounds and the intensity of the auditory stimulus producing a reaction depends very much on the psychophysiological state of the child. For this reason it is not possible, at this stage, to assess accurately a child's hearing threshold by behavioural techniques.

Responses of the infant aged under 4 months

As the infant matures he/she begins to notice sounds and to respond by stilling and listening. By 4 months of age an infant stills and smiles to a parent's voice, even when the source is not in visual range, and obviously vocalizes in response to voice in a communicative way. The response is mainly seen to louder sounds and there is no consistent response to quieter sounds that could reliably be used for threshold estimations.

Responses at age 4–6 months

At this age the infant is beginning to turn its head to the source of a sound with increasing consistency. Not only is the response more reliable, but it also occurs to sounds of lower intensity, so that estimates of the threshold of hearing using behavioural techniques are sometimes possible. However, because the localization of sound is still developing at this age, the response often varies from the prompt localization of a sound in an older child.

The turn to an auditory stimulus is often delayed and a longer presentation of the stimulus is necessary prior to a response, without raising the intensity of the sound. The sound may also need to be presented closer to the child than the usual 1 m distance. A child of this age may learn to localize sound to the first side tested but then only turn to this direction, wherever the source of sound. This could lead to a suspicion of a unilateral hearing loss if the child's developmental age is not taken into account. The child may also turn to the correct side but with a half turn that does not visualize the sound source, or may assume the sound to generate from the first object or person identified on turning, again not recognizing the actual source of sound. These are the normal responses for many children of this age. Children of this developmental age respond best to the more traditional testing sounds and do not turn to warble tones at the same quiet levels, which could lead to a suspicion of hearing impairment if only the latter are used.

Responses at age 7–9 months

At this age a child can localize accurately quiet sounds on a horizontal plane, although many children still have some problems in identifying a source of sound below and, in particular, above their heads on testing. A child will turn readily to a parent's voice across the room and search for the source of interesting sounds. The child should also be babbling tunefully and during this time may begin more noticeably to copy sounds.

Responses at 10–12 months

At this age a child can localize quiet sound on any plane when not otherwise occupied. Verbal comprehension is developing for single words, such as his/her name, 'no' and well-known objects. The range of vocalizations increases and by their first birthday a few children are attempting to say and repeat one or two words.

Responses at 13–24 months

A child of this age localizes sounds readily but begins to anticipate and search for the sound source during testing, so that more active distraction may be necessary. Understanding of words

increases so that by 18 months many children will respond readily to questions such as 'Where's your nose?' or 'Where's the cat?'. By the age of 2 years children will often pick out toys when requested, and simple speech tests can be introduced into the assessment. The child's vocabulary increases over the second year of life and many children are joining two words together by 18–21 months. Even before speech is heard the vocalizations should show good intonation patterns with speech like rhythms.

Responses over the age of 2 years

As the child gets older, he/she becomes increasingly able to inhibit the earlier, ready response to sound. Such a child will usually turn to a particular stimulus on the first presentation only, and will subsequently appear to ignore the sound. There is a developing ability to recognize background sounds without visual confirmation, so that many sounds do not seem to be registered at a conscious level. At the same time there develops an ability consciously to avoid turning to sounds when anticipated, for example during testing. Sometimes a response may be seen as an eye-glide, but as many parents will testify, an older child can appear to be completely unaware of unwelcome requests and demands. As this stage is reached simple distraction techniques of testing become more difficult and eventually impossible to carry out reliably.

Testing

There are various factors which have to be taken into consideration if accurate results are to be obtained on testing a young child.

Environment

The environment in which the testing of a young child takes place is vitally important if the results are to be accurate. The room must be not only acoustically acceptable, but must also be a comfortable, inviting place, where a child can relax. An insecure, worried child is not going to cooperate fully in the necessary assessment, and anything which may help such a child to enjoy the session is invaluable.

While older children and adults may perform hearing tests seated in small, sound-treated booths, the testing of the younger child and infant should take place in a normal-sized room. There needs to be space for the child and care-giver to sit in the centre of the room with a distractor up to

2 m (6 feet) in front and a tester moving freely behind.

The room, as for a booth, should be extremely quiet and the design of audiometric rooms is a very specialized area. Such rooms are expensive to provide and a reasonable compromise for diagnostic audiometric testing is an overall sound level not exceeding 30 dB(A). However, the testing of very young children is normally carried out in free field and, ideally, even lower background sound levels are necessary in these conditions. A full discussion of the design of such rooms to meet recommended standards acoustically would be out of place in this chapter, but certain other features are worthy of consideration. For example, the sound absorbent lining to the walls of audiometric rooms is often finished with acoustic tiles, but a more welcoming environment may be created by the use of a fabric finish.

In addition to reducing the acoustic interference with testing, consideration has to be given to the visual aspects of the test room. The lighting of an audiometric room is extremely important when carrying out free field testing. There should be even illumination, with no possibility of shadows alerting a hearing impaired child to the test procedure. There should not be large windows overlooking interesting, and in particular moving, objects that may distract the child and make testing unreliable, and in the room itself there should be no distracting features such as pictures, attractive toys or equipment within the child's visual field during testing. When testing a child it is important that there are no reflective surfaces, particularly two-way mirrors for observation, which are in visual range, as again this would invalidate test results. This should be considered when designing the layout of the room, also remembering that a window becomes a mirror after dark, but suitable blinds or curtains may solve the problem.

Stimulus

Frequency

In the past a wide variety of uncalibrated sounds were used to assess hearing. These included such items as squeaky toys, musical boxes, crinkled paper from a number of sources, and bells. While some of these may still have a place during assessment, it is now recognized that sounds for testing have to be far more frequency specific if accurate and meaningful hearing levels are to be obtained. When testing, the most important point is that the tester should be aware of the frequency spectrum of the sounds, so that an overall pattern of hearing can be deduced from the results. The aim is to build up information about a child's hearing at various frequencies in the same way that one carries out an audiogram in the older child. During the test for threshold levels the minimum requirement should be an assessment of hearing at a low, medium and high frequency.

Many different test sounds are used in different centres. One traditional test sound which gives a wide frequency spectrum (*Figure 6.1*) and thus remains effective as part of a test battery is the cup/spoon combination. The sound must be produced by lightly rubbing the back of the spoon around the rim of the cup, as any clinking sound will change the flat frequency spectrum.

Test sounds include the human voice, and although the frequency may be less exact, the sound 'oo' is usually about 500 Hz, the hummed 'mm' about 1 kHz and the sound 's' is usually about 3 kHz. The traditional, and still very practical instruments for assessing high frequency hearing, in the UK are the Manchester and Nuffield rattles (*Figures 6.2* and *6.3*).

More recently, instruments producing warble tones have been introduced to the assessment procedure. These have the advantage of a reproducible and frequency-specific stimulus that will

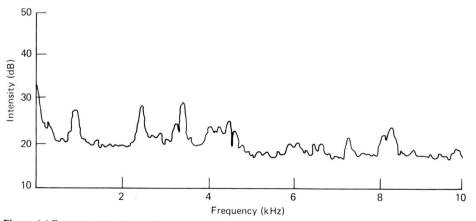

Figure 6.1 Frequency spectrum of cup/spoon

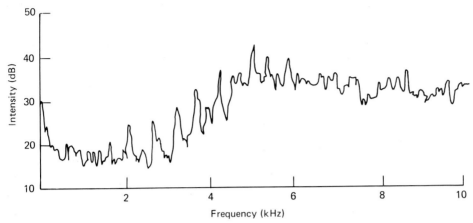

Figure 6.2 Frequency spectrum of Manchester rattle

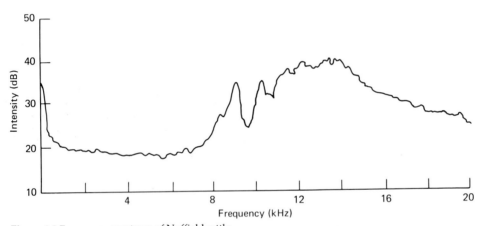

Figure 6.3 Frequency spectrum of Nuffield rattle

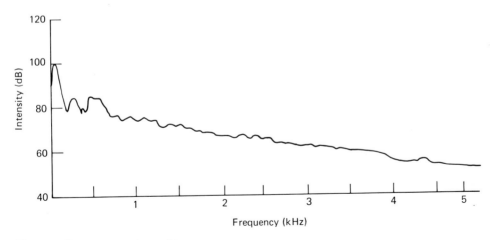

Figure 6.4 Frequency spectrum of drum

not give standing waves, with variation in intensity, while testing. Some are small devices designed for screening, but others are more powerful, delivering sound up to 120 dB(A) SPL in free field, with adjustable modulation of the warble, based on frequencies from 125 Hz–8 kHz. Some also produce other stimuli such as narrow band sound. For a hearing-impaired child the drum is still used to test low frequency hearing on occasions (*Figure 6.4*) but frequency specific information from tests using warble tones is preferable particularly for fitting of a hearing-aid.

Intensity

During an assessment of hearing, it is essential to know not only the frequency of the sound to which the child responds, but also the intensity of the quietest sound responded to at each frequency. The only accurate way of monitoring the delivery of these sounds is with a sound level meter. Sounds used for testing in free field are normally measured in dB(A) SPL. An experienced tester may be able to produce sounds of minimal intensity reliably, making regular checks on delivery with the sound level meter. However, when a tester is relatively inexperienced, or the sound is above normal threshold levels, each needs to be checked against a sound level meter. The distance from the ear at which the sound is produced has a marked effect on its intensity, the diminution in intensity following the inverse square law, so that the testing distance must be scrupulously observed on each occasion.

Subject

When testing children it is very important to use the appropriate method for the child's overall developmental stage (*Table 6.1*), and this must be roughly assessed prior to starting the test. Application of a wrong method will lead to lack of cooperation from the child and unreliable results. Some measure of a child's developmental level can

be obtained by providing suitable toys for the child to play with while taking a history from the care-giver, and observing the use of these toys. A child who has developed an understanding of miniature toys and shows reasonable play with these items is usually able to condition to sound in free field, and may accept headphones and proceed to an audiogram. A child who only understands the use of real objects and does not have any concept of the symbolic significance of a miniature toy is likely to need testing by distraction techniques.

Distraction tests of hearing

This technique, which requires two trained testers, was originally described by Ewing (1957) and later in greater detail by Sheridan (1968). One tester remains in front of the child and is responsible for maintaining the child's attention in the correct state for testing and is able to observe the reactions of the child. The other tester is behind the child and produces the test sounds when the child's attention is in the appropriate state. This requires good coordination between the testers, which is best achieved when the two concerned are used to working as a pair.

The test lay-out is demonstrated in *Figure 6.5* with the test sounds being produced 1 m from the child's ear (apart from the Nuffield rattle, which is used at 30 cm), and on a horizontal plane. The sounds are produced behind the child, and it is

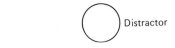

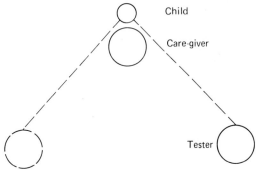

Table 6.1 Clinical testing in children

Test	Developmental age
Startle reaction to speech (65 dB)	Any age from birth
Stilling to sound	6–16 weeks
Distraction tests	4–30 months
Visual reinforcement audiometry	6–30 months
Conditioning audiometry	From 2 years
Pure tone audiometry (air and bone)	From 30 months
Audiometry with masking	From 5 years
Speech tests (of increasing complexity)	From 21 months

Figure 6.5 Lay-out of room for distraction testing

important that the tester and equipment do not come into visual range and that the distractor does not look at the tester at any time. There should also be no chance of tactile stimulation, which can occur if the tester is too close to the child, particularly with vigorously shaken rattles producing air currents. It is also important that the distractor should be experienced in judging the attention levels of young children. The younger the infant the easier it is to attract and fix the attention visually, so overdistraction, which parents commonly quote as a problem during testing, must be avoided. As a child gets older, and in particular over the age of 12–15 months, continuous distraction varying in degree may become necessary, as these children start to look around when there is nothing of interest to watch in front.

The distraction technique is most sensitive at 7–10 months of age, and some of the problems that may be encountered on testing children of different developmental levels are mentioned previously. Thompson and Weber (1974) reported median thresholds to noise through a loud speaker of 45–55 dB at 3–5 months, 35–45 dB at 6–11 months and 35–40 dB at 12–17 months, when testing normal hearing infants by behavioural observation audiometry. In practice, slightly lower thresholds are observed with 'live' presentation of the sound.

Visual reinforcement audiometry

In some centres, this method is used in addition to the normal distraction techniques, in particular to test the hearing of children over the age of 1 year. This method is said to reduce the habituation to sound seen in this age group, and to reinforce the localization of a sound stimulus. The sound stimulus is presented through loud speakers accompanied by a visual stimulus, such as a flashing light or animated toy near to or above the loud speaker. Moore and Wilson (1978) reported less habituation when using an animated toy for reinforcement. They felt this approach was reliable from 5 months of age, and after using a complex sound at 70 dB SPL for conditioning they reported thresholds of under 20 dB SPL at 500 Hz, 1 kHz and 4 kHz on testing the older infant. The 'distractor' is still essential during this test to control the prestimulus level of activity and attention.

Conditioning audiometry

This is also known as performance testing and play audiometry as the child is taught to join in a 'game' with the tester. Although some children

below the age of 2 years can carry out this type of task, and many 2 year olds are able to cooperate reasonably in the test, it is most useful in children aged 30 months and over. Basically, the child is taught to carry out some simple task in response to a sound stimulus, for example putting a brick in a box, a wooden man in a bus, or a peg in a board. The task is first taught with visual reinforcement, either using the word 'go' with visible mouth movements and facial expressions, or using a free field audiometer with the stimulus button visible. The visual stimulus is then withdrawn and the minimum response level obtained for the test sounds. Thompson and Weber (1974) reported median thresholds to noise, on using play audiometry, of 26 dB SPL at 24–29 months, and 13 dB SPL at 30–35 months of age.

With the younger child there are various strategies that may be necessary during testing in order to complete the task. Several different play activities may be used in succession, and obvious suprathreshold stimuli may be interspersed to reinforce the conditioning when attention flags. The crucial ability in the child is that of being able to wait and make no response when there is no stimulus present. The younger child or those with attention problems may respond after a certain time regardless of any stimulus, and this activity needs to be discouraged without losing the child's confidence in his ability to play the game.

Once children are able to condition reliably to sound the only factor preventing them from carrying out an unmasked pure tone audiogram is the acceptance of headphones. With modern technology, many young children have seen or even used headphones for stereo radios and hi-fi units and will happily cooperate at around 30 months of age. However, some children do take longer to accept strange instruments and may be over 3 years of age before they will carry out an audiogram. Warren (personal communication) has suggested the use of an earphone on a wall-mounted Flexarm to overcome the difficulty in accepting headphones. Some children will accept a bone vibrator more readily, and bone conduction thresholds may be obtained first. Many children can cope with masking from the age of 4–6 years and, from the age of 7 years, virtually all normal children are able to be tested for hearing thresholds in the same way as adults.

Testing the 'difficult' child

The decision as to which test is appropriate in a particular child to estimate the hearing thresholds and speech discrimination ability depends on the overall developmental age of the child, and not the chronological age. Thus, for example, a child of any age who is developmentally at the 9-month level would be best tested by distraction techniques. The validity of this approach was assessed by Flexner *et al.* (1985) who tested children with different degrees of mental handicap and found comparable results with children of the similar developmental levels.

When a child's developmental level is below 3–4 months, behavioural methods of testing are not sufficiently reliable for accurate assessment of hearing. Under these circumstances, one of the so-called 'objective' methods of assessing hearing is necessary, for example electrocochleography or auditory brainstem evoked responses. Although such tests do have their limitations (*see below* and Chapter 7), they may be the only available method of gaining any information on the hearing ability of a very young or handicapped child.

Children with visual impairment may respond differently to sound from their normal-sighted peers, and this must be taken into account when testing their hearing. A young child with very poor vision is unable to relate a sound to a source and will react to sounds by stilling and listening. If the sound appears to be that of an object with which he is familiar, he may reach out a hand for the object, while keeping the body and head still and continuing to listen. Many visually-impaired children respond reasonably reliably to voice at minimal intensities, but do not respond to other test sounds, particularly warble tones, unless presented at suprathreshold levels. It can be difficult with some of these children to be sure that they can hear to minimal levels, and if there is any doubt at all, 'objective' tests of hearing should be used as optimal hearing is essential in a child with a visual loss to achieve the maximum sensory input.

Once partially-sighted children are able to use their residual vision effectively, following either correction or training, they will attempt to localize a sound source and also start to respond at lower intensities. When using distraction techniques large, brightly-coloured objects are required, and on occasions a torch light may be helpful to attract the attention to the front. When a visually-handicapped child has reached the age where conditioning tests are more suitable the task chosen must be appropriate to the child's visual-motor skills. This usually includes larger objects and a simple task, such as dropping a brick into a basket, rather than fitting tasks.

Some children, particularly those with various forms of cerebral palsy, may be difficult to test because of the limitations they have in carrying out voluntary movements. This problem may also occur against a background of involuntary movement, making the presence or absence of a response difficult to assess with certainty. Even when a child can localize a sound by head or eye movement, the response may be slow and require prolonged presentation of the stimulus. The older child may understand the task during conditioning tests, but only be capable of one or two different movements in response. A familiar care-giver is essential to interpret the child's communications. Again 'objective' tests are needed when there is any doubt about the hearing levels. Some of these children may have been affected by perinatal problems, for example severe asphyxia or hyperbilirubinaemia, and be thus at high risk of hearing impairment.

Children with autistic features can be difficult to test if there are problems in gaining their attention. They may show only fleeting regard for a distractor and any objects being used, and are sometimes very difficult to keep in one area for testing. These children may also show little interest in voice, although many will respond very promptly to warble tones and rattles. If there are persistent problems in obtaining reliable results due to a child's behaviour, 'objective' tests may be necessary, but experienced testers can usually obtain hearing levels in these children.

In a similar way, a hyperactive child or any child with attention problems may be difficult to test and may require a variety of different techniques to complete a hearing assessment. Again, in some children, it may be necessary to resort to 'objective' tests, but this is not normally the case.

Speech tests

From a functional point of view the most important measure of a child's hearing is the ability to hear and discriminate speech. If children have hearing difficulties it may be helpful to gain a measure of their discrimination of speech sounds not only in optimal conditions, in a sound-treated room, but also in the presence of background noise, such as their normal school environment. This is also an important aspect in monitoring the function of a child with hearing aids.

In the older child, speech detection and discrimination tests can be carried out in a similar way to tests on adults. This is by presentation of phonetically balanced words through headphones with the instruction to the child to repeat the word/sound that they hear, with scoring for correctly heard phonemes. The word lists for younger children may have to be simplified, and suitable material in the UK would include the Manchester junior word lists. However, such tasks are not possible for routine use in children under the age of 7–8 years. Even above this age there may be some problems in testing. The younger the child the more likely it is that he/she will give no response if unable to recognize a complete word, thus giving an underestimate of ability, and some children may have articulatory problems that make it difficult to score the response accurately.

For the younger child different approaches are needed to estimate speech discrimination thresholds. (In practice, the parameters measured are the optimal discrimination score, and the sound level at which this is achieved.) Tests at this age are generally more acceptable if delivered live rather than through loud speakers, and involve the use of closed sets, that is a finite number of objects or pictures are presented and the child's response is limited to picking out one of these (as pass or fail). The results are not directly comparable to open methods, and are influenced by set size. The task needs to be presented as a game, and it is important that children should not feel that they are failing, as they will cease to cooperate. Thus the approach used must be appropriate to the child's developmental level. The vocabulary also needs to be appropriate to the child's level of verbal comprehension, and this cannot be predicted from the general level of abilities and has to be gained from the history. A hearing-impaired child will probably have a smaller vocabulary than his/her peers, limiting the items that can be used for testing, and he may, in fact, not recognize any words using hearing alone, so that a speech discrimination test is not possible.

From the age of 18 months a rough measure of speech discrimination may be obtained in a cooperative child by using toys and a parent (for example daddy, teddy and dolly) as recipients, and items such as a cup, spoon or shoe. The child can then be asked to give the cup to teddy, and the quietest level at which this can be carried out accurately, as measured on a sound level meter, recorded. The game, as with all tests for the younger age groups, needs to be carried out first with lip-reading and facial expression visible and a normal intensity of voice, and only when the child can reliably perform the task under these circumstances should the mouth be covered and the voice dropped.

As children get older, toys from an established test such as the Kendal toy test or the modification by McCormick (1977), used in the UK, can be introduced gradually. These tests contain items that have similar vowel sounds but different consonants, for example cup/duck, cow/house, shoe/spoon. Suitable words would obviously vary in different countries and cultures. A child aged around 2 years may only be able to cope with a limited number of items, which must be used in pairs, but by 3 years of age most children can cope with the whole test, containing 15 items, without difficulty. The child is asked to identify the item,

and when the task is understood the minimum level at which all the items can be successfully identified is recorded. In a normal hearing child under optimal conditions this test can be completed at 35–40 dB(SPL). If a raised level of speech is needed for discrimination, the level is recorded and any particular word confusions noted, as they may give additional evidence as to the type of hearing problem being encountered.

Older children learn to relate pictures to objects, and picture tests can be used instead of the above toy tests. In a child with a short attention span, the two approaches can be combined as a way of varying the game, to obtain reliable results. As school age approaches the range of vocabulary suitable for the speech tests increases (a discussion on suitable word pairs for screening and testing English speaking 5 year olds can be found in Haggard, Wood and Carroll, 1984). In the older child, it may be possible to extend the testing session long enough to record the percentage of correct responses at various intensities, as well as the level needed for 100% accuracy, whereas in a younger child the latter may be the only level obtainable within a test session.

During tests for speech discrimination a child may have other problems that necessitate a modification to the test procedure. For example if a child has visual problems, the objects or pictures used may have to be larger than usual and a smaller number of items may be dictated by available space. The child will also need to become familiar with the layout of the objects, so that they can be identified easily without prolonged scanning of the whole field.

A child who has difficulty in controlling voluntary movements accurately enough to pick out the requested object will need fewer objects with wide spacing to make the task physically possible. For a child who can only use eye pointing as a form of identification, the objects need to be well spread out so that there is no confusion over that chosen.

Speech perception in the hearing impaired

The hearing impaired are a special group with respect to speech discrimination tests, and a full coverage of such a specialized field is not appropriate in this chapter. Hearing-impaired individuals gain their information on speech content from both visual and auditory inputs, and a full assessment should encompass the use of both modalities separately and in combination. This section will cover only the simpler aspects of the assessment of the level of auditory input.

On initial assessment some children may be able to carry out a speech discrimination task using a limited number of known items, with a measurable response when a raised intensity of voice is used. Other children may have insufficient understanding of words to carry out such a task at all. A further group may be able to pick out items correctly when they are also allowed to use lip or speech-reading, but cannot carry out the task using auditory input alone.

Further information is required regarding the speech reception skills of these groups of children, but for testing to take place, the children need to develop an appropriate vocabulary. The first information required is some measure of the child's ability to distinguish words under optimal conditions. One such test was designed for hearing-impaired children by Ross and Lerman (1970) using monosyllabic word lists, with the response identified on picture plates. Further information on the hearing of children who have low scores on this test can be obtained using a spondee-recognition score as described by Cramer and Erber (1974). Children fall into two groups – those who can distinguish the words accurately and those who only have the ability to perceive the time and intensity patterns of speech. Another test, using a combination of monosyllables (for example bed), trochees (for example table), and spondees (for example toothbrush), can differentiate those children who are able to recognize words accurately, those who can recognize stress patterns, and those who cannot use their hearing to recognize either. Although these types of tests are not helpful in isolation, they do give information which can then be applied to modify hearing aid fittings and rehabilitative programmes.

Objective tests of hearing

Impedance audiometry

This is covered fully in Chapter 8, but some aspects of its applicability are worth emphasizing again in relation to the testing of hearing in young children. There are three measurements used in impedance audiometry, the middle-ear compliance, the tympanogram and acoustic reflex measurements. In isolation all these measures are of limited value, but a good deal of information can be obtained, particularly from the latter two, when they are viewed in combination. When taken in conjunction with other tests of hearing and otoscopy they contribute significantly to the overall picture.

Many young children do have middle ear abnormalities, the most common being the temporary presence of fluid. Impedance audiometry gives particularly useful information on middle ear function, which can aid diagnosis, and also monitor progress in young children with conductive hearing losses.

Acoustic reflex measurements are used in the more detailed assessment of a sensorineural hearing loss, to distinguish a cochlear from a neural lesion. In an ear with a cochlear disorder, Jerger and Hayes (1984) demonstrated the decline in the acoustic reflex sensation level in proportion to the degree of hearing loss. The reflex threshold remains at around 85 dB (a normal level) until the hearing loss exceeds 40–50 dB HL and may still be elicited at 110 dB with hearing losses of 80 dB HL. A combination of acoustic reflex threshold measurement and reflex decay was felt to be reasonably sensitive in eighth nerve lesions (Olsen, Noffsinger and Kurdziel, 1975). This aspect of impedance audiometry may be of help in the investigation of a hearing-impaired child.

In addition, Jerger *et al.* (1974) have suggested that, in the presence of normal middle ear function, the acoustic reflex can predict the sensorineural hearing level. This prediction is based on the relationship between the acoustic reflex hearing threshold level to pure tone signals and broad band noise. In ears with a sensorineural hearing loss the reflex threshold level for noise becomes elevated, whereas that for pure tones remains relatively stable, declining as described previously. This has been suggested as a further method of testing hearing in the young infant and difficult to test child, although other workers have not found this technique to be helpful.

One of the problems in carrying out impedance audiometry in young children is that some will not tolerate the probe for a sufficient time to complete the necessary measurements. This also occurs in difficult to test children, who are often fairly strong and active. The more modern screening tympanometers, although easier to handle in these groups of children, do not have broad band sound as a stimulus and can give unreliable reflex thresholds (Bennett and Mowat, 1981; Wood, Lutman and Fernandes, 1982).

Evoked response audiometry

This is fully covered in Chapter 7, but some points are worth repeating in the context of testing of hearing. The usual aim of such tests in children is to gain an indication of hearing threshold in those who are too young or handicapped to be tested by 'subjective' methods. There is no place for these tests in estimating thresholds in children who can cooperate with other forms of testing, as both distraction and conditioning methods give more information regarding the hearing levels at a wider range of frequencies.

The ideal test for use in children, based on evoked responses, would be of short duration, reliable during sleep or sedation, and would predict accurately the thresholds of hearing at a range of frequencies. In practice, such a test is not yet available, although research is continuing. Present techniques include electrocochleography and auditory brainstem evoked responses, while the SN10 response, middle latency responses and the 40 Hz test, first described by Galambos, Makeiz and Talmachoff (1981), continue to be evaluated. These latter techniques appear to be affected by sleep and sedation, and use in children will be restricted by this.

Both electrocochleography and auditory brainstem evoked responses are applied clinically, each having different advantages and disadvantages. Electrocochleography requires general anaesthesia and is an invasive technique, but while the child is asleep, a good view of the tympanic membrane can be obtained, with minor procedures, such as removal of wax, myringotomy and even the insertion of ventilation tubes also being carried out. It is also possible to make ear moulds, if required, before a difficult to test child awakes. The testing can also be carried out over a more prolonged period of time, if necessary, without fear of the child waking in the middle of the procedures.

Auditory brainstem evoked responses require a still child, and young infants are often in a suitable state for testing following a feed. Older and more disturbed children require sedation if they are to stay still for testing, and children of any age are liable to wake after 45–60 minutes, thus limiting the testing that can be carried out in any one session. This test gives more information regarding the auditory pathways, but neurological abnormalities may affect later waves in such a way as to make threshold estimation unreliable.

Historically, the stimulus used in both auditory brainstem evoked responses and electrocochleography has been a click, with reasonable correlation found between the thresholds obtained in children and their behavioural thresholds to frequencies of 2–3 kHz. The use of tone pips and filtered clicks to gain more frequency specific information has been disappointing (Kileny, 1981; Sohmer and Kinarti, 1984). One promising method is the use of tone bursts in notched noise or high pass noise, but problems still occur with frequencies below 1 kHz.

In practice, the results of electrophysiological tests, although not giving an exact measure of hearing, are invaluable when combined with other tests of hearing to build up an overall picture of a child's auditory function.

Screening

Screening programmes to identify children who have abnormal hearing are in use in many countries. The early screen is normally carried out at some time during the first year of life, and the aim of this programme is to identify at an early age children who are hearing impaired, and in particular those who need amplification, in order to start the rehabilitative programme as soon as possible. This is then supplemented in many areas by preschool screening, which should identify any children who may have been missed at the earlier screen, particularly those with mild losses, high-frequency losses and persistent middle ear effusions. Further screening is frequently carried out at school entry and at intervals during school life, and the aim of these screens is predominantly to identify those children with middle ear disease, although some sensorineural hearing losses are first identified at this time.

Identification of hearing loss by infant screening

Screening of hearing by the distraction method (*see above*), has been carried out in infancy for many years in the UK. The EEC study reported by Martin and Moore (1979) highlighted the disappointing results of this programme, with only 55% of those children with a loss of 50 dB or greater being identified by the age of 3 years. Local authorities in the UK have attempted to improve the screening, so that hearing-impaired children are identified in the first year of life, but although in some districts the results of screening are said to be satisfactory, the most recent figures from Newton (1985) in Manchester revealed that the mean age at identification of presumed congenital hearing loss was 23.3 months. These figures would be typical of the results of screening in many districts in the UK. Two main problems are encountered, the first being the initial passing on screening of many children with hearing impairment, the proportion in Manchester being 44%, and the second being the low attendance rate for screening in many districts. The children who are not brought for screening are a particular worry because according to the law of inverse care (Brimblecombe, 1975) these children may be at higher risk of handicap than those who attend relevant screening.

These problems are also encountered in screening programmes in other countries. For example Tell, Levi and Feinmesser (1977) documented the results of the screening programme in the well-baby clinics in Jerusalem, with 85% of infants attending a check at 7 months. Of the 28 known deaf children who should have been identified in infancy only 24 had actually been screened and of these 10 had passed the initial screen.

These figures become more alarming when

placed alongside the report of the Saskatoon conference (1978) which recommended that hearing-impaired children should be identified and remediation started in the first 6 months of life. Workers with hearing-impaired children have subjectively noted the improvement in vocalizations and language development of these children and Markides (1986) has demonstrated the significantly superior speech intelligibility of children fitted with hearing aids in their first 6 months compared with those fitted in the second half of the first year or the second and third years of life, who all performed very similarly. The aim of a modern screening programme should thus be, to identify children with hearing impairment within the first 6 months of life, so that the majority of these children can have hearing aids fitted by 3–4 months of age. Present infant screening programmes alone are unable to meet these aims.

Routine infant screening in the USA has been discouraged because of the poor results, with the emphasis being placed on testing of high-risk infants (*Table 6.2*). This has been effective in identifying 65–70% of infants with a congenital hearing loss in their first few months (Mencher, 1977), but the remaining infants with no risk factors need to be identified by an alternative method.

Table 6.2 High risk factors for hearing impairment

(1) Positive family history of childhood hearing impairment
(2) Intrauterine infections (for example rubella, cytomegalovirus, syphilis, toxoplasmosis)
(3) Anatomical abnormalities of the ears, head and neck
(4) Birthweight less than 1500 g
(5) Severe neonatal asphyxia
(6) Hyperbilirubinaemia of 342 µmol/l or over (less in preterm)
(7) Bacterial meningitis
(8) Ototoxic drug administration

Neonatal screening

The time at which infants are most accessible for screening is in the neonatal period. Where there is a hospital-based obstetric service the majority of neonates could be screened, if an effective method were available. However, in areas where many babies are born at home or taken home within a few hours, any neonatal screening programme must rely on motivating the parents sufficiently to attend a hospital or clinic for the hearing test. When the aim of a programme is to identify hearing impairment before 6 months of age, neonatal screening is theoretically the most efficient way of reaching the target population.

If such a screening programme is to be implemented it is essential that facilities are available to help those infants identified as a result of the programme. When the screening is carried out at 7–9 months the fitting of hearing aids following a fuller assessment is reasonably easy, and in many countries there are rehabilitative programmes available for children of this age and their parents.

However, the position is not so straightforward if some form of neonatal screening is used. Following the screening there need to be facilities for assessing the babies in more detail, and this involves electrophysiological testing, particularly auditory brainstem evoked responses, in addition to careful behavioural observation to estimate the hearing thresholds. There also need to be facilities for investigation and rehabilitation of those infants found to be hearing impaired. Hearing aids can be fitted to these young babies, but this requires far more skill and experience than in the older child, both in estimating the desirable degree of amplification and in ear mould fitting (Seeward *et al.*, 1985; Nolan *et al.*, 1986). The personnel involved in working with the families in rehabilitation programmes must also be experienced in the development of very young infants, and this expertise is not widely available because training has previously concentrated more on the older infant and toddler. Without the necessary back-up facilities neonatal screening is not a viable proposition.

Behavioural screening in neonates

Various studies have been carried out to evaluate screening programmes that use observation of a neonate's behaviour in response to sound to identify those with a possible hearing impairment. The Nova Scotia conference on early identification of hearing loss recommended that the sound applied should be random noise with low-frequency attenuation of 30 dB/octave below 750 Hz, a rise-decay time of 5 ms and duration of 0.5–2.0 s. The interval between test presentations should be a minimum of 15 s and the sound intensity should not exceed 90 dB SPL at the pinna. It was also recommended that there should be two independent observers for each test.

It was pointed out by Gerber, Jones and Costello (1977) that such a test would only pick up those who are profoundly deaf and these reservations were confirmed by Downs (1978), who found that screening in this way only identified 60% of those later found to be hearing impaired, missing mild and moderate losses with average hearing levels better than 75 dB.

The false positive rate using behavioural observation following the recommended protocol is high, so that many infants need referral for further evaluation. The Halifax study, reported by Durieux-Smith and Jacobson (1985), observed a false positive rate of around 50% in normal and at-risk neonates, rising to 86% in babies from the neonatal intensive care unit.

Various methods have been tried to improve the reliability of behavioural testing by eliminating observer error and measuring the reactions to sound using instrumentation. These modifications use body and head movements and changes in respiration or heart rate as parameters of response, and not the aural-palpebral reflex which is the most consistent behaviour observed.

The first instrument, the Crib-o-gram, (Simmons, 1978) is in use in parts of North America. Early reports suggested that the test had a false positive rate of 9% and only missed one in 29 children with confirmed moderate/severe hearing loss. However, many children who failed the test were lost to follow-up.

The study reported by Durieux-Smith and Jacobson (1985) also compared the results of the Crib-o-gram with auditory brainstem evoked responses in a neonatal intensive care unit (the Ottawa study). At 38 weeks' gestational age or greater, 72.4% of infants with normal auditory brainstem evoked responses were correctly identified by the Crib-o-gram, with the figure falling to 63.8% in infants of 31–37 weeks' gestational age. Only one of the three infants in the 31–37 week group having auditory brainstem evoked responses thresholds of 50 dB HL or greater was identified by the Crib-o-gram, whereas in the full-term group the Crib-o-gram identified all those with thresholds on auditory brainstem evoked responses of 60 dB HL or greater. It thus appears that the Crib-o-gram has a high false positive rate, particularly in terms of the further evaluation needed by infants who fail the test, but does identify term babies with hearing losses of 60 dB or greater.

In the UK, the Linco Bennett or auditory response cradle was developed, and the results of the preliminary trial, involving 6000 neonates were reported by Bhattacharya, Bennett and Taylor (1984). Of those babies screened, 8% failed the first screen, 1.7% failed two screens and following auditory brainstem evoked responses there was said to be a false positive rate of 1.2%. Eighteen neonates were found to be hearing impaired and three have later been found to have hearing problems, presumed to be progressive in nature, but follow-up was limited in that it was only available on two-thirds of those tested at 3 years of age.

The auditory response cradle is designed for use on full-term babies but, with some modifications (Davis, 1984), it can be used on neonates in a special care baby unit, where the incidence of hearing impairment is higher than in the normal nursery. The false positive rate has varied in different units, rising to 20% in the special care babies, but seems consistently lower than that achieved with the Crib-o-gram. However, longer term follow-up is needed to confirm the number of hearing-impaired children not identified by the screen.

Electrophysiological methods of screening

The test that has been evaluated for screening a newborn population is auditory brainstem evoked response. Different figures emerge from different centres, which may well reflect differences in the infants tested as well as methodology used. In the UK, Bradford *et al.* (1985) screened special care babies using 100 dB SPL clicks, and reported absent responses in 8.2%, that is 10 babies, with nine of these having sensorineural hearing loss. So far no false negatives have been reported.

In Canada, the results from a number of centres are reported by Sanders *et al.* (1985). Their criteria for failing auditory brainstem evoked responses are taken as absent response at 30–40 dB, often combining with abnormal morphology at 60–70 dB. Using these more stringent criteria, 10–30% of babies in neonatal intensive care units will fail the first auditory brainstem evoked response screen. When retested 2–4% of the high-risk infants and those in the intensive care units are found to have a moderate to profound sensorineural hearing loss, with a further 6–8% having unilateral or conductive losses. These results are similar to figures reported by Galambos, Hicks and Wilson (1984).

All reports agree that auditory brainstem evoked responses provide overall accurate diagnostic information on hearing levels in almost all newborns tested. However, the test is time consuming and requires experienced personnel as well as specialized equipment. Because of the high cost and lower yield it is difficult to justify screening the whole neonatal population by this means. However, in the at-risk group, including those babies in the special care unit, screening by auditory brainstem evoked responses is justifiable because of the higher yield of hearing-impaired children within this much smaller population.

Within the special care unit, behavioural testing is being evaluated, the main justification being that less skilled personnel are needed to carry out these forms of screening. There is a high false positive rate with many infants needing follow-up by auditory brainstem evoked responses. In view of the relatively high incidence of hearing loss and the additional information available regarding neurological function when using auditory brain-stem evoked responses, this latter technique would seem a more sensible tool to use for the primary screen.

7–9 months screen

Whether or not neonatal screening is being used in a community, the hearing screen at 7–9 months of age continues to play a role in the identification of hearing-impaired children. In areas where the technology needed to carry through a neonatal programme is not available, this later screen provides the first opportunity to identify affected children. Even when children have undergone an earlier screen it is possible that they have a hearing loss, either progressive in nature, or missed by the earlier test because it is a mild loss or because of administrative errors. The screen at 7–9 months is also an opportunity to identify those children with middle ear disease, who can then be followed-up in case intervention is needed later.

However, if this screen is to play an important part in identifying hearing impairment, the testing needs to be improved so that more reliable results are obtained than those documented previously. It is important that those who carry out the screening are both well trained and regularly assessed to ensure accuracy of the test method. The rooms used for testing must be reasonably quiet and the background noise and the level of screening sounds should be monitored with a sound level meter. The test sounds should cover the full range of frequencies, with different programmes employing a variety of noise makers.

It is also important, if the screen is to be of value, that it reaches as many infants as possible. Attempts are being made to educate professionals and parents regarding the importance of hearing loss in the young child, and the range of normal development. In Canada, the task force on Childhood Hearing Impairment (1984) has prepared information kits designed to increase the knowledge of health care professionals regarding hearing loss, to promote awareness of the preventative aspects and encourage earlier referral for diagnosis and management. This is to be distributed principally to primary care physicians, paediatricians and otolaryngologists. A speech and hearing check list modified from one produced by the Alexander Graham Bell Association for the Deaf is used as a guide to normal development.

In the UK, a checklist of normal hearing behaviour has been designed by McCormick (Nottingham) to be given to parents following delivery. It is designed to encourage parents to seek advice from their health visitor if they are concerned about their child's hearing, and an open access audiology service is provided to test infants at any age, with routine health visitor screening to supplement this. McCormick *et al.* (1984) have documented identification of hearing loss at a much lower age following this approach.

Experimental methods of screening in the first year

Assessment using the postauricular myogenic response

This response was first described by Kiang *et al.* (1963) and recently a new instrument for detecting the response has been suggested as suitable for use in an 'objective' test for infant screening (Flood *et al.*, 1982). This test was evaluated using a portable instrument on infants at around 6 months of age. Such a test was suggested because it was said to be easy to carry out and did not need the quiet conditions and skilled personnel of the routine distraction tests. A click stimulus was used at 60 dB HL and, if necessary repeated at 80 dB HL. Children who did not pass the test were further assessed using conventional methods. The place of such a method in screening infants is still being assessed, and it is suggested that it may be suitable for a wide age range, excluding neonates following a feed, for whom it is unreliable. The preliminary trials were said to demonstrate that a positive response, while not giving a precise hearing threshold, does indicate that the infant has adequate hearing to develop normal speech.

Otoacoustic emissions

These emissions were first described by Kemp (1978) following acoustic stimulation, and trials are being undertaken to evaluate the detection of such emissions as a means of screening for hearing impairment (Johnsen, Bagi and Alberling, 1983). Use of this technique remains experimental at this time.

Preschool screening

Screening of hearing between the ages of 1 and 5 years is not universal, but is carried out in individual areas at various ages. In practice, it is often combined with an assessment of language development and the age chosen is around the third birthday, because children of this age are more cooperative in both aspects of the assessment. However, it could be argued that the screening should be carried out earlier so that remediation can be started in those who need help.

The tests used to screen hearing are usually a conditioning technique in free field using 'go', 's' or a range of pure-tone or warble-tone stimuli, plus a test of speech discrimination, as described previously. This is supplemented in some areas by tympanometry. This screen is carried out in order to identify those children with sensorineural losses missed by earlier screens, particularly those with mild or high-frequency losses, and also those children with persistent middle ear effusions, with resultant hearing problems.

School screening

Screening of children for hearing problems has been carried out for over 50 years in schools in various countries, but the distribution of screening is patchy. Reports on the results of screening consistently show that 4–6% of those tested have hearing impairment and Fisch (1981) argued that school screening was very effective and should be extended to all areas. A sweep test is frequently employed using a stimulus of 20–25 dB HL at frequencies 250 Hz–4 kHz, and this is supplemented in some areas by speech tests and tympanometry.

Bennett and Mowat (1981) reported on the validity of impedance measures in school screening and found that moderate sensorineural losses were not identified by impedance studies including stapedial reflex thresholds, as might be expected, and that tympanometry failed a significant number of children who passed a sweep test carried out at the same time. The two procedures took the same length of time. Tympanometry alone thus appears to be too sensitive as a tool for routine screening, particularly in view of the fluctuant nature of many middle ear effusions, although if repeated it will identify those children with persistent problems. Bluestone *et al.* (1983) felt that screening tympanometry was best confined to the high-risk groups, such as children with Down's syndrome, cleft palates or language delay.

Haggard, Wood and Carroll (1984) argued that the best combination of tests for school screening would be otoadmittance measures to identify pathological problems, and a speech test in noise on those who failed the first screen to identify those with hearing disability. These latter children would then be referred for further assessment, plus a few referred directly following the otoadmittance screen because of abnormalities such as very high compliance. This was felt to be an economic method that would identify virtually all children with problems, with the assumption that children with congenital and severe, acquired hearing losses should already have been identified.

Whichever method of screening is favoured, and at whatever age, there is agreement between the professionals involved that it continues to be an essential tool in identifying hearing impairment in infants and children, so that the adverse consequences of hearing loss can, so far as possible, be averted.

References

BENNETT, M. and MOWAT, L. (1981) Validity of impedance measurements and referral criteria in school hearing screening programmes. Research report. *British Journal of Audiology*, **15**, 147–150

BHATTACHARYA, J., BENNETT, M. J. and TUCKER, S. M. (1984) Long term follow-up of newborns tested with the auditory response cradle. *Archives of Disease in Childhood*, **59**, 504–511

BLUESTONE, C. D., KLEIN, J. O., PARADISE, J.L., EICHERWALD, H., BESS, F. H., DOWNS, M. P. *et al.* (1983) Workshop on effects of otitis media on the child. *Pediatrics*, **71**, 639–652

BRADFORD, B. C., BAUDIN, J., CONWAY, M. J., HAZELL, J. W. P., STEWART, A. L. and REYNOLDS, E. O. R. (1985) Identification of sensorineural hearing loss in very pre-term infants by brainstem auditory evoked potentials. *Archives of Disease in Childhood*, **60**, 105–109

BRIMBLECOMBE, F. S. W. (1975) In *Bridging in Health*, edited by G. McLachlan, p. ix. London: Oxford University Press

CHILDHOOD HEARING IMPAIRMENT (1984) *Report of Task Force*. Ottawa: Minister of National Health and Welfare

CRAMER, K. D. and ERBER, N. P. (1974) A spondee recognition test for young hearing-impaired children. *Journal of Speech and Hearing Disorders*, **39**, 304–311

DAVIS, A. (1984) Detecting hearing impairment in neonates – the statistical decision criterion for the auditory response cradle. *British Journal of Audiology*, **18**, 163–168

DOWNS, M. A. (1978) Auditory screening. *Otolaryngologic Clinics of North America*, **11**, 611–629

DURIEUX-SMITH, A. and JACOBSON, J. T. (1985) Comparison of auditory brainstem response and behavioural screening in neonates. *Journal of Otolaryngology*, Suppl. 14, 47–53

EWING, I. R. (1957) Screening tests and guidance clinics for babies and young children. In *Educational Guidance of the Deaf Child*, edited by A. W. G. Ewing, p. 21. Manchester: Manchester University Press

FISCH, L. (1981) Development of school screening audiometry. *British Journal of Audiology*, **15**, 87–96

FLEXNER, C. and GANS, D. P. (1985) Comparative evaluation of the auditory responsiveness of normal and profoundly multihandicapped children. *Journal of Speech and Hearing Research*, **28**, 163–168

FLOOD, L. M., FRASER, J. G., CONWAY, M. J. and STEWART, A. (1982) The assessment of hearing in infancy using the post-auricular myogenic response: evaluation of an instrument which simplifies its detection. *British Journal of Audiology*, **16**, 211–214

GALAMBOS, R., HICKS, G. E. and WILSON, M. J. (1984) The auditory brain stem response predicts hearing loss in graduates of a tertiary intensive care nursery. *Ear and Hearing*, **5**, 254–260

GALAMBOS, R., MAKEIZ, S. and TALMACHOFF, P. J. (1981) A 40 Hz auditory potential recorded from the human scalp. *Proceedings of the National Academy of Science*, **78**, 2643–2647

GERBER, S. E., JONES, B. L. and COSTELLO, J. M. (1977) Behavioural measures. In *Audiometry in Infancy*, edited by S. E. Gerber, pp. 85–97. New York: Grune and Stratton

HAGGARD, M. P., WOOD, E. J. and CARROLL, S. (1984) Speech, admittance and tone-tests in school screening. Reconciling economics with pathology and disability perspectives. *British Journal of Audiology*, **18**, 133–154

JERGER, J., BURNEY, P., MAULDIN, L. and CRUMP, B. (1974) Predicting hearing loss from the acoustic reflex. *Journal of Speech and Hearing Disorders*, **39**, 11–22

JERGER, J. and HAYES, W. (1984) Clinical use of acoustic impedance testing in audiological diagnosis. In *Audiology and Audiological Medicine*, vol. 2, edited by H. A. Beagley, p. 716. Oxford: Oxford University Press

JOHNSEN, N. J., BAGI, P. and ALBERLING, C. (1983) Evoked emissions from the human ear. III Findings in neonates. *Scandinavian Audiology*, **12**, 17–24

KEMP, D. T. (1978) Stimulated acoustic emissions from within the human auditory system. *Journal of the Acoustical Society of America*, **64**, 1386–1391

KIANG, N. Y. YS., CRIST, A. H., FRENCH, M. A. and EDWARDS, A. G. (1963) Postauricular electrical response to acoustic stimuli in humans. *Quarterly Progress report no. 68*. MIT Cambridge, Massachusetts: Research Laboratory of Electronics

KILENY, P. (1981) The frequency specificity of tone-pip evoked auditory brain stem responses. *Ear and Hearing*, **2**, 270–275

McCORMICK, B. (1977) The toy discrimination test: an aid to screening the hearing of children above a mental age of two years. *Public Health (London)*, **91**, 67–73

McCORMICK, B., WOOD, S. A., COPE, Y. and SPAVINS, F. M. (1984) Analysis of records from an open access audiology service. *British Journal of Audiology*, **18**, 127–132

MARKIDES, A. (1986) Age at fitting of hearing aids and speech intelligibility. *British Journal of Audiology*, **20**, 165–168

MARTIN, J. A. M. and MOORE, W. J. (1979) *Childhood Deafness in the European Community*. EUR6413. Luxembourg: Commission of the European Communities

MENCHER, G. T. (1977) Screening the newborn infant for hearing loss: a complete identification program. In *Childhood Deafness: Causation Assessment and Manage-ment*, edited by F. H. Bess, pp. 107–116. New York: Grune and Stratton

MOORE, J. M. and WILSON, W. R. (1978) Visual reinforcement audiometry (VRA) with infants. In *Early Diagnosis of Hearing Loss*, edited by S. E. Gerber and G. T. Mencher, pp. 177–213. New York: Grune and Stratton

NEWTON, V. (1985) Aetiology of bilateral sensorineural hearing loss in young children. *Journal of Laryngology and Otology*, Suppl. 10

NOLAN, M., HOSTLER, M., TAYLOR, I. G. and CASH, A. (1986) Practical considerations in the fabrication of earmoulds for young babies. *Scandinavian Audiology*, **15**, 21–30

OLSEN, W., NOFFSINGER, D. and KURDZIEL, S. (1975) Acoustic reflex and reflex decay. Occurrence in patients with cochlear and eighth nerve lesions. *Archives of Otolaryngology*, **101**, 622–625

ROSS, M. and LERMAN, J. W. (1970) A picture identification test for hearing-impaired children. *Journal of Speech and Hearing Research*, **13**, 44–83

SANDERS, M. A., DURIEUX-SMITH, A., HYDE, M., JACOBSON, J., KILENY, P. and MURNANE, O. (1985) Incidence of hearing loss in high risk and intensive care nursery infants. *Journal of Otolaryngology*, Suppl. 14, 28–33

SASKATOON CONFERENCE (1978) Early diagnosis of hearing loss. *Proceedings of the Saskatoon Conference on Early Diagnosis of Hearing Loss*, edited by S. E. Gerber and G. T. Mencher, pp. 1–32. New York: Grune and Stratton

SEEWARD, R. C., SEEWARD, R. C., ROSS, M. and SPIRO, M. K. (1985) Selecting amplification characteristics for young hearing impaired children. *Ear and Hearing*, **6**, 48–53

SHERIDAN, M. D. (1968) *Manual for Stycar tests of vision and hearing*. Windsor: National Foundation for Educational Research

SIMMONS, F. B. (1978) Identification of hearing loss in infants and young children. *Otolaryngologic Clinics of North America*, **11**, 19–28

SOHMER, H. and KINARTI, R. (1984) Survey of attempts to use auditory evoked potentials to obtain an audiogram. *British Journal of Audiology*, **18**, 237–244

TELL, L., LEVI, C. and FEINMESSER, M. (1977) Screening infants in baby clinics. In *Childhood Deafness: Causation, Assessment and Management*, edited by F. H. Bess, pp. 117–126. New York: Grune and Stratton

THOMPSON, G. and WEBER, B. A. (1974) Response of infants and young children to behavioural observation audiometry (BAO). *Journal of Speech and Hearing Disorders*, **39**, 140–147

WOOD, E. J., LUTMAN, M. E. and FERNANDES, M. A. (1982) Validation of a screening oto-admittance instrument. *British Journal of Audiology*, **16**, 273–276

7

Evoked potential audiometry

Martyn L. Hyde

When conventional behavioural audiometry is difficult or impossible, or when its results are inaccurate or suspect, there is a need for more objective hearing tests. Candidates for such tests include young infants, uncooperative, hyperactive, or neurologically impaired children, and those suspected of non-organic hearing loss. The usual goal is to approximate pure tone thresholds, using some measure other than conditioned or voluntary behaviour. The accuracy and extent of the required audiometry range from simple screening to a complete 'diagnostic' audiogram.

A very important class of objective tests is based upon auditory evoked potentials (AEPs). The general term used for such tests is evoked potential audiometry, more widely known as electric response audiometry (ERA). Electric response audiometry is applicable, at least in principle, regardless of the age of the patient or of the audiometric precision and detail required. Introductory articles are available (Davis, 1976; Beagley, 1981; Jacobson and Hyde, 1985). Some alternatives to electric response audiometry are discussed in Chapter 6, and the topic of objective audiometry in adults is covered in Volume 2, Chapter 8.

Over the last 10–15 years, auditory evoked potential tests have had a major impact in both paediatric and adult audiology, and they are now of proven clinical value for both estimation of hearing sensitivity and for assessment of cochlear and retrocochlear pathology. It is now clear that many auditory evoked potentials can be used audiometrically, and electric response audiometry has emerged as a substantial sub-discipline within audiology. The field is evolving dynamically, and various auditory evoked potentials wax and wane in popularity. Indeed, there is an unfortunate

tendency among clinicians and researchers alike to become absorbed with a particular tool, such as the auditory brainstem response, to the detriment of a broad-minded approach to the key question: what techniques will obtain the desired results in the particular patient? In fact, no single auditory evoked potential is always best, and electric response audiometry must be viewed as an integrated testing scheme which should take account of the goals and exigencies of the individual patient.

Many aspects of electric response audiometry are imperfectly understood, and both research and clinical experience are accumulating rapidly. The field is broad, both in clinical application and in terms of its base within several disparate areas of knowledge. Therefore, it is essential that the clinician should grasp the underlying technical principles and should appreciate the roles, strengths and weaknesses of several techniques. Here, a cookbook approach is inappropriate. This chapter contains a brief review, with emphasis on rationale and comparative merits of procedures.

A brief history of auditory evoked potentials

The history of auditory evoked potentials has been well-reviewed by Davis (1976), the father of the field. Developments in auditory electrophysiology and electroencephalography converged in a report of human scalp auditory evoked potentials to single sounds (Davis, 1939), but despite many microelectrode studies of electrical activity in the cochlea and auditory nerve (Davis, Fernandez and McAuliffe, 1950), there was little systematic study of scalp auditory evoked potentials until the development of the electronic averager (Dawson, 1954). This device extracts the minute auditory evoked potentials from the much larger spontaneous EEG activity, by summating responses to many stimuli.

The averaging computer precipitated massive research into averaged evoked potentials elicited by many modalities of stimuli (for example auditory, visual, somatosensory), which continues to this day. The 1960s saw rapid and diverse development. Geisler (1960) described click-evoked average auditory evoked potentials from the human scalp, and a Toronto symposium on the deaf child yielded a major report on the audiometric application of scalp auditory evoked potentials arising from the cerebral cortex (Davis, 1965). Ruben (1967), Sohmer and Feinmesser (1967), Yoshie, Ohashi and Suzuki (1967), Aran and LeBert (1968), and many others applied averaging to the potentials of the cochlea and auditory nerve, and introduced electrocochleography (ECochG) as a clinical tool. Others explored audiometric uses of responses from higher parts of the auditory system (Rapin and Graziani, 1967; Mendel and Goldstein, 1969), and the first reports appeared of long-latency evoked potentials related to cognitive processes such as expectancy and decision-making (Walter, Cooper and Aldridge, 1964; Sutton, Braren and Zubin, 1965).

A landmark of the 1970s was the definitive description of the auditory brainstem response (ABR) by Jewett and Williston (1971); the curious and instructive history of the discovery of the auditory brainstem response has been reviewed by Jewett (1983). Audiometric applications were described by Hecox and Galambos (1974), and applications to acoustic tumour diagnosis were reported by Selters and Brackmann (1977). In recent years, the auditory brainstem response has achieved prominence as a tool for audiometric assessment of infants (Fria, 1980; Galambos, Hicks and Wilson, 1984), and many neurological applications have emerged (Fria, 1980; Stockard, Stockard and Sharbrough, 1980). A comprehensive description of the auditory brainstem response and its clinical applications is given by Jacobson (1985).

An overview of auditory evoked potentials

Recording electrodes placed in the ear or on the scalp register a summation of electric events in many active cells, and the resulting auditory evoked potentials are called 'gross' or 'compound'. The key to their development at recording sites 'remote' from their sources is *synchrony* of the many elementary events, which must have timing such that they can summate constructively at the recording site.

There are numerous gross auditory evoked potentials arising from many parts of the auditory pathway from the cochlea to the cerebral cortex. There have been various attempts to classify these potentials into distinct groups (Davis, 1976; Picton and Fitzgerald, 1983; Davis and Owen, 1985), and while there is no particularly elegant or complete classification, consideration of certain important auditory evoked potential attributes introduces some useful terminology and brings a limited degree of order. Factors of particular interest are: physiological source, relationship to the stimulus, latency, and anatomical source (*Table 7.1*).

Table 7.1 A classification of auditory evoked potentials*

Main attribute	*Subclasses*

Physiological source	Neurogenic
	    receptor potentials
	    action potentials
	    postsynaptic potentials
	Myogenic

Stimulus relationships	Exogenous
	    transient
	        onset responses
	        offset responses
	    steady-state responses
	    sustained responses
	Endogenous

Latency	First (0–1 ms) Fast (1–10 ms) Middle (10–75 ms) Slow (75–300 ms) Late (300+ ms)
Anatomical source	Cochlea Cochlear nerve Auditory brainstem pathways Cerebral cortex

* Attempts at auditory evoked potential classification are merely guidelines. The reader should assess carefully the differences between various proposals, for example the above, Davis (1976), Picton and Fitzgerald (1983), Davis and Owen (1985)

Physiological sources

The auditory evoked potentials of primary interest here are *neurogenic*, that is they arise from activity in neurons of the auditory pathway (*see* for example Tsuchitani, 1983). There are also *myogenic* auditory evoked potentials associated with reflex activation of scalp musculature (Picton *et al.*, 1974; Davis, 1976), which are highly variable and have little audiometric value; they may contaminate recordings of neurogenic auditory evoked potentials, but usually only at stimulus levels well above threshold. Myogenic potentials will not be discussed further. The important neurogenic potentials are of three main types: the term *receptor potentials* is often applied to electrical activity in the cochlear hair cells; *action potentials* (APs) are large, rapidly propagated all-or-none phenomena, and *postsynaptic (dendritic) potentials* (PSPs) are small, localized and graded potentials associated with synaptic transmission (Davis, 1976; Tsuchitani, 1983).

It is fairly clear that summated receptor potentials from the cochlear hair cells underlie gross cochlear auditory evoked potentials, and that the gross response of the cochlear nerve comprises summated action potentials; indeed, the latter is known as the cochlear nerve *compound action potential* (CAP). It is also clear that responses from highest parts of the auditory pathways, for example the cerebral cortex, comprise summated postsynaptic potentials (Davis, 1976). On the other hand, the relative contributions of action potentials and postsynaptic potentials to potentials from intermediate levels, such as the auditory brainstem response, is still a matter of debate (Picton, Stapells and Campbell, 1981; Buchwald, 1983; Moller and Jannetta, 1985). In the author's view, it is probable that action potentials are the main source of brainstem responses, but it is possible that postsynaptic potentials also contribute and their relative importance may depend upon the stimulation and recording conditions.

Stimulus relationships

Neurogenic auditory evoked potentials can be differentiated by how strongly their properties (shape, size, etc.) depend upon physical parameters of the stimulus, such as its frequency, intensity, duration, repetition rate. Any auditory evoked potential which depends primarily on the physical stimulus is *exogenous,* and those from the auditory periphery tend to be of this type. Any auditory evoked potential which is strongly dependent on cognitive function is *endogenous,* and these arise from the highest parts of the auditory pathway. Also known as 'cognitive' or 'perceptual' responses (Callaway, 1975; Picton and Stuss, 1980), they reflect functions such as anticipation of a stimulus or attribution of meaning to it. The very subtlety of endogenous auditory evoked potentials leads to dependency on patient cooperation and to high variability, which limit their audiometric application, especially in children.

Exogenous auditory evoked potentials are most important for audiometry. The major types of exogenous auditory evoked potential are *transient, steady-state* and *sustained* responses. Transient auditory evoked potentials are associated with certain epochs of the stimulus, especially its beginning (*onset* responses). The steady-state responses are essentially transient responses elicited in such rapid succession that they overlap to form a quasi-continuous response waveform. Sustained responses are quite different, in that they are generated throughout the entire duration of the stimulus, even if it is very long.

Latency

This term refers to the interval between a response feature (for example a waveform peak or trough) and a reference point on the stimulus (usually its onset). Latency is a very important quantitative response parameter for transient responses, and gross latency categories can be used to classify both transient and sustained responses. Some common latency-based categories are indicated in *Table 7.1.* The ranges shown are only guidelines, being 'typical' for a normal adult. The actual latency of any auditory evoked potential may vary greatly, depending on many aspects of the stimulus, the recording conditions, and the patient.

Anatomical sources

The anatomical origins of many auditory evoked potentials are uncertain, but when there is reasonable evidence, the site name is used, for example in such terms as cochlear microphonic potential (CM), cochlear summating potential (SP), auditory brainstem response, cortical response, etc. Many of these terms are imprecise; for example, the auditory brainstem response includes components (waves I and probably II) which do not come from the brainstem, and the term 'cortical response' is insufficient because there are many auditory evoked potentials of presumed cortical origin. In general, it is simplistic to expect a one-to-one correspondence between auditory evoked potentials and specific anatomical sites. The various component waves of any auditory evoked potential may have different sources, and the complexity of the ascending auditory pathway is such that even a single auditory evoked potential wave may have several concurrent sources, for example for the auditory brainstem response (Picton, Stapells and Campbell, 1981). The present author follows Moller and Jannetta (1985) in the opinion that the auditory brainstem response wave V has sub-collicular origin in man; the reader may have encountered a more 'classical' view that the auditory brainstem response wave V comes from the inferior colliculi,

Table 7.2 Important neurogenic auditory evoked potentials and their characteristics

Exogenous transient responses
Cochlear nerve compound action potential
    Action potentials; fast; cochlear nerve
Auditory brainstem response*
    Action potentials; fast; cochlear nerve (waves I and II), cochlear nucleus (III), superior olivary complex (IV), lateral lemniscus (V), inferior colliculus (VI and VII)*
Middle-latency response
    Postsynaptic potentials; middle; thalamus/primary auditory cortex
Slow vertex response
    Postsynaptic potentials; slow; cerebral cortex (probably primary auditory)

Exogenous steady-state responses
40 Hz middle-latency response
    Postsynaptic potentials; thalamus/primary auditory cortex

Exogenous sustained responses
Cochlear microphonic potential
    Receptor potentials (AC); first; cochlear hair cells
Cochlear summating potential
    Receptor potentials (DC); first; cochlear hair cells
Frequency-following response
    Action potentials; fast (AC); auditory brainstem pathways
Sustained cortical potential
    Postsynaptic potentials; slow (DC); cerebral cortex

Endogenous responses
P300 (P3) and the contingent negative variation
    Postsynaptic potentials; late; cerebral cortex

---

* See, for example, Moller and Jannetta (1985), regarding this recent formulation of human auditory brainstem response sources

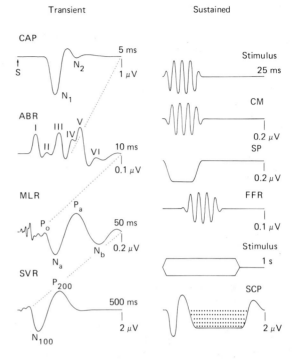

Figure 7.1 Diagrammatic examples of various auditory evoked potentials. CAP: compound action potential; ABR: auditory brainstem response; MLR: middle latency response; SVR: slow vertex response; CM: cochlear microphonic; SP: cochlear summating potential; FFR: frequency-following response; SCP: sustained cortical potential. Transient responses (left column) are as elicited by a click stimulus (S) at moderate intensity; for sustained responses (right column) the stimuli are brief tonepips (for cochlear microphonic, cochlear summating potentials and frequency-following response) or long tonebursts (for sustained cortical potential), and the stimulus waveforms are shown to emphasize the close relationship between stimulus and response. The compound action potential, cochlear microphonic and cochlear summating potential are recorded best with a transtympanic needle electrode on the middle-ear promontory; the polarity shown is promontory-negative downward. Other potentials are as recorded with a vertex-mastoid electrode derivation, with vertex positive upward. Note carefully the various amplitude and time scales.

but the weight of recent evidence leans against this.

In *Table 7.2*, some important auditory evoked potentials are listed together with attribute data along the lines developed above. It is desirable that the reader be at least aware of this diversity of auditory evoked potentials, although as will be clarified later, only a few of the available responses are widely accepted as current audiometric tools. The most useful tools are neurogenic, exogenous, and either of the transient (onset) or steady-state types.

Wave nomenclature

Figure 7.1 shows schematically some common auditory evoked potential waveforms and nomenclature. The wave labels usually reflect typical order within a latency category. Use of the symbols N (negative) or P (positive) to denote

wave polarity is superficially attractive, but has caused confusion in the past; for example, the auditory brainstem response wave V is scalp-positive, but it has been called N_4 or NV. It has also been called P_6, reflecting a typical latency of 6 ms, although its actual latency can be anything from 5 to 15 ms.

Overall, there is no entirely satisfactory and standard nomenclature; attempts to standardize usually founder. Indeed, *ad hoc* terminology and a plethora of abbreviations litter the auditory evoked potential field, whether for wave peaks, entire response complexes, or procedures based upon them. The reader must be very careful to identify precisely what is being referred to by any particular piece of jargon. Furthermore, the understanding of published waveforms can be hampered by plotting of voltages as either positive-up or positive-down, often without specification of which convention was used.

The technical basis of auditory evoked potential measurements

Overview

Some basic technical aspects are crucial and common to all procedures falling under the penumbra of electric response audiometry. The major functional components of an auditory evoked potential measurement system are shown in *Figure 7.2*. Commercial instrumentation can accommodate all the tests discussed here, merely by changing the stimulation and recording parameters.

The essential principle is straightforward. Briefly, recording electrodes monitor the random net result (electrical 'noise') of spontaneous neurogenic and myogenic electrical activity from a myriad of sources. Following delivery of a controlled acoustic stimulus, a segment of the ensuing activity (a sweep) will be the sum of the noise and evoked potentials (signal) which may be

at least an order of magnitude smaller than the noise. If many stimuli are delivered, and all the sweeps are summed (or averaged) in a computer memory, the elementary evoked potentials are superimposed and the resultant will grow in proportion to the number of sweeps, whereas partial cancellation of the random noise will occur. As the number of sweeps increases, the auditory evoked potential becomes increasingly clear.

To overcome low signal-to-noise ratio (SNR) is the dominant technical problem in auditory evoked potential measurement, and some of the steps will now be examined in a little more detail. The auditory stimulus is also crucial. More complete discussions of various technical aspects are available (Davis, 1976; Coats, 1983; Durrant, 1983; Hyde, 1985a), and only major points are covered here.

Stimulation

Most of the practice of electric response audiometry in children is directed towards estimating hearing thresholds, with testing of integrity of the central auditory pathways as a secondary matter. To estimate the pure tone audiogram, it is logical to use a stimulus which excites a very narrow frequency region of the cochlea, that is one which is *frequency-specific*. Stimuli must be repeated rapidly, to achieve the summation of sweeps, so pure tones are approximated by brief tonebursts (tonepips). Tonepips are usually described in terms of their nominal frequency and some

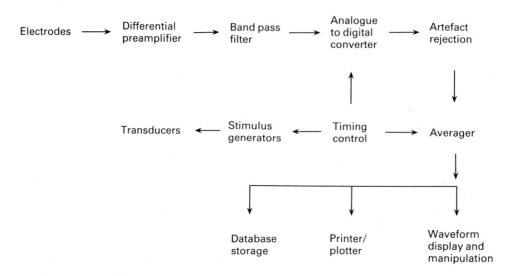

Figure 7.2 A block diagram of typical instrumentation for auditory evoked potential measurement

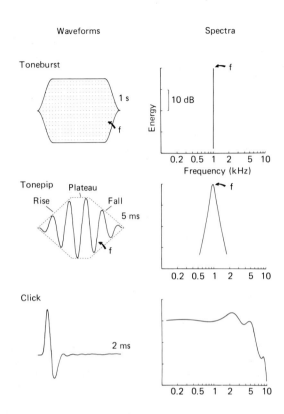

Waveforms   Spectra

Toneburst

1 s

Energy

10 dB

0.2 0.5 1 2 5 10
Frequency (kHz)

Tonepip   Plateau

Rise   Fall

5 ms

0.2 0.5 1 2 5 10

Click

2 ms

0.2 0.5 1 2 5 10

Figure 7.3 Common stimuli and their energy spectra. A very long tone, as used in conventional audiometry, has all its energy at a single frequency, so its spectrum is a line at that frequency. For brief, shaped tonebursts (tonepips), the shorter the duration and the rise/fall times, the wider the energy spread away from the nominal frequency, as dictated by Fourier analysis. The click is the briefest stimulus possible, and has energy over a very wide range of frequencies, that is, it has a wide bandwidth

parameters of their envelope. Often, the envelope is trapezoidal, with linear rise and fall, and a plateau. Some stimulus waveforms are illustrated in *Figure 7.3*.

The most appropriate choice of tonepip parameters depends upon the auditory evoked potential which is to be used, and here there is a dilemma. The more peripheral auditory evoked potentials such as the compound action potential and auditory brainstem response have latencies of only a few milliseconds, and it makes little sense to use a tonepip with duration longer than the latency of the auditory evoked potential, because all the response-generating events within the cochlea will be completed within the first few milliseconds of the stimulus. Also, stimuli with long rise times induce poorer neural synchrony than do stimuli with abrupt onset. Neural synchrony is especially important for eliciting clear responses from the more peripheral parts of the auditory pathway, for example for the compound action potential and auditory brainstem response.

Unfortunately, the use of brief stimuli with rapid onset has undesirable consequences for audiometry. Consider the spectrum of the stimulus, that is its distribution of energy over

frequency. As shown in *Figure 7.3*, the long tone with gradual onset which is the standard for conventional audiometry is carefully selected so that almost all of its energy is at a single frequency, which is the nominal frequency to be tested. The spectrum of a stimulus generated by a tuning fork has similar appearance. However, very brief stimuli with rapid onset do not have this simple 'line' spectrum; rather, there is a 'splash' or spread of energy to other frequencies, also shown in *Figure 7.3*. This increase in bandwidth for brief stimuli is explained by an area of mathematics known as Fourier analysis. The concept is introduced at this point, and some of the consequences are dealt with later.

The acoustic click stimulus, produced by exciting the headphone with a simple rectangular voltage pulse (usually of length about 100 μs) is the briefest stimulus and has the most rapid onset possible. Accordingly, it usually elicits good neural synchrony and clear transient auditory evoked potential waveforms, but it has a very wide bandwidth. The click is not a good stimulus for electric response audiometry, although the elicitation of particularly clear peripheral auditory evoked potentials is a point in its favour, and it can be used to give a rough estimate of average hearing in the region between 1 kHz and 4 kHz. It should be stressed that auditory evoked potentials of relatively rostral origin, such as the middle-latency response (MLR) or the slow vertex response (SVR), are less dependent on neural synchrony than are the compound action potential and auditory brainstem response, and can be elicited quite well with both click and fairly long tonepip stimuli.

To assess the integrity of the central auditory pathways, especially within the auditory brainstem, the general concept is that central lesions may alter the responsiveness of particular sites in the pathway, and this will manifest itself as a change in response waveform. The auditory brainstem response is particularly sensitive, and the lesion effect is usually a depression or delay of later auditory brainstem response waves. For this application, it is desirable that the auditory system be stimulated with a click, or some comparable stimulus which normally elicits excellent neural synchrony.

For eliciting exogenous auditory evoked potentials, there is usually a simple sequence of repeated stimuli which are identical or which differ only in that their polarity is alternated throughout the sequence in order to cancel electromagnetic artefacts associated with transducer excitation. This also has the effect of cancelling out the cochlear microphonic which is a polarity-dependent response. For endogenous auditory evoked potentials, the stimulus sequencing is more complex, but these responses will not be discussed further.

Lastly, in electric response audiometry the stimuli are transduced most commonly by standard headphones, and usually monaurally. Bone conduction transducers can also be used, but special care is required if very brief stimuli such as clicks are to be delivered; the frequency response of ordinary bone conductors is markedly inferior to that of headphones, so the effective stimulus may differ significantly, for the two types of transducer.

Differential recording

The recording electrodes are the 'front line' in auditory evoked potential measurement. More problems are caused by bad electrode contact than by any other technical matter, and a mechanically and electrically adequate connection to the patient is essential. Needle electrodes are rarely used, exept for measurement of the cochlear microphonic, cochlear summating or compound action potentials (electrocochleography). Transtympanic electrocochleography involves a needle electrode

through the tympanic membrane onto the middle-ear promontory (Eggermont *et al.*, 1974). For endomeatal (extratympanic) electrocochleography, the electrode is usually a silver ball in the ear canal (Coats, 1983). Other auditory evoked potentials are recorded using disc or cup electrodes on the scalp (Kriss, 1982).

The largest potentials registered are usually caused by external electromagnetic sources such as radio stations, power lines and outlets, etc., the patient and the electrodes acting as an antenna. Sometimes, it is necessary to place the patient inside an electrically shielded, grounded enclosure (a Faraday cage), but even then, there will usually be large potentials (biological noise) caused by cardiac and gross muscular activity. To focus upon signals generated in the head, it is necessary to use *differential* recording, wherein the potential at one electrode is subtracted from that at another, and then the difference is amplified by a gain between 10 000 and 50 000. Fortunately, many of the sources of interference cause similar potentials at many sites on the head, that is the noise is common to the two electrodes, so the subtraction reduces (rejects) it. This rejection is imperfect and is expressed by the common-mode rejection ratio (CMRR), the ratio of gain for activity at one input versus that for the same activity at both inputs. A typical value is 80 dB (10 000). High common-mode rejection ratio is essential for enhancement of auditory evoked potentials, and a loss of a few dB can degrade the auditory evoked potential record; common-mode rejection ratio is reduced by large or unequal electrode impedances.

Electrode position is governed by the topography of the auditory evoked potential, conceived as an evolving contour map of potentials. One electrode is placed near the site of highest potential and the other near a site of minimum potential. Cochlear and auditory nerve auditory evoked potentials are largest when recorded transtympanically, the other electrode being elsewhere on the head. The other auditory evoked potentials discussed here have broad topographies, usually with maxima at or near the scalp vertex. Thus, one electrode is placed near the vertex, and it is usually convenient to place the other on an earlobe or mastoid. This 'vertex-mastoid derivation' is the most common (Davis, 1976), although others are possible. The two electrodes form a differential pair, one being non-inverting and the other the inverting electrode. The terms 'active' and 'reference' are misleading because, often, both electrodes register part of the auditory evoked potential. A third electrode acts as a ground and is needed for correct preamplifier function.

It is important to remember that recorded auditory evoked potentials are not absolute potentials but differences. If the non-inverting electrode is at the vertex, and the inverting electrode is on the mastoid, a net positive potential at the amplifier output might be the result of excess positivity at the vertex, or excess negativity at the mastoid. For example, auditory brainstem response wave I (the compound action potential) appears to have the same polarity as the later auditory brainstem response waves, yet wave I is mainly the result of excess periauricular negativity whereas the later waves are mainly scalp-positive at the vertex (*see* for example Parker, 1981). Of course, rejection of common activity applies to the auditory evoked potential as well as the noise; if the auditory evoked potential were the same at the two electrode sites, the net result would be zero.

Filtering

Following differential amplification, filtering (filtration) of the activity is the next step in enhancing the auditory evoked potential relative to the noise.

The goal is selectively to attenuate frequency components which are rich in noise energy. Examples of filters and their effects are shown in *Figure 7.4*. The terms high-pass, low-pass, etc., are perfectly descriptive of the filter action. Bandpass and band-reject (band-stop, notch) filters can be thought of as combinations of high-pass and low-pass units. Real filters do not stop energy perfectly, but progressively, and the steepness of this 'cut-off slope' is usually expressed in multiples of 6 dB attenuation per octave (doubling) of frequency. Filtering works well if the energy spectra of the auditory evoked potential and noise are different, but often there is much overlap, so filtering usually achieves limited but important gains in auditory evoked potential clarity.

Auditory evoked potential and noise spectra differ greatly for various potentials, so a filter suitable for one auditory evoked potential may be entirely inappropriate for another. In general, the more rostral the auditory evoked potential source the slower the voltage fluctuation is over time, and in the frequency domain this constitutes a shift of

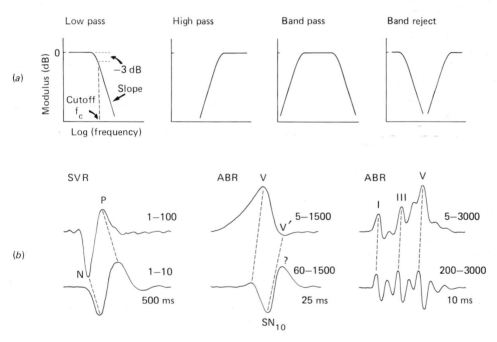

Figure 7.4 Common filters and their effects on auditory evoked potential waveforms. (*a*) Filter frequency responses (moduli). The attenuation of input signal energy varies with frequency, as shown, zero dB corresponding to no attenuation. The corner or cutoff frequencies are defined as the -3 dB points; the roll-off slopes are usually multiples of 6 dB attenuation per octave (doubling) of frequency. (*b*) In the three pairs of auditory evoked potential waveforms, the upper traces are the true, essentially unfiltered, waveforms. Filter pass-bands are indicated numerically (Hz). (1) Low pass filtering of a slow vertex response (SVR). (2) High pass filtering of an auditory brainstem response (ABR) elicited by a low-frequency, low-intensity stimulus. Only wave V is seen under these stimulus conditions; the filtering enhances the vertex-negative wave V', giving the potential known as SN_{10}. (3) High pass filtering of an auditory brainstem response elicited by a high-intensity click stimulus

the spectral maximum towards lower frequency. For example, the auditory brainstem response for a high-intensity click looks like an oscillation at about 1 kHz, and as expected, its spectrum has a maximum at about that frequency; the slow vertex response, on the other hand, usually looks like one cycle of a sinusoid at about 5 Hz, corresponding to a spectral maximum at about that frequency. Myogenic noise activity has much energy in the 50–200 Hz region, so it constitutes a low-frequency noise in an auditory brainstem response recording, but a high-frequency noise in a slow vertex response recording. The appropriate filters reflect these considerations.

Filters are often contained within the EEG amplifier. They operate on input signals that vary continuously, and are called analogue filters. An unfortunate by-product of analogue filtering is that the frequency components of the input activity are not only attenuated but also are displaced in time relative to each other. This *phase distortion (see Figure 7.4)* may alter drastically the filtered auditory evoked potential waveform, even to the extent that entirely artefactual peaks are produced (Doyle and Hyde, 1981). When the primary goal is to determine the presence or absence of an auditory evoked potential, phase distortion may be unimportant or even helpful in clarifying the auditory evoked potential. For otoneurological assessment, the precise waveform may be important, so all sources of distortion must be considered carefully.

It is possible to filter by using mathematical formulae operating on digitized activity stored in a computer memory. This digital filtering is far more powerful and flexible than analogue filtering, and can be done in such a way that phase distortion is much less of a problem. It is becoming widely available in the latest instrumentation for auditory evoked potential measurement.

Analogue to digital (A/D) conversion

The continuously variable (analogue) output of the amplifier/filter is converted electronically into a sequence of digits for computer processing, by means of rapid, periodic sampling. The A/D convertor must sample at a rate exceeding twice the highest frequency component present in the activity, to avoid distortions caused by an effect known as 'aliasing'; provided this is undertaken, there are usually no significant practical problems associated with digitization.

Summation or averaging

As introduced earlier, the next step in enhancement of auditory evoked potential is summation,

or averaging, of n digitized sweeps in a columnwise fashion, corresponding points of each sweep being added to produce a sum or average array of the same length as each sweep. Then, defining the signal-to-noise ratio as the ratio of auditory evoked potential amplitude to noise standard deviation, elementary statistics reveals that the initial signal-to-noise ratio in a single sweep is increased by a factor $\sqrt{n}$ in the resultant record. This is the case, regardless of whether the sum or average is used, although the statistical argument and the appearance of the process on the computer display screen differ slightly. *Figure 7.5* illustrates the averaging process for the auditory brainstem response.

The number of sweeps needed differs drastically for various auditory evoked potentials, depending

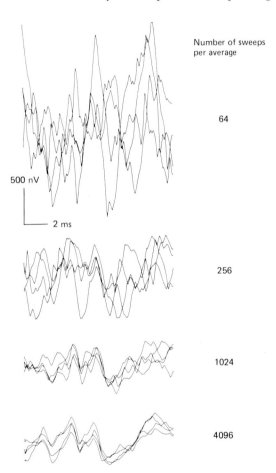

Number of sweeps per average

64

500 nV

2 ms

256

1024

4096

Figure 7.5 Extraction of the auditory evoked potential, in this case an auditory brainstem response, from spontaneous electrical noise, by averaging. The groups each contain four replicated averages, each with the number of sweeps indicated. The sweep numbers quadruple, so the signal to noise ratios double, from group to group

on the auditory evoked potential and noise size. A final signal-to-noise ratio of at least two is desirable, in the sum or average record, and it is easily shown that *n* must be at least four divided by the square of the single-sweep signal-to-noise ratio. For the auditory brainstem response for example, the initial signal-to-noise ratio might be 0.05, so *n* must be at least 1600, whereas for the slow vertex response the corresponding numbers are roughly 0.5 and 16.

There are two very important points about averaging. First, noise is *never* totally abolished: part of the sum or average record may be real auditory evoked potential, but part of it will definitely be noise. Second, averaging yields diminishing returns of signal-to-noise ratio enhancement per unit time. For example, it takes four sweeps to double the signal-to-noise ratio, 16 to double it again, 64 to double it again, and so on. Most auditory evoked potential tests consist mainly of waiting for averages to accumulate, and so averaging time is an important determinant of how much can be accomplished in a given test time. A mere doubling of the initial signal-to-noise ratio cuts the averaging time by 75%, so it is important not to regard averaging as a panacea, and to optimize the initial signal-to-noise ratio (*see* Picton, *et al.*, 1983 for a useful discussion of averaging.)

Artefact rejection

The $\sqrt{n}$ law is based on the assumption that the noise has constant properties over time, that it is *stationary*. Often, though, the activity contains large voltage transients caused by sporadic myogenic activity or by movement of the electrode/skin interface. These transients are not governed by the $\sqrt{n}$ law. For example, a transient of $200\,\mu V$ will have a size of $0.2\,\mu V$ after 1000 sweeps, which is about the size of an auditory brainstem response. These artefacts can simulate, distort, or abolish real auditory evoked potentials. A method of reducing this problem is to acquire each sweep to a temporary 'buffer', test the buffer for large values, and discard it if an artefact is found. Most commercial systems have this facility, which helps to obtain good auditory evoked potential records under poor conditions.

General principles of electric response audiometry

The basic rationale

Regardless of the auditory evoked potential used, the usual electric response audiometry test is a series of pure tone threshold estimations for various frequencies and routes of stimulation. For each frequency and route, the goal is to find the auditory evoked potential threshold, that is the lowest intensity at which the auditory evoked potential is just detectable. The curve relating stimulus level to response size is known as the intensity-amplitude function (also the amplitude-intensity function); it is one of many functions which relate a stimulus property, such as intensity, frequency, repetition rate, etc., to a response property, such as amplitude or latency. The generic term is the *input-output* (I-O) function. Particularly important here are the intensity-amplitude function, which underlies the existence of the auditory evoked potential threshold and the precision with which it can be determined, the intensity-latency function, which is helpful in determining at what place in the record the auditory evoked potential should be found, and the rate-amplitude function, which is especially influential in selection of a stimulus repetition rate which is efficient in terms of maximizing the signal-to-noise ratio gain per unit test time. Examples of these functions are given in *Figure 7.6*.

Each auditory evoked potential threshold is estimated by a bracketing method analogous to that used in conventional audiometry, involving determination of the presence or absence of response at various intensities. Several averages at several intensities are usually required to estimate a single auditory evoked potential threshold, and since each average may take several minutes to accumulate, it follows that, in general, electric response audiometry is time-consuming; every effort to optimize efficiency and to seek the most critical information is required. This is especially important when available test time is severely limited or is unpredictable, as is usually the case.

A practicable bracketing procedure will rarely yield the exact auditory evoked potential threshold. Interpolation may be required, and there will be errors in response detection decisions, so the auditory evoked potential threshold obtained is a statistical approximation of the true threshold. Also, even if the latter were known exactly, many technical and pathophysiological variables cause it to have only a *probabilistic* correspondence to the true perceptual threshold. Thus, in the individual patient, the only recourse is to statistical estimation, based on normative studies of the relationships between the two kinds of threshold. This is contingent upon the procedures and patient characteristics in the norms being applicable to the clinical case at hand. It would be unwise, for example, for an inexperienced tester to apply the normative results published by an experienced group.

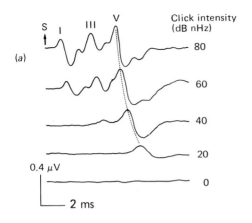

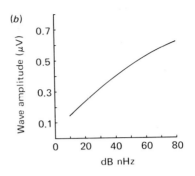

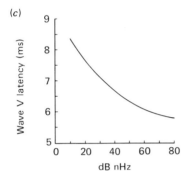

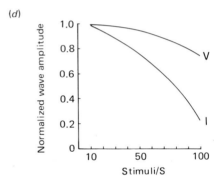

Figure 7.6 Illustrative input-output functions for the auditory brainstem response. (*a*) An intensity series, showing progressive changes of amplitude, latency and waveform. (*b*) The intensity-amplitude function for wave V. (*c*) The intensity-latency function for wave V.

(*d*) The rate-amplitude functions for wave I and V. Note that the effects of various stimulus parameters may interact; for example the intensity-amplitude function may depend upon stimulus rate or nominal frequency

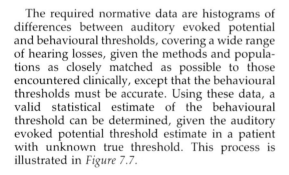

The required normative data are histograms of differences between auditory evoked potential and behavioural thresholds, covering a wide range of hearing losses, given the methods and populations as closely matched as possible to those encountered clinically, except that the behavioural thresholds must be accurate. Using these data, a valid statistical estimate of the behavioural threshold can be determined, given the auditory evoked potential threshold estimate in a patient with unknown true threshold. This process is illustrated in *Figure 7.7*.

Dimensions of electric response audiometry test performance

There are several performance criteria which underlie selection of one or more types of auditory evoked potential for use in the individual patient (Davis, 1976, 1981; Picton *et al.*, 1977). Six important factors are: validity, objectivity, accuracy, frequency-specificity, efficiency and convenience.

Validity

Any attempt to approximate a psychoacoustic measure such as the pure tone threshold by an objective phenomenon such as an auditory evoked potential has an intrinsic validity problem. The correspondence between auditory evoked potential detectability and stimulus audibility is imperfect for many reasons. The auditory system has scant functional resemblance to an EEG amplifier and averager. Neither audition nor auditory evoked potentials has a well-understood neurophysiological basis, so their relationship is analytically obscure even in the normal case, and even more so in the presence of dysfunction. In fact, auditory evoked potentials are best regarded as epiphenomena of auditory processing.

Some auditory evoked potentials, such as the auditory brainstem response, may be mediated by neural pathways which are different from, or are a subset of, those which mediate perceptual events. Also, the neural synchrony requirement for auditory evoked potentials does not apply to the

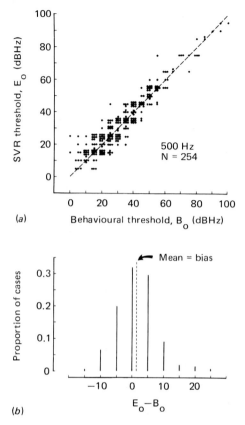

(a)

(b)

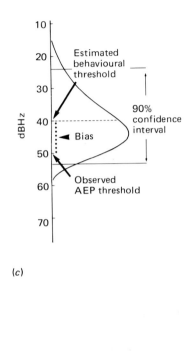

(c)

Figure 7.7 Estimation of auditory threshold using auditory evoked potential methods. (*a*) A scattergram relating auditory evoked potential and behavioural thresholds in a normative population. The data shown are for the slow vertex response at 500 Hz, for adults with various degrees of cochlear hearing loss. (*b*) The differences between the auditory evoked potential and behavioural thresholds are collapsed into a histogram; the mean difference should be called the 'bias' of the auditory evoked potential threshold. (*c*) In any patient with unknown true threshold, first the auditory evoked potential threshold (E_0) is estimated by a bracketing procedure. Then, the normative difference distribution (shown as smoothed and accentuated, for clarity) is used to estimate the true threshold (E_0 minus the bias, also accentuated) and to construct a confidence interval for it

same degree for perception. In patients with brainstem neuropathy, for example, neuronal desynchronization may abolish the auditory brainstem response yet the pure tone audiogram may be normal. As well, idiopathic absence or depression of the auditory brainstem response has been reported in children (Worthington and Peters, 1980). The thresholds of high-level auditory evoked potentials such as the middle latency response and slow vertex response appear to be less sensitive to neuropathy, partly because they are less dependent upon neural synchrony.

The situation in which the auditory evoked potential threshold is much better than the *true* behavioural threshold is rarer, but disorders located more rostrally than the generator site of the chosen auditory evoked potential may cause hearing loss without affecting the evoked potential

thresholds. An example of discrepancy between auditory evoked potential and behavioural thresholds, and of the use of more than one auditory evoked potential to localize a lesion, was reported by Ozdamar, Kraus and Curry (1982). The (adult) patient had bilateral temporal lobe lesions, severe pure tone hearing loss, normal auditory brainstem response thresholds and absent middle latency response. This situation is uncommon because most disorders causing pure tone hearing loss are peripheral to the auditory nerve, and because lesions at a high neuronal level usually do not affect pure tone thresholds drastically, unless they are bilateral and extensive.

All in all, it is prudent to consider any method of electric response audiometry to be valid only in an empirical and probabilistic sense. However, serious discrepancies between electric response audiometry and behavioural tests should not be dismissed lightly. If there is no traceable error in either procedure, the case must be monitored until the cause of divergence is revealed, or it resolves, or the behavioural data become indisputable.

Objectivity

None of the tests discussed here even requires that the patient attend to the stimulus. In a sense, however, the subjectivity is transferred to the tester, and auditory evoked potential threshold estimation can require great skill. The key decisions concern the presence or absence of auditory evoked potential, and averages are often contaminated with residual noise or artefacts. Errors by inexperienced testers can give wildly inaccurate thresholds. Interpretation is best done on-line; clues such as the trend of response development, and EEG characteristics, can improve judgements and are not apparent in the final tracings. *Post hoc* interpretation can be very unreliable, especially by the inexperienced.

Techniques which assist or replace subjective interpretation can improve the objectivity of electric response audiometry. Computer-based interpretation of auditory evoked potential records is an important goal (Beagley, 1981; Don, Elberling and Waring, 1984; Mason and Adams, 1984), but is neither straightforward nor yet widely implemented. It is easy to formulate algorithms which avoid the blatant errors committed by inexperienced testers, or which perform very well in situations for which they are entirely unnecessary, but it is difficult to imitate the performance of a skilled interpreter in a taxing situation. This area is one of active research and development.

Accuracy

From *Figure 7.7*, it is apparent that for a given true threshold, the auditory evoked potential threshold is distributed in a statistical manner over quite a large range. Reversing this view, and using the auditory evoked potential threshold as an estimator of the true (unknown) threshold, statistical theory distinguishes two components of estimation accuracy: bias and precision. Bias is the overall expected difference between a quantity and its estimates, while precision reflects random variation from estimate to estimate.

Auditory evoked potential threshold bias is approximated by the large-sample average difference between the auditory evoked potential and behavioural thresholds in the normative population, as illustrated in *Figure 7.7*. In the literature, bias has been loosely expressed as 'sensitivity', in the sense that a method with large positive bias

will tend to produce auditory evoked potential thresholds much higher (worse) than the behavioural thresholds, and is therefore 'insensitive'. One effect of large bias is that it restricts the range of hearing losses which can be estimated, because of limits on maximum stimulus levels.

For any auditory evoked potential, bias is affected by many physical and physiological factors. For example, it may vary with stimulus frequency, or differ between sleeping and awake children. Normative studies of bias must take into account the host of variables to be specified or controlled. Thus, while such data are available for many auditory evoked potentials, there is frequently a lack of consensus, attributable to variations in procedures and in test populations. For most of the auditory evoked potential procedures in common use, typical bias is within the range 5–25 dB.

While bias can be compensated by using correction factors, precision of threshold estimates is more problematic. The typical normative difference distribution has a standard deviation of about 10 dB, and skewness towards positive differences (higher auditory evoked potential thresholds). Breakdown of validity is a source of occasional large errors, but the bulk of the errors is attributable to incorrect threshold detection decisions, caused by summated noise. In general, precision is more difficult to quantify than bias; large samples are required in normative studies, to ensure that all sources of variation are represented. Published norms are of limited relevance, because their use requires emulation of all aspects of the procedures and populations to which they refer.

The history of electric response audiometry indicates that those who are experienced with a particular auditory evoked potential often report greater accuracy than that achieved by others in 'replication' studies. Comparative evaluations often appear to be based on limited experience in each of several auditory evoked potential procedures; they may produce poor results on each test and either a 'battery' is proposed or all the tests are denigrated. This pattern suggests that skill and experience are critical for accurate electric response audiometry, regardless of the auditory evoked potential. Those wishing to introduce electric response audiometry should obtain the best possible advice and training for the testers, and should develop their own substantial norms. The case load should be sufficient to maintain skills, once acquired; in routine clinical operation, testers can become complacent about their ability to judge thresholds, and occasional monitoring with blind trials on hearing-impaired subjects with reliable behavioural thresholds can have very salutary effects on test precision.

Because there are several auditory evoked potentials which might be tried, and options such as whether or not to use sedation, the accuracy of any particular procedure is influenced by the overall electric response audiometry strategy. For example, the accuracy of auditory brainstem response audiometry in the awake child depends on the point at which it is decided that the observed level of EEG noise is unacceptable, and sedation or anaesthesia must be used. The effect of these decisions is to increase the precision associated with each technique.

The auditory evoked potential threshold minus the bias gives a *point* estimate of the true threshold, but no clue as to the range within which it might reasonably be expected to lie (*interval* estimate). Confidence intervals for the true threshold can be constructed, using normative difference distributions. If electric response audiometry results routinely were to include confidence statements, there would be fewer cases of apparent conflict with other tests.

Frequency-specificity

The ideal electric response audiometry method should reproduce the pure tone audiogram accurately, whatever its shape. If frequency-specificity were poor, there would be no problem with flat audiograms, but sloping or notched audiograms will not be estimated correctly (*see* for example Davis *et al.*, 1984). For the electric response audiometry to be frequency-specific, a necessary *but not sufficient* condition is that the stimulus should be frequency-specific.

The relationship between stimulus waveform and bandwidth was introduced earlier. Because of the brevity and short rise-times of tonepips suitable for use with short-latency auditory evoked potentials, a problem with frequency-specificity is to be expected. Another concern, with these auditory evoked potentials, is that to excite low-frequency cochlear regions, the travelling wave must pass through basal regions where it may also elicit neural activity which is picked up by the recording electrode. For example, auditory brainstem response latencies for low-frequency tonepips are prolonged by high-pass filtered ipsilateral masking noise (Kileny, 1981), which suggests basal spread of cochlear excitation. This problem may be compounded in patients with cochlear hearing impairment, where the normal ability of primary neurons to respond preferentially to a very narrow range of stimulus frequencies, known as 'tuning' or 'frequency selectivity,', is often markedly degraded (Salvi *et al.*, 1983). This increases the likelihood of contribution to the auditory evoked potential from cochlear regions

other than those normally associated with the nominal stimulus frequency.

The problem of frequency-specificity is not resolved (Gorga and Worthington, 1983; Sohmer and Kinarti, 1984; Stapells *et al.*, 1985), and its severity is unclear. In the author's opinion, this matter has not yet been investigated definitively, and the cautious view is that adequate frequency-specificity cannot be guaranteed for the compound action potential and auditory brainstem response, using tonepips alone.

Cochlear excitation can be controlled using masking noise in the same ear as the click or tonepip. The principle is that masked cochlear regions will not be available to respond to the transient stimulus. The so-called 'derived response' and 'band-reject masking' methods depend on this concept. These methods have been reviewed in detail by Stapells *et al.*, (1985). In the derived-response method, the stimulus is a click in high-pass filtered masking noise; the response arises from the unmasked region of the cochlea. A second determination with lower filter cut-off frequency will yield response from a smaller region. If the auditory evoked potential contributions from various cochlear regions are linearly additive, subtraction of the second response from the first gives the derived response from the region between the cut-off frequencies. This may be the best way to achieve frequency-specificity for peripheral auditory evoked potentials, but is time-consuming.

The band-reject (notch) masking method is quicker: masking noise is filtered to remove a narrow band of energy about the frequency of interest. The stimulus must excite this unmasked region, and is usually a tonepip with frequency at the centre of the notch. This procedure limits the spread of activity, and may give adequate specificity, but extra instrumentation is needed and its use is not yet widespread. Further research is required, to clarify problems of masking spread and interactions between the masking and the stimulus.

Efficiency

The less time it takes to estimate thresholds with a specified accuracy, the better. There is a trade-off between accuracy and the number of stimulus frequencies and routes. Two important factors are the number of averages and the test time per average. For any threshold search, a progressive and generally efficient approach is to select stimulus levels which roughly bisect the current range of uncertainty about the threshold. The time per average is determined mainly by the number of stimuli and their repetition rate, and for any auditory evoked potential there is a most efficient repetition rate. The more rapid the stimulation, the less the response amplitude per stimulus, but the more sweeps can be averaged in a given time. There is an optimal compromise between these competing effects on the signal-to-noise ratio in the average record; the preferred rates differ drastically between auditory evoked potentials, generally decreasing, the more rostral the auditory evoked potential source.

Convenience

Most electric response audiometry tests involving scalp electrodes pose comparable demands in terms of test facilities, staffing and tester skills; for electrocochleography, the transtympanic electrode must be placed by a physician. The other major factor is whether or not there is a need for sedation or anaesthesia.

A comparison of selected auditory evoked potentials

Several auditory evoked potentials which are the primary candidates for objective threshold estimation will now be reviewed briefly, in the light of the performance aspects introduced above. Auditory evoked potentials not selected here, for example the frequency following response and sustained cortical potential, are used in some centres, but attention is focused upon the tools which are applied most widely, at least in the author's experience.

The reader will observe that detailed comparison of the audiometric performance of various auditory evoked potentials is quite a complicated matter, each auditory evoked potential having its own strengths and weaknesses. Much further research is needed and, unfortunately, most published comparative studies are lacking either in breadth or in terms of the optimization of technique for each auditory evoked potential to be compared.

The cochlear nerve compound action potential

This transient response can be recorded from many sites in and around the ear. It comprises wave I of the auditory brainstem response complex recorded with vertex/periauricular derivations, but is much larger using a transtympanic needle electrode resting on the bony promontory of the middle ear. Recordings from the external meatus yield intermediate amplitudes. The classic treatise on electrocochleography is

given by Eggermont *et al.* (1974), and Beagley (1981) reviewed its role in the broader context of electric response audiometry as a whole.

The usual waveform recorded endomeatally or transtympanically is a composite of the cochlear microphonic, summating and compound action potentials, although the action potential is usually the most prominent at typical stimulation rates of about 10/s. To remove the microphonic and summating potentials, a recording is made using the same stimulus at a very high repetition rate, about 100/s. Here, the compound action potential is almost zero, due to adaptation, whereas the other potentials do not adapt. Subtraction of the second waveform from the first will yield the true action potential waveform. If alternating stimulus polarity is used, the microphonic potential will not be apparent in any average, because it will cancel. To isolate the microphonic, separate averages must be accumulated for the two stimulus polarities; subtraction of one average from the other will then cancel the summating and action potentials, and reveal the microphonic potential. Thus, by these various manipulations, it is possible to separate all of the components in the composite recorded waveform.

Validity of electric response audiometry with the compound action potential is a concern as a consequence of its peripheral origins. Objectivity is relatively good with transtympanic recording, because the signal-to-noise ratio is relatively high. Bias is small and precision is good, for the same reason, except possibly for low-frequency stimuli, for which published reports are inconsistent. Another advantage of electrocochleography is that it is entirely ear-specific, whereas for all other auditory evoked potentials considered here, cross-hearing can affect the measured response waveform so contralateral masking may be required.

Frequency-specificity of the compound action potential is not firmly established for simple tonepip stimuli, and opinions vary. The derived response method is the safest approach but is time-consuming in spite of the good signal-to-noise ratio. The notch-masking method requires further validation. The efficiency of transtympanic electrocochleography is good, again as a result of the relatively high signal-to-noise ratio. Thus, averaging time is usually less than for the other auditory evoked potentials discussed here.

While most adults can tolerate the moderate discomfort of transtympanic electrode insertion with, at most, local anaesthesia, general anaesthesia is required in children (*see* for example Hutton, 1981). Infection or other problems resulting from electrode insertion are actually extremely rare, but the invasiveness of the procedure has certainly influenced its acceptance in medicolegal climates such as exist in the USA.

The V–V′ complex of the auditory brainstem response

In electric response audiometry, the concern is primarily with auditory evoked potential characteristics for tonepip stimuli close to threshold. Here, and especially for low-frequency stimuli, the appearance of the auditory brainstem response is very different from that normally illustrated (*see Figure 7.4*). The waveform loses its fine structure; the most prominent features are a vertex-positive wave V, and an ensuing negative peak, wave V′. Latencies may be as long as 10–15 ms, especially at low frequencies. Wave V′ has also been called SN_{10} (Davis and Hirsh, 1979), and it may be enhanced by using strong high-pass filters which phase-distort the wave complex (*see Figure 7.4*). In the author's view, waves V, V′ and SN_{10} can be treated as a single entity, in terms of audiometric performance.

Validity of electric response audiometry with the auditory brainstem response suffers the same caveats as for the compound action potential, perhaps more acutely because of the opportunity for response depression by even subtle disorders affecting the auditory brainstem pathways. With regard to objectivity, the auditory brainstem response is extremely susceptible to contamination by myogenic noise artefact, and under these conditions the problem of response detection is severe. This is also a serious impediment to accuracy, especially for low-frequency stimuli which elicit relatively poor neuronal synchronization. Indeed, the accuracy of auditory brainstem response audiometry is enhanced when the patient is asleep or anaesthetized. If that is undertaken, it is much improved, even at low frequencies (Davis *et al.*, 1985).

Frequency-specificity is a problem, as noted earlier. Signal-to-noise ratios are much poorer, per unit test time, than for the compound action potential, so the derived response method is totally impractical. Notch masking is viable, but requires further validation (Hyde, 1985b). Davis *et al.* (1985) considered that 'adequate' frequency-specificity is obtainable with the V-SN_{10} complex, using suitable tonepips, so the real question concerns the degree of specificity needed. This depends on the patient and the management decisions to be made. To the author's knowledge, there have been no definitive studies of the limits of auditory brainstem response frequency-specificity.

With regard to efficiency, while the V-V′ complex can be elicited at very high stimulus repetition rates, up to the bound imposed by the sweep length, this does not appear to outweigh the intrinsically poor signal-to-noise ratio and susceptibility to myogenic noise. Electric response audiometry with the auditory brainstem response is non-invasive in terms of the electrodes, but this is offset by the frequent need for sedation or general anaesthesia, to obtain adequate EEG noise characteristics.

The middle latency response or its 40 Hz variant

The middle latency response has received comparatively little attention as an audiometric tool, as a consequence of preoccupation with the auditory brainstem response and of an early misconception that the middle latency response is of myogenic origin. Certainly, it is neurogenic at stimulus levels close to threshold (*see* Mendel (1980) and Ozdamar and Kraus (1983) regarding middle latency response properties and clinical applications). With regard to validity, the middle latency response threshold is less sensitive to auditory nerve and brainstem neuropathy than is that of the auditory brainstem response, but more research is needed into effects of cortical lesions on middle latency response–pure tone threshold relationships. Subjective detection of the middle latency response is similar in difficulty to that for the auditory brainstem response, and there is comparable vulnerability to myogenic noise. Unlike the auditory brainstem response, the middle latency response is particularly clear at low stimulus frequencies, although whether this makes it a superior tool is debatable, because the middle latency response waveform is more variable across subjects than is that of the auditory brainstem response. Also, the middle latency response is more affected by sleep (Osterhammel, Shallop and Terkildsen, 1985) and anaesthesia.

The frequency-specificity of the middle latency response is almost certainly superior to that of the compound action potential and auditory brainstem response, using simple tonepip stimuli; these can have rise times and durations of up to about 10 ms and 20 ms respectively, without substantial response degradation as a result of loss of synchrony. These parameters should give adequate specificity for all but the most demanding audiometric tests.

The so-called 40 Hz middle latency response is closely related to the ordinary middle latency response. The latter is a discrete transient auditory evoked potential, whereas the 40 Hz response is a steady-state potential. The difference is not profound: whereas the regular middle latency response is recorded with sweep lengths of up to 100 ms, and repetition rates of about 10/s, the essence of the 40 Hz procedure is that the rate is increased further, so that the responses to successive stimuli overlap. The middle latency response is itself oscillatory, with an interpeak interval of about 25 ms, so if stimuli are delivered at about 40/s the response peaks may overlap and augment each other. Provided that this constructive superposition offsets the response adaptation caused by rate increase, the net effect should be a gain in efficiency and accuracy. This technique is relatively new (Galambos, Makeig and Talmachoff, 1981), and further study is required to clarify its power relative to the other methods presented here, especially in children. It appears to be an accurate tool in awake subjects, provided myogenic interference is minimal (Sammeth and Barry, 1985). The efficiency advantage over the ordinary middle latency response may be lost if the patient is asleep (Österhammel, Shallop and Terkildsen, 1985). In other respects, such as validity and frequency-specificity, one would expect no difference from the ordinary middle latency response. There is a concern, however, that for some stimulus and recording conditions, part of the 40 Hz middle latency response is, in fact, auditory brainstem response; this requires further clarification.

The slow vertex response

This response is the basis for so-called 'cortical electric response audiometry' or 'cortical audiometry', which term is to be discouraged on the grounds that it is vague: the middle latency response and many other auditory evoked potentials, such as all the cognitive auditory evoked potentials, are also of cortical origin. Because it is the most rostral of all the auditory evoked potentials considered here, the slow vertex response might be expected to have the highest validity. Certainly, in many thousands of cases, the author has not seen a case in which the true hearing levels were proven to be much worse than those indicated by the slow vertex response. Occasionally, slow vertex response threshold estimates are much worse than the volunteered thresholds, but usually there is an obvious technical cause.

Concerning objectivity, the major problem occurs when the patient's EEG contains high-amplitude rhythmic activity (θ, 5–8 Hz, and α, 9–13 Hz). These can abolish or obscure genuine slow vertex responses. Alpha rhythm is suppressed by visual attention, such as by reading, but not necessarily abolished. The extent of this problem varies greatly across subjects. Accuracy of slow vertex response audiometry is dependent on tester skill, especially in cases of strong rhythms or marginal cooperation, but given the skills and appropriate test conditions it is almost always possible to estimate the true threshold within 10 dB. Frequency-specificity is excellent, and tonebursts comparable to those of conventional audiometry may be used. Efficiency is comparable to

that of the middle latency response, the larger response being offset by the need for repetition rates no greater than one per second.

The slow vertex response is very variable during sleep, and is depressed or abolished by common anaesthetic agents. It can be used under light sedation (Davis, 1976), but this requires much skill and the current trend is towards the use of other techniques, when sedation is needed. Accurate slow vertex response audiometry is straightforward only in the passive, alert patient.

General strategy of electric response audiometry

Clearly, there are many options within electric response audiometry. The natural tendency to specialize in a single procedure is clinically suboptimal. Electric response audiometry is a scheme within which several auditory evoked potentials may be used in the individual patient. The procedure of initial choice depends primarily upon the behavioural state of the patient; this first choice may give entirely satisfactory results but if it does not, subsequent events are dictated primarily by the observed deficiencies and their probable causes. The performance aspects and response properties discussed above suggest how the scheme can be organized. The strategy suggested below is only a general guide, and many local variables may require changes

(1) If the patient is passively cooperative and alert, unusual in children, the slow vertex response is the tool of initial choice. The test should be discontinued if averages are excessively contaminated by rhythmic EEG activity.
(2) If the slow vertex response fails as a result of EEG rhythmicity, the 40 Hz middle latency response may be tried. The test should be discontinued if averages are highly contaminated by myogenic activity.
(3) If the patient is active or uncooperative, or if myogenic noise levels are very high (which they can be even in the apparently relaxed and passive patient), the slow vertex response is a possible tool, but its use demands great skill and patience. Usually, in such circumstances, sedation or general anaesthesia will be needed, for accurate audiometry.
(4) If light sedation is used, the auditory brainstem response is probably a superior tool to the middle latency response. The consistency of the auditory brainstem response waveform outweighs concerns of frequency-specificity. However, if the auditory brainstem response waveform suggests brainstem neuropathy and thresholds are abnormal, verification with the middle latency response is desirable.

(5) If general anaesthesia is used, electrocochleography is of particular value when there is no auditory brainstem response at the highest stimulus levels, or when a pattern of bilateral hearing loss renders the ear-specificity of the compound action potential crucial.

Some specific clinical applications

Neonates and infants

Early detection of hearing loss is a goal which is widely-espoused (Swigart, 1986). According to the American Academy of Pediatrics (1982), the aim is to quantify hearing loss and initiate management at or before the age of 6 months, so as to optimize communicative development. There is ample evidence that in general, current detection and management of hearing loss falls short of these goals (Ruben, 1978; Martin, 1982). It is becoming apparent that impairments which are less than moderate-severe, or are unilateral or purely conductive, may also warrant greater detection and management efforts (Ruben, 1984). Furthermore, early audiometric assessment can be an important contributor to the management of the multiply-handicapped infant (Stein and Kraus, 1985).

Behavioural screening, whether subjective or automated, is limited in sensitivity and reliability in the neonate and young infant (Jacobson and Morehouse, 1984; Durieux-Smith and Picton, 1985). Electric response audiometry is considered by many to be very useful (Galambos, Hicks and Wilson, 1984; Alberti et al., 1985; Swigart, 1986). It is impractical to screen every live birth with electric response audiometry and registers of high-risk factors for hearing loss, such as low birthweight or severe asphyxia, are helpful in selection of the population most in need of testing (American Academy of Pediatrics, 1982), although such registers have far from perfect sensitivity. Many neonates receiving intensive care are at risk for hearing loss, and in some centres, all intensive care nursery graduates are screened.

Neonatal screening with electric response audiometry during the postpartum hospital stay has the advantage of assured access to the child, assuming logistical difficulties can be overcome. Neonates spend most of their time asleep, giving excellent EEG conditions for auditory brainstem response testing, which is feasible within a few hours of birth. Auditory brainstem response screening is fairly quick and effective with click stimuli at about 40 dB (Fria, 1985), although such a screen may miss deficits at low or high frequency (Hyde, 1985b). Auditory brainstem response results may be affected by acute illness or maturational delay, and hearing losses may develop or resolve (Stockard and Stockard, 1983; Alberti et al., 1985), so neonatal electric response audiometry screening failure is not definitive but is a flag for follow-up testing.

Electric response audiometry with the auditory brainstem response is particularly useful for detailed audiometric evaluation of infants under the age of 6 months. The target group includes neonatal screening failures, babies with risk factors associated with congenital or early-onset hearing loss, and those showing delayed development. In some centres, assessment of high-risk babies is deferred until 3 or 4 months of age, mainly on the grounds that, at that time, recovery from neonatal illness, maturation, resolution and expression of hearing loss are likely to give better and more relevant results (Alberti et al., 1985). Most babies under 6 months can be tested while asleep, if proper account is taken of natural feeding and sleeping habits. Beyond the age of 6 months, natural sleep is increasingly difficult to orchestrate; these older infants can often be tested, at least crudely, while awake, but success requires much skill and patience. At some point which depends upon resources and attitudes, testing under sedation or general anaesthesia must be considered.

Efficient, progressive test protocols are of paramount importance in the sleeping infant. A click-based categorization of hearing sensitivity is appropriate as a first step. Any abnormality may lead to more accurate click threshold measurements, although there is an increasing trend towards the use of more quantifiable and frequency-specific stimuli. Click electric response audiometry can miss both low- and high-frequency losses, and the detailed audiometric contour is useful both diagnostically and for defining appropriate hearing aids.

It is desirable to exclude significant neurological abnormality which may affect the auditory brainstem response and compromise the accuracy of threshold estimates. Brainstem status may be inferred from the auditory brainstem response waveform for clicks which are well above threshold; if the interpeak latency interval between waves I and V is not prolonged, then neural conduction within the brainstem is normal and confidence in auditory brainstem response thresholds increases. Sometimes it is difficult to confirm brainstem normality because severe, high-frequency or mixed hearing losses may also affect the auditory brainstem response waveform (Stockard and Stockard, 1983; Stein, Ozdamar and Schnabel, 1981). When the auditory brainstem response is absent at the highest stimulus levels, the most probable cause is severe hearing loss; if anaesthesia is feasible, then electrocochleography may be useful because of its low bias and the absence of crossed-response problems. If, however, there is auditory brainstem response evidence of neurological abnormality, then the value of using a more peripheral auditory evoked potential is questionable, and the middle latency response is probably the last resort.

Having detected a hearing loss and excluded gross neurological disorders of the auditory brainstem, the differentiation of conductive and sensory loss by auditory brainstem response measurements is not a simple matter. Otomicroscopy can rule out gross middle-ear disease, but a normal tympanogram or absent acoustic reflexes are not sensitive or specific findings in infants under 6 months of age (Paradise, 1982). Bone conduction auditory brainstem response testing can be useful (Weber, 1983), but there are problems of large stimulus artefact, consistency of transducer coupling to the head, and restricted transducer frequency response (Schwartz and Berry, 1985). Further research is needed to validate bone-conduction electric response audiometry with the auditory brainstem response.

The wave V intensity-latency function may help to differentiate the lesion site, because the slope may be larger in recruiting sensorineural hearing loss (Stapells *et al.*, 1985). However, some cochlear deficits, especially sloping high-frequency losses, do not give this effect; also, accuracy of latency measurement is an issue, and careful attention is required to age-related latency norms. Overall, the predictive utility of slope in the individual case is questionable (Eggermont, 1982). Certainly, however, marked prolongation of wave I latency, which does not return to normal at high stimulus levels, suggests conductive pathology. Wave I is recordable at much lower sensation levels in infants than in adults, and its latency matures and stabilizes much earlier than that of wave V (Fria and Doyle, 1984).

The difficult-to-test child

This population includes children with physical, intellectual, neurological or multiple deficits, and those who are hyperactive or uncooperative. The demand for electric response audiometry is inversely related to the availability and competence of behavioural testing, but there is always a core group that defies even the most skilled behavioural testing.

The choice of initial electric response audiometry procedure depends on why the child is difficult to test. Unless the child is very uncooperative or continuously moving, slow vertex response testing should be tried. Toleration of electrodes and periods of relative inactivity are essential, and quiet play is acceptable. With the slow vertex response, entirely conventional audiometric management of stimulus conditions, transducers and contralateral masking are appropriate. If headphones are not tolerated, sound-field slow vertex response testing is perfectly feasible, but is obviously more limited in scope.

The most common cause of slow vertex response test failure in this population is low-frequency artefact, especially arising from movement of the electrode or its interface with the skin. The second most common cause is a rhythmic EEG, especially strong θ-rhythm (5–8 Hz). Proper EEG filtering (for example 24 dB/octave, bandwidth from 2 to 15 Hz) can ameliorate the first problem but not the second, and commercial units may not include adequate filters for slow vertex response testing.

It is difficult to define hard and fast rules about when the slow vertex response testing will work well and when it will not. There is a continuum of difficulty, related largely to behaviour, and the more active the child, the more skill and time are required, just as in conventional audiometry. Often, even with uncooperative or active children, there are brief periods in which the EEG conditions are favourable; making the best use of these opportunities, and making reliable response judgements with frequently insufficient data, are decidedly an art.

Even if behaviour is adequate, the slow vertex response thresholds may be difficult to judge because of rhythmic activity. In this case, the situation is unlikely to improve and an alternative method should be tried. The 40 Hz middle latency response may still be useful so long as there is not much high-frequency electromyogenic activity. On the other hand, if slow vertex response test failure is the result of excessive movement, then it is unlikely that waking-state middle latency response or auditory brainstem response testing will be successful.

It is worth noting that response to commonly used sedative agents is often unpredictable in children with neurological or behavioural disorders. Indeed, mild sedatives may even produce anomalous excitability. In addition, a complete electric response audiometry test usually requires at least one hour of satisfactory conditions, and it can be difficult to maintain adequate conditions for this length of time, under sedation. All in all, general anaesthesia merits strong consideration, and the anaesthesia need not be deep in order to give excellent conditions for auditory brainstem response audiometry.

Non-organic hearing loss

The problem of non-organic hearing loss (pseudohypacusis) has long been recognized, and the topic has been reviewed in detail recently by

Martin (1985). Of primary concern is the patient who wishes to feign or exaggerate hearing loss; more rarely, there is an attempt to conceal a genuine loss. There is no clear audiometric demarcation between deliberate exaggeration, unconscious exaggeration associated with physical or emotional disorders, and inaccuracies that arise from poor understanding of the test procedure or poor motivation. While non-organic hearing loss is particularly common in adult groups seeking material gain, as in compensation assessment for noise-induced hearing loss (*see* for example Alberti, 1981), it occurs sufficiently often in children to warrant concern. The causes may include stress of family conflict, a desire to seek attention or an attempt to explain poor scholastic performance. There may be a non-organic overlay on a genuine organic hearing loss.

There is a host of techniques to detect non-organic hearing loss, including informal clinical observations, characteristic findings on conventional audiometric tests, and an array of special tests (Alberti, 1981; Martin, 1985). While most of these techniques are orientated towards the adult patient, many can also be applied to the older child of primary concern here. Electric response audiometry is an obvious candidate procedure, and is of particular value in this population because, unlike most tests for non-organic hearing loss, it not only detects the phenomenon but also provides quantitative estimates of both the non-organic component and the true hearing levels. Another factor is that the objective nature of electric response audiometry is disconcerting for the patient, and may promote better behavioural performance. Alberti (1981) has noted the value of the technique in adults, and also that, at least in the USA, electric response audiometry has not yet achieved the widespread application that it merits. It can no longer be argued that instrumentation for electric response audiometry is particularly expensive, so the deterrent is perhaps a combination of misconceptions about the accuracy of the technique, and the fact that considerable expertise is required to achieve reliable results. The author considers electric response audiometry to be very useful indeed, in this population.

The basic rationale for the electric response audiometry scheme in a child suspected of non-organic hearing loss follows the arguments outlined earlier. The patients are often, at least superficially, cooperative so they are good candidates for slow vertex response testing, and a reliable audiogram can usually be obtained. In most cases, this will be accurate within 10 dB, for air and bone conduction between 500 Hz and 4 kHz. Indeed, patients who are exaggerating hearing loss often give remarkably clear slow vertex responses, probably because their anxiety promotes stimulus-orientated attention. This effect can be enhanced by instructing the patient to ignore the stimuli, whereupon he may promptly begin to count them.

The slow vertex response test should start at 500 Hz or 1 kHz, because at these frequencies the slow vertex response is clearest and non-organic components are often larger. If there is any difficulty in obtaining reliable slow vertex response thresholds, it pays to spend more time seeking a definitive answer for only a few stimulus conditions, rather than obtaining a complete but questionable audiogram. If the results are clear and 10 dB or more better than the behavioural thresholds, exaggeration is highly likely. If the slow vertex response results are clear and consistent with conventional results, the latter will be strongly supported. If the slow vertex response thresholds are worse than the conventional audiogram, the electric response audiometry is usually considered to be non-contributory. As noted earlier, the relationship between conventional and auditory evoked potential thresholds is one of correlation, not identity, and there are many reasons why an electric response audiometry threshold may be higher than a behavioural threshold. Thus, *concealment* of hearing loss is difficult to confirm by electric response audiometry, unless the threshold difference is large and supported by other evidence.

When the final outcome of the electric response audiometry scheme is that the thresholds are much better than those obtained earlier by behavioural means, every effort should be made to obtain plausible behavioural data which are consistent with the electric response audiometry. Usually, of course, there will be audiometric grounds for suspicion, which prompted the electric response audiometry in the first place. Often, the slow vertex response thresholds will be more consistent with conventional speech or bone conduction data, or with the clinical impression of the skilled audiologist. In general, if the slow vertex response test fails, subsequent procedures with other auditory evoked potentials are similar to those indicated earlier for the difficult-to-test child, and depend on the cause of failure.

Retrocochlear dysfunction

Auditory evoked potentials are windows onto neural function, and as such they are tools which are complementary to structural investigative methods such as conventional radiography. The use of auditory evoked potentials to detect retrocochlear disorders in adults is well established, as outlined in Volume 2, Chapter 8. The auditory brainstem response is by far the most powerful tool for disorders affecting the cochlear nerve and auditory brainstem pathways, although combinations of auditory evoked potentials can reveal lesions at higher levels. These techniques can be applied in children without substantial modification, except for the need to account for maturational factors in the very young. (*See*, for example, the text by Jacobson (1985), for comprehensive information on the auditory brainstem response and its clinical application in various populations.)

In paediatric assessment with auditory evoked potentials, while detection of neuropathy is usually secondary to estimating hearing loss, the problem of unravelling auditory and neurological aspects of the auditory evoked potential can be acute. Gross abnormalities of auditory brainstem response indicating brainstem dysfunction are not common, even in children with multiple neurological disorders, so electric response audiometry is usually helpful in this population. An example of a problematic record of auditory brainstem response is shown in *Figure 7.8*. This was obtained from a high-risk infant who suffered severe perinatal asphyxia. The record shows clear and objective evidence of neuropathy in the caudal brainstem, which helps to clarify the extent of neurological damage, but what are its implications audiometrically? It was noted earlier than an abnormal auditory brainstem response morphology casts doubt upon the validity of threshold estimates, especially when neurological disorders are suspected, and this is a very clear example.

At present, there are insufficient data to justify concrete statements, although several follow-up studies of such material are in progress. Neverthe-less, it may be useful to outline some possibilities. In spite of the absence of wave V, which may be the result of disruption of neural synchrony at about the level of the cochlear nucleus, it is feasible that the child could have normal sensitivity to pure tones. In the early years, it may be very difficult to establish this unequivocally, because other electric response audiometry tests with more rostral auditory evoked potentials may be unreliable and behavioural tests may suffer the same fate, especially if there are other neurological sequelae.

Another possibility is that there is indeed a pure tone deficit commensurate with the observed auditory brainstem response wave V threshold, but that neural recovery, plasticity and development may resolve the problem, at least in part. There is an obvious need for careful audiometric monitoring of such a child, and for integration of this information into a multi-faceted developmental assessment. A third possibility is that even if there is no pure tone deficit, or if there is one but it resolves, there may be a residual deficiency in auditory signal processing which is not necessarily apparent from basic audiometry. This could underlie subtle perceptual disorders which might manifest themselves in language delay or other developmental abnormalities. These speculations touch upon areas of obvious importance and considerable difficulty, requiring much research.

The reader will doubtless have already inferred, correctly, that a record such as that shown in *Figure 7.8* is basically useless audiometrically, except that it indicates the need for close monitoring. It should be noted that any devotee of electrocochleography would probably obtain

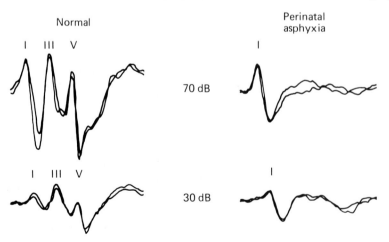

Figure 7.8 The effect of brainstem dysfunction on the auditory brainstem response. On the left, normal waveforms are shown. On the right are the records from a 4-month old infant who had suffered severe perinatal asphyxia. Wave I is remarkably clear at low click intensities, but subsequent waves are essentially absent; the same pattern is seen at higher intensities. In such a case, neuropathy of the caudal brainstem is confirmed, but audiometric inference is extremely difficult

normal compound action potential thresholds in such a patient, wave I being clear at low intensities even in the auditory brainstem response record.

More generally, at present there is little quantitative information concerning auditory evoked potential correlates of so-called central auditory disorders in children, although it is an area of active investigation. Given the current, undoubtedly crude, methods of measuring auditory evoked potentials, only the auditory brainstem response has demonstrably marked sensitivity to neuronal dysfunction; many central lesions may have a higher locus in the auditory system, and for these, the sensitivity of present-day middle latency response and slow vertex response analysis technique is limited. Also, it is quite possible that some so-called 'central' disorders actually have their origins in subtle cochlear dysfunctions which are not revealed by present behavioural or auditory evoked potential measures.

Summary

Electric response audiometry is certainly a major advance in audiological technique, and has matured to the point of unquestionable clinical utility in a wide variety of patients, both child and adult. Electric response audiometry should be viewed as a scheme of related procedures which must be adapted flexibly to the needs and exigencies in the individual patient. Electrophysiological and behavioural testing are not in competition; rather, they are complementary tools in the overall assessment, and their relative roles and utility depend strongly upon expertise and facilities in each domain.

Instrumentation for electric response audiometry is not prohibitively costly, but the need for adequate tester training, case load and performance monitoring is emphasized; failure to recognize this can lead to results which are worse than useless clinically, and has contributed in the past to gross misconceptions about the accuracy and clinical value of electric response audiometry. Given adequate facilities, skill and strategy, there are now few patients in which audiometric uncertainty need be tolerated.

Much further research into electric response audiometry is needed. In particular, computer-based automatic test control and interpretive decision support will help to improve accuracy and efficiency, and to reduce the dependency on individual skills. Except for the slow vertex response, frequency-specificity in particular requires further study, and all techniques require further optimization and assessment of their comparative performance and relative roles.

While electric response audiometry is an established tool for pursuit of the pure tone audiogram, that goal is a restricted one. More subtle indices of auditory performance and its development are required, an important example being cochlear frequency-selectivity. In children especially, for whom difficult psychoacoustic tasks are largely impracticable, auditory evoked potentials are likely to be a major tool in such a thrust. It is also likely that present methods of auditory evoked potential recording and analysis can be refined substantially, permitting improved audiological and neurological inference, as well as better understanding of their interactions.

References

ALBERTI, P. W. (1981) Non-organic hearing loss in adults. In *Audiology and Audiological Medicine*, volume 2, edited by H. A. Beagley, pp. 910–93. Oxford: Oxford University Press

ALBERTI, P. W., HYDE, M. L., RIKO, K., CORBIN, H. and FITZHARDINGE, P. M. (1985) Issues in early identification of hearing loss. *The Laryngoscope*, **95**, 373–381

AMERICAN ACADEMY OF PEDIATRICS (1982) Joint committee on infant hearing: position statement 1982. *Pediatrics*, **70**, 496–497

ARAN, J-M. and LEBERT, G. (1968) Les réponses nerveuses cochleaires chez l'homme, image du fonctionnement de l'oreille at nouveau test d'audiometrie objective. *Revue de Laryngologie, Otologie, Rhinologie (Bordeaux)*, **89**, 361–378

BEAGLEY, H. A. (1981) (Editor). Electrophysiological tests of hearing. In *Audiology and Audiological Medicine*, volume 2, pp. 781–808. Oxford: Oxford University Press

BUCHWALD, J. S. (1983) Generators. In *Bases of Auditory Brain-Stem Evoked Responses*, edited by E. J. Moore, pp. 157–196. New York: Grune and Stratton

CALLAWAY, E. C. (1975) *Brain Electrical Potentials and Individual Psychological Differences*. New York: Grune and Stratton

COATS, A. C. (1983) Instrumentation. In *Bases of Auditory Brain-Stem Evoked Responses*, edited by E. J. Moore, pp. 197–220. New York: Grune and Stratton

DAVIS, H. (1965) The young deaf child: identification and management. *Acta Oto-Laryngologica Supplementum*, **206**, 1–258

DAVIS, H. (1976) Principles of electric response audiometry. *Annals of Otology, Rhinology and Laryngology*, **85** (suppl. 28), 1–96

DAVIS, H. (1981) Electric response audiology: past, present, and future. *Ear and Hearing*, **2**, 5–8

DAVIS, H. and HIRSH, S. K. (1979) A slow brainstem response for low-frequency audiometry. *Audiology*, **18**, 445–461

DAVIS, H. and OWEN, J. (1985) Auditory evoked potentials. In *Evoked Potential Testing. Clinical Applications*, edited by J. H. Owen and H. Davis, pp. 55–108. Orlando: Grune and Stratton

DAVIS, H., FERNANDEZ, C. and McAULIFFE, D. R. (1950) The excitatory process in the cochlea. *Proceedings of the National Academy of Sciences*, **36**, 580–587

DAVIS, H., HIRSH, S. K., POPELKA, G. R. and FORMBY, C. (1984) Frequency selectivity and thresholds of brief stimuli suitable for electric response audiometry. *Audiology,* **23,** 59–74

DAVIS, H., HIRSH, S. K., TURPIN, L. L. and PEACOCK, M. E. (1985) Threshold sensitivity and frequency specificity in auditory brainstem response audiometry. *Audiology,* **24,** 54–70

DAVIS, P. A. (1939) Effects of acoustic stimuli on the waking human brain. *Journal of Neurophysiology,* **2,** 494–499

DAWSON, G. D. (1954) A summation technique for the detection of small evoked potentials. *Electroencephalography and Clinical Neurophysiology,* **6,** 65–84

DON, M., ELBERLING, C. and WARING, M. (1984) Objective detection of averaged auditory brainstem responses. *Scandinavian Audiology,* **13,** 219–228

DOYLE, D. J. and HYDE, M. L. (1981) Analogue and digital filtering of auditory brainstem potentials. *Scandinavian Audiology,* **10,** 81–89

DURIEUX-SMITH, A. and PICTON, T. W. (1985) Neonatal hearing assessment by auditory brainstem response – the Canadian experience. *Journal of Otolaryngology,* **14** (suppl. 14), 3–55

DURRANT, J. D. (1983) Fundamentals of sound generation. In *Bases of Auditory Brain-Stem Evoked Responses,* edited by E. J. Moore, pp. 15–50. New York: Grune and Stratton

EGGERMONT, J. J. (1982) The inadequacy of click-evoked auditory brainstem responses in audiological applications. *Annals of the New York Academy of Sciences,* **388,** 707–709

EGGERMONT, J. J., ODENTHAL, D. W., SCHMIDT, P. H. and SPOOR, A. (1974) Electrocochleography: basic principles and clinical application. *Acta Oto-Laryngologica Supplementum,* **316,** 1–84

FRIA, T. J. (1980) The auditory brain stem response: background and clinical applications. *Monographs in Contemporary Audiology,* **2,** 1–44

FRIA, T. J. (1985) Identification of congenital hearing loss with the auditory brainstem response. In *The Auditory Brainstem Response,* edited by J. T. Jacobson, pp. 317–336. San Diego: College-Hill Press

FRIA, T. J. and DOYLE, W. J. (1984) Maturation of the auditory brain stem response (ABR): additional perspectives. *Ear and Hearing,* **5,** 361

GALAMBOS, R., HICKS, G. E. and WILSON, M. J. (1984) The auditory brainstem response reliably predicts hearing loss in graduates of a tertiary intensive care nursery. *Ear and Hearing,* **5,** 254–260

GALAMBOS, R., MAKEIG, S. and TALMACHOFF, P. J. (1981) A 40-Hz auditory potential recorded from the human scalp. *Proceedings of the US National Academy of Science,* **78,** 2643

GEISLER, C. D. (1960) Average responses to clicks in man recorded by scalp electrodes. *Massachusetts Institute of Technology, Technical Report 380*

GORGA, M. P. and WORTHINGTON, D. W. (1983) Some issues relevant to the measurement of frequency-specific auditory brainstem responses. *Seminars in Hearing,* **4,** 353–362

HECOX, K. and GALAMBOS, R. (1974) Brain stem auditory evoked responses in human infants and adults. *Archives of Otolaryngology,* **99,** 30–33

HUTTON, J. N. (1981) Sedation and anaesthesia in audiological medicine. In *Audiology and Audiological Medicine,* volume 2, edited by H. A. Beagley, pp. 809–815. Oxford: Oxford University Press

HYDE, M. L. (1985a) Instrumentation and signal processing. In *The Auditory Brainstem Response,* edited by J. T. Jacobson, pp. 33–48. San Diego: College-Hill Press

HYDE, M. L. (1985b) Frequency-specific BERA in infants. *Journal of Otolaryngology,* **14** (suppl. 14), 19–27

JACOBSON, J. T. (1985) (Editor). *The Auditory Brainstem Response.* San Diego: College-Hill Press

JACOBSON, J. T. and HYDE, M. L. (1985) An introduction to auditory evoked potentials. In *Handbook of Clinical Audiology,* 3rd edn, edited by J. Katz, pp. 496–533. Baltimore: Williams and Wilkins

JACOBSON, J. T. and MOREHOUSE, C. R. (1984) A comparison of auditory brainstem response and behavioural screening in high risk and normal newborn infants. *Ear and Hearing,* **5,** 247

JEWETT, D. L. (1983) Introduction. In *Bases of Auditory Brain-Stem Evoked Responses,* edited by E. J. Moore, pp. xxi–xxx. New York: Grune and Stratton

JEWETT, D. L. and WILLISTON, J. S. (1971) Auditory-evoked far fields averaged from the scalp of humans. *Brain,* **94,** 681–696

KILENY, P. (1981) The frequency specificity of tone-pip evoked auditory brainstem responses. *Ear and Hearing,* **2,** 270–275

KRISS, A. (1982) Setting up an evoked potential (EP) laboratory. In *Evoked Potentials in Clinical Testing,* edited by A. M. Halliday, pp. 1–12. New York: Churchill Livingstone

MARTIN, F. N. (1985) The pseudohypacusic. In *Handbook of Clinical Audiology,* 3rd edn, edited by J. Katz, pp. 742–768. Baltimore: Williams and Wilkins

MARTIN, J. A. M. (1982) Aetiological factors relating to childhood deafness in the European Community. *Audiology,* **21,** 149–158

MASON, S. M. and ADAMS, W. (1984) An automated microcomputer based electric response audiometry system for machine scoring of auditory evoked potentials. *Clinical Physiology and Physiological Measurement,* **5,** 219–222

MENDEL, M. I. (1980) Clinical use of primary cortical responses. *Audiology,* **19,** 1–15

MENDEL, M. I. and GOLDSTEIN, R. (1969) Stability of the early components of the averaged electroencephalic response. *Journal of Speech and Hearing Research,* **12,** 351–361

MOLLER, A. R. and JANNETTA, P. J. (1985) Neural generators of the auditory brainstem response. In *The Auditory Brainstem Response,* edited by J. T. Jacobson, pp. 13–32. San Diego: College-Hill Press

OSTERHAMMEL, P. A., SHALLOP, J. K. and TERKILDSEN, K. (1985) The effect of sleep on the auditory brainstem response (ABR) and the middle latency response (MLR). *Scandinavian Audiology,* **14,** 47–50

OZDAMAR, O. and KRAUS, N. (1983) Auditory middle-latency response in humans. *Audiology,* **22,** 34–49

OZDAMAR, O., KRAUS, N. and CURRY, F. (1982) Auditory brain stem and middle latency responses in a patient with cortical deafness. *Electroencephalography and Clinical Neurophysiology,* **53,** 224–230

PARADISE, J. L. (1982) Tympanometry. *New England Journal of Medicine,* **307,** 1074–1076

PARKER, D. J. (1981) Dependence of the auditory brainstem response on electrode location. *Archives of Otolaryngology,* **107,** 367

PICTON, T. W. and FITZGERALD, P. G. (1983) A general description of the human auditory evoked potentials. In *Bases of Auditory Brain-Stem Evoked Responses,* edited by E. J. Moore, pp. 141–156. New York: Grune and Stratton

PICTON, T. W. and STUSS, D. T. (1980) The component structure of the human event-related potentials. In *Progress in Brain Research, vol. 54. Motivation, Motor and Sensory Processes of the Brain: Electrical Potentials, Behaviour and Clinical Use,* edited by H. H. Kornhuber and L. Deecke, pp. 17–49. Amsterdam: Elsevier

PICTON, T. W., HILLYARD, S., KRAUSZ, H. and GALAMBOS, R. (1974) Human auditory evoked potentials. I. Evaluation of components. *Electroencephalography and Clinical Neurophysiology,* **36,** 179–190

PICTON, T. W., LINDEN, R. D., HAMEL, G. and MARU, J. T. (1983) Aspects of averaging. *Seminars in Hearing,* **4,** 327–341

PICTON, T. W., STAPELLS, D. R. and CAMPBELL, K. B. (1981) Auditory evoked potentials from the human cochlea and brainstem. *Journal of Otolaryngology,* **10** (suppl. 9), 1–41

PICTON, T. W., WOODS, D., BARIBEAU-BROWN, B. and HEALEY, T. M. G. (1977) Evoked potential audiometry. *Journal of Otolaryngology,* **6,** 90–119

RAPIN, I. and GRAZIANI, L. J. (1967) Auditory-evoked responses in normal, brain-damaged, and deaf infants. *Neurology,* **17,** 881–894

RUBEN, R. J. (1967) Cochlear potentials as a diagnostic test in deafness. In *Sensorineural Hearing Processes and Disorders,* edited by A. B. Graham, pp. 313–337. Boston: Little, Brown

RUBEN, R. J. (1978) Delay in diagnosis. *Volta Reviews,* **80,** 201–202

RUBEN, R. J. (1984) An inquiry into the minimal amount of auditory deprivation which results in a cognitive effect in man. *Acta Oto-Laryngologica Supplementum,* **414,** 157–164

SALVI, R. J., HENDERSON, D., HAMERNIK, R. and AHROON, W. A. (1983) Neural correlates of sensorineural hearing loss. *Ear and Hearing,* **4,** 115–129

SAMMETH, C. A. and BARRY, S. J. (1985) The 40-Hz event-related potential as a measure of auditory sensitivity in normals. *Scandinavian Audiology,* **14,** 51–55

SCHWARTZ, D. M. and BERRY, G. A. (1985) Normative aspects of the ABR. In *The Auditory Brainstem Response,* edited by J. T. Jacobson, pp. 65–98. San Diego: College-Hill Press

SELTERS, W. A. and BRACKMAN, D. E. (1977) Acoustic tumor detection with brain stem electric response audiometry. *Archives of Otolaryngology,* **103,** 181–187

SOHMER, H. and FEINMESSER, M. (1967) Cochlear action potentials recorded from the external ear in man. *Annals of Otology, Rhinology and Laryngology,* **76,** 427–435

SOHMER, H. and KINARTI, R. (1984) Survey of attempts to use auditory evoked potentials to obtain an audiogram. *British Journal of Audiology,* **18,** 237–244

STAPELLS, D. R., PICTON, T. W., PEREZ-ABALO, M., READ, D. and SMITH, A. (1985) Frequency specificity in evoked potential audiometry. In *The Auditory Brainstem Response,* edited by J. T. Jacobson, pp. 147–180. San Diego: College-Hill Press

STEIN, L. K. and KRAUS, N. (1985) Auditory brainstem response measures with multiply handicapped children and adults. In *The Auditory Brainstem Response,* edited by J. T. Jacobson, pp. 337–348. San Diego: College-Hill Press

STEIN, L. K., OZDAMAR, O. and SCHNABEL, M. (1981) Auditory brainstem responses (ABR) with suspected deaf-blind children. *Ear and Hearing,* **2,** 30–40

STOCKARD, J. E. and STOCKARD, J. J. (1983) Recording and analyzing. In *Bases of Auditory Brain-Stem Evoked Responses,* edited by E. J. Moore, pp. 255–286. New York: Grune and Stratton

STOCKARD, J. J., STOCKARD, J. E. and SHARBROUGH, F. W. (1980) Brainstem auditory evoked potentials in neurology: methodology, interpretation, clinical application. In *Electrodiagnosis in Clinical Neurology,* edited by M. J. Aminoff, pp. 370–413. New York: Churchill Livingstone

SUTTON, M., BRAREN, M. and ZUBIN, J. (1965) Evoked potential correlates of stimulus uncertainty. *Science,* **150,** 1187–1188

SWIGART, E. T. (1986). (Editor). *Neonatal Hearing Screening.* San Diego: College-Hill

TSUCHITANI, C. (1983) Physiology of the auditory system. In *Bases of Auditory Brain-Stem Evoked Responses,* edited by E. J. Moore, pp. 67–108. New York: Grune and Stratton

WALTER, W. G., COOPER, R. and ALDRIDGE, V. J. (1964) Contingent negative variation: an electric sign of sensori-motor association and expectancy in the human brain. *Nature,* **203,** 380–384

WEBER, B. A. (1983) Masking and bone conduction testing in brainstem response audiometry. *Seminars in Hearing,* **4,** 343–352

WORTHINGTON, D. W. and PETERS, J. F. (1980) Quantifiable hearing and no ABR: paradox or error? *Ear and Hearing,* **1,** 281–285

YOSHIE, N., OHASHI, T. and SUZUKI, T. (1967) Non-surgical recording of auditory nerve action potentials in man. *The Laryngoscope,* **77,** 76–85

8

Impedance studies

Denzil Brooks

Evaluating auditory function in adults is normally a reasonably straightforward procedure. Except where deliberate efforts are made to deceive, or where the subject is seriously ill or mentally incapable, cooperation can be depended on even in complex and time-consuming listening tests.

With children, especially babies and infants, even passive toleration of simple test procedures cannot be presumed or relied upon. Consequently, for many years there has been a search for so-called 'objective methods' of assessing hearing and auditory status that require no voluntary involvement of the test subject.

Almost 200 years ago, changes of infant behaviour in response to sound were reported by Tiedeman (1789), whose 13-day-old son was observed to give attention to those who spoke to him and whose 'crying could be somewhat hushed by soothing speech'. Charles Darwin (1877) wrote, of his son born in 1840: 'He often started on hearing sudden sound, and blinked his eyes'. Two responses to acoustic stimulation are noted here: startle and eye-blink. Until relatively recently, detection of hearing loss in infants has depended upon such involuntary responses. These tend to be inconsistent and the differentiation of a sound-provoked response from an adventitious movement is extremely difficult even with highly skilled and adequately self-critical observers. Today the trend is to transfer the decision-making process to a microprocessor, as in the auditory response cradle (Bennett and Wade, 1980). Where there is suspicion of hearing loss, estimation of hearing level may be obtained by non-invasive, objective techniques such as electric response measurement.

However, such sophisticated evaluative methods are not really practicable in the clinical setting. Faced with a small, distressed child and a worried and perhaps equally distressed mother, what can the clinician employ for evaluating the auditory system? Traditionally there have been two basic approaches: visual examination and the use of some type of sound–response assessment. Looking at the ears has limitations; the tympanic membrane is almost opaque, and although inferences may be made about middle ear conditions, virtually nothing can be deduced about the inner ear status by direct vision down the external canal. Response to sound is subject to the limitations noted above for babies, and children up to the age of 2.5–3 years are difficult to assess accurately, even by skilled personnel.

It was probably with some such thoughts in mind that a German otologist, Dr August Lucae, investigated an alternative method of auditory examination. In 1867, he published a paper describing the use of the 'interference otoscope', a device that employed sound itself as the investigating medium. From these pioneering studies has developed the modern range of acoustic impedance measuring systems that can be found in routine use in every otolaryngology department.

Rationale of acoustic impedance/admittance measurement

Underlying Lucae's observations was the concept that the normal ear efficiently absorbs the acoustic energy falling on it and that any malfunction in the mechanical system of the middle ear would affect the efficiency of absorption. To a substantial degree, the same concept lies at the heart of the current techniques for assessing auditory function by evaluating the acoustic impedance of the ear.

The middle ear is an impedance matching device for optimizing the transfer of acoustic energy from the gaseous medium of sound transmission, air, to the much denser fluid medium of the inner ear. Without the middle ear, at least 97% of the incident energy would be reflected at the oval window. The mechanism by which the middle ear reduces this potential loss of energy is primarily by gathering sound at low pressure over the relatively large area of the tympanic membrane and transmitting it into the cochlea over a much smaller area, at higher pressure through the footplate of the stapes. The tympanic membrane has an effective area which is about 18 times that of the footplate. Furthermore, there is a beneficial lever effect due to the malleus being longer than the incus. This leverage ratio is about 1.3:1, so in total the middle ear has an amplification factor of 18 × 1.3 – approximately 23 times, equivalent to 27 dB, that is 20 log 23.

This basic view of the function of the middle ear assumes that the tympanic membrane operates as a simple piston. In fact its operation is far more complex, especially at frequencies higher than 2 kHz, since above this frequency progressively less of the membrane is coupled to the manubrium. Hence the efficiency of the middle ear system varies according to the frequency of the incident sound. It is also highly dependent on the condition of the many component parts that make up the middle ear transmission system.

An impaired middle ear will function differently from normal in relation to the sound incident upon it. If the impairment is one that causes an increase in stiffness, then the tympanic membrane will be less able to respond to the pressure changes that constitute a sound stimulus. It will, relative to a normal ear, present a greater impedance to the passage of sound to the cochlea and it will effect a lower admittance of sound. Conversely, an abnormally mobile system, for example that occurring when the incudostapedial joint is disrupted may absorb or admit proportionately more energy than a normal middle ear, although this will not be transmitted to the cochlea because of the break in the ossicular chain. Lucae hypothesized, and indeed established, that some indication of the status of the middle ear might be made by examining the manner in which the tympanic membrane admits or impedes sound falling on it.

Principles of acoustic impedance/ admittance measurement

The middle ear is a mechanical system and can, from a mechanical standpoint, be regarded as consisting of three component types: mass, elasticity and friction.

In the middle ear the major components involving mass are the ossicles, in particular the malleus and incus, with lesser contributions coming from the tympanic membrane, the suspensory ligaments of the ossicles and the stapes.

Elasticity is provided by (a) the tympanic membrane, essentially from its radial fibres, (b) the volume of gases contained in the middle ear cleft which is compressed on inward movement of the drum and rarefied by outward movement such that it always acts to restore equilibrium, (c) by the suspensory ligaments, and (d) to a lesser extent by the incudostapedial joint and the cochlear windows.

Friction is inevitable in all dynamic systems, human as well as purely mechanical. It occurs throughout the middle ear mechanism.

The three types of mechanical component react differently to an applied oscillating force such as sound. Friction or resistance is responsible for energy loss and is virtually constant regardless of the frequency of the excitation. The mass and elasticity and stiffness components do not cause the loss of energy; instead they convert motion into kinetic or potential energy depending on the phase relationship with the stimulus. At low frequencies the elasticity is dominant, at high frequencies mass dominates.

Pathologically the mass elements of the middle ear are rarely altered. The ossicles rarely change appreciably in size or weight. The tympanic membrane may become thickened, but the overall change in the mass of the middle ear system is small. The situation is very different with regard to the elasticity elements. In otosclerosis the elasticity of the stapedial footplate is effectively reduced to zero. With the stapes immobile, movement of the incus/malleus is greatly inhibited, and this inhibition of movement is transferred to the tympanic membrane. Incident sound energy is then less freely admitted into the middle ear system. Likewise, in adhesive otitis, ossicular movement is restricted by the fibrous tissue, and the capacity of the tympanic membrane to move freely is reduced; the impedance it presents to incident sound energy is increased. An opposite effect is observed when the incudostapedial linkage is severed. Under such circumstances the incus/malleus is less constrained in its movement than in the normal ear, and the tympanic membrane is therefore more compliant than normal. If the eustachian tube is functioning poorly and the gas pressure within the middle ear is below normal, the tympanic membrane will be indrawn and the fibres will be stretched so stiffening the membrane. An opposite effect occurs if, through long-standing disease, the tympanic membrane loses its radial fibres. It then becomes flaccid and abnormally compliant.

Changes in mass are rare; changes in stiffness or

elasticity are common. In order to maximize the efficiency in detecting disorders of the middle ear by examination of the system's response to acoustic stimulation, the most useful information will, therefore, be obtained by employing sounds in the low auditory frequency range.

The basic layout of an acoustic device for assessing efficiency of sound reception of the middle ear is shown in *Figure 8.1*. A low frequency tone is generated by an oscillator and, after amplification, is introduced into the ear canal.

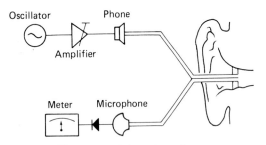

Figure 8.1 Electroacoustic impedance instrument

Here some energy will be absorbed and some reflected and, if the middle ear is efficient, the amount reflected will be low. It will be raised if the tympanic membrane is stiffened thereby presenting a greater impedance to the ingress of sound and it will be reduced below the normal level if the tympanic membrane is flaccid or hypermobile. Hence, the sound pressure level in the ear canal will depend on the impedance or admittance of the middle ear detected at the tympanic membrane. This level can be detected and measured by means of a microphone, the output from which will indicate the status of the middle ear in terms of its elasticity.

Such a simple system has a number of limitations. If the tympanic membrane is highly absorbent, the sound pressure level in the canal may be so low that other physiological noises interfere with the accurate measurement of the 'reflected' sound. If, to overcome this difficulty, the input sound level is raised, the possibility of stimulating the stapedius muscle arises. However, should this happen, the stiffness of the system will be increased and the measured status will then not represent the normal condition of that ear.

To overcome these measurement difficulties, it is now the practice to maintain the ear canal sound pressure level at a constant value high enough to avoid interference from physiological noise, but not so high as to trigger a contraction of the stapedius muscle. In such a system, the input level is closely related to the impedance/admittance of the middle ear. If the tympanic membrane is

stiffened (of itself, or in response to conditions within the middle ear), it will present a high impedance to sound. The admittance of sound into the middle ear will be low and hence, to reach the chosen sound pressure level in the ear canal, it will be necessary to provide only a small amount of amplification. The opposite will apply when the tympanic membrane is flaccid and absorbent, much more energy having to be provided by the amplifier to maintain the chosen sound pressure level in the ear canal. Thus, a direct relationship exists between the gain of the amplifier and the impedance/admittance to the middle ear measured at the tympanic membrane.

Up to this point the terms 'impedance' and 'admittance' have been employed without clear definition. Acoustic impedance refers to the inhibition of acoustic energy flow. Admittance is the reciprocal and indicates the readiness of the system, the middle ear in this situation, to allow the flow of acoustic energy. Both terms appear in the voluminous literature, often seemingly in an almost interchangeable fashion. Historically 'impedance' was the first term to gain acceptance, but 'admittance' is now becoming the accepted term, and will be used hereafter in this text.

Tympanometry – basic principles and classification

One of the functions of the eustachian tube is to maintain the pressure in the middle ear at, or very close to, atmospheric pressure. Only when the pressure is the same on both sides of the tympanic membrane will the membrane be completely free from stress and hence at its most efficient. It will then, and only then, admit the maximum amount of acoustic energy to the middle ear. If the pressure either in the middle ear or in the external meatus changes, tensions will arise in the radial fibres. The membrane will stiffen and the admittance of acoustic energy will diminish. Observations indicate that a pressure differential across a normal tympanic membrane of 0.5% of atmospheric pressure ($50\,mmH_2O$ or 50 decapascals (daPa)) will almost halve the admittance. A pressure differential of 2% is sufficient to render the tympanic membrane effectively acoustically rigid.

In the majority of modern electroacoustic impedance measuring instruments, means are provided to alter the pressure in the ear canal in a controlled and quantified manner. Tympanometry is the graphical representation of the admittance (or impedance, or compliance) of the middle ear as a function of the pressure load applied to the tympanic membrane. There is an almost infinite range of variation of shape in tympanograms, but certain patterns tend to be associated with specific middle ear conditions.

The normal middle ear produces a peaked curve that is almost symmetrical about the point of maximum admittance. A typical tympanogram obtained from a normal middle ear is shown in *Figure 8.2*. The abscissa indicates the pressure in

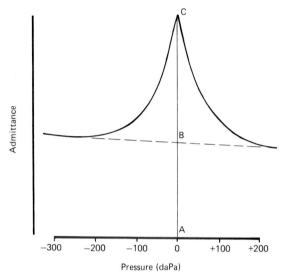

Figure 8.2 Typical normal tympanogram. 1 daPa = 1 mmH₂0

the ear canal relative to the ambient (atmospheric) pressure and the ordinate shows the magnitude of the acoustic admittance detected by the instrument at the tip of the probe which is hermetically sealed into, or at the entry to, the ear canal. Between the probe tip and the tympanic membrane is a volume of air, the magnitude of which will depend on the size of the individual's ear canal and the depth of insertion of the probe. This air has an elasticity which is directly related to its volume, and which 'adds on' to the elasticity of the middle ear. However, when the air pressure in the ear canal is more than 2% different from the pressure in the middle ear, the tympanic membrane is, as noted above, effectively rigid. The admittance of sound into the middle ear is reduced to almost zero. Under these circumstances the admittance measured by the instrument is attributable to the air in the ear canal. Its effect can be estimated in this manner and, by subtraction, the true admittance of middle ear can be derived.

Thus, from a tympanogram, one can calculate:

(1) the volume of the ear canal medial to the probe tip (A–B in *Figure 8.2*)
(2) the admittance of the middle ear, that is the difference in admittance from the stressed to

the completely unstressed condition of the tympanic membrane (B–C in *Figure 8.2*)
(3) the middle ear pressure, which is the same as the ear canal pressure for maximum admittance.

If a middle ear with otosclerosis is considered, when the pressure differential across the tympanic membrane is more than 2% the tympanic membrane is, as in a normal ear, effectively stiff and the admittance falls to almost zero. If the pressure differential is removed, the admittance rises to a maximum, but this will not be as great as for a normal ear due to the loading imposed on the tympanic membrane by the fixation of the stapes and the consequent reduced mobility of the major ossicles. The result is a smaller, shallower tympanogram (*Figure 8.3* (B)). Conversely, in an ear where the incudostapedial joint is disrupted, the tympanic membrane may be more than normally mobile. The resulting tympanogram may be higher than normal (*Figure 8.3* (C)) and a similar tympanogram may be obtained from an ear where the tympanic membrane is hypertrophic.

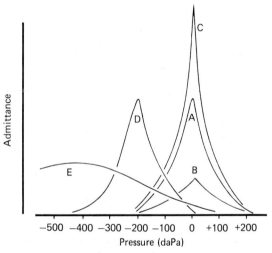

Figure 8.3 Typical tympanograms. (A) Normal; (B) otosclerosis; (C) hypermobility; (D) retracted tympanic membrane; (E) middle ear effusion

Caution needs to be exercised in drawing conclusions from the size of tympanograms. Otosclerosis tends to produce shallower curves and thinning of the tympanic membrane tends to produce deeper curves. Thus an ear in which the two conditions coexist may produce a tympanogram that is normal in size.

If the eustachian tube is underfunctioning so that the gas pressure in the middle ear falls below normal, then the tympanic membrane is stiffened.

The stress on the tympanic membrane is completely removed only when the pressure in the external ear canal is exactly equal to the pressure in the middle ear. The tympanogram for an ear with this condition has the same shape as that for a normally functioning ear except that the peak admittance is displaced in the direction of reduced pressure to a degree that indicates the reduction in pressure in the middle ear (*see Figure 8.3* (D)). In children, negative pressure in the middle ear is frequently followed by effusion. The whole of the middle ear cleft may be filled with a fluid that severely damps movement of the tympanic membrane. The tympanogram produced by an ear with effusion is typically low and flat with a maximum admittance at some degree of negative pressure (*see Figure 8.3* (E)).

When the tympanic membrane is not intact, a pressure differential cannot be created and maintained between the ear canal and the middle ear. A virtually flat tympanogram is then obtained. This can be valuable in indicating a perforation not visible to the naked eye. It can also be employed to assess the status of a ventilation tube, that is whether it is patent or blocked.

Tympanograms that vary over short periods of time can have diagnostic significance. If the variation is synchronous with respiration, the most probable cause is a patent eustachian tube. The air pressure in the middle ear then varies according to whether the subject is inhaling or exhaling: the pressure differential across the tympanic membrane similarly varies, and the admittance rises and falls in time with the breathing. A faster variation, synchronous with the pulse, is sometimes seen where there is some acute inflammation of the middle ear or tympanic membrane. More rarely it may indicate a glomus tumour (Black *et al.*, 1979).

In an effort to improve the diagnostic potential of tympanometry, Brooks (1968) quantified tympanograms using three parameters: these were *compliance* (the height of the tympanogram: equivalent to the admittance), the *middle ear pressure* indicated by the peak of the curve, and the *shape*, this being defined in terms of the 'gradient' of the tympanogram around the point of inflection. With these three measurements almost any tympanometric curve could be numerically defined and, if so desired, reconstituted graphically.

Jerger (1970) devised a different classification system that was based essentially on subjective judgement of the shape of the curve. He divided tympanograms into three basic shapes: that obtained from a normal ear was designated 'type A'. The flat curve typical of an ear loaded with effusion was designated 'type B'. The curve of normal shape, but displaced in terms of reduced pressure, was designated 'type C'. After a little experience with these limited options, it was recognized that the range of variation of tympanograms was such that further subdivision was needed. Exceptionally deep tympanograms were therefore designated as 'type A_d', and very shallow ones as 'type A_s'. The Jerger classification has been widely adopted in the USA; it has a simplicity that is superficially appealing, but it is imprecise and does not lend itself to mathematical analysis.

Middle ear muscle reflexes: basic principles

Tensor tympani muscle

The role of the tensor tympani muscle in audition is still largely conjectural, despite much research. Contraction in response to sound only occurs when the intensity is such as to cause a generalized startle reaction (Djupesland, 1965). The effect of contraction of the tensor tympani on the admittance of the middle ear is inconsistent both between and within subjects. Consequently evaluation of tensor tympani function has very limited diagnostic potential.

Stapedius muscle

Contraction of the stapedius muscle produces a stiffening of the ossicular chain observable as a decrease in the admittance of sound at the tympanic membrane. In the mid-frequency range a sound of 85 dB ($\pm$10) above the normal hearing threshold is sufficient to elicit a detectable response, and this sound level is defined as the acoustic reflex threshold (ART). Contraction can be elicited by a variety of forms of stimulation. Touching the skin close to the auricle elicits a homolateral contraction that fatigues rapidly (Djupesland, 1965). Low voltage electrical pulses applied to the ear canal also result in stapedius muscle contraction in most normal middle ears, but the stimulus tends to be at least uncomfortable and sometimes painful; hence this is not a procedure that is acceptable for the testing of children.

Acoustic stimulation has proved to be a simple, effective and acceptable method of eliciting reproducible responses from the stapedius muscle. The reflex centre is believed to be in the superior olivary complex. Afferent signals from the cochlea are assessed and, when certain conditions are met, efferent signals pass by way of the seventh nerve to the stapedius muscle to initiate a response. The conditions for emission of efferent signals in response to acoustic stimulation appear to be dominantly related to the loudness of the sound – the subjective correlate of intensity.

Klockhoff (1961) stated that a detectable stapedius reflex indicated a middle ear free from mechanical defect, that is free of conductive dysfunction. Otosclerosis, fibrosis, middle ear effusion, atelectasis, ossicular discontinuity, even quite small degrees of reduced middle ear pressure will normally stiffen the middle ear system so much that no stapedius muscle reflex can be detected. According to Jerger *et al.* (1974a) an air–bone gap of only 5 dB in the ear in which the muscle response is being observed will, in about 50% of subjects be sufficient to suppress the reflex. An air–bone gap of 10 dB reduces the likelihood of a reflex to less than 25%. However, in a very small number of middle ears, acoustically induced reflexes can be elicited even in the presence of a substantial conductive hearing loss. Subsequent observations have largely, but not entirely, confirmed Klockhoff's original statement. The situation now is that a detectable stapedius reflex indicates with a better than 95% probability that the middle ear is within normal limits.

Absence of stapedial reflex does not, however, necessarily indicate a middle ear lesion. It is possible that: the stimulus may not be adequate, the ascending tract of the eighth nerve may be impaired, there is some central lesion, the descending motor channel via the seventh nerve may be malfunctioning, or the stapedius muscle is non-functioning, a condition that appears to exist in a small percentage of otherwise completely normal individuals.

Limitations of admittance measurement

Keith (1973) tested 40 normal babies from 36 to 151 hours of age with an admittance system with a probe frequency of 220 Hz. In the ears of seven infants he observed 'W'-shaped tympanograms which are rarely seen in older individuals, and are almost invariably associated with an abnormally compliant system. It seems probable that the external canal of the infant lacks the rigidity of the more mature child or adult and consequently the acoustic characteristics of the meatal walls alter during the pressure changes employed in tympanometry. Paradise, Smith and Bluestone (1976) studied the correlation between tympanometry and otoscopy in infants. Agreement was good in older subjects, but below 7 months of age correlations were poor. Of 40 ears with effusion confirmed later by myringotomy, 24 displayed normal tympanograms. The conclusion drawn from these findings is that tympanometry on subjects under 7 months of age is of doubtful reliability.

Early studies on the acoustic stapedial reflex in infants seemed to indicate similar problems. One of the earliest published studies on admittance measurement in children (Robertson, Peterson and Lamb, 1968) was concerned with the acoustic reflex. At the age of 12 months, only three out of 10 children tested produced stapedius reflex responses to acoustic stimulation. In older children (from 18 to 36 months), stapedial reflex responses were obtained in about 70% of those tested. Bennett (1975) tested 98 babies ranging in age from 5 to 218 hours and was able to obtain acoustic stapedial reflexes from only 16%. Newman, Stream and Chesnutt (1974) reported that in many infants the stapedial reflex did not emerge until as late as age 9 weeks, a supposition receiving support from Keith and Bench (1978) who suggested that the reason for lack of reflexes in such a high proportion of neonates was immaturity of the neurological mechanism. However, Bennett and Weatherby (1980) in a study of 44 neonates aged from 10 to 169 hours indicated that absence of measurable response was more likely to be a function of the probe frequency of the admittance measuring system. Prior to this study, researchers had used a conventional admittance measuring system with a probe frequency of around 220 Hz. Bennett and Weatherby employed a detection system having a variable probe frequency. As the frequency was raised from 400 to 800 Hz, the percentage of observable reflexes increased, reaching 100% at 800 Hz. The most probable reason for the lack of acoustic reflexes at 220 Hz is, as with the 'W'-shaped tympanograms, that the middle ear of the neonate is markedly more flaccid than that of the older child or adult.

There are few other limitations to admittance measurement in children. Atresia of the external auditory meatus renders the test ineffective. Perforation of the tympanic membrane rules out tympanometry in that no pressure differential can be maintained across the membrane. For the same reason no acoustic reflexes can be detected.

Hyperactive children are difficult to test even with modern high-speed automatic recording admittance equipment. It may prove impossible to insert the probe into the ear or even hold it against the ear for the 3–4 seconds required for the instrument to gather and store the data. For such children, the acoustic reflectometer (Teele and Teele, 1984) may be appropriate, providing some basic data about middle ear status in about one-tenth of a second and without the need for airtight sealing of the probe tip into the ear canal.

Admittance measurement: evaluation of conductive disorders
General

In congenital disorders of the conductive mechanism, admittance measurement has limited value due to the gross abnormalities in the middle ear structures. Fortunately, such disorders are rare and the abnormalities, if not obvious otoscopically or physically, may often be inferred from external manifestations.

Otosclerosis, neoplasm, fibrosis and disruption of the ossicular chain occur very infrequently in children. Where they do occur, admittance measurement may add to the information gathered from the history and clinical examination.

Otitis media

Unquestionably the commonest condition affecting the middle ear system that results in a conductive dysfunction is otitis media. This may be acute or chronic: with or without perforation. The acute condition is usually seen and treated at the level of primary medical care. Perforation in children is no longer a common occurrence. But chronic otitis media with effusion (*see* Chapter 12) is a very common condition and admittance measurement has a significant role to play in the detection and treatment of this condition.

How can otitis media with effusion best be detected?

Admittance measurement appears at present to be the technique possessing the best potential for identifying children with otitis media with effusion. In 1977, a Symposium on Impedance Screening was held at Nashville, Tennessee (Harford *et al.*, 1978). A task force of 28 experts considered the state of the art and strongly encouraged the use of the technique for research studies. The majority did not advocate the immediate introduction of mass screening, partly because screening should not be introduced until adequate support services are available and partly because of uncertainties about the effectiveness of treatment and possible risks of overaggressive treatment (Black, 1985). However, even though the effectiveness of medical or surgical intervention may be in doubt, early detection is desirable in order that parents and teachers may know that a child is hearing impaired, albeit only slightly, and not lazy, inattentive or naughty. Simple remedial action can then be taken to minimize the effects of the hearing loss. A single admittance screening in schoolchildren would, however, not only identify children with chronic otitis media with effusion, but also those with transient conditions that will recover spontaneously. To overcome the otherwise excessive rate of over-referral, a two-tier screening system is desirable (Brooks, 1978). Such a scheme has been employed

and shown to be highly effective in identifying children in need of attention without causing overload of the otolaryngological services (Ferrer, 1983).

When should admittance screening be performed?

In the long-term studies on otitis media with effusion carried out by the author (Brooks, 1976), it was noted that the children who had the most persistent middle ear effusions had, in contradistinction to all the other children in the study, clear indications of otitis media with effusion at the first admittance test which was carried out within days of their entry into full-time schooling. In other words, these children already had chronic otitis media with effusion. It seems quite likely that they belong to the group of children described by Howie, Ploussard and Sloyer (1976) as 'otitis prone'. This condition appears to develop very early, certainly during the first 2 years of life. Whether screening could be effectively employed to identify 'otitis-prone' children at this early stage, and whether this would improve prognosis remains to be established. The logistic problems of such an early screening programme are certainly formidable.

Special need groups

Children with severe sensorineural hearing loss

There has been an assumption for many years that the worst possible auditory condition a child can experience is severe or profound sensorineural hearing loss, and undoubtedly this does present enormous problems to the educator and can greatly affect the quality of life of the individual.

Early identification and remediation with high quality amplification systems greatly improves the prognosis. Conversely anything that reduces the speed or effectiveness of remediation will diminish the prospects of effective habilitation. The additional hearing loss associated with otitis media with effusion is a factor that professionals involved with the severely hearing impaired have, in the past, tended to overlook.

Brooks (1974) employed admittance measurement to test 306 children who were in residential schools for the deaf in 1969. The prevalence of otitis media with effusion at age 5 was the same as in normally hearing children of the same age, that is about one child in five had otitis media with effusion on the day of test, the child otherwise appearing to be in good health. As with normal hearing children, the prevalence diminished with increasing age, but the rate at which it diminished was slower, and at age 11 approximately 7% of the children still had tympanograms that strongly suggested effusion in the middle ear. This compares with only 2% in normal hearing children of the same age.

A number of other studies (Porter, 1974; Mehta and Ehrlich, 1978; Newall and Campbell, 1978; Stool, Craig and Lord, 1980) support the finding of high prevalence of middle ear disorders in children with severe sensorineural hearing loss. Inevitably the hearing levels of children with otitis media with effusion will be further depressed. Even without any middle ear dysfunction the hearing levels of many children in such an educational setting is such that hearing aids and earmoulds are working at the very limit of performance. The added loss occasioned by otitis media with effusion is likely to diminish substantially the effectiveness of the aid, probably resulting in acoustic feedback, high levels of distortion and gross loss of performance.

Hence for children with known severe/profound hearing loss, regular monitoring with admittance measurement is advisable, and early referral for management vital (Milner, Weller and Brenman, 1985).

Down's syndrome

For all Down's syndrome patients with hearing loss, especially those with intractable middle ear dysfunction, hearing aids should be considered as a practicable and beneficial option. As Balkany *et al.* (1979) stated, retarded children use aids well and are helped by them as much or more than otherwise normal children.

Likewise, admittance testing should be a regular feature of the management of Down's syndrome children, in order that middle ear malfunctions can be identified as soon as possible and treatment provided and monitored.

Cleft palate children

According to Doyle *et al.* (1984): 'Children with cleft palate are considered to be at risk for the development of otitis media with effusion with an incidence approaching 100 per cent.' An inevitable consequence of this will be a high incidence of hearing loss, and this is confirmed by Jarvis (1976) who, in a study of 350 children with cleft palate, found that at least half the children had a hearing loss in one ear exceeding 20 dB at some time, and that 35% were likely to have a permanent defect. Bess, Schwartz and Redfield (1976) showed that admittance measurement was effective in identifying middle ear dysfunction in cleft palate children, correlating highly with otoscopy.

Others

The truly autistic child is, fortunately, rare as are children with central nervous system disorders. In such children admittance measurement can add to the diagnostic information (Petersen, 1978). It bears repeating that children with severe physical or mental disorders are not precluded thereby from the additional difficulties imposed by otitis media with effusion. Where cooperation in testing is not readily forthcoming, admittance testing will normally provide accurate, repeatable information on middle ear function with the minimum of difficulty.

Monitoring of treatment

Insertion of ventilation tubes in the tympanic membrane is the most frequent surgical procedure employed in the treatment of otitis media with effusion (Black, 1985). Postoperative tympanometry can be helpful in determining the effectiveness of the ventilation tube. In an ear with an intact tympanic membrane the compliance or admittance measurement obtained with the membrane fully stressed with either positive or negative pressure, is the volume of the ear canal. In children this is usually less than 1 ml. Only rarely will it exceed 1.5 ml. If, when testing an ear with a ventilation tube, a straight-line tympanogram is obtained with, at the same time, indications of a larger than normal volume (over 1.5 ml), then the probability is that the ventilation tube is in place and functioning as a perforation. The large volume is due to the coupling of the middle ear space to the ear canal through the ventilation tube.

If the ventilation tube is blocked and there has been recurrence of the effusion then a typical flat (type B) tympanogram will be obtained. If the ventilation tube has been extruded and the tympanic membrane has healed the tympanogram patterns will be the same as with an intact tympanic membrane.

Evaluation of eustachian tubal function

If tympanoplasty is being considered, it may be helpful to have some indication of the functional state of the eustachian tube. It is possible to apply positive pressures from the admittance instrument to the sealed ear canal and to observe at what pressure the tube is forced open to allow the passage of air into the nasopharynx. However, this is not a physiological test. The eustachian tube normally operates against a negative pressure gradient. A more realistic approach is, therefore, to reduce the pressure in the ear canal to, say,

−200 daPa (or −200 mmH$_2$0) and then ask the subject to swallow. If the tubal function is good, then with each swallow the negativity of the pressure is reduced. In perhaps four or five swallows the pressure is restored to normal atmospheric pressure.

Sometimes, although the tube opens and more air enters initially, a plateau is reached beyond which no further normalization occurs. The nearer this plateau is to atmospheric pressure, the more normal the function of the tube is likely to be.

Admittance measurement: evaluation of sensorineural disorders

Identification of sensorineural hearing loss

Norris, Stelmachowicz and Taylor (1974) studied the response of the stapedius muscle to pulsed auditory stimulation in a series of normal and sensorineurally hearing impaired children. A difference in the pattern of response between the two groups was identified. The normally hearing ears followed the modulation of the stimulus, but the stapedius muscles in the sensorineurally impaired ears tended to remain contracted in the inter-stimulus intervals. Parameters for the stimulus were suggested that would assist objectively in determining from admittance measurement of the acoustic reflex whether an ear under test was close to the normal limit for hearing, or whether there was a substantial degree of hearing loss. The test procedure did not give any finer degree of resolution of hearing loss, and so appeared to have limited applicability.

In the same year, Niemeyer and Sesterhenn (1974) demonstrated that some estimate of degree of hearing loss might be made by measuring the reflex threshold for pure tones and for broad band noise. Earlier research had shown that the threshold for band noise was lower (quieter) than the threshold for pure tones in normal hearing subjects. Niemeyer and Sesterhenn observed that, as the severity of the sensorineural hearing loss increased, the difference between the thresholds of the acoustic reflex to tones and noise diminished.

The basis for this phenomenon is thought to be related to the number of critical bands stimulated by the broad band noise. It is conjectured that, in the impaired ear, the number of bands is reduced due to the widening of the individual bands.

Jerger *et al.* (1974b) used this technique to predict hearing levels in 1043 subjects ranging in age from 3 to 91 years. No attempt was made to determine the actual hearing level in decibel terms, but hearing loss was categorized as either normal, mild to moderate, severe or profound.

Correct assignment to category was achieved in just over 60% of subjects. A one-category error was made in approximately 35% of subjects. In just over 4% of those tested a two-category error was made designating severe losses as normal or *vice versa*. Fortunately, the majority of the errors were such as to overestimate the degree of impairment – a 'safer' type of error than the reverse whereby the parents of a child with a severe loss might be falsely reassured as to the degree of hearing ability. Efforts were made to add information about the shape of the audiogram as well as the degree of loss, but these proved to be of little value.

Several other attempts have been made to assess hearing level from the acoustic reflex to tones and noise bands (Popelka, 1981). No one method stands out as being superior in its ability to predict the actual level of hearing.

In 1977, Sesterhenn and Breuninger described a new method of assessment wherein a high frequency (8000 Hz) tone was used to 'pre-activate' the stapedius muscle. The reflex-eliciting threshold for this tone is first determined and then the intensity of the tone is reduced to just below that level. A second tone of lower frequency (between 250 and 4000 Hz) is then introduced at the same time and into the same ear as the pre-activating tone.

The reflex-eliciting threshold is determined by adjusting the intensity of the low frequency tone while maintaining the intensity of the pre-activating tone at the just-subthreshold level. Under this condition of two-tone stimulation, the level of the lower tone is found to be somewhat below the intensity required to elicit a reflex when that tone is presented alone. The difference between the thresholds under the two test conditions can be related to the hearing threshold at the frequency of the lower tone. The single frequency accuracy obtained by Sesterhenn and Breuninger was such that 65–79% of the results were within 10 dB of the true threshold and 87–98% were within 20 dB. Brooks and Ghosh (1982) produced results of similar accuracy employing this technique. For the five frequency average (250–4000 Hz) 89% of results were within 10 dB of true threshold.

However, Brooks and Ghosh (1982) expressed reservations about the clinical applicability of this test. The procedure is time consuming, taking around 15 minutes per ear. The signal levels are high and may temporarily cause tinnitus. The test would not be tolerated by young children or the mentally subnormal, two of the groups for whom such a test would be most applicable. Refinements may be possible to improve the test procedures but, at present, application seems to be limited to evaluation of non-organic hearing loss.

Assessment of recruitment

Recruitment of loudness is generally regarded as indicating the probable locus of pathology in the cochlea. Dix, Hallpike and Hood (1948) suggested that patients with sensorineural hearing loss without recruitment had a retrocochlear lesion and those with recruitment had a lesion that was essentially cochlear in origin.

Thus the presence or absence of recruitment was perceived as a vital factor in the differential diagnosis of cochlear *versus* retrocochlear hearing loss. The classical test for recruitment of loudness is the alternate binaural loudness balance (ABLB) test in which a series of loudness balances is obtained between the two ears of the subject. The ABLB test depends on the willingness and ability of the patient to make the series of judgements of loudness, this often being made more difficult by the presence of diplacusis.

As early as 1952, Metz proposed the use of acoustic reflex measurements for assessing recruitment. He observed that in normal hearing subjects the threshold of the reflex for contralateral stimulation was around 85 ± 10 dB. In patients with sensorineural hearing loss the reflex could be elicited with little elevation of the intensity of the stimulus, despite the reduction of threshold sensitivity in hearing. Metz suggested that, if the difference between pure tone hearing threshold and acoustic reflex threshold was less than 60 dB, then recruitment of loudness was present.

One merit of the acoustic reflex test for recruitment as compared to the ABLB test is objectivity. The patient no longer has to make difficult loudness judgements. The reflex response is automatic and repeatable. The test is quick and easy to employ. It can also be employed in cases of bilateral hearing loss where the ABLB test may be difficult or even impossible to apply.

Time and experience have shown that the simple association of recruitment with cochlear pathology and absence of recruitment with neural pathology is invalid. There appears rather to be a continuum between the extremes. Measurement of recruitment is now seen as one of a number of tests that helps in localizing a lesion rather than as a definitive diagnostic tool.

Acoustic reflex decay

The phenomenon of tone decay has been known and investigated for upwards of 30 years. The perceived loudness of a sustained tone just above the threshold remains virtually constant over time for an individual with normal hearing. In an individual with a *retrocochlear lesion,* a tone at the same level may fade into inaudibility in seconds.

Anderson, Barr and Wedenberg (1970) reported an equivalent effect in the acoustic reflex. In an individual with normal auditory function a low frequency, 500 or 1000 Hz, stimulus tone at an intensity 10 dB above the stapedial reflex threshold will produce a contraction of the stapedius muscle that is sustained over many seconds or even minutes. In individuals with tumours of the eighth nerve they observed that the response decayed rapidly. A decay to half of the initial magnitude of contraction in 4 seconds or less was found to be strongly associated with retrocochlear pathology.

As with recruitment testing, a major benefit of this type of test, especially in children, is that it does not involve the subject in difficult decision making: it is objective. The time course of the reflex response can be recorded and the rate of decay observed.

Non-organic hearing loss

Non-organic hearing loss is a not uncommon phenomenon in children, particularly girls, between the ages of 8 and 14 (McCanna and DeLapa, 1981; Ward, 1984). Measurement of acoustic reflex thresholds may help in demonstrating a non-organic element in a presenting hearing loss. As previously noted, the acoustic reflex threshold (ART) for a normal hearing individual is 85 ± 10 dB. With increasing sensorineural hearing loss, the difference between auditory threshold and ART diminishes, but does not normally fall below 10 dB except for very severe losses.

A non-organic hearing loss may be suspected if the ART is less than 10 dB above the air conduction threshold. It is almost certainly established if the ART is at a lower intensity level than the pure tone threshold.

Hearing aid fitting

Establishing correct gain and output levels for hearing aids on infants and young children is fraught with difficulty. McCandless and Miller (1972) suggested that since the ART and loudness discomfort level for some types of acoustic stimuli – especially speech – were at approximately the same levels, the ART might be used as an objective method of indicating the upper limit of usable amplification from a hearing aid. The technique employed in this procedure is to place the subject in front of a loudspeaker (at, say, 1 metre distance) and stimulate with continuous speech at a level of approximately 70 dB. The aid is placed in the ear in which it is to be worn, complete with individual earmould and with the controls of the aid in the intended settings.

The probe of the admittance measuring system is placed in the opposite ear after verifying that there is no conductive loss and that stapedial reflexes can be elicited. The gain of the aid is then increased until the intensity peaks of the speech just begin to produce stapedial muscle contraction. If further gain is needed, then peak clipping or compression can be introduced such that the peaks of speech activity remain just at the level of reflex elicitation.

Tonisson (1975) described how the effective gain of a hearing aid could be measured from reflex data. In the first stage of testing the subject faces a loudspeaker at a distance of approximately 1 metre. The hearing aid is not worn and an admittance probe is placed in the ear opposite to the potentially aided ear. The ARTs are measured in this free-field situation for a range of frequencies spanning the amplification range of the aid. The aid is then fitted and adjusted to normal level and the measurement of the ARTs is repeated. The reduction in gain of the loudspeaker amplifier is the same as the gain *in situ* of the aid.

Unfortunately, the technique is time consuming and demanding on the subject's patience. In-the-ear pressure measurements, while not exactly indicating the insertion gain of an aid, are so much simpler to effect, especially with children, that the Tonisson method is now used only rarely.

Summary

Admittance measurement has been the most important development in audiology in the last 20 years. Used as a test battery comprising tympanometry and acoustic reflex measurements, both contra- and ipsilaterally elicited and measured, it is a source of valuable information in virtually every type of auditory disorder. It is a simple, quick procedure to employ. It is non-invasive. It is readily acceptable to the great majority of subjects from infancy to old age. The importance and value of admittance measurement in children was stated by Jerger *et al.* (1974c) as 'the single most powerful tool at our disposal in pediatric evaluation. It cannot, however, stand alone. It can be interpreted successfully only in combination with some independent assessment of sensitivity level. When this condition is met, the combination leads to a significant advance in the sophistication of pediatric audiologic assessment.'

References

ANDERSON, H., BARR, B. and WEDENBERG, E. (1970) Early diagnosis of VIII nerve tumours by acoustic reflex tests. *Acta Oto-Laryngologica Supplementum*, **263**, 232–237

BALKANY, T. J., DOWNS, M. P., JAFEK, B. W. and KRAJICEK, M. J. (1979) Hearing loss in Down's syndrome. *Clinical Pediatrics*, **18**, 116–118

BENNETT, M. J. (1975) Acoustic impedance bridge measurements with the neonate. *British Journal of Audiology*, **9**, 117–124

BENNETT, M. and WADE, K. (1978) Automated newborn screening using the auditory response cradle. In *Disorders of Auditory Function III*, edited by I. Taylor and A. Markides, pp. 59–69. London: Academic Press

BENNETT, M. J. and WEATHERBY, L. A. (1979) Multiple probe frequency acoustic reflex measurements. *Scandinavian Audiology*, **8**, 233–239

BESS, F. H., SCHWARTZ, D. M. and REDFIELD, N. P. (1976) Audiometric, impedance and otoscopic findings in children with cleft palates. *Archives of Otolaryngology*, **102**, 465–469

BLACK, N. (1985) Glue ear; the new dyslexia? *British Medical Journal*, **290**, 1963–1965

BLACK, M. J., BERGER, H., TRITT, R. A. and SCHLOSS, M. D. (1979) Impedance audiometry: its use in the diagnosis of glomus tympanicum tumors. *Journal of Otolaryngology*, **8**, 360–366

BROOKS, D. N. (1968) An objective method of detecting fluid in the middle ear. *International Audiology*, **7**, 280–286

BROOKS, D. N. (1974) Impedance bridge studies on normal hearing and hearing impaired children. *Acta Oto-rhino-laryngologica Belgica*, **28**, 140–145

BROOKS, D. N. (1976) Middle ear effusion in children. *Journal of Otolaryngology*, **5**, 453–458

BROOKS, D. N. (1978) Impedance screening for school children. State of the art. In *Impedance Screening for School Children*, edited by E. R. Harford, F. H. Bess, C. D. Bluestone, and J. O. Klein, pp. 173–180. New York: Grune & Stratton

BROOKS, D. N. and GHOSH, S. (1982) Assessment of hearing level by means of the acoustic reflex. *Ear and Hearing*, **3**, 320–324

DARWIN, C. (1877) A biographical sketch of an infant. *Mind*, **2**, 286–294

DIX, M. R., HALLPIKE, C. S. and HOOD, J. D. (1948) Observations upon the loudness recruitment phenomenon. *Proceedings of the Royal Society of Medicine*, **41**, 516–526

DJUPESLAND, G. (1965) Electromyography of the tympanic muscles in man. *International Audiology*, **4**, 34–41

DOYLE, W. J., REILLY, J. S., STOOL, S. E. and CANTEKIN, E. I. (1984) Eustachian tube function in children with unrepaired cleft palates. In *Recent Advances in Otitis Media with Effusion*, edited by D. J. Lim, C. D. Bluestone, J. O. Klein and J. D. Nelson, pp. 59–62. Philadelphia: B. C. Decker Inc.

FERRER, H. P. (1983) The use of impedance measurements in the diagnosis of serous otitis media. *International Journal of Pediatric Otorhinolaryngology*, **5**, 243–250

HARFORD, E. R., BESS, F. H., BLUESTONE, C. D. and KLEIN, J. O. (1978) (Editors) *Impedance Screening for Middle Ear Disease in Children*. New York: Grune & Stratton

HOWIE, V. M., PLOUSSARD, J. H. and SLOYER, J. (1976) Natural history of otitis media. *Annals of Otology, Rhinology and Laryngology*, Suppl. 25, 18–19

JARVIS, J. F. (1976) Audiological status of children with cleft palate. *Audiology*, **15**, 242–248

JERGER, J. F. (1970) Clinical experience with impedance audiometry. *Archives of Otolaryngology*, **92**, 311–324

JERGER, J. F., ANTHONY, L., JERGER, S. and MAULDIN, L. (1974a) Studies in impedance audiometry. III. Middle ear disorders. *Archives of Otolaryngology*, **99**, 165–171

JERGER, J., BURNEY, P., MAULDIN, L. and CRUMP, B. (1974b) Predicting hearing loss from the acoustic reflex. *Journal of Speech and Hearing Disorders*, **39**, 1–11

JERGER, S., JERGER, J., MAULDIN, L. and SEGAL, P. (1974c) Studies in impedance audiometry. II. Children less than 6 years old. *Archives of Otolaryngology*, **99**, 1–9

KEITH, R. W. (1973) Impedance audiometry with neonates. *Archives of Otolaryngology*, **97**, 465–467

KEITH, R. W. and BENCH, R. J. (1978) Stapedial reflex in neonates. *Scandinavian Audiology*, **7**, 187–191

KLOCKHOFF, I. (1961) Middle ear muscle reflexes in man. *Acta Oto-laryngologica, Supplementum*, **164**, 83

LUCAE, A. (1867) Ueber eine neue Methode zur Unterzuchung des Gehoerorgans zu physiologischen und diagnostischen Zwecken mit Huelfe des Interferenz-Otoscopes. *Archiv fur Ohren, Nasen und Kehlkopfheilkunde*, **3**, 186–225

McCANDLESS, G. A. and MILLER, D. L. (1972) Loudness discomfort in hearing aids. *National Hearing Aid Journal*, **25**, 7–32

McCANNA, D. L. and DeLAPA, G. (1981) A clinical study of twenty-seven children exhibiting functional hearing loss. *Language, Speech and Hearing Service for Schools*, **12**, 26–35

MEHTA, D. and ERLICH, M. (1978) Serous otitis media in a school for the deaf. *Volta Review*, **80**, 75–80

METZ, O. (1952) Threshold for reflex contraction of the muscles of the middle ear and recruitment of loudness. *Archives of Otolaryngology*, **55**, 536–543

MILNER, R. M., WELLER, C. R. and BRENMAN, A. K. (1985) Management of the hearing impaired child with serous otitis media. *International Journal of Pediatric Otorhinolaryngology*, **9**, 233–239

NEWALL, P. and CAMPBELL, G. B. (1978) Acoustic impedance audiometry in a school for hearing impaired children. *Journal of the British Association of Teachers of the Deaf*, **2**, 136–140

NEWMAN, R., STREAM, R. and CHESNUTT, B.(1974) Application of the Niemeyer method of predicting hearing loss in neonates. *American Speech and Hearing Association*, **16**, 564

NIEMEYER, W. and SESTERHENN, G. (1974) Calculating the hearing threshold from the stapedius reflex threshold for different sound stimuli. *Audiology*, **13**, 421–427

NORRIS, T. W., STELMACHOWICZ, P. and TAYLOR, D. (1974) Acoustic reflex relaxation to identify sensorineural hearing impairment. *Archives of Otolaryngology*, **99**, 194–197

PARADISE, J. L., SMITH, C. G. and BLUESTONE, C. D. (1976) Tympanometric detection of middle ear effusion in infants and children. *Pediatrics*, **58**, 198–210

PETERSEN, K. M. (1978) Impedance audiometry and the brain damaged child. *Developmental Medicine and Child Neurology*, **20**, 800–802

POPELKA, G. R. (1981) (Editor) *Hearing Assessment with the Acoustic Reflex*. New York: Grune & Stratton

PORTER, T. A. (1974) Otoadmittance measurements in a residential population. *American Annals of the Deaf*, **119**, 47–52

ROBERTSON, E. O., PETERSON, J. L. and LAMB, L. F. (1968) Relative impedance measurements in young children. *Archives of Otolaryngology*, **88**, 162–168

SESTERHENN, G. and BREUNINGER, H. (1977) Determination of hearing threshold for single frequencies from the acoustic reflex. *Audiology*, **16**, 201–214

STOOL, S. E., CRAIG, H. B. and LAIRD, M. A. (1980) Screening for middle ear disease in a school for the deaf. *Annals of Otology, Rhinology and Laryngology*, Suppl. 68, 172–177

TEELE, D. W. and TEELE, J. (1984) Detection of middle ear effusion by acoustic reflectometry. *Journal of Pediatrics*, **104**, 832–838

TIEDEMAN, D. (1789) Cited by M. A. Bradford. *Neonatal Auditory Testing*. Maico Audiological Library, **XIII**, 9

TONISSON, W. (1975) Measuring in-the-ear gain of hearing aids by the acoustic reflex. *Journal of Speech and Hearing Research*, **18**, 17–30

WARD, H. (1984) Non-organic hearing loss in a sample of schoolchildren in Manchester. Unpublished MSc dissertation, University of Salford

9

Management of the hearing impaired child

David A. Adams

Man is a social creature; he derives his livelihood and his pleasure from communication, through sight and hearing, with others and with his environment. Deafness will impair this communication and, if present from birth, may hinder or even prevent its development. Children born with a hearing loss – the prelingual deaf – have a much greater problem than those who acquire deafness after language development. Furthermore, children with mild or moderate degrees of hearing impairment do not usually present as many management problems as those born with a severe or profound loss.

The importance of early detection

Fisch (1983) published a fascinating review of the development and maturation of the hearing system in normal infants and in those with a hearing loss. The hearing impaired child will have difficulty with speech perception and may therefore have delayed or absent speech and language development. There is no doubt, however, that many severely hearing impaired children do learn to understand speech well in spite of the restricted function of the auditory channel. It is known that much of the information contained in speech is redundant, since it contains more information than is needed to understand the message. In a deaf child, much of this redundancy is eliminated since it is not heard, although sufficient auditory information does reach the higher centres to allow adequate speech discrimination. Fisch postulated that, for optimum development of speech and language, the auditory pathway must be stimu-

lated from a very early age to allow it and the higher centres to mature properly. The effects of auditory deprivation and poor communication ability on the child's social, psychological and educational development are well recognized (Boothroyd, 1982).

The benefits of early detection and initiation of management of deafness have been known for many years (Ewing, 1957). A survery of the countries of the European Economic Community (EEC) demonstrated that achievements in these fields are far from adequate (Martin, 1982). Only one-quarter of the children in the survey were suspected of being deaf (usually by their parents) during the first year of life. Ninety per cent of children had not been diagnosed by their first birthday and as many as 50% had still not been detected until 3 years of age. In most cases, *even after diagnosis*, there was a delay in the provision of aids, with 60% waiting up to 12 months or more.

This study also demonstrated that more than one-half of the children were unable to carry on meaningful conversation with strangers.

The importance of mild degrees of deafness, either conductive or sensorineural is not yet fully understood. Acute otitis media and secretory otitis media are common and many otologists have long lists of children waiting for the insertion of ventilation tubes. Some authors have suggested that children with recurrent or chronic middle ear problems show evidence of delayed language development and educational achievement (Hamilton, 1972; Rapin, 1979; Bergstrom, 1980). Others have advocated caution in attributing language disorders and learning disabilities to middle ear problems (Leviton, 1980; Ventry, 1980).

Present detection policies

Deafness in children is discovered in one of the following ways:

(1) the child fails a screening test of hearing
(2) the child is known to be 'at risk' of having a hearing loss
(3) parental suspicion
(4) the child fails to develop speech and language in the normal way.

Screening tests of hearing

These are discussed in full in Chapter 6. They are performed in an attempt to identify those children in need of further investigation.

At risk children

A family history of deafness, exposure of the fetus to a known pathogen, or a difficult birth increase the possibility of a child having a hearing loss. It is generally accepted that most at risk registers are incomplete for many reasons and there is doubt as to the usefulness of such a register (Parving, 1984; Riko, Hyde and Alberti, 1985).

Parental suspicion

If parents suspect their child to be deaf they are rarely wrong. Parving (1984) found that, in more than one-half of the hearing impaired children in his study group, the parents were the first to suspect the hearing loss. Parving also found a profound sense of bitterness in parents towards the health personnel who did not believe them or take their suspicions seriously.

Children who fail to develop speech

Clinicians occasionally see a child who, by the age of 2 or 3 years, has no speech or very indistinct speech. Some of these children have a hearing loss, although others have specific language disorders, emotional problems or mental retardation. There may be complex combinations of these disorders. There is also no doubt that some of these children have been missed by the earlier screening test.

Future detection policies

At present, considerable research is directed towards improving the early detection of deafness. This must use objective electrophysiological methods, since reliable behavioural responses are not usually present until 6 months of age. Techniques described include the Crib-o-gram (Simmons, McFarland and Jones, 1979), the auditory response cradle (Bennett, 1979), and auditory brainstem responses (Alberti *et al.*, 1983; Galambos, Hicks and Wilson, 1984; Durieux-Smith and Picton, 1985).

Management of the child referred for assessment

Children who fail screening tests or are otherwise suspected of having a hearing loss should be referred to an otolaryngologist or audiological physician for further assessment. The aims of this should be as follows:

(1) to determine if a hearing loss is present. Many children referred are found to have normal hearing
(2) to determine the severity of the hearing loss
(3) to decide on the type of deafness, whether conductive or sensorineural
(4) to determine, if possible, the age of onset of deafness. Prelingual deafness has more serious implications for the child
(5) to look for other relevant handicaps.

It is the author's practice to send the parents a questionnaire with the initial appointment. This asks the parents to state their main worry about the child and what they think of the child's hearing. There are sections dealing with the pregnancy, postnatal development, ear, nose and throat symptoms and family history. Questionnaires are a notoriously unreliable means of gathering information, although they do give parents forewarning of the type of questions that will be asked during the visit to the clinic.

The first part of the assessment must be spent taking a brief, relevant history about the child's hearing. The author feels that it is better to move quickly on to the audiological assessment since children become restless and anxious very quickly in unfamiliar surroundings. If necessary a full history, including family history, exposure to pathogens and speech development may be obtained later.

The diagnostic test used depends on the child's chronological and developmental age. The tests are discussed in full in Chapter 6, and include:

(1) distraction test, children 6–18 months
(2) cooperative test, children 8–30 months
(3) performance test (conditioning), children older than 30 months
(4) pure-tone audiometry.

It is usually possible with these techniques to establish reliable hearing thresholds at different frequencies. Evoked (electric) response audiometry is useful in children under the age of 6 months or in those who are handicapped and will not or cannot respond to auditory stimuli in the usual way.

All children should have impedance audiometry (tympanometry), especially if free-field tests of hearing are used since the free-field test may not detect mild conductive hearing loss. Free-field speech discrimination tests are used with children under the age of 5 years. Older children will cooperate for more sophisticated tests of speech discrimination.

The greatest number of children with hearing impairment tested in outpatient clinics have conductive deafness, usually caused by otitis media with effusion. The management of these children is discussed in Chapter 12. It is sometimes necessary to fit children with a conductive loss with hearing aids, particularly if there is a middle or outer ear problem not immediately amenable to surgical or medical treatment (Bergstrom, 1980).

Children with sensorineural hearing impairments present much greater management problems. Modern techniques including evoked response audiometry, tympanometry and radiology, make possible a reliable identification of sites of lesions and hearing thresholds (Parving, 1983, 1985). Accurate identification of hearing thresholds is particularly important when deciding which type of hearing aid to fit.

The investigation of the cause of deafness, while not having immediate implications with respect to management of the child's hearing loss, is important. Parents want to know about the risk of subsequent children being born with a hearing loss, and also the risk to future generations. This investigation involves a multidisciplinary approach.

Serological investigations

Deafness as a result of maternal rubella may be diagnosed from the history and also the presence of specific antibodies, IgM or IgG, dependent on the child's age. It must not be forgotten that rubella antibodies may be present as a result of a postnatal infection in 5–10% of children under 4 years of age.

Serological tests for cytomegalovirus, toxoplasmosis and syphilis should be routinely performed.

Other laboratory tests

The urine of children under the age of 6 months may be examined for cytomegalovirus. Renal disease is sometimes associated with sensorineural deafness. It is therefore useful to screen the urine for blood cells, protein or sugar. Congenital hypothyroidism and Pendred's syndrome are associated with hearing loss. Fisch (1981) pointed out that effective screening of neonates for congenital hypothyroidism could virtually eliminate this as a cause of deafness. A simple means of doing this would be to check the serum thyroxine, although this test is not performed routinely in most centres.

Radiology

Intracranial calcification is sometimes found on skull X-rays in children with toxoplasmosis.

Tomography and computerized tomographic (CT) scanning techniques have limited usefulness in the identification of aetiology in sensorineural deafness, but can help to localize the lesion and demonstrate structural abnormalities. Lund, Phelps and Beagley (1982) found that a combination of evoked response audiometry and tomography of the ear were useful with reference to surgical reconstruction of the middle ear.

Frazer *et al.* (1986) discussed the role of hypocycloidal tomography in assessing the suitability of patients for cochlear implants. Most of their patients had a radiologically normal cochlea, although a few had 'cochlear otosclerosis' or labyrinthitis obliterans which precluded insertion of a cochlear implant.

Electrocardiography

In some disorders, such as the rare Jervell and Lange-Nielsen syndrome, there are characteristic electrocardiographic findings with prolongation of the QT interval and abnormal T waves (Fisch, 1981). Beighton and Sellars (1982) pointed out that this investigation had only a very limited place in the assessment of deaf children.

Assessment by other specialists

Ophthalmological examination is essential in children with sensorineural deafness. The fundus changes in rubella retinopathy are characteristic and have been described as a 'pepper and salt' appearance. They may be located in the macular area or at the periphery of the fundus (Wolff, 1973). Parving (1985) stated that combined serological and ophthalmological examination is necessary for the assessment of rubella deafness.

Fisch (1981) summarized the ocular findings in Usher's, Cockaynes, Laurence-Moon-Biedl and Refsum's syndromes.

Assessment of visual acuity may also be important when considering the education and management of the hearing impaired child.

The hearing impaired child may be referred for further assessment either to a paediatrician or paediatric neurologist, especially if there is evidence of head and neck abnormalities or of delayed growth and development in any sphere.

If the hearing loss is not caused by an obvious environmental factor, it should be assumed, until proven otherwise, that it has a genetic basis. These children and the parents should be referred to a medical geneticist, although all medical personnel dealing with these children should have a working knowledge of genetically transmitted deafness. The genetic basis of deafness is discussed in Chapter 3.

Parents' reactions to the diagnosis

Much has been written about parents' responses to the diagnosis (Boothroyd, 1982; Tucker and Nolan, 1984). The impact is usually devastating and the sequence of reactions is sometimes similar to that in mourning.

Shock

This is a natural defence mechanism and protects the individual from information which he or she does not want to hear. There is a profound sense of loss – the child is handicapped and abnormal. There is very little point in giving detailed information to parents in this state. They cannot take any of it in. It is important that the parents are shown that there is a team of professional people immediately available to help and support them through this difficult time. In Belfast this is achieved by having a peripatetic teacher and a social worker with the deaf at the diagnostic clinic.

Denial

The protective effects of shock wear off. Parents question the diagnosis and produce 'evidence' that their child can hear. Some parents seek second, third, or even fourth opinions, taking the child to many different clinics in the hope that someone will say that the child's hearing is normal.

Anger

Parents sometimes ask why this disaster should have happened to them. Tucker and Nolan (1984) cited an example in which the mother blamed her husband for the child's hearing impairment. Some parents become hostile and bitter and their anger may be directed at the clinician. Patient support and willingness to listen often helps parents through this stage.

Acceptance and constructive action

Eventually the parents acknowledge the child's hearing loss and accept that the child, although handicapped, must and can be helped. This involves the parents learning about deafness and how it affects the child's development and education.

Other reactions

The author would agree with Tucker and Nolan's observation that parent adaptation does not always follow a predictable sequence of events as outlined above. Most parents do eventually adapt to the child's deafness. Some continue to deny the existence of the handicap and others remain angry and bitter.

Other parental responses are observed. Parents may have suspected for some time that the child is deaf and with the diagnosis comes a sense of relief that at last their suspicions are believed and action will be taken to help their child. There is also relief that the child does not have brain damage.

Parents of deaf children often feel isolated and inadequate. This can be lessened by immediate contact with counselling and supporting services who should provide ready access for help and information as required. Local parent support groups allow the parents of newly diagnosed children to discuss their problems with others who have been through the initial traumas. Branches of various organizations such as the Royal National Institute for the Deaf and the National Deaf Children's Society have regular educational meetings for parents, and act as a forum for exchange of information and ideas.

Tucker and Nolan (1984) discussed the theory and practice of counselling and pointed out that the counsellor's professional background is unimportant. The essential quality in any person undertaking this task is that they be knowledgeable in all aspects pertaining to the child's management. Parents come into contact with many different professionals – otologists, audiological physicians, peripatetic teachers, audiological scientists, physiological measurement technicians, social workers with the deaf, hearing therapists, speech therapists and educational psychologists. Each has expertise in some aspects of management of the hearing impaired child and often this expertise overlaps. It is important that each understands their own role and also the role of the others. Parents must be given sufficient information which is intelligible and relevant. Enright and O'Connor (1982) emphasized the importance of peripatetic teacher counselling families of pre-school children. Good relationships between teachers and parents may contribute significantly towards making more effective the educational guidance provided. This relationship allows the parents to exercise a central role in their child's progress.

Parents, unfortunately, are often given conflict-ing advice, especially about forms of education, whether oral or total communication. Some professionals have fixed ideas about which type of hearing aid is best and refuse to have anything to do with the others. Such conflicts should be avoided since they merely add to the parents' sense of insecurity and may cause a lack of confidence in the professionals involved.

The medical profession have, in general, a reputation for being abrupt and of having little time to spare to discuss problems with parents. Tucker and Nolan pointed out that medical people are usually trained to an action-orientated approach and sometimes lack the skills in other essential areas such as giving information and support.

There is a need for a team approach and there must be a flexible interchange of ideas and information. It is essential that the parents are seen as part of the team and that management decisions are not made without full consultation and explanation. Once the parents' confidence has been lost it is difficult to regain.

Having a deaf child causes enormous stress within the family. Other children may feel that they are being ignored, and sometimes one parent may feel neglected. Worries about the child's education are very real since there may not be a suitable local school. There is no doubt that having a deaf child throws a considerable financial burden on the family. These parents need good counsell-ing and support throughout the child's develop-ment.

Concern has been expressed about interference with parent–child bonding, especially in neonates and young babies. Taylor (1985) emphasized the fine balance between the need to have parental awareness when hearing loss is suspected and a fear of interference with bonding. He reported the results of a questionnaire sent out to families of hearing impaired children. About 20% of parents who replied would rather not have known about the child's hearing loss within the first week of life. The most common reason given was that parents would have preferred to establish a bond with the baby before undertaking the task of managing a deaf child. Some parents felt that they would rather not know because they thought that nothing could be done for the child at such an early age. There is clearly a need for improved awareness and better education of both parents and professionals if deafness is to be detected early.

Subsequent management of the deaf child

The mainstays of management of the child with sensorineural deafness are:

(1) appropriate hearing aid selection
(2) promotion of the development of language and communication skills.

It is rare for a child to be born totally deaf and every attempt should be made to reach any residual hearing by the use of the high powered hearing aids which are currently available. Com-monly, the only residual hearing is for low frequency sounds and hearing aids with extended low frequency responses can be used.

Every effort must be made to encourage the child to develop intelligible speech. The term auditory training has been used to describe techniques by which the child is taught to listen and hopefully to copy speech. This will be discussed later in this chapter.

Hearing aids

Sensorineural hearing loss in children cannot be corrected by any form of medical or surgical treatment. The role of cochlear implants will be discussed later. Similarly, some conductive losses caused by congenital abnormalities of the external or middle ear are not suitable for surgical treatment. These children should be considered for the fitting of hearing aids.

A full discussion of hearing aids is to be found in Volume 2. The following is limited to the particular problems found with children.

Types of hearing aids

Two types of hearing aids are currently available – personal aids and hearing aid systems (Tucker and Nolan, 1984).

Personal hearing aids

A variety of different personal hearing aids can be bought from several commercial firms. In the UK, the National Health Service (NHS) supplies a wide range of such aids free of charge. It is, however, possible for an NHS consultant to prescribe certain aids outside this range if it is considered that there is no NHS aid sufficient to meet the child's needs.

There are two groups of NHS aids, the body worn (BW) aids and the behind the ear (BE) aids.

Body worn aids
    BW 60 series – low/medium power
    BW 80 series – high power
Behind the ear aids
    BE 10 series – low power
    BE 30 series – medium power
    BE 50 series – high power.

The range of aids is such that a suitable aid can be found to fit most children's requirements. However, it must not be forgotten that the NHS range has been designed chiefly for adults and the powerful BE aids are too big for most small children's ears.

Bone conduction hearing aids are available for children with deformed external ears or severe, recurrent ear infections which prohibit the insertion of ear moulds. The bone conductor can be used in conjunction with a conventional body worn aid, although a better cosmetic result is achieved by using a postaural aid on a head band with the output receiver wired to the bone conductor (*Figure 9.1*).

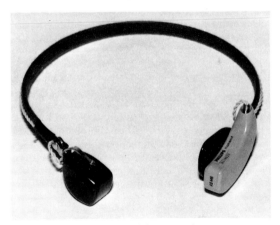

Figure 9.1 Postaural aid with bone conductor on headband

Hearing aid systems

The greatest disadvantage of conventional hearing aids is their inability to distinguish between speech sounds and the unwanted background noise which tends to mask speech. This is referred to as the signal-to-noise ratio of the system. The problem is made worse by reverberation caused by sound reflections off walls, ceilings, floors and furnishings and will cause the relatively strong vowel sounds to persist and mask the weaker consonants which contain most of the information in speech (John, 1957).

With most hearing aids the signal-to-noise ratio is a function of the distance between the signal source and the listener. Classrooms tend to be very noisy so that children seated away from the teacher will be at a disadvantage in that the background noise will mask the teacher's voice. This problem can be overcome in a variety of ways by using aids primarily supplied by education authorities.

Speech trainer

The child wears headphones connected to an amplifier, and controls on the amplifier allow adjustment of gain and frequency response. The teacher or parent uses a microphone connected directly to the amplifier. This useful device has a low signal-to-noise ratio since the microphone is close to the speaker's mouth. In addition, since feedback is reduced because of the distance between microphone and headphone, it is possible to achieve high levels of amplification with profoundly deaf children. It is most useful for short periods of intensive speech and language teaching.

Group hearing aid

The principle is very similar to that of the speech trainer except that several children are connected to one teacher and to each other. Each child's 'station' has an amplifier which allows individual adjustment of output and frequency response. Tucker and Nolan (1984) described this system's benefits and drawbacks, the chief drawback being lack of mobility of both children and teacher.

Radio hearing aids

Frequency modulated (FM) radio systems allow the child to be fully mobile within a fairly large area while retaining the good signal-to-noise ratio of group aids. The teacher or parent wears a microphone transmitter and the child a receiver so that no matter where the child is in a room the person using the microphone will seem to be speaking almost directly into the child's ears.

There are two types of radio aid (Nolan, 1983a):

(a) the body worn receiver/hearing aid. This can be used either as an ordinary body worn aid or as an FM system
(b) the audio-input system, used in conjunction with the child's personal hearing aids. This

type of FM system can be plugged into the child's personal BW or BE aids as required. The advantage of this system is that the child need only wear one set of aids and will not have to change between the body worn receiver/aid and personal aids.

The chief drawback of both types of FM system is that only the teacher has a radio transmitter and therefore interaction between pupils is limited. In the UK one-third of these radio aids are supplied by charitable sources or paid for by parents (McCormick, Bamford and Martin, 1986). The NHS has no policy of central provision for radio aids, although a recent circular (C331) does allow an otologist or audiological physician to supply these aids if money is available locally within the health system.

Infra-red hearing aid systems

The FM radio signals from the teacher's transmitter pass easily through walls and doors into adjacent areas. This gives rise to problems if children in a nearby classrooms are using a system on the same frequency. The infra-red system overcomes this difficulty since the infra-red waves are contained by the boundaries of any room in which the system is used. Problems do occur in bright sunlight which can produce noise in the system.

Loop system

Input from the teacher's microphone is amplified and transmitted either directly around an electromagnetic loop installed on the classroom walls, or by means of an FM system to a loop worn around the child's neck. Tucker and Nolan (1984) listed the drawbacks of the loop system, including spill-over into adjacent classrooms, unpredictable frequency response and weak or dead spots with the classroom loop. These authors pointed out that most of the drawbacks are eliminated by using the personal neck loop with an FM receiver.

Problems with hearing aid selection in children

There are two main areas of difficulty with hearing aid fitting:

(1) there is often limited information about the extent of the child's hearing loss
(2) young children cannot say which aid, or settings on the aid, they prefer.

Young children present particular problems with respect to information about the hearing loss.

Standard free-field distraction test stimuli give a reasonable estimate of thresholds at different frequencies. These stimuli can be supplemented by using warble tones or narrow band noise. Information about children too young for distraction testing can be obtained by evoked response audiometry, although it is usually difficult to obtain measurements of low frequency thresholds by this technique.

It is important to estimate the dynamic range of the residual hearing. This is the difference between threshold and loudness discomfort level. If the child receives frequent aided stimulation greater than the loudness discomfort level, there is a risk that the aids might be rejected. One means of estimating loudness discomfort level is to examine the stapedial reflex, although in many cases this is not present because of the severity of the deafness. Tucker and Nolan (1984) described an electroacoustical method of estimating loudness discomfort using an earmould receiver and watching the child's responses to increasing stimulation at different frequencies.

Most profoundly deaf children do have some residual hearing, usually for the low frequencies. In the newly diagnosed child there is no way of predicting how useful this will be, if at all, in helping speech discrimination. Every effort, however, must be made to use this residual hearing in an attempt to obtain communication.

Having obtained as much information as possible about the child's hearing it is then essential to select appropriate aids and to adjust their output and frequency responses as necessary to suit the child's needs. As with adults there are two main ways of choosing an aid.

The empirical (selective) method

The child is given several different aids in turn for trial. The problem with this method is that young children cannot say which aid is best. It is possible, by carrying out free-field tests including speech if the child is old enough, to gain a partly subjective impression of the relative merits of each aid.

The theoretical (prescriptive) method

Information about various parameters such as the child's thresholds at each frequency, most comfortable listening level and speech discrimination scores, allows a prediction of the best amplification characteristics for that child. This allows a suitable hearing aid to be chosen. Many different formulae are available which calculate theoretical settings for the frequency response and gain of the aids. It must not be forgotten that the hearing aid performance in a test box with a 2 ml coupler is not an accurate reflection of the aid's performance in the human ear. Modifications to the frequency response occur as a result of variations in earmould parameters and the resonance effect of the ear canal.

As the child becomes older the hearing aids, or the settings of the controls may need to be changed as more information about the child's hearing becomes available. There are also children, particularly those with hereditary deafness, in whom the hearing may deteriorate.

Hearing aids are usually fitted to each ear, except when low and middle frequency hearing are normal or only slightly impaired. Amplification of these frequencies may introduce distortion of the perceived speech signal.

There are many advantages to binaural fitting:

(1) improved localization of the sound source
(2) improved hearing in background noise
(3) a binaural summation effect giving better amplification.

There has been some controversy over the relative merits of behind the ear and body worn aids. The power outputs of both types are equivalent. It is generally agreed that BE aids give a more natural sound environment because sound reception is at ear level. In addition, they are free from the rubbing of clothes, give improved localization over the BW aids, and are cosmetically more acceptable. It has been argued that they are more easily removed and thrown away by young children. This can be avoided by taping the aid to the back of the ear or by using double-sided sticky tape. Children with a body worn aid can pull the cord and displace the receiver from the ear. The body baffle effect with BW aids improves the frequency response below 600 Hz by 5 dB (Wald, 1976). This may be useful in children with residual low frequency hearing only, but can be a disadvantage in a child with a flat loss. In these children the masking effects of the powerful low frequency vowel sounds on the weaker consonants will be enhanced by the body baffle effect.

The most significant limitation of all types of powerful hearing aids is acoustic feedback (Nolan, 1983b). This is most likely to occur when the microphone of the hearing aid is close to the receiver or earmould. Body worn aids are therefore less susceptible to this problem since they are worn on the chest. Good fitting earmoulds are essential if powerful BE aids are to be used. The impression should be obtained by the syringe technique after putting a small sponge tamp into the child's external ear. Children need to have their earmoulds renewed at regular intervals as the external auditory canal grows.

It is important that parents and teachers check the child's hearing aids daily. This is most easily carried out using a stethoclip. The hearing aid is attached either by hollow plastic tubing (BE aid) or by plugging the receiver into the stethoclip (BW aid). This permits detection of low battery power and other faults in the aid. Many schools and peripatetic teachers of the deaf have access to a hearing aid test box and can more accurately assess the aid's performance.

Cochlear implants

Considerable interest has been focused on the possibility of directly stimulating the cochlea or auditory nerve to help speech discrimination in the profoundly deaf. In the UK children are not, at present, considered for implantation (Frazer *et al.*, 1986). There are ethical problems with informed consent. In addition, there is a risk of further damage to the ear with subsequent limitation of hearing aid benefit. Extracochlear implants are not without risk since middle ear infection is common in children.

The education of hearing impaired children

The ideal outcome is a child with good speech who can progress normally through the education system and integrate fully into a society which communicates mainly by the oral-aural channel. In the author's experience, this is possible, even with profoundly deaf children, although with this group it is the exception rather than the rule.

Conrad (1980) investigated the reading, lip reading, speech intelligibility and 'inner speech' in a large group of 15–16.5 year olds with either partial or severe hearing losses. He found that 50% of children with a severe loss and 25% of the partially hearing had no reading comprehension at all. In addition, the severely deaf had poor lip reading ability, poor speech and poor 'inner speech'. A survey of children in the European Economic Community with an average loss of greater than 50 dB showed that more than one-half of these children were unable to carry on meaningful conversation with strangers (Martin, 1982).

A child's ability to acquire normal, or intelligible speech depends on several factors.

(1) The extent of the hearing loss. This must take into account the pattern of the hearing loss, whether flat or ski-slope shaped.
(2) The child's ability to use the residual hearing. In some cases the residual hearing, even with amplification, is insufficient for speech discrimination.

(3) The time of onset of the hearing loss, whether present at birth, or developing later in childhood.
(4) The child's personality and motivation.
(5) The child's intelligence.
(6) Sufficient exposure to communication systems, especially speech. This requires considerable motivation on the part of the parents.

Preschool children

Enright and O'Connor (1982) examined the role of peripatetic teachers of the deaf in preschool education of hearing impaired children. A major part of their task involves giving information, support and encouragement to parents, in addition to teaching language skills to the child. Parents are shown how to develop these skills and how best to use the child's residual hearing.

Kernohan, Lucas and Muter (1981) listed the information that should be given to parents:

(1) an explanation of the child's hearing loss, with special reference to the frequencies involved
(2) the differences between vowels and consonants and the importance of each to speech
(3) the effects of amplification on speech and which parts of speech the child is likely to receive
(4) the effects of background noise
(5) how to look after the hearing aids
(6) the importance of talking normally to the child.

Much of the information in speech is contained in transitions between phonemes, speech rhythm and intonation patterns. In the hearing impaired child this information is vital and is lost if the child is spoken to in an artificial or exaggerated manner.

School-age children

There is a move towards integrating hearing impaired children into ordinary schools. At present hearing impaired children may be placed in one of several types of school situation:

(1) ordinary classroom, using hearing aids
(2) ordinary classroom, with hearing aids and regular help from a peripatetic teacher of the deaf
(3) ordinary classroom for part of the day, the remainder of the time being spent in an attached partially-hearing unit
(4) partially-hearing unit only, staffed by specialist teachers of the deaf
(5) school for the profoundly deaf
(6) other schools, such as speech and language units, for children with additional handicaps.

Legislation in the UK

The Education Act of 1976 amended the Act of 1944. It required local education authorities to make provision for the education of handicapped pupils in ordinary county or voluntary schools as well as in special schools. The trend towards integration was further encouraged by a report from the Department of Education and Science (The Warnock Report, 1978). This provided an overview of the then existing provisions and made proposals for future policy. It highlighted the importance of parental involvement in the general management of the hearing impaired child, especially in the preschool years.

The Education Act (1981) is based largely on the proposals of the Warnock Report. The Act abolished the use of existing categories of handicap (educationally subnormal, maladjusted, partially hearing, and deaf) and replaced them with a 'statement'. A statement is produced for each affected child and details the child's needs. It also lists the facilities and resources, including school placement, necessary to meet these needs. The statement is prepared from evidence submitted by the various people in contact with the child, including the parents, teachers of the deaf, educational psychologists, clinical medical officers, otologists and audiological physicians. The Act encourages the trend towards integration of the handicapped into ordinary schools.

The 1981 Act has been criticized by many. It introduces complex referral, assessment and appeal procedures which increase administrative time and costs. With resources already stretched this reduces the amount of time spent in educating these children (Reeves, 1983).

Communication methods in the education of deaf children

Arguments about which method of education is best for severely hearing impaired children have been continuing for many years. Llewellyn-Jones (1986) gave a brief account of the history. In the early 1800s the predominant method of communication was the combined system using speech, finger-spelling and signing simultaneously. By the 1870s, oralism was being used increasingly in Europe and, at the International Congress on the Education of the Deaf in Milan in 1880, oralism was endorsed as the method of choice. In Britain in 1889 a Royal Commission recommended that every child should have the full opportunity of being educated in the oral system. The move towards oralism in schools was resisted by the British Deaf and Dumb Association (now the British Deaf Association) who fought to retain the combined system in schools.

The Lewis Report in 1968 found that, although British schools claimed to prefer pure oralism, over three-quarters of them used some form of signs or manual communication. As a result of this report some schools in the late 1960s and early 1970s began to use a variety of sign systems as educational aids. This move towards a combined system has continued.

Recent figures published by the National Deaf Children's Society shows that, in the UK, 47% of special schools and 13% of partially hearing units now nominally use a combined speech and signing system.

Oralism

Children educated in this system use only speech and lip reading as a means of communication. Signing of any sort is strongly discouraged or even prevented. Listening and speaking require considerable effort and concentration by the severely hearing impaired child, signing is much easier. Oralists argue that the ability of a child to develop speech is inhibited if the child is allowed to communicate by signing. The normal hearing child is thought to understand a significant amount of language at about the age of 12 months and 80% of his language development has occurred by 3 years of age. Oralism assumes that the brain of the hearing impaired child remains capable of learning speech and language at least to puberty, and perhaps beyond (Lenneberg, 1967). Many others subscribe to the view that there is a 'critical period' for most children during the first few years of life during which language development is at a premium. If these children are not taught communication skills within this period they may never acquire them.

Finger spelling

This, on its own, is a slow means of communication.

Cued speech

Some speech sounds, such as M, P, B or K, D, L, cannot be distinguished by lip reading alone. Cued speech uses eight different hand shapes in four different positions close to the speaker's mouth to enable the child to discriminate the lip movement. It was developed as an aid to teaching English to deaf children, and not as an exclusive signing system.

Signing systems (manualism)

British sign language

This is the communication system favoured by most profoundly deaf adults. It is a completely separate language since it does not follow the rules of English grammar.

Paget-Gorman sign system

This was developed as a means of accurately reflecting spoken and written English. It has a large vocabulary of inverted signs with provision for indicating grammatical structures such as word endings and tenses. It is rarely used in schools for the deaf.

Signed English

True (exact) signed English uses signs taken from British sign language with artificially developed 'sign markers' to indicate tense, word endings, etc. Another more popular version, Signs Supported English, uses signings in English word order, without sign markers, together with speech.

Makaton

This signing system, based largely on gestures and simple signs, is used with mentally handicapped patients.

Total communication

Total communication involves using a combination of speech, gestures, formal signing, finger spelling, speech reading (lip reading), reading and writing. Conrad (1980) postulated that, in very deaf children, exclusive use of spoken language fails to provide sufficient linguistic stimulation to the child's brain, parts of which may then undergo functional and perhaps even physical atrophy.

Supporters of total communication argue that providing sensory input through different channels – auditory and visual – enhances the possibility of language development. This must be understood as being language in its widest sense, since language may be thought of as a system of symbols and rules for communication.

Speech is one mode of language. It has been argued that total communication impairs speech development. Taylor (1985), in a survey of different schools, produced evidence that oral-only schools are more likely to succeed in developing the most normal speech aspects of language. Nix (1983) reviewed various studies of communication systems and suggested that simultaneous oral/manual communication is beneficial, but that stimulation of the two channels together did not produce such good results as oralism alone. On the other hand, Dee, Rapin and Ruben (1982) demonstrated that total communication facilitated speech development and did not inhibit it.

There are problems in comparing results claimed for oralism and total communication. It is often difficult to know which parameters are being assessed, since intelligible speech is not always a measure of language development. There is no standardization of teaching practice. In many schools total communication is not total, but sacrifices speech in the interests of signing. One of the difficulties encountered with total communication is that total synchrony of speech and signing is impossible. It is difficult to sign quickly enough so as not to interrupt normal speech flow. Normal speech patterns contain information which is highly redundant to the normal hearing person, but essential to those with a hearing loss.

Total communication aims not only to stimulate language development, but also to provide a reliable system by which the child can communicate with teachers, parents, classmates and an increasing number of the population who are learning to sign. The child is hopefully 'bilingual' and has a flexible means of communication for use in different situations.

Arnold (1982), in a reply to Conrad's paper, pointed out that there was no evidence that any approach yet devised has successfully been used to educate the majority of severely deaf children.

Recent legislation gives parents a central role in the education of their hearing impaired child. Parents must therefore be given a balanced and informed view of the different communication methods available. Professionals must not force their opinions on parents.

There are many problems in the management of the deaf child. There is a need for more information about the extent of the child's hearing loss and the implications of this in the selection of suitable amplification. It is obvious that no single type of education system meets the needs of all deaf children. How can the decision be made about which type is best for a particular child? Is it reasonable to insist that oralism be used until it becomes obvious that the child cannot develop useful speech? Does total communication impair speech development? Objective research may answer some of these questions.

References

ALBERTI, P. W., HYDE, M. L., RIKO, K., CORBIN, H. and ABRAMOVICH, S. (1983) An evaluation of BERA for hearing screening in high risk neonates. *The Laryngoscope*, **93**, 1115–1121

ARNOLD, P. (1982) Oralism and the deaf child's brain: a reply to Dr Conrad. *International Journal of Paediatric Otorhinolaryngology*, **4**, 275–286

BEIGHTON, P. and SELLARS, S. (1982) Inherited deafness – diagnostic evaluation, screening and genetic management. In *Genetics and Otology*, pp. 98–104. Edinburgh: Churchill Livingstone

BENNETT, M. J. (1979) Trials with the auditory response cradle. I – Neonatal responses to auditory stimuli. *British Journal of Audiology*, **13**, 125–134

BERGSTROM, L. (1980) Continuing management of conductive hearing loss during language development. *International Journal of Paediatric Otorhinolaryngology*, **2**, 3–9

BOOTHROYD, A. (1982) *Hearing Impairments in Young Children*. Englewood Cliffs: Prentice Hall

CONRAD, R. (1980) Let the children choose. *International Journal of Paediatric Otorhinolaryngology*, **1**, 317–329

DEE, A., RAPIN, I. and RUBEN, R. J. (1982) Speech and language development in a parent-infant total communication programme. *Annals of Otology, Rhinology and Laryngology*, **91**, (suppl. 97), 62–72

DEPARTMENT OF EDUCATION AND SCIENCE (1978) Special Educational Needs. Report of the Committee of Enquiry into the education of handicapped children and young people (Warnock Report). London: HMSO

DURIEUX-SMITH, A. and PICTON, T. W. (1985) Neonatal hearing assessment by auditory brainstem response– the Canadian experience. *Journal of Otolaryngology*, **14**, (suppl. 14), 5–15

ENRIGHT, F. P. and O'CONNOR, D. J. (1982) A profile of counselling skills applied in the pre-school setting by peripatetic teachers of the deaf. *Journal of the British Association of Teachers of the Deaf*, **6**, 94–100

EWING, I. R. (1957) Screening tests and guidance clinics for babies and young children. In *Educational Guidance and the Deaf Child*, edited by A. W. G. Ewing, pp. 21–43. Manchester: Manchester University Press

FISCH, L. (1981) Syndromes associated with hearing loss. In *Audiology and Audiological Medicine*, Volume II, edited by H. Beagley, pp. 595–639. Oxford: Oxford University Press

FISCH, L. (1983) Integrated development and maturation of the hearing system. A critical review article. *British Journal of Audiology*, **17**, 137–154

FRAZER, J. G., COOPER, H. R., HAZEL, J. W. P., PHELPS, P. D. and LLOYD, G. A. S. (1986) The UCH/RNID cochlear implant programme. *British Journal of Audiology*, **20**, 9–17

GALAMBOS, R., HICKS, G. E. and WILSON, M. J. (1984) The auditory brainstem response reliably predicts hearing loss in graduates of a tertiary intensive care nursery. *Ear and Hearing*, **5**, 254–260

HAMILTON, P. (1972) Language and reading skills in children with impaired hearing in ordinary schools. *MSc Thesis*, University of Manchester, Manchester

JOHN, J. E. J. (1957) Acoustics in the use of hearing aids. In *Educational Guidance and the Deaf Child*, edited by A. W. G. Ewing, pp. 160–175. Manchester: Manchester University Press

KERNOHAN, G., LUCAS, G. and MUTER, V. (1981) Education of the hearing-handicapped child. In *Audiology and Audiological Medicine*, Volume II, edited by H. Beagley, 663–684. Oxford: Oxford University Press

LENNEBERG, E. H. (1967) *Biological Foundations of Language*. New York: Wiley

LEVITON, A. (1980) Otitis media and learning disorders. *Journal of Developmental and Behavioural Paediatrics*, **1**, 58–63

LLEWELLYN-JONES, P. (1986). *A Language for Ben. Early Communication – a Parent's Choice*. London: Tyne Tees Television

LUND, V. J., PHELPS, P. D. and BEAGLEY, H. A. (1982) Evoked response audiometry and tomography – complementary procedures for the assessment of the deaf infant. *International Journal of Paediatric Otorhinolaryngology*, **4**, 95–106

McCORMICK, B., BAMFORD, J. and MARTIN, M. (1986) *The Provision of Radio Hearing Aids for Children*. London: RNID

MARTIN, J. A. M. (1982) Diagnosis and communicative ability in deaf children in the European Community. *Audiology*, **21**, 185–196

NIX, G. W. (1983) How total is total communication? *Journal of the British Association of Teachers of the Deaf*, **7**, 177–181

NOLAN, M. (1983a) Radio hearing aid systems. *Journal of the British Association of Teachers of the Deaf*, **7**, 105–121

NOLAN, M. (1983b) Acoustic feedback – causes and cures. *Journal of the British Association of Teachers of the Deaf*, **7**, 13–17

PARVING, A. (1983) Aetiological diagnosis in the hearing impaired child – clinical value and application of a modern examination programme. *International Journal of Paediatric Otorhinolaryngology*, **5**, 159–165

PARVING, A. (1984) Early detection and identification of congenital/early acquired hearing disability. Who takes the initiative? *International Journal of Paediatric Otorhinolaryngology*, **7**, 107–117

PARVING, A. (1985) Hearing disorders in childhood, some procedures for detection, identification and diagnosis

evaluation. *International Journal of Paediatric Otorhinolaryngology*, **9**, 31–57

RAPIN, I. (1979) Conductive hearing loss. Effects on children's language and scholastic skills. *Annals of Otology, Rhinology and Laryngology*, **88**, (suppl. 60), 3–12

REEVES, K. (1983) The Education Act, 1981. The influence of government and legislation on the education of the hearing impaired. *Journal of the British Association of Teachers of the Deaf*, **7**, 170–197

RIKO, K., HYDE, M. L. and ALBERTI, P. W. (1985) Hearing loss in early infancy: incidence, detection and assessment. *The Laryngoscope*, **95**, 137–145

SIMMONS, F. B., McFARLAND, W. H. and JONES, F. R. (1979) An automated hearing screening technique for newborns. *Acta Otolaryngologica*, **87**, 1–8

TAYLOR, I. G. (1985) Hearing impaired babies and methods of communication. *Ear and Hearing*, **6**, 25–28

TUCKER, I. and NOLAN, M. (1984) *Educational Audiology*. Beckenham: Croom Helm

VENTRY, I. M. (1980) Effects of conductive hearing loss: fact or fiction. *Journal of Speech and Hearing Disorders*, **45**, 143–156

WALD, Z. J. (1976) The coupler measurement of hearing aid gain – some reservations: *MSc Thesis*, University of Manchester, Manchester

WOLFF, S. M. (1973) The ocular manifestations of congenital rubella. *Journal of Paediatric Ophthalmology*, **10**, 101–141

10

Development and disorders of language

L. Rosenbloom

Language can perhaps be most simply defined as the capacity to generate and transmit symbolic or coded communication (Sheridan, 1961). Although demonstrable in some other mammals, language appears to be only well developed as a facet of human behaviour.

Linguistic symbols or codes can be words used in speech or in writing or some other forms of signing, for example those used by the deaf. Their fundamental characteristic is that particular symbols consistently represent particular concepts whether these are concrete objects or abstract ideas.

It is useful to regard language as having three functional components: first as a tool for thinking, most commonly termed 'inner language'; second as a capacity for understanding others; and third as an instrument for expressing thoughts. The development of inner language implies that the individual has acquired an internal store of coded concepts that can readily be drawn upon in cognitive processes. It is elegantly illustrated in children by their symbolic play, for example how they use miniature toys such as dolls' house furniture as representative of the real thing. In an activity such as this, and without necessarily a word being uttered, children by their complex and imaginative play indicate that they can both understand and systematically apply the principles of using symbols in thought.

The ability of children to understand others' language, that is their comprehension, emerges in parallel with their inner language and clearly each reinforces the other. Both comprehension and inner language are more fundamental to cognitive and linguistic competence than is the expressive function of language and perhaps as a result they normally develop considerably ahead of children's expressive abilities. Nevertheless, it is the way that children communicate with others that most readily brings them to attention or is a cause of concern to their parents. It is not surprising, therefore, that at a lay level 'speech' and 'language' are terms that are used interchangeably.

However, the term 'expressive language' implies both the capacity to organize one's thoughts prior to expressing them, that is an encoding function, well illustrated by the task of preparing in one's mind a sentence in a foreign language, and also the motor functions involved in communication, best exemplified by the word and sound production of speech. Speech can be regarded, therefore, as the capacity and ability to express verbal symbols and is largely a motor function. Its development and disorders are considered in detail elsewhere in this volume (*see* Chapter 11).

The development of language

The newborn infant has a remarkable social competence both in reacting to and initiating contacts with adults. These behaviours include a variety of facial expressions, cries and other sounds and the ability to take turns with an adult in interactive situations. Although such behaviours are not truly linguistic within the context of the definitions given above as symbolic communication is not being used, they nevertheless indicate that social interaction is an innate human ability.

Linguistic competence is built onto this social behaviour. Although it has been postulated that inherent within the brain is a language acquisition device, this is best regarded not as a localizable anatomical region within one or both temporal lobes, but more as an indication that the acquisition of language is inherently determined as a cerebral cortical function with the details of an individual's subsequent performance being then shaped by environmental experiences.

In the first year, children demonstrate little in the way of symbolic performance. Instead they show situational understanding, for example by appropriate excitement or distress in particular circumstances. At the same time, their expressive abilities are limited to a multisyllable babble and, in spite of the optimistic interpretation of parents and the obvious foundations of prosody (speech rhythms) in babble, clear words do not normally emerge at this stage.

Genuine symbolic skills emerge during the second year. Verbal comprehension increases from an ability to cope with single concepts, for example, 'where are your *shoes*?' at 12 months to two linked items at 24 months, for example 'put the *cup* on the *table*'. Inner language can be demonstrated in play with toys but is still immature and most play at this age is constructive rather than symbolic or imaginative. The rate of development of expressive abilities at this age is enormously variable with girls usually being so considerably in advance of boys that different age norms for the relevant standardized tests are used (Reynell, 1977). It is nevertheless customary to expect children to have two word utterances by the time they are 2 years old, the corollary being that any child who by this age has no clear words must be referred for further evaluation.

Between 2 and 5 years of age comprehension extends progressively to include complex sentences involving abstract concepts and the various parts of speech. Inner language can be demonstrated in detailed imaginative play and expressive abilities are such that by age 5, most parts of speech are normally used and articulation is clear.

Beyond 5 years of age the further development of linguistic skills is seen in such diverse ways as reading and writing, the understanding of grammatical rules and the use of language in problem solving. Language at this stage is very much an integral part of higher cognitive functioning.

Factors influencing language development

Cerebral functioning

As has already been discussed, children have an innate capacity to acquire and use language. It follows that any abnormality of the brain, whether this is a developmental anomaly or a disorder acquired pre-, peri- or postnatally, can delay or retard linguistic competence specifically or as part of a more generalized neurological disorder such as is seen in global developmental retardation.

Sensory experiences

Consistently normal hearing is a prerequisite for normal language development and the effects of hearing loss on language are considered presently. In addition, however, the ability to see is obviously of great importance in, for example, associating objects with their labels. Visually impaired children commonly have significant language problems.

Emotional status

Given the social functions of language, it is not surprising that behavioural or emotional disorders that lead to some failure of adaptation of a child are frequently reflected in delayed or deviant linguistic function.

Environmental experiences

To communicate normally, children need both appropriate linguistic experiences to stimulate development and also the opportunity to express themselves. Environmental deprivation is a potent cause, therefore, of developmental and linguistic delay.

Disorders of speech and language

Speech and language disorders are not specific disease entities. Instead, when a child's speech or language deviates sufficiently far from that which is conventional and acceptable for a child of similar age and causes overt communication, intelligibility or social adaptation difficulties or alternatively parental concern, then it might reasonably be considered that he/she has a significant functional disorder of speech or language.

Incidence

Both the pattern and severity of communication disorders vary with children's age and state of language development. As a result, prevalence studies in populations have used different criteria for assessment and have been difficult to compare. As an approximate indication of the size of the problem, however, some 4% of 4 year olds have sufficient difficulty, for whatever reason, with their intelligibility to bring them to notice (Morley, 1965). About one in a 100 children have more severe, long-standing or refractory communication disorders.

130

Table 10.1 Medical and linguistic classification of language disorders

Patterns of language impairment	Defects of speech apparatus	Hearing loss	Pre- or perinatal brain damage or dysfunction	Acquired brain damage or dysfunction	Emotional or behavioural disorder	Environmental deprivation	Unknown aetiology: developmental language disorder
			Medical factors				
Abnormal speech	Dysphonia Dysarthria	Deafness acquired after language development			Elective mutism		Stuttering
Generalized language delay		Chronic conductive hearing loss	Intellectual retardation			Neglect	Delayed language acquisition
Abnormal syntax or phonology		?With high frequency loss		Left hemisphere lesions			Phonological syntactic syndrome
Semantic or pragmatic problems			Cocktail party syndrome				Semantic pragmatic disorder
Poor comprehension and limited expression		Prelingual deafness	Mental handicap	Landau–Kleffner syndrome			Congenital auditory imperception
Severe non-verbal and verbal impairment			Severe mental handicap, autism	Degenerative disorders			

Causes

At a broad level these are abnormalities of the factors listed above that influence normal language development:

(1) neurological abnormalities – either developmental or acquired
(2) sensory impairments of hearing or vision
(3) emotional disorders
(4) environmental deprivation.

Unfortunately specific language abnormality syndromes correlate poorly with their underlying causes even when these are definitely known. Frequently, also, the cause of a language problem has to be assumed or considered as unknown even after relevant investigations. This is especially so for what have been termed 'developmental language disorders'. Moreover, it is more likely that the problems of individual children will have multiple causes.

It follows, therefore, that aetiological considerations are relatively minor when language disorders are classified and when analysis is made of specific clinical problems.

Classification (Bishop and Rosenbloom, 1986)

Historically, medical classifications based on a mixture of aetiological and clinical considerations and linguistic classifications have competed. It is probably best, however, to combine medical and linguistic criteria and *Table 10.1* summarizes this approach.

It can be seen in *Table 10.1* that individually identifiable disorders of language have both linguistic and medical parameters and, far from competing, both are necessary for a full description of the disorder. In the following discussion, each of the conditions identified in *Table 10.1* are considered by taking each of the vertical columns in turn.

Defects of speech apparatus

These include congenital structural abnormalities, for example cleft palate, and neuromotor disorders, as shown in suprabulbar palsy. 'Dysarthria' refers to speech problems associated with weakness, spasticity or incoordination of the speech musculature and 'dysphonia' to abnormalities of voice control. Defective speech sound production can also occur in the absence of obvious physical handicap. Investigation in such cases may provide evidence of minor physical problems of oromotor control, for example a history of feeding difficulty or drooling. It is important also to examine oral sensory skills (Martin, 1981).

When children present with speech disorders, it is important to recall that language disorders can coexist especially in children with cerebral palsy or those with cleft palate with an associated hearing loss.

Hearing loss

Sensorineural deafness

When this is acquired after language has fully developed, there may be comprehension difficulty and voice and articulation deterioration but little effect on linguistic skills. By contrast, deafness that is congenital or acquired prelingually has profound consequences even after early diagnosis and amplification. The majority of deaf children have limited or abnormal speech and frequently their problems extend to writing and signing which are also limited in linguistic terms. Given the controversies that exist about how best to teach language to deaf children, it is disappointing that there is no research evidence to support either the concept that signing interferes with speech acquisition or that it fosters it (Bishop, 1983).

Selective high frequency hearing loss can also seriously affect language development and is often missed, children being considered to have a developmental dysphasia. The voice quality in affected individuals is not characteristically 'deaf'.

Conductive loss

It is likely, although conclusive evidence is lacking, that children who sustain several episodes of otitis media in the preschool years are at risk of language disorder with poor listening skills, phonological problems and persistent educational handicaps.

Congenital brain damage or dysfunction

Sparks (1984) has recently reviewed the many patterns of speech and language disorder resulting from a variety of birth defects and, although slow speech development may be the first indication of developmental disorder, fuller assessment quickly reveals more pervasive problems. Medical investigation in such circumstances is often unrewarding, even when a disciplined approach using modern investigative methods is used. Nevertheless, a search for an underlying cause in an attempt to demonstrate the site and nature of the lesion, to suggest treatment and to indicate a prognosis are prerequisites for helping affected children and their families.

In mentally retarded children, language tends to be delayed in proportion to their intellectual difficulties rather than to be deviant, but norms for what is appropriate language in this group have never really been defined.

Chromosomal disorders

In Down's syndrome, (trisomy 21), the most common chromosomal disorder, language is frequently disproportionately impaired so that verbal attainments are poor even when compared to other children of similar non-verbal ability. It is likely that a higher incidence of conductive hearing loss and specific motor disorders of speech are contributory factors to this situation.

More generally there appears to be an increased incidence of language disorders in children with chromosomal problems (Friedrich *et al.*, 1982) and this includes boys with the sex-linked variety of mental retardation (the fragile X syndrome).

Hydrocephalus and the cocktail party syndrome
(Hadenius *et al.*, 1962)

Some hydrocephalic children of low intelligence seem to have disproportionately good language. However, although they have a sophisticated vocabulary, there is poor content to what they say and formal testing reveals poor comprehension.

Infantile autism

Here there is a major cognitive disturbance characterized by marked impairment in the development of social relationships, many and varied obsessional characteristics and a constellation of linguistic abnormalities ranging at their most severe from mutism through poor comprehension to abnormal speech, for example pronoun reversal. Detailed analysis of the language of autistic children demonstrates impairment for all modalities including gesture and other forms of signing.

The ultimate ability of autistic children to live independently is determined primarily by their intellectual limitations. For those who are autistic, but less severely mentally handicapped, and these are the minority, language acquisition can lead to a superficial competence although problems with social and personal relationships remain.

Acquired brain damage or dysfunction

The effects of localized brain lesions on language are very different for children and adults. In the adult, damage to circumscribed areas of the left hemisphere is associated with dysphasia and there is a close relationship between the locus of injury and the type of language problem. In children the effects of similar lesions depend on age. In infants, left hemisphere lesions typically depress general intelligence without causing dysphasia. This reflects the immature brain's plasticity of function which enables language to develop in the right hemisphere following early left-sided damage. Persistent dysphasia may, however, be found after bilateral lesions in infancy.

When left hemispheric lesions are acquired after a child has learned to speak, language impairment frequently develops resulting in word finding and phonological problems rather than the typical features of adult dysphasia.

Acquired aphasia with convulsive disorder – Landau–Kleffner syndrome

Rarely, previously normal children acquire very severe language comprehension problems in association with epilepsy (Landau and Kleffner, 1957). Affected children develop normal language for their first 4–8 years but then regress either suddenly or over a period of weeks or months. The vast majority have convulsions around the time of onset of their aphasia; the remainder have abnormal electroencephalograms with seizure discharge, usually from both temporal lobes. Some affected children recover fully, others continue with language problems which may fluctuate and a few remain subject to epilepsy. Conventional tests of hearing including evoked response audiometry in children with this disorder, show no abnormality; however, a central (cortical) auditory origin is postulated because the children respond best to language presented in a visual modality and also some individuals do appear to have abnormal auditory adaptation to cortical auditory evoked responses with frequency modulated stimuli.

Degenerative disorders

Speech and language can be lost progressively as part of the more generalized loss of psychosocial skills that is seen in a variety of degenerative brain disorders. The causes, clinical features and differential diagnosis of these uncommon conditions are described by Rosenbloom (1981). Deterioration is often slow. As with other disorders in which cognitive functions are globally impaired, retardation of linguistic progress may be the first indication that anything is wrong. More comprehensive assessment then indicates the widespread range of disabilities.

Unusually a severe form of acquired autistic behaviour with loss of language, social isolation and obsessional characteristics can be the presenting feature of degenerative brain disorders in childhood.

Emotional and behavioural disorders

Emotional disorders may make children reluctant to communicate. However, when there are no or few other signs of psychological disturbance, emotional and behavioural disorders are an implausible explanation for delayed language acquisition and great care is needed in assuming this aetiology in individual cases.

Elective mutism

This term is used to describe children who refuse to speak in all but a few situations and appear excessively shy. A significant proportion of electively mute children also have articulatory or language defects. In such cases reticence may be an understandable reaction to being teased, criticized or not understood. Others can speak normally but fail to do so. Such individuals do not have a language disorder but they may have other features of psychiatric disability.

Environmental deprivation

Environmental deprivation can be due to physical factors, for example poverty, malnutrition and poor housing, or to social factors, for example a lack of a caring relationship between children and their caretakers or inadequate linguistic stimulation. When severe, both forms of deprivation tend to occur at the same time and, in such circumstances, children do show global developmental delay but with particular impairment linguistically. Similar findings have been demonstrated in institutionalized children suggesting that, even when children's physical needs are reasonably catered for, severe and continuing social deprivation in itself can adversely affect the development of language.

In less extreme situations, however, there is no evidence that children of working class mothers have significantly depressed linguistic attainments when compared with middle class children (Tizard *et al.*, 1983). It has also been demonstrated that placing children in a day nursery may well be counterproductive from the language development viewpoint for the vast majority of children who have conventional rearing experiences.

Unknown aetiology – developmental language disorders

Many children present with language disorders for which there is no obvious explanation. Peripheral hearing is normal, non-verbal intelligence is good, the family home adequate and there is no sign of genetic, physical or psychiatric abnormality. These can be termed for the time being the 'developmental language disorders', although it is reasonable to assume that in due course their specific causation will become clearer.

Stuttering

Here speech is dysfluent and individual words are disrupted by syllable or sound repetition or sound prolongation. Stuttering is more common in boys than girls and tends to run in families. It is presumed that both genetic and environmental factors contribute to its presentation in individual children. Most young children go through a period of dysfluency as they learn language and parental anxiety may exacerbate or prolong the problem. Specific and direct help to affected children from speech therapists is usually best delayed, however, until children themselves are aware of their having a significant problem.

Delayed language acquisition

This term is often used loosely about any language difficulty; however, it should really be reserved for those children whose overall development is normal but whose language development progresses at a slow rate with essentially normal language nevertheless appearing by the age of about 6 years. This development pattern can be regarded as a normal biological variant rather than evidence of a neurodevelopmental disorder.

The problem for clinicians in such cases is how to distinguish language delay and language disorder in practice. One clue to outcome is the severity of the problem especially if it is monitored over a period of time. As a rule of thumb, there should be cause for concern if a child has only a handful of words at 3 years, speaks in single words at 3½ years or in two word utterances at 4 years.

It may also be that the pattern of a child's immature language can also give a guide to the prognosis. Thus, those who have a phonological system resembling that of younger normal children are likely to have a better outcome than those with deviant characteristics.

Phonological syntactic syndrome (Rapin and Allen, 1983)

This is the most common variety of developmental language disorder in which otherwise normal children have selective difficulties with language form but have normal language content. There is a normal urge to communicate and sensible and appropriate things are said but in a phonologically inappropriate or unintelligible way. There is a wide range of severity in this disorder ranging from total unintelligibility to relatively minor deviations in individual children's sound systems.

Parents typically report slow language development from birth and there is often a positive family history of language or reading difficulties. Boys are two to three times more likely to be affected than girls. In addition to their phonological problems, affected children may also have oromotor dysfunction including a history of difficulty in swallowing, sucking or chewing.

As time proceeds, there is usually slow resolution of this disorder, but not infrequently children are significantly behind in their basic school attainments and social adjustment by the time that reasonable expressive language is acquired.

Semantic pragmatic disorder

In this condition, children have difficulty in using language as a social tool. As a result they demonstrate a literal and rigid use of language, have major comprehension difficulties, for example of abstract concepts, and have problems in initiating and maintaining social contacts and understanding the rules of social behaviour. As a result, many become socially isolated. The term to describe such children was first used by Rapin and Allen (1983). In their mildest forms semantic and pragmatic problems, especially in older children, may be subtle and difficult to distinguish from normality, but detailed language testing reveals comprehension problems. More severely affected children clearly overlap those who can be labelled as autistic. Social skill training programmes rather than conventional language therapy appears to effect improvement in individuals with this disorder.

Congenital auditory imperception

Very rarely indeed, children appear to be born with normal peripheral hearing but an inability to make sense of spoken language. Affected individuals make very slow linguistic progress and frequently have to be provided in due course with alternative communication systems, for example with signing. It may very well be that affected children have a defect in auditory cortical functioning but the methodology to confirm this is not yet available.

Assessment and management of childhood language disorders

In promoting children's optimal functioning it is reasonable to surmise that early detection, full assessment, relevant treatment programmes and appropriate advice to parents contribute significantly.

Screening programmes for developmental abnormalities in childhood include linguistic items and it is appropriate that language be seen in the context of overall child development, rather than that abnormalities of language should be separately sought. Similarly, when children are found to have developmental problems and are referred for comprehensive assessment evaluation, their linguistic functioning needs to be set within this context if only because of the interaction that exists between linguistic and other developmental parameters. It cannot be emphasized too strongly, however, that accurate and detailed evaluation of auditory functioning in children who present with developmental or linguistic delay is fundamental.

When, following comprehensive assessment, children are found to have language disorders, the detailed analysis needs to be multidisciplinary and based on the children's perceived developmental and educational needs. Full description of therapy and educational programmes for language disordered children is beyond the remit of this discussion. The points can nevertheless be made that not only do relevant therapy and educational resources need to be made available for language disordered children but also that their parents need appropriate counselling and advice.

References

BISHOP, D. V. M. (1983) Comprehension of English syntax by profoundly deaf children. *Journal of Child Psychology and Psychiatry*, **24**, 415–434

BISHOP, D. V. M. and ROSENBLOOM, L. (1986) Childhood language disorders; classification and overview. In *Language Development and Disorders*, edited by W. Yule, M. Rutter and M. Bax. *Clinics in Developmental Medicine* Nos. 99/100. Oxford: MacKeith Press/Blackwell

FRIEDRICH, U., DALBY, M., STAEHELIN-JENSEN, T. and BRUUN-PETERSEN, G. (1982) Chromosomal studies of children with developmental language retardation. *Developmental Medicine and Child Neurology*, **24**, 645–652

HADENIUS, A. M., HAGBERG, B., HYTHAS-BENSCH, K. and SJOGREN, I. (1962) The natural prognosis of infantile hydrocephalus *Acta Paediatrica*, **51**, 117–118

LANDAU, W., KLEFFNER, F. (1957) Syndrome of acquired aphasia with convulsive disorder in children. *Neurology*, **7**, 523–530

MARTIN, J. A. M. (1981) *Voice, Speech and Language in the Child: Development and Disorder*. Vienna: Springer-Verlag

MORLEY, M. (1965) *The Development and Disorders of Speech in Childhood*, 2nd edn. London: Churchill Livingstone

RAPIN, I. and ALLEN, D. (1983) Developmental language disorders; nosologic considerations. In *Neuropsychology of Language, Reading and Spelling*, edited by U. Kirk. New York: Academic Press

REYNELL, J. K. (1977) *Manual for the Reynell Developmental Language Scales (Revised)*. Windsor: NFER

ROSENBLOOM, L. (1981) Chronic central nervous system disease in childhood. In *Recent Advances in Paediatrics 6*, edited by D. Hull. Edinburgh: Churchill Livingstone

SPARKS, S. N. (1984) *Birth Defects and Speech-Language Disorders*. San Diego: College-Hill Press

SHERIDAN, M. D. (1961) Disorders of spoken language in young children. *Archives of Disease in Childhood*, **36**, 11–16

TIZARD, B., HUGHES, M., CARMICHAEL, H. and PINKERTON, G. (1983) Language and social class; is verbal deprivation a myth? *Journal of Child Psychology and Psychiatry*, **24**, 533–542

11

Disorders of speech

Debbie Sell

The aim of this chapter is to describe the range of paediatric speech disorders that may present to the otolaryngologist. It is hoped that by providing the otolaryngologist with insight into speech therapy, it will promote effective teamwork between the disciplines involved as emphasized by Bull and Cook (1976).

Speech is arguably the most interesting and certainly one of the most complex and highly skilled learned behaviours of which man is capable (Code and Ball, 1984).

Speech is viewed here as a generic term to cover the complex motor activity of the vocal tract in the production of spoken language. However, it is more than just motor activity. Speech is intimately involved with language, and is dependent on maturation and intelligence, and audiological, physiological, environmental and psychosocial factors.

The distinction between speech and language has been described elsewhere (Crystal, 1980). It is important to appreciate this dichotomy. It is also possible to view the relationship between language and speech as a hierarchy of interacting levels from semantic, syntactic (language) to phonetic (speech) with the phonological level acting as a bridge between the two (Lyons, 1968).

It can be appreciated therefore that a disorder of speech implies that the formulation of meaning is not affected, but the transmission of messages through the medium of sound is in some way impaired. The production of speech requires the controlled integration of the respiratory-phonatory, resonatory and articulatory musculature. These three muscular systems of the vocal tract are inextricably interwoven and interrelated, but for simplicity, each system will be discussed separately.

A disorder can occur in one or more systems. Alternatively a problem in just one system may be reflected in another system as a consequence of the development of compensatory gestures in the vocal tract. For this reason the aetiology of a speech disorder may not be easy to identify (Crystal, 1980).

In broad terms, the causes of speech disorders can be *organic* or *functional*, but are very often a combination of the two. Therefore, the severity of the speech disorder may not be directly related to the degree of organic involvement. Functional causes include faulty learning, habit, imitation, environmental or psychological factors.

Furthermore, in paediatrics, any communication disorder must be considered within the context of the normal processes and sequences of development generally. Therefore the speech disorder is evaluated taking into account the maturation of the relevant skills in the individual child, and with regard to the possibility of delay in this maturational process.

The speech therapist considers the whole range of communication abilities of the child referred with a speech disorder and not just his speech production. Where appropriate, the following may be investigated: feeding history, prelanguage skills, communicative competence, play and non-verbal skills, the child's level of understanding, his use and content of language, stage of development in grammatical structures, and his attention and listening skills.

In considering appropriate intervention and management strategies, the speech therapist selects from a range of possibilities, including referral to other agencies, instigation of a therapy programme, and the possible prescription of alternative or augmentative communication systems.

Table 11.1 Classic areas of speech disorders

	Disorders	*Classification*		
	Disorders of articulation	Phonetic Phonological		
Speech	Disorders of resonance	Hypernasality e.g. velopharyngeal insufficiency Hyponasality Mixed nasality		
	Disorders of phonation/respiration	Organic	Congenital e.g. structural anomalies Acquired	
		Functional/psychogenic e.g. vocal abuse and vocal nodules, mutational falsetto		

Combined disorders of articulation, resonance, phonation-respiration
Hearing impairment
Craniofacial abnormality
Long-term tracheostomy
Stammering

This chapter, however, focuses on the classic area of speech disorders. Disorders of *articulation, resonance* and *phonation-respiration* are each considered. This is followed by a discussion of complex speech disorders found in association with *hearing impairment, craniofacial abnormality,* and *long-term tracheostomy.* Finally the disorder of *stammering* is covered (*Table 11.1*).

Disorders of articulation

An articulation disorder exists if there is a failure to communicate effectively using spoken language, resulting from abnormal pronunciation. It is intended for this discussion to focus on the impairment at the segmental level, that is individual phonemes or speech sounds. A discussion of the suprasegmental features of speech, including intonation, stress, rhythm and phrasing is considered below under hearing impairment.

The nature and severity of articulation disorders is highly variable, and ranges from complete unintelligibility to a mild error in speech, such as a difficulty with a particular sound or group of sounds, as with lisping or a 'weak' r. Aetiology of articulation disorders is often multifactorial.

Traditionally the phonetic aspect of an articulation problem was stressed but, with the recent contributions of linguistics, there have been considerable advances made in the understanding of articulation disorders such that it is now possible to view articulation as both physiological and linguistic in nature. It is therefore important to appreciate the complex relationship between phonetics and phonology, to understand fully the nature of speech disorders.

The phonetic aspect of articulation refers to the physical adjustments and movements of the speech articulators (lips, tongue, and palate being the primary articulators), in the modification of the air stream for the production of individual speech sounds. The phonological aspect refers to the way in which the sound system of a language is organized into a system of contrasts that has the role of distinguishing meanings in a language. For example, in the words – sea, key, bee, me – the initial sounds /s, k, b, m/ function contrastively with each other to distinguish the different word meanings. When the child is limited in his ability to signal these contrasts, he has a problem at the phonological level. It should be noted, however, that phonological disorders are not satisfactorily classified as disorders of articulation but for logistic reasons will be dealt with in this way.

Classification of articulation disorders

Two groups can be identified:

(1) phonetic disorders
(2) phonological disorders.

Phonetic disorders

A disorder leading to a speech disability at the phonetic level, involves an inability or difficulty in the physical production of speech. The phonological sound system may or may not be complete. There is some kind of physical distortion in sound production. A common example is the variation heard in the production of /r/ or /s/ speech sounds. A phonetic disorder is usually a result of an organic deficiency in the speech mechanism, such as a structural abnormality, sensory impairment, or impairment of neurophysiological functioning.

Two distinct types of phonetic disorders that are distinguished using a medical classification are *articulatory dyspraxia* and *dysarthria*.

Articulatory dyspraxia occurs when the child knows what he wishes to say but exhibits great difficulty in achieving the intended pronunciation. The controlled coordinated sequence of articulatory movements that is required, presents major difficulties. The child frequently has a generalized oral-motor problem that affects non-speech oral activities including feeding. There is no paralysis, and the disorder is distinguished by its variability so that a movement that may be presenting difficulties on one occasion may be adequately performed at another time (Grunwell, 1982).

Dysarthria reflects a neuromuscular involvement of the articulators, characterized by muscular weakness and lack of muscular control. There is a disturbance in the execution of the motor patterns for speech and feeding, due to paralysis or incoordination of the speech musculature. This is often seen in children with cerebral palsy.

Phonological disorders

A disorder leading to a speech disability at the phonological level, involves the use of an abnormal, inadequate, or disorganized system of sound patterns. The child is usually able to make articulatory movements and most speech sounds can be easily elicited in isolation or non-meaningful speech. In other words the child is able to make all the sounds required, but has difficulty organizing these sounds into a system for signalling differences in meaning. For example, a common phonological problem is one where in speaking, the child only makes lingual sounds at one place in his mouth, despite the ability to produce a full range of tongue movements, and the individual speech sounds, in isolation. The usual wide range of tongue placements used in speech is reduced to one. Continuing the example above, if /s,k,t,/ were all produced at the alveolar ridge as a /d/ sound, this would result in the words sea, key, tea all being pronounced dee. The child would thus have a severely reduced sound system. The cause of a phonological disability is not fully understood, but appears to be a neurolinguistic dysfunction at the phonological level of cortical representation, and organization of the language system (Grunwell, 1982).

Some patients have these disorders despite having normal hearing, with no detectable neurological, physiological or anatomical deficit. Comprehension of speech is normal, intelligence is within the average range, and often expressive language appears to be developing along normal lines, although this is difficult to assess as the children often have reduced intelligibility.

Although much remains unknown about these problems, several types of phonological disorders can be distinguished. Children with developmental phonological disorders may exhibit delayed or deviant pronunciation patterns. The delayed phonological pattern follows the normal sequence of development but is appropriate for a younger child. The deviant pattern is characterized by features not seen in normal phonological development.

It is possible to have either a phonetic or a phonological disorder, but the majority of articulation problems are a combination of the two.

Aetiology of phonetic and phonological disorders

Organic and functional factors may be identified as causes of articulation disorders, although very often the aetiology is unknown or a result of a combination of factors.

Organic causes

Structural deviations

Structural deviations of the oral cavity, such as malocclusion, abnormalities of dentition, microglossia or macroglossia, tongue tie, tongue thrust and repaired cleft palate, may or may not affect speech. A simple one-to-one relationship does not exist between structural deficits and defective speech characteristics. There is also much individual variation, as described below under craniofacial abnormality. Here, a discussion of two of the more common conditions follows.

Tongue thrust

Often tongue thrust may be seen in association with mouth breathing and enlarged tonsils, such that the latter may be an aetiological factor in the development of tongue thrust (Hanson, Barnard and Case, 1969). This may or may not be associated with an articulation problem, but when it is, may well present as an interdental /s/. The sounds /sz/ normally made at the alveolar ridge are produced with the tongue between the teeth resulting in the sound /th/.

Tongue tie or ankylossia

It is often thought that tongue tie may be the cause of speech difficulties. Research has failed to prove a positive relationship between tongue tie and speech disorders, or other oral motor dysfunction (Bloomer, 1971). In practice, it is seldom the case that a tongue tie is the cause of a speech difficulty. In a child presenting with tongue tie and a speech problem all the factors that may impinge on the speech disorder should be taken into account in assessing each child. A speech therapy assessment will determine the degree to which the tongue tie and the speech disorder are related.

If the child is able to protrude his tongue beyond his central incisors, or there is some evidence of the use of alveolar placements in his speech, such as the sounds /t, d, l, s/ it is unlikely that the tongue tie is significantly affecting his speech and its release is unnecessary (McEnery and Gaines, 1941). Speech therapy is recommended to establish a full sound system.

The situation may arise, however, when a child consistently fails to maintain the use of these sounds in conversation or alternatively it may not be possible to elicit alveolar sounds. This may occur where the child has additional problems. There then may be an argument for releasing the tongue tie, but this decision should be based on the speech therapist's assessment and knowledge of the child's progress in therapy.

Williams and Waldron (1985) described a method of clinical measurement in an attempt to obtain a more objective system for evaluating lingual function.

Hearing impairment

This is discussed more fully below.

Neuromotor pathology

This has been briefly discussed in the preceding section and further discussion is not pertinent to the concerns of this chapter. The reader is referred elsewhere for information on speech disorders associated with neurophysiological deficits (Darley, Aronson and Brown, 1975).

Functional causes

Research has been directed to the role of auditory perceptual skills as a causal factor, and although it has been found that a relationship does exist between speech sound discrimination and impaired phonology, the precise nature of this relationship is not fully understood (Winitz, 1969).

Research has failed to demonstrate a significant and consistent relationship between oral sensory function, or depressed oral motor skills, and speech disorders (Bernthal and Bankson, 1981). Acquisition of the adult sound system is positively related to maturation and problems in language acquisition, and later difficulties in reading and writing. Many diverse environmental influences, such as poor speech models, sibling status, lack of stimulation, inappropriate reinforcement, or the child's emotional reaction to the speech difficulty are often felt to be significant in the development and maintenance of a disorder. Such factors are not easily verified by research.

Assessment of articulation disorders

The speech therapist assesses the child's speech, using principles of phonetic and phonological analysis, and standardized test procedures that give quantitative and qualitative evaluations. In addition, the therapist fully assesses the speech mechanism and oral-motor skills, language, and other aspects of speech production. Referral for audiological assessment should be considered. The listening skills involving auditory memory, discrimination and sequencing are all evaluated, and may be a focus for remediation. It is then possible to differentiate between the different types of disorder, that is phonological, phonetic, or both. This information is added to that gained from the case history, and assessments of other aspects of the child's abilities and related behaviour.

Traditionally, an articulation disorder was assessed in terms of omissions, substitutions, or distortions of speech sounds. This is now regarded as an inadequate framework, in that it considers each mispronounced sound separately and not in relation to each other. Instead the aim of the phonological analysis is to compare patterns of contrast used in the child's system with those used in the adult system.

Management of articulation disorders

The focus of therapy in a phonological disorder is to facilitate change in the child's patterns, so that the child can be assisted to acquire the missing phonological contrasts together with the required motor movements to signal them. The focus of therapy in a phonetic disorder is directed at the mechanics of articulation often aimed towards developing compensatory movements.

Referral guidelines

The following are broad guidelines for referral:

(1) the child who presents to the otolaryngologist with no words at 20–24 months
(2) the child who is not speaking in phrases at 28 months
(3) the child who is unintelligible at 3 years or above.

Early referral to the speech therapist is essential in the long-term management of the speech-impaired child (Byers Brown, 1981). Any suggestion of parental concern should be investigated thoroughly by a speech therapist.

Disorders of resonance

Normal resonance

Resonance is a complex attribute of speech that is not completely understood. It refers perceptually to the overall tone or timbre of the voice. In physical terms it may be defined as the vibratory response of a body or air-filled cavity to a frequency imposed upon it (Wood, 1971). The resonating cavities anatomically consist of the supraglottic larynx, the hypopharynx, the oropharynx and nasopharynx, and the oral and nasal cavities.

Resonance depends primarily on the size and shape of the pharynx as altered by the pharyngeal muscles, and on the patency of the oral and nasal cavities. In the normal speaker there is a balance between nasal and oral resonance and in English the balance is primarily oral. Resonance is further influenced by the extrinsic laryngeal muscles, which affect not only the shape of the pharyngeal resonators, but also the mode of vocal fold vibration (MacCurtain and Fourcin, 1982). Movement of the articulators, especially the tongue, also affects resonance.

Almost all sounds in the English sound system are characterized by oral resonance. Plosives /p,b,t,d,k,g/, fricatives /s,z,f,v/, affricates /ch,ge/, all require varying degrees of intraoral pressure, and are dependent on effective velopharyngeal closure for their adequate production (*Figure 11.1*). The only exceptions are the nasal continuants /m,n,ng/. These sounds are produced by the lowering of the velum, effectively coupling the nasal and oral resonators (*Figure 11.2*). A certain amount of nasal resonance may also be normally heard in vowels that occur adjacent to the nasal continuants. In other languages, different situations may be observed. In French, for example, oral vowels function contrastively with nasalized vowels to signal different word meanings.

Disordered resonance

Resonance is deviant when there is an imbalance in the overall harmonic spectrum of the voice leading to abnormal tone. This occurs when the usual size or shape of the resonators is changed significantly in some way. There are two distinct causes.

(1) Abnormal coupling of the nasal and oral cavities as a result of structural abnormalities, such as cleft palate, or oral or nasal obstruction
(2) non-structural deficits, such as abnormal articulatory postures, excessive muscular tension in the vocal tract, and habitual poor oral opening.

The fine line between normal and pathological conditions is often a matter of the listener's preference, affected by linguistic factors, and emotional reactions to speech.

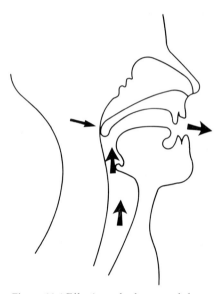

Figure 11.1 Effective velopharyngeal closure

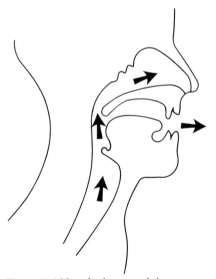

Figure 11.2 No velopharyngeal closure

Classification of disorders

Resonance disorders can be classified into three main types:

(1) hypernasality
(2) hyponasality
(3) mixed nasality.

Hypernasality (rhinolalia aperta, hyper-rhinolalia, and open nasality)

Hypernasal resonance refers to a type of abnormal tone characterized by excessive nasal resonance of voiced sounds, particularly vowels and the voiced consonants. The anatomical-physiological basis is faulty velopharyngeal function resulting in a failure of the velopharyngeal port to attain and maintain sufficient closure. Nasal escape and nasal grimacing are often associated with hypernasality. Nasal escape refers to an audible or inaudible, abnormal escape of air from the nostrils. This accompanies or replaces the target sounds, in particular fricatives. This is also sometimes referred to as nasal snort. A mirror clouding test can be used to test for nasal escape. The patient should repeat a sentence that is free of all nasal sounds, for example 'Katy's sister was six yesterday', with a mirror placed under the nares. Fogging may indicate velopharyngeal incompetence. It may help to identify hypernasality by asking the patient to repeat the test sentence above with nostrils pinched and unpinched.

Nasal grimacing refers to occlusion of the nares by contraction of the alae, and in its more severe form, may include the forehead too, resulting in facial grimace. It occurs as an unconscious attempt to effect velopharyngeal closure.

Hypernasality and nasal escape associated with velopharyngeal incompetence, is the major type of resonance disorder. This is partly because of their high association with cleft lip and palate, and their far-reaching effects on speech and language. It is a complex problem to manage, and requires a multidisciplinary team approach often involving the plastic surgeon, orthodontist, radiologist and speech therapist.

Hyponasality (denasality, rhinolalia clausa, and closed nasality)

This refers to speech in which there is reduction or absence of normal nasal resonance of the nasal continuants and a loss of normal nasal assimilation. It is also detectable in the production of vowels. In common everyday terms, it is called adenoidal speech, and usually has an organic basis.

Two subtypes of hyponasality are defined.

Rhinolalia clausa posterior

When there is an obstruction in the posterior region of the nasal cavities or nasopharynx, the nasals /m,n,ng/sound more like their voiced oral plosive equivalents /b,d,g/. In a sentence loaded with nasal sounds such as 'Mummy and Nanny are mending', the /m,n,ng/ sound more like /b,d, g/, that is 'bubby and daddy are bedding'. Using the mirror clouding test while saying such a sentence may indicate that the normal fogging that the nasal sounds produce may be prevented or reduced.

Rhinolalia clausa anterior, cul de sac

This type of hyponasality is detectable when all the vowels and nasals are produced with a muffled, hollow sounding resonance, owing to an obstruction in the anterior region of the nasal cavities. This sounds equivalent to the resonance produced when the nose is pinched.

Mixed nasality (rhinolalia mixta)

This refers to the coexistence of hyper- and hyponasality and reflects simultaneously velopharyngeal incompetence and nasal obstruction. There is fluctuating resonance, which the listener perceives as abnormal.

Aetiology of resonance disorders

Aetiology can be broadly classified as organic or functional. Organic causes include structural abnormalities, congenital, or acquired neurological conditions. Functional factors include poor learning, habit, imitation, poor motivation, immature, or improper use of the articulators (*Table 11.2*). A resonance disorder may be exacerbated by intellectual and environmental factors.

Assessment of resonance disorders

Correct identification of nasality type is not easy for the untrained listener. Aronson (1985) described how many professional people in medicine and allied health fields, as well as parents, often describe hyponasal speech erroneously as nasal, inferring velopharyngeal insufficiency instead of nasopharyngeal obstruction. A study by Razzell, Anthony and Watson (1983) however, demonstrated the accuracy of the trained ear of the speech therapist in the assessment of nasal air escape and resonance. The speech therapist's role in dealing with resonance problems is to identify type, degree, consistency, and severity of disordered resonance.

Table 11.2 Aetiology of resonance disorders

Organic
Hypernasality
  history of repaired cleft palate
  submucous cleft palate
  occult cleft palate
  congenitally short soft palate
  large nasopharynx
  post adenoidectomy
  trauma
  severe hearing loss
  following midfacial osteotomy
  neuromuscular impairment e.g. palatal paresis,
    cerebral palsy
Hyponasality
  deviated nasal septum
  space-occupying lesion
  construction of a pharyngeal flap
Mixed nasality
  combination of aetiologies of hyper- and hyponasality
Functional
Habit ⎫
Imitation ⎪
Poor motivation ⎬ Hyper- and hyponasality
Poor learning ⎭
Inappropriate tongue postures ⎫
Degree of mouth opening ⎬ Hypernasality
Rate of speech ⎭

Hypernasality

In addition to assessing hypernasal resonance, the therapist detects nasal air escape, and describes fully the range of phonetic contexts in which it occurs. Velopharyngeal incompetence not only causes hypernasality and nasal escape, but is often associated with articulation problems.

When the velopharyngeal port is left open, air escapes through the nose and the necessary oral air pressure required for plosives, fricatives and affricates is then either reduced or absent. This may lead to a weak nasally distorted production of the target sound, or the development of compensatory articulation patterns. One example of this is the use of laryngeal sounds or pharyngeal sounds, such as the glottal stop or pharyngeal fricative (*Figure 11.3*). Another compensatory pattern is the excessive use of velar placement referred to as tongue bunching (*Figure 11.4*).

The presence of these abnormal articulation patterns may complicate the evaluation of the velopharyngeal mechanism. In a tongue bunching pattern the back of the tongue may habitually force air through the velopharyngeal area with the resulting impression of velopharyngeal incompetence (Huskie, 1983). The opposite may arise when speech is characterized by an excessive amount of glottal stops. Since these sounds are

released well before air can be lost at the velopharyngeal sphincter, it may sound as if there is a competent sphincter mechanism.

In addition, velopharyngeal insufficiency may encourage the development of dysphonia from compensatory vocal abuse, and abnormal use of tongue patterns.

The speech therapist makes a detailed oral examination of structure and function, and performs a full phonetic and phonological analysis. The ease with which resonance, nasal escape or

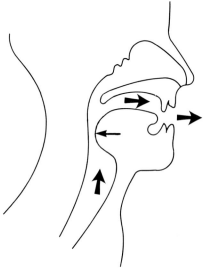

Figure 11.3 Pharyngeal fricative – fricative produced by constriction of the pharyngeal walls and the posterior elevation of the tongue

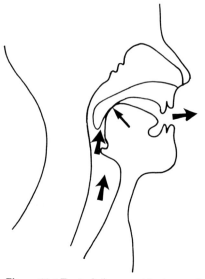

Figure 11.4 Typical placement for tongue bunching

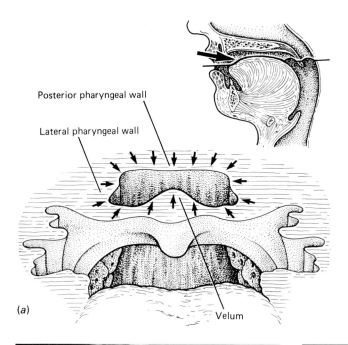

Posterior pharyngeal wall

Lateral pharyngeal wall

Velum

(a)

Figure 11.5 (*a*) Three-dimensional view of section through the velopharyngeal port; (*b*) lateral upper airways – X-ray showing quiet breathing; (*c*) lateral upper airways – X-ray showing patient with velopharyngeal incompetence saying the vowel 'ee'

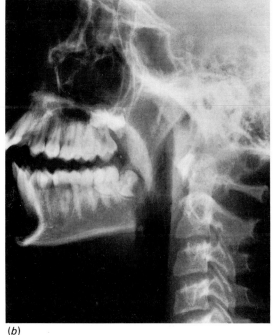

(b)

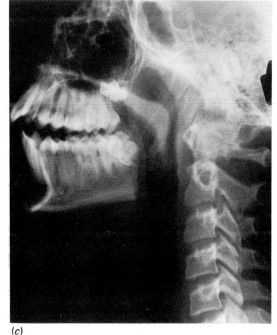

(c)

defective articulation may be modified is ascertained. This perceptual assessment is supplemented by the objective techniques of nasoendoscopy and multiview videofluoroscopy which provide invaluable information about velopharyngeal structure and function and are essential for determining appropriate management (*Figure 11.5*). These techniques determine the nature of

and contexts in which velopharyngeal closure can be achieved. Furthermore, the reasons for incompetency and the potential for closure can be identified. The speech therapist should be present during these procedures, so that the nature of the speech sample elicited can be determined according to the individual child's speech problem. All the assessments are discussed with the surgeon and future management is then decided. Other information may be gained from nasal anemometry (Ellis, 1979) (*Figures 11.6, 11.7, 11.8 and 11.9*). This investigates abnormal nasal air flow, its instant of occurrence, and its peak value during speech. Although equipment has been designed to measure the area of velopharyngeal opening and resistance to airflow during speech, as a method of assessment of the velopharyngeal port (Warren, 1964), this is not readily available for routine clinical use.

Management of hypernasal resonance

The speech therapist contributes to a differential diagnosis identifying the organic, functional and

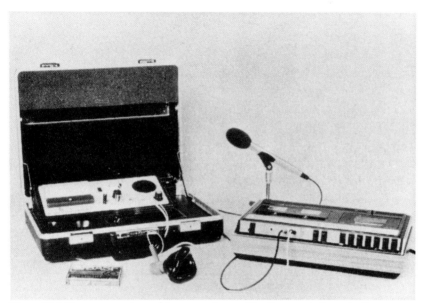

Figure 11.6 The anemometer and tape recorder used by the speech therapist (by permission of the College of Speech Therapists)

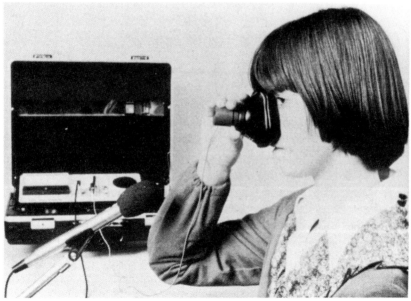

Figure 11.7 Patient holding mask in correct position for recording (by permission of the College of Speech Therapists)

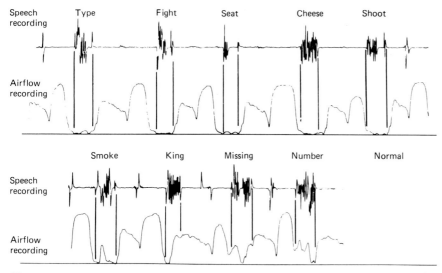

Figure 11.8 Typical anemometry chart produced from recordings of a normal speaker (by permission of the College of Speech Therapists)

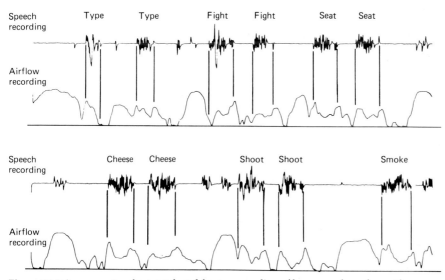

Figure 11.9 Anemometry chart produced from a recording of hypernasal speaker with velopharyngeal incompetence (by permission of the College of Speech Therapists)

other contributory factors and recommending therapy where appropriate.

Speech therapy may be sufficient in some cases, but if surgery is required, this should always be supported by pre- and postoperative speech therapy assessment.

In velopharyngeal incompetence, where the disorder is purely one of resonance, speech therapy is unsuccessful (McWilliams, 1983). Surgical intervention is indicated, although obturation may be an alternative method of management.

However, when velopharyngeal incompetence is associated with other articulation problems, there is a case for speech therapy directed at these while waiting definitive assessment and surgery. Indeed, sometimes a course of therapy, aimed at eliminating erroneous tongue patterns, may be an essential precursor to allow for the accurate assessment of the sphincter mechanism on endoscopy. Furthermore, parents sometimes accept more easily that a surgical procedure is required to achieve normal speech if a course of speech therapy has been followed, and been only partially successful. This group of children usually requires postoperative therapy.

Speech therapy is appropriate when closure at the velopharyngeal sphincter is achieved on some sounds, but not others. Here, habit may be a factor. These cases underline the importance of the speech therapist's presence at endoscopy and multiview videofluoroscopy, so that the best possible oral speech sample is used. Otherwise the child could be submitted to unnecessary surgery.

Children may present with inconsistent nasal escape and hypernasality. This variation may be related to phonetic context, rate of speech, length, spontaneity of utterance, or psychosocial factors such as fatigue or stress. A timing defect of closure may account for this, reflecting poor coordination. In borderline cases of incompetency it is not always straightforward to determine if physical management or speech therapy is required (McWilliams, Morris and Shelton, 1984). In the first instance speech therapy is indicated. Such cases may be appropriate for a palatal training device in collaboration with the orthodontist, for example as developed by Selley (1979). This possibly assists the relaxation of the palatoglossus muscle which may in turn allow the levator palati to be more efficient. It encourages dorsal tongue relaxation, thereby reducing hypernasality by increasing oral patency. This aid alone may be sufficient, but it may be necessary to improve the timing defect with the help of a visual speech aid (*Figure 11.10*). This provides immediate visual feedback of soft palate movement in therapy.

Acquired hypernasality

One of the most worrying problems for any otolaryngologist is when an apparently normal child develops hypernasal speech following adenoidectomy. Excessive nasality and nasal escape may develop temporarily, but this usually does not persist for longer than a few days or weeks at the most. A study by Neiman and Simpson (1975) concluded that the velopharyngeal mechanism normally compensates for the imbalance between pharyngeal dimensions and velar length caused by adenoidectomy.

When, however, there is a deficit in the velopharyngeal valving mechanism, and the adenoids are removed, hypernasality will persist. Assessment and management of this disorder are then indicated. A brief period of therapy should be tried, aimed at encouraging oral resonance and preventing the development of nasal grimace. Usually this condition responds poorly to therapy. Objective investigations are then instigated, and surgery is frequently indicated.

The patients at greatest risk for this outcome postadenoidectomy are those where there is a history of cleft palate, submucous cleft palate, congenital short palate, large nasopharynx, motor deficits, or scarring from tonsillectomy producing a stiff immobile palate. Adenoidectomy should actively be avoided in these cases. Possible predictive factors for incompetency have been described (Mason, 1973; Morris, Krueger and Bumsted, 1982). They stated that evidence of any

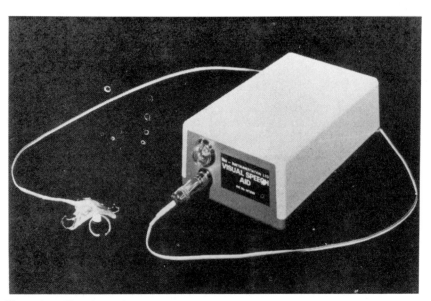

Figure 11.10 Visual speech aid with palatal training appliance (by permission of the College of Speech Therapists)

structural or neurological abnormality of the velopharyngeal structures, family history of cleft lip, cleft palate, congenital velopharyngeal insufficiency, or related disorders, especially nasalization, and nasal leakage during feeding in infancy all appear to be relevant.

Careful joint assessment, if there is any doubt, with the speech therapist and radiologist is recommended. Croft *et al.* (1978) described indications of potential velopharyngeal incompetence that can be seen on multiview videofluoroscopy, in particular any sign of borderline valving.

Functional hypernasality

Speech therapy is appropriate when no demonstrable organic deficit is found, and faulty learning or psychological factors are the cause (Peterson, 1975).

Hyponasality

Hyponasality is almost always organically based, although occasionally it may have a functional basis, such as imitation or habit. For example, the voice may continue to be hyponasal following tonsillectomy or adenoidectomy. Therapy may be indicated.

Disorders of phonation

Normal phonation

Perkins (1971) described as efficient, a voice that yields maximum acoustic output, flexibility and pleasant tonal qualities, with minimal effort in phonation. Wilson (1979) considered that the rate of speech is also an important factor in normal voice production.

Adequate voice production depends on a finely balanced interaction in the vocal tract between airflow, vocal fold tension, and supraglottic gesture, that is changes in size, and/or shape of the oropharynx, nasopharynx, hypopharynx, and oral cavity. It demands adequate breath control and capacity, combined with relaxed musculature and good posture, efficient use of the articulators and forward tone. Van Deinse (1982) stated that the whole of the vocal tract is involved in the production of voice.

Disorders of phonation

A disorder of phonation, often referred to as dysphonia, exists when the abnormality of voice production is located at the laryngeal level. The psychoacoustic or perceptual parameters of voice, that of quality, pitch, and intensity, deviate from that expected for the age, sex and cultural group of the child.

These parameters and their potential abnormalities are outlined below.

Voice quality

Voice quality is the perception of the physical complexity of the laryngeal tone, modified by resonance. Disturbed voice quality caused by laryngeal dysfunction is usually described using terms such as harsh, breathy, or hoarse. Such terminology has its limitations as rarely is the disordered voice characterized by only one type of quality. Studies have also found that there is inconsistency among speech therapists in their choice of labels (Wynter, 1974). However, as voice quality cannot yet be measured through instrumentation this descriptive terminology is still used.

Harshness is characterized by abrupt voice onset, low pitch, weak intensity, and overadduction of the vocal cords. There is frequent excessive tension of the laryngeal musculature involving a constricted vocal tract. It is often associated with generalized upper body tension.

Breathiness is a combination of phonation and the whispery noise components of turbulent air. It occurs when the vocal folds are not fully approximated, as in bowing, or vocal cord palsy, and unvibrated air is audible. In its more extreme form, when no air is set in vibration, the resulting voice is produced without phonation, and is described as aphonic. The breathy voice is characterized by limited intensity, and low pitch.

Hoarseness combines the acoustic characteristics of harshness and breathiness and usually results from laryngeal pathology. Pitch is usually low, restricted in range with pitch breaks. Aphonic episodes may also be observed.

Pitch

Pitch can be inappropriately high, low, uncontrolled, or restricted in range. Glottal fry is a term used to describe the creaky voice associated with the inappropriate use of lower pitch range.

Intensity

Intensity, or volume can be inappropriately soft or loud, or uncontrolled.

Rate of utterance and resonance, need to be considered, because of the important role they play in the overall voice as highlighted by Perkins (1971).

Taking an overall view, although pitch and intensity can be measured objectively with instrumentation, such as electrolaryngography, quality relies on the subjective impression of the listener. This lack of measurement means the decision that the voice is abnormal is culturally and environmentally determined, and relies upon the orientation of the listener. Most studies quote the incidence of phonatory disorders as approximately 6–9% of the school-aged population, and yet probably a significant number of these children are not referred for investigation. This is reflected in a study by Wertz and Mead (1975) showing how phonatory disorders were rated by teachers as the least handicapping communication difficulty compared with other disorders. Parents are often unaware of the voice disorder, in that they have never known their child to sound any different.

As some authors claim that the disordered voice in adults may have its roots in childhood (Ellis, 1959), it is very important for the paediatric voice disordered population to be treated. Ellis identified the particular risk factors in children as vocal strain, habitual shouting, screaming, or singing in an unnatural pitch range.

Assessment of phonation

The aim of the speech therapist's assessment, which usually takes at least one hour, is to provide the otolaryngologist with a detailed description of the patient's voice characteristics, and the significant psychosocial factors. A voice case history is obtained, such that environmental, physical, personality and emotional factors are explored. The voice history examines onset, duration, variability, severity of the voice disorder and patterns of voice use.

The therapist considers posture and respiratory function. Restricted thoracic movement or poorly coordinated movement of the muscles of respiration may lead to inadequate control of the expiratory air stream. This results in irregularities of vocal fold function, particularly affecting intensity and strength of glottal closure. However, for the majority of voice disordered patients, respiration is anatomically and physiologically normal. Compromised breathing patterns are probably due to anxiety and tension, or faulty habits, causing shallow upper chest and clavicular breathing, and inadequate control of the air stream.

The therapist subjectively evaluates different parameters of voice production: pitch range, optimal pitch, habitual pitch, pitch discrimination, intensity, voice quality, maximum phonation time, and sites of musculoskeletal tension. Often rating scales are used, such as the Buffalo voice profile, designed by D. K. Wilson (1979) (*Figure 11.11*). This allows the therapist to make several simultaneous severity evaluations on different

Name ______ Birth Date ______ Age ____ Sex ____

Rater ______ Date ______ Time of Day ______ Place ______

1. *Laryngeal Tone* Normal Breathy Harsh Hoarse	1	2	3	4	5	6	7
2. *Laryngeal Tension* Normal Hypertense Hypotense	1	2	3	4	5	6	7
3. *Vocal Abuse* No Yes	1	2	3	4	5	6	7
4. *Loudness* Normal Too loud Too soft	1	2	3	4	5	6	7
5. *Pitch* Normal High Low	1	2	3	4	5	6	7
6. *Vocal Inflections* Normal Monotone Excessive	1	2	3	4	5	6	7
7. *Pitch Breaks* None Amount	1	2	3	4	5	6	7
8. *Diplophonia* None Amount	1	2	3	4	5	6	7
9. *Resonance* Normal Hypernasal Hyponasal	1	2	3	4	5	6	7
10. *Nasal Emission* No Yes	1	2	3	4	5	6	7
11. *Rate* Normal Fast Slow	1	2	3	4	5	6	7
12. *Overall Voice Efficiency* Adequate Inadequate	1	2	3	4	5	6	7

Circle the appropriate descriptive term under *each* item. For each item *not* normal or adequate, circle a number on the scale for that item. Do *not* mark between numbers.
Key: 1 = slight deviation 4 = moderate deviation 7 = severe deviation
COMMENTS:

Figure 11.11 Buffalo voice profile rating scale (from Wilson, 1979, *Voice Problems of Children*, 2nd edn, Baltimore: Williams and Wilkins, by kind permission of the author and publishers)

aspects of voice. An assessment of the potential to change individual vocal parameters is also made.

It is important to assess the child's awareness of the problem and to explore the ways in which the voice disorder may limit his activities, or alternatively be of benefit to him. For example he may be excluded from a disliked activity on the basis of his voice problem. Parental attitudes, and those of significant persons need also to be taken into account. The detailed case history allows the therapist to identify potential aetiology, and perpetuating factors. The original causes are often different from the factors maintaining the disorder. The therapist judges if the child would benefit from voice therapy.

It is vital for the results of the assessment to be coordinated with the findings of the other team members. Indeed, many researchers advocate a team approach as the most effective for treating children with voice disorders (Wilson, 1979).

Classification of voice disorders

One method of classifying disorders is on the basis of aetiology. Voice disorders exist on a continuum, with structural disorders at one end, and functional or psychogenic at the other (Wilson, 1979). There is an intimate relationship between the two. In practice, it is often not possible to separate organic from psychogenic factors. For example, a psychologically based voice disorder can lead to organic changes, conversely an organic condition can engender in a patient a psychological reaction which may persist after the organic condition has been medically treated. However, for ease, in this discussion, voice disorders are classified aetiologically into organic or functional.

Aetiology of voice disorders

Organic disorders

(1) *Congenital:* these include stenosis, web, vocal fold paralysis, laryngeal cyst, chromosomal defects, neurological disorders (Aronson, 1985).
(2) *Acquired:* these include neurological disease, papillomata, inflammation, or trauma, particularly long-term intubation, resulting in acquired stenosis, web formation, or cricoarytenoid fixation. Occasionally laryngeal candidiasis may complicate steroid therapy for asthma.

Psychogenic or functional disorders

This term is used when the degree of pathology, if any, is disproportionately small compared to the severity of the voice problem. The vocal folds commonly appear normal, mildly inflamed, or fail to adduct completely as in bowing.

Brodnitz (1965) has observed how often the dysphonia persists long after any organic involvement disappears, highlighting the importance of the case history seeking out psychological factors. Some patients have long-standing emotional difficulties while, in others, the voice disorder may occur as an acute reaction to a stressful situation. In some patients, the psychogenic nature of the disorder is less clear, and these patients may seem to have a purely habitual voice disorder. Research into adult voice disorders has shown that there is frequently a physiological basis to these problems. The extrinsic and intrinsic laryngeal muscles are so sensitive to emotional stress that their overcontraction may be observed resulting in measurable tension in the muscles of the vocal tract (Berry *et al.*, 1982) and hyperfunctional voice disorders (Aronson, 1985). The whole vocal tract is frequently involved, so that the shape of the supralaryngeal resonators is aberrant and inadequate air pressure is characteristic (Berry *et al.*, 1982). Therefore there would appear to be a relationship between functional dysphonia, musculoskeletal tensions, and environmental factors.

Management of organic disorders

One of the commonest organically based paediatric voice disorders results from prolonged intubation secondary to airway problems. Possible sequelae are anterior commissure webbing and posterior glottic stenosis (Dejonckere, 1984). In a study by Hengerer, Strome, and Jaffe (1975) persistent breathiness and hoarseness were observed in postintubation cases with a history of aphonia at extubation, caused by cricoarytenoid fixation. They observed that children who are not aphonic at extubation, but hoarse, usually have a normal voice at one year of age. They concluded that the degree of phonatory problem at extubation relates to the degree of damage to the larynx.

In congenital or acquired laryngeal problems such as laryngeal web, or stenosis, the voice is often characterized by excessive contraction of all the muscles participating in phonation, with observable excess tension and effort (Luchsinger, 1965). The voice of a child with laryngeal web is typically high-pitched and weak. Other structural anomalies, for example stenosis, are usually characterized by a low-pitched, hoarse voice. When a tracheostomy is required, reconstructive laryngeal procedures are aimed at improving the airway as a primary objective, such that some children manage to be decannulated at the expense of their voice.

Sometimes, if the surgical management leaves a roughened free margin on the vocal folds, for example following the removal of papillomata, dysphonia may persist and voice therapy is advocated (Prater and Swift, 1984).

The speech therapist determines if the dysphonia is of a greater severity or different in character than that warranted by the lesion, in which case a functional element is suspected. The aim of therapy is to obtain the best voice possible within the patient's anatomical and physiological capabilities, by developing compensatory phonatory and respiratory patterns, or muscle strengthening techniques, for example in vocal cord palsy.

The voice disorder found in association with neurological and developmental problems, such as cerebral palsy or Down's syndrome may play a relatively minor part in the total communication disorder, when there is impairment of the respiratory, resonatory and articulatory systems, and language skills. Sometimes, however, the abnormal voice may be causing concern, and it then becomes the focus of therapy.

Psychogenic or functional disorders
Vocal abuse and vocal nodules

Dysphonias in school-aged children are mostly a result of vocal abuse, and vocal misuse, which frequently lead to mucosal changes, and vocal nodules. The dysphonia associated with vocal nodules is often breathy or husky in quality, with a tendency towards low pitch. The mass results in reduced glottal resistance, increased airflow, and a shortened phonatory time. Patterns of vocal abuse such as shouting, yelling, excessive talking, can often be identified (Toohill, 1975) and associated with a marked degree of musculoskeletal tension.

It is logical to consider these disorders as organic, and yet more properly they should be classified as psychogenic. It is important to appreciate the significance of this. These disorders are the result of abnormal speaking behaviour, frequently associated with personality or emotional factors, so that vocal nodules were described by Brodnitz and Froeschels (1954) as 'visible organic changes that are the consequence of a functional disorder'.

Children who develop nodules differ in personality and family history from those who do not. Nemec (1961) found that children with vocal abuse, including vocal nodules, were more aggressive, less mature, and had more difficulty in managing stressful situations than children with normal voice. These personality traits have been supported by other studies (Aronson, 1985). Other causal factors, such as chronic upper respiratory tract infections in association with allergies, have been described in the literature, but basic to all, is a constitutional tendency in these children towards the development of nodules (Luchsinger, 1965).

Management

Previously speech therapy was not advocated (Greene, 1972), but therapy is now considered not only appropriate but essential (Wilson, 1979). Surgery alone is insufficient – if the aetiological factors are not changed, there will be a recurrence of nodules. Therapy aims to eliminate vocal abuses, to attend to the personality and environmental problems, and thereby reduce the stress factors that created the patterns of vocal abuse, and where appropriate, work directly at modifying individual vocal parameters. It is frequently unsuccessful however to instruct the mother to tell her child to stop a specific abusive pattern. This usually fails and is frustrating for the parent and the child.

Instead the effective management of vocal abuse is through a carefully structured behavioural programme that extends into the child's home environment, school, and clubs. This is achieved through reinforcing desirable behaviour patterns using charts, with an individually designed reward system built into them. Parental and teacher cooperation is an integral part of therapy.

Mutational falsetto (puberphonia, disturbed mutation)

The majority of male adolescents have uneventful voice change. However, the period of voice change can be stormy, with sudden voice breaks from high to low pitch, or the reverse, with a marked degree of hoarseness or huskiness. When the voice fails to change from the higher pitched voice of prepubescence to the lower pitched voice of adolescence and adulthood, the pathological condition of mutational falsetto or puberphonia exists. This condition can be found in patients of all ages, some as young as 14 or 15 years. The voice is characterized by high pitch, with pitch breaks, and restricted pitch range. It is often thin, weak, and breathy, and gives the impression of an immature and effeminate personality.

During phonation, the larynx is characteristically held high in the neck; the vocal folds are lax and stretched thin, with the body of the larynx tilted downwards. Respiration is often shallow, with inadequate subglottal air pressure so that only the medial edges of the folds vibrate (*Figure 11.12*).

Puberphonia may have a neurological basis, or may be associated with severe hearing impairment or an endocrine disorder. In the absence of these conditions it is considered a psychogenic disorder. The voice disorder may signal the rejection of the responsibilities and roles of adulthood. The patient may be embarrassed by his low pitched voice among his peers, or may unconsciously want to retain his higher-pitched singing voice. He may attend as a teenager motivated by teasing, or brought by his parents, or as a young adult tired of being taken for a woman on the telephone, or not achieving job expectations.

It is relatively easy to elicit and establish the appropriate voice in therapy. It is much more difficult to maintain the use of the new voice outside the clinic. Counselling and a carefully structured maintenance programme may be required in order to achieve long-term success.

Hypofunctional voice disorders

Bowing of the vocal folds seen on direct laryngoscopy may occur as a result of prolonged hyperfunctioning.

Psychogenic aphonia

Children fortunately rarely present with conversion voice disorders. The possibility of elective mutism should be considered in making a differential diagnosis. In severe cases if there are deep-seated emotional problems, referral to a psychologist or psychiatrist is indicated.

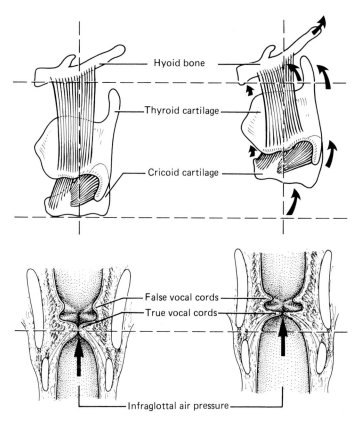

Figure 11.12 Comparison of normal laryngeal position with that of mutational falsetto. Normal phonation: relatively low position of larynx, ample thyrohyoid space blunt edges of vocal folds, high infraglottal pressure. Mutational falsetto: relatively high position of larynx, narrow thyrohyoid space, thin edges of vocal folds, low infraglottal pressure

Hearing impairment

The speech of the deaf differs from normal speech as a result of the altered sensory conditions under which speech is learnt. The deaf individual has to rely on imitating and reproducing an incoming signal which he hears in a distorted manner (Monsen, 1983). The important factors that affect the eventual quality of speech achieved include date of diagnosis, use made of residual hearing, age of onset of hearing loss, family support and quality of the language environment, individual differences, and speech training where necessary.

All forms of deafness can affect speech production. Even intermittent otitis media may affect not only speech and language development, but also cognitive, and educational achievements (Klein, 1984; Needleman, 1977; Paradise, 1981; Penniceard, 1981). There is also some suggestion of a link between early middle ear disease that subsequently resolves, and later language and educational difficulties (Penniceard, 1981).

The speech of the hearing impaired may show abnormalities in each of the systems of the vocal tract previously outlined – respiratory control, phonation, resonance, and articulation.

Segmental features

The speech of the hearing impaired characteristically shows disordered patterns in both consonant and vowel usage. The consonant system is frequently reduced, for example, high frequency sounds are often not established. The system is often characterized too by sounds that are visually distinct as these are easily learnt. In the vowel system, diphthongs are typically reduced or neutralized to a central vowel. It is important to appreciate that the deaf child may be using phonological contrasts in a highly individual way. For example, instead of using the consonant contrast /m,b/ to differentiate meaning in a pair of words such as 'me' and 'bee', the deaf child uses a /mb,b/ contrast to mark this distinction. A traditional way of viewing this would be to classify /mb/ as a distortion of /b/. It would then appear logical to eliminate the distortion therapeutically as not being a meaningful phoneme of English, but that would ignore that individual child's way of making a meaningful phonological contrast. If eliminated the individual's ability to signal the contrast between the words 'me' and 'bee' may be lost so rendering the person more unintelligible!

The speaker needs to retain his individual method of making these contrasts even though the distortion at the phonetic level is abnormal (Fisher *et al.*, 1983).

Suprasegmental features

The suprasegmental features, or prosodic features are those characteristics that relate to entire phrases or sentences. Such features include intonation, stress, rhythm, and phrasing. They have a very important function in normal speech in that they signal differences in meaning. These features are not usually markedly affected unless the degree of deafness is severe.

Inaccurate duration of phonemes may lead to stress distortion. All the syllables may be equally stressed, or the wrong stress pattern used. This is partly because the hearing impaired person maximizes his articulatory feedback, and in so doing exaggerates articulatory movement. This leads to slow speech often with extra vowels inserted. Intonation may be flat and monotonous, or characterized by one favourite intonation pattern.

With regard to resonance and phonation there are a variety of different manifestations of the hearing impaired speakers difficulty in controlling his speech output. Concerning resonance, there may be hypernasality. With respect to other aspects, frequency is often too high with wide pitch range. Voice quality may be abnormal. With regard to respiratory control, talking, on an inspiratory air stream or inappropriate phrasing may be observed.

Poor suprasegmental features can not only mask intelligibility but may be socially unacceptable (for example inappropriately high overall pitch). Currently, visual feedback such as the electrolaryngograph is extensively employed in therapy to help the child monitor certain suprasegmental features, such as pitch changes (Abberton and Fourcin, 1984).

Craniofacial abnormalities

These patients present the speech therapist with an interesting problem caused by the interaction between structure and function. Bloomer (1971) stated: 'The correspondence between structure and function is imperfect because some speakers are capable of compensating for seemingly unsurmountable handicaps of orofacial deformity, whereas other speakers whose structures are anatomically satisfactory reveal handicapping effects of function'.

The commonest abnormality is cleft lip and palate.

Cleft lip and palate

It is well recognized that children with cleft lip and palate risk developing problems with speech and language development, facial growth, dentition, hearing and psychosocial well-being.

This condition illustrates the complex nature of speech and language development. Its adequate development is related, not just to the type and degree of cleft but many other factors.

These include conductive hearing loss, and its treatment, the timing and nature of surgical intervention, effective velopharyngeal closure, the presence of palatal fistulae, occlusion and dentition, neuromotor ability, and oral-motor perception. If intelligence is limited, this may affect the child's ability to compensate for an anatomical defect.

The importance of regular audiological and otolaryngological review cannot be overemphasized, since all children with cleft palate are born with fluid in their middle ears. They are at increased risk for conductive hearing loss in the preschool years which, combined with the other risk factors for speech development, has serious implications.

Psychosocial and environmental factors may be significant, for example if there is a family history of clefting. Early counselling by the therapist in the first few months is important to influence any preconceived notions regarding future speech and language development.

Resonance

Resonance is at risk not only from velopharyngeal insufficiency but also the frequent high association of deviant structures of the nasal cavity. The role of the velopharyngeal valve may possibly be obscured until the nasal airway is corrected.

The primary speech disorder of hypernasality and nasal escape may need to be managed as previously described.

Articulation

This may be characterized by weakness of plosives, fricatives and affricates, compensatory articulatory placement patterns as described above, and nasal escape and nasal grimace. Sometimes these occur alongside developmental phonological delay or disorder, or phonological patterns associated with hearing loss. In addition, phonetic defects directly attributable to abnormal occlusion and dentition may be operating. For example, rotated or supernumerary teeth will distort the production of fricatives. Maxillary hypoplasia, resulting in a class three malocclusion, restricts tongue movement for the anterior lingual consonants. Palatal fistulae may lead to phonetic distortions although usually small fistulae do not affect resonance or cause nasal escape.

The speech therapist's differential diagnosis identifies the exact nature of the articulatory defects. This diagnosis will change over time altered by factors, such as facial growth, maturation and age, the state of hearing, and surgical intervention at the velopharyngeal sphincter.

Phonation

Phonatory disorders are also found in association with cleft lip and palate. They occur as the result of efforts to compensate for excessive nasality, and the child's unconscious effort to overcome unintelligibility. Breathy voice quality and reduced intensity have been reported. The need for higher intraoral pressures and for increased loudness causes the compensatory development of excessive tensions throughout the vocal tract. A phonatory disorder is easily overlooked when there are severe defects of resonance and articulations. Auditorily it may not be perceptible because of the masking effect of nasality (Edwards, 1980). McWilliams, Bluestone and Musgrave (1969) documented a high incidence of vocal nodules in patients with cleft palate.

Language

These children are at risk of delayed language development, especially in the preschool years. In school-aged children, expressive language is at greater risk than receptive language, but generally improves with age. It is quite probable that in adulthood the cleft population is less verbal than the non-cleft population (McWilliams, Morris and Shelton, 1984).

Research into speech disorders associated with clefting has focused on the velopharyngeal mechanism, and yet this discussion highlights the complex nature of the total speech disorder and the involvement of the whole vocal tract. Many of the coexisting characteristics described interact and alter each other in an individual who is growing and changing. This group must be managed from birth to maturity by a multidisciplinary team, of which the otolaryngologist and speech therapist are integral members (McWilliams, 1983).

Rare craniofacial syndromes

Major craniofacial malformations, such as Apert's and Crouzon's syndromes, are replete with features that affect the acquisition of speech and language, for example structural anomalies, frequent association of depressed hearing levels, mental retardation, and the profound psychosocial effect of craniofacial anomaly (Elfenbein, Wazim and Morris, 1981). Patients with these syndromes are specifically at risk for phonetic distortions related to severe malocclusion, and multiple intraoral anomalies. Resonance may be affected due to abnormalities of the velopharyngeal sphincter, either incompetency or nasopharyngeal obstruction. Since palatal clefts occur in approximately 154 syndromes, all the features of speech disorders associated with velopharyngeal incompetence need to be considered (Cohen, 1978).

Morrees *et al.* (1971) stated that the likelihood of defective speech increases as the number of structural deviations increases, but there is no direct relationship implying that the more severe anatomical deformity causes more severe speech problems. Many authors attest to the remarkable ability of speakers to compensate within limits in the vocal tract (Bloomer, 1971).

It is the role of the speech therapist to determine if the patient is speaking to his potential. Therapy is usually recommended if there is evidence that structure is compatible with better speech than is actually being produced. Furthermore, Witzell (1983) also maintains that it is the responsibility of the speech therapist to document speech problems in rare craniofacial syndromes, to record changes in articulation and resonance after craniofacial surgery and predict changes that may occur due to specific operative procedures. This is due to the lack of studies in this area and therefore it is important to begin to build a data base of detailed case studies and their profiles.

Communication and the long-term tracheostomy child

Tracheostomy in early childhood is often followed by aphonia so that even the cry is lost. This may be unavoidable if there is severe laryngeal obstruction, but even in children with an apparently normal larynx (for example in sleep apnoea), the voice may be absent. As a result, the infant experiences little, if any, auditory-vocal feedback, and a decrease in oral behaviour is seen. If aphonia extends into the child's second year, this inevitably leads to a potentially severe delay in the development and use of expressive language, with delay in the acquisition of phonology. The child's own lack of voice often renders him less attentive to other speakers over a period of time, such that attention and listening skills become disrupted and poorly developed so that receptive language skills are affected (Kaslon and Stein, 1985).

It is therefore important to strive for vocalization in any tracheostomized child. A close working relationship between the surgeon and the speech therapist is advocated. Fortunately, many children find the airleak around the tube sufficient to produce voice, while others require a fenestrated tube. This can either be a silver Alder Hey pattern with a speaking valve, or a Great Ormond Street (GOS) pattern tube fenestrated, using a lateral neck X-ray as a template and employing a silver di-santi valve.

Unfortunately, accurately maintaining the fenestration in line with the tracheal lumen is a constant problem, and some children are reluctant to tolerate a valved tube. This leads to a group of children who are aphonic, or have insufficient vocalization to support the development of expressive language.

Speech therapy management

The importance of early intervention by the speech therapist has been advocated by Harlor (1980), Tucker (1982), and Simon and Handler (1981). The review by Kaslon, Grabo and Ruben (1978) showed that in the past, these children were rarely referred. Handler, Simon and Fowler (1983) outlined reasons for this lack of referral.

If phonation is not possible the therapist focuses her intervention on fostering the development of the child's early communicative intent, normal gesture, and the development of prelanguage skills. Once the child reaches 12–18 months, the use of sign language as an alternative method of communication, is advised (Simon, Fowler and Handler, 1983). In this way, the child has a structured means of expression, as an interim measure, before oral language is possible. Research has proven that the use of signing augments the rate of language acquisition (Kiernan and Reid, 1984).

If the tracheostomized child is able to vocalize, language development should proceed normally. However, it may not necessarily do so, especially if there has been some months of aphonia, during which the tracheostomized child typically develops a sophisticated non-verbal communication system which persists and reduces his need to develop oral language.

In older children, when vocalization is not possible, and expressive language and speech are developed, the child is aphonic, and mouths his words. This has been referred to as buccal speech or 'Donald Duck' voice. The air stream appears to be created by the larynx acting as the initiator which is indicated by the production of ejectives for target plosives. Very occasionally the speech therapist may recommend an electrolarynx.

By providing speech therapy during cannulation, the child's predicted delay in language acquisition is minimized and the child is stretched to communicate to his potential. Frustration due to a lack of systematized communication system is lessened, and therefore the risk of emotional problems, well documented to occur in association with speech and language delay, are reduced (Rutter and Martin, 1972).

Stammering (stuttering)

Definition

Stammering is a disorder of the rhythm of speech in which the speaker knows precisely what he wishes to say but cannot for the moment say it, because of involuntary repetitions, prolongations, or cessation of sounds (World Health Organization, 1978). It is more than just a disruption in the smooth flow of words, as the syndrome is typically characterized by emotional reactions to the trouble experienced in speaking. Therefore it should be viewed as a disorder of communication rather than purely a speech symptom. If it persists into adolescence or adulthood it frequently becomes a major obstacle to the formation of close relationships and careers.

Onset

Stammering is a disorder of childhood often occurring between the ages of 2 and 10 years, but more commonly between 2 and 5 years (Bloodstein, 1960). It is at exactly this time when non-fluency may be observed as a normal stage in language development. The child has ideas which he wishes to communicate, but his expressive language has not developed sufficiently to allow him to do so and therefore there are hesitancies as he plans his utterances. It is vital that a differential diagnosis between normal non-fluency and the onset of stammering is made, to prevent the development of a chronic handicap.

Normal non-fluency consists mainly of whole word or phrase repetitions (for example it's . . . it's . . . cold today, or put the . . . put the . . . ball there), interjections, and revisions (the man . . . the boy is happy) with occasional partword repetitions. The stammering child is characterized by an increase in partword repetitions (bbbbbbball), sound prolongation (b . . . ball) and the insertion of the schwa vowel after the initial sound (tu-tu-tu-today). Sometimes the child may be seen to struggle to get the word out, disrupting the expiratory airflow. Variations of the pitch, intensity and rate of the voice may be observed. Concomitant movements of the head and trunk and word and situation avoidance may develop.

Part of the reason that this disorder is so complex, is due to its variability in severity and frequency with time and circumstance.

Aetiology

Many theories as to aetiology have been proposed from organic, psychogenic to viewing stammering as a learned behaviour. Despite much research, however, the aetiology is still not fully understood. It is known, however, that there is often a familial pattern. The risk of stammering among first degree relatives exceeds the population risk by a factor of three, and this risk is increased for the offspring of female stammerers. It is quite probable that environmental factors do play a part in the development and maintenance of the syndrome, and that possibly the psychogenic aspects, in particular difficulties with social adjustment, develop as a learned reaction to the handicap. Stammerers often demonstrate poor interpersonal skills, avoid social contact, and do not initiate communication.

Current research is studying neurophysiological theory on the supposition that there is a neurological inadequacy.

Incidence

In childhood, the prevalence in the prepubertal population is 1% dropping to 0.8% at 16 years of age. The distribution of stammerers between males and females is three to one. This disproportion increases with age, and the remission of stammering is more common in girls than boys. This has been attributed to differences in constitution, in particular physical maturation and speech and language development, and to the different parental attitudes and expectations of boys and girls (Andrews *et al.*, 1981).

Management

The speech therapist's assessment of stammering is complex. A quantitative and qualitative assessment of the overt behavioural manifestations of dysfluency is made. Other aspects of speech and language behaviour are assessed and information on educational achievements sought. Environmental factors including the child's and parents' attitudes, and other significant persons, are all carefully explored.

Current approaches to therapy can take widely different forms, and is determined by the assessment. Treatment usually is based on three main principles.

(1) Modification of the environmental factors that are contributing to the development and maintenance of stammering may be indicated.

(2) Therapy may be needed to modify directly aspects of speech production, with attention to the effective carryover and maintenance of fluency (Rustin and Cook, 1983).

(3) The importance of changing the child's perception of himself as a stammerer, sometimes needs to be worked upon in therapy.

This developmental disorder should never be ignored on the assumption that it will go away, especially if parental concern is expressed. The earlier the problem is identified and the factors contributing to it understood, the better the prognosis (Shine, 1980).

Appendix 11.1: Glossary

(Nicolosi, Harryman and Kreschek, 1983)

Affricate: consonant sound beginning with a stop closure which is released as a fricative.

Articulation: the physical production of speech sounds.

Consonant: a speech sound that is produced when the expired air stream, with or without voice, passes through a stricture of either complete closure or close approximation.

Fricative: consonant sound made by forcing the air stream through a narrow opening, resulting in audible high frequency sounds.

Glottal stop: a plosive sound produced by a tight closure of the vocal folds followed by the sudden release of subglottic air pressure.

Hyperfunction: excessive forcing and straining, usually at the level of the vocal folds, but which may occur at various points along the vocal tract.

Hypernasality: excessive amount of perceived nasal resonance on voiced consonants and vowels.

Hypofunction: reduced vocal capacity resulting from prolonged overuse, muscle fatigue, tissue irritation, or general laryngeal or specific problems relating to the opening and closing of the glottis. It is characterized by air loss and sometimes hoarseness and pitch breaks.

Hyponasality: reduction or absence of nasal resonance especially of the nasal consonants.

Intensity: force or stress with which a sound is produced by a speaker, equivalent to the loudness perceived by the listener.

Pharyngeal fricative: a fricative produced by constriction of the pharyngeal walls and the retraction of the root of the tongue towards the back wall of the pharynx.

Phonation: physiological process whereby the energy of moving air in the vocal tract is transformed into acoustic energy within the larynx.

Phoneme: sound segment in a given language that can be recognized as being distinct from other sounds in the language. It is the minimal distinctive unit used to signal a meaning difference.

Phonetics: study of the production and perception of speech.

Phonology: study of the structure and function of speech sounds in a language.

Pitch: perception of an aspect of the voice related to its fundamental frequency.

Plosive: consonant sound produced by stopping the air flow in the mouth and then suddenly releasing it, while there is velopharyngeal closure.

Resonance: the vibratory response of an air-filled cavity to a frequency imposed upon it.

Semantics: the study of meaning.

Suprasegmental: the characteristics that span linguistic units longer than a phonetic segment such as intonation, voice quality, stress and rhythm.

Syntax: the study of phrase, clause and sentence structure.

Vocal abuse: mistreatment usually by overuse of the laryngeal and pharyngeal musculature.

Vocal misuse: incorrect use of pitch, quality, volume, breath support, or rate, singularly or in combination.

Voice quality: the perception of the physical complexity of laryngeal tone, modified by resonance.

Voiced/voiceless consonant: speech sounds produced with the vocal cords vibrating or not.

Vowel: a voiced speech sound produced when the vocal tract, primarily the oral cavity, changes shape producing change in the resonance of the tract.

References

ABBERTON, E. and FOURCIN, A. (1984) Electrolaryngography. In *Experimental Clinical Phonetics*, edited by C. Code and M. Ball, pp. 62–78. London: Croom-Helm

ANDREWS, G., CRAIG, A., FEYER, A. M., HODDINOTT, S., HOWIE, P. and NEILSON, M. (1983) Stuttering: a review of research findings and theories circa. *Journal of Speech and Hearing Disorders*, **8**, 226–246

ARONSON, A. E. (1985) *Clinical Voice Disorders*, 2nd edn. New York: Thieme Inc.

BERNTHAL, J. E. and BANKSON, N. W. (1981) *Articulation Disorders*. Englewood Cliffs: Prentice-Hall

BERRY, R. J., EPSTEIN, R., FOURCIN, A. J., FREEMAN, M. and MacCURTAIN, F. M. (1982) An objective analysis of voice disorder. *British Journal of Disorders of Communication*, **17**, 67–83

BLOODSTEIN, O. (1960) The development of stuttering: II development phases. *Journal of Speech and Hearing Disorders*, **25**, 366–376

BLOOMER, H. H. (1971) Speech defects associated with dental malocclusions and related abnormalities. In *Handbook of Speech Pathology and Audiology*, edited by L. E. Travis, pp. 715–767. New York: Appleton-Century-Crofts

BRODNITZ, F. S. (1965) Vocal rehabilitation. 4th edn. *American Academy of Ophthalmology and Otolaryngology*, Rochester, Minnesota

BRODNITZ, F. S. and FROESCHELS, E. (1954) Treatment of vocal nodules by chewing method. *Archives of Otolaryngology*, **59**, 560–565

BULL, T. R. and COOK, J. R. (1976) *Speech Therapy and ENT Surgery*. Oxford: Blackwell Scientific Publications

BYERS BROWN, B. (1981) *Speech Therapy: Principles and Practice*. London: Churchill Livingstone

CODE, C. and BALL, M. (1984) Editors. *Experimental Clinical Phonetics*. London: Croom-Helm

COHEN, M. M. (1978) Syndromes with cleft lip and palate. *Cleft Palate Journal*, **15**, 306–328

CROFT, C. B., SHPRINTZEN, R. J., DANILLES, A. and LEWIN, M. L. (1978) The occult submucous cleft palate and the musculus uvulae. *Cleft Palate Journal*, **15**, 150

CRYSTAL, D. (1980) *Introduction to Language Pathology*. London: Edward Arnold

DARLEY, F. L., ARONSON, A. E. and BROWN, J. R. (1975) *Motor Speech Disorders*. Toronto: W. B. Saunders Co.

DEJONCKERE, P. H. (1984) Pathogenesis of voice disorders in childhood. *Acta-Oto-Rhino-Laryngologica*, **38**, 307–314

EDWARDS, M. (1980) Speech and language disability. In *Advances in the Management of Cleft Palate*, edited by M. Edwards and A. C. H. Watson, pp. 83–96. Edinburgh: Churchill Livingstone

ELFENBEIN, J. L., WAZIRI, M. and MORRIS, H. L. (1981) Verbal communication skills of six children with craniofacial anomalies. *Cleft Palate Journal*, **18**, 59–64

ELLIS, M. (1959) Remarks on dysphonia. *Journal of Laryngology and Otology*, **73**, 99–103

ELLIS, R. E. (1979) The Exeter nasal anemometry system. In *Diagnosis and Treatment of Palato Glossal Malfunction*, edited by R. E. Ellis and F. C. Flack, pp. 31–36. London: The College of Speech Therapists

FISHER, J., KING, A., PARKER, A. and WRIGHT, R. (1983) Assessment of speech production and speech perception as a basis for therapy. In *Speech of the Hearing Impaired*, edited by I. Hochberg, H. Levitt and M. J. Osberger, pp. 195–214. Baltimore: University Park Press

GREENE, M. (1972) *The Voice and its Disorders*. London: Pitman Medical

GRUNWELL, P. G. (1982) Principles of clinical phonology. In *Clinical Phonology*, pp. 197–207. London: Croom-Helm

HANDLER, S. D., SIMON, B. and FOWLER, S. (1983) Speech and the child with a long-term tracheostomy – the problem and the otolaryngologist's role. *Transactions of the Pennsylvanian Academy of Ophthalmology and Otolaryngology*, **36**, 67–71

HANSON, M., BARNARD, L. and CASE, J. (1969) Tongue-thrust in preschool children. *American Journal of Orthopsychiatry*, **56**, 60–69

HARLOR, M. (1983) Communication strategies for a child having total laryngeal stenosis: a case report. *Journal of the Development of Speech, Language and Hearing*, **16**, 2–9

HENGERER, A. S., STROME, M. and JAFFE, B. F. (1975) Injuries to the neonatal larynx from longterm endotracheal tube intubation and suggested tube modification for prevention. *Annals of Otology, Rhinology and Laryngology*, **84**, 764–770

HIRANO, M. (1981) *Clinical Examination of Voice*. Vienna, New York: Springer-Verlag

HUSKIE, C. (1983) Velopharyngeal incompetence versus tongue patterns: surgery or speech? In *Proceedings of the 19th Congress of the International Association of Logopaedics and Phoniatrics* (Edinburgh, 1984), edited by M. Edwards, vol. 2, pp. 227–229. Perth: Danscot Print Ltd

KASLON, K. W., GRABO, D. E. and RUBEN, R. J. (1978) Voice, speech, and language habilitation in young children without laryngeal function. *Archives of Otolaryngology*, **104**, 737–739

KASLON, K. W. and STEIN, R. E. (1985) Chronic paediatric tracheotomy: assessment and implications for habilitation of voice, speech, and language in young children. *International Journal of Paediatric Otorhinolaryngology*, **9**, 165–171

KIERNAN, C. and REID, B. (1984) Augmentative communication systems in the UK. *British Journal of Disorders of Communication*, **19**, 47–61

KLEIN, J. O. (1984) Otitis media and the development of speech and language. In *Paediatric Infectious Disease*, vol. 3 no. 4 pp. 389–390. Baltimore: Williams & Wilkins

LUCHSINGER, R. (1965) *Voice-Speech-Language. Clinical Communicology: Its Physiology and Pathology*. Belmont: Wadsworth

LYONS, J. (1968) *Introduction to Theoretical Linguistics*. London: Macmillan

MacCURTAIN, F. and FOURCIN, A. J. (1982) Applications of the electrolaryngograph wave form display. In *Transcripts of the Tenth Symposium Care of the Professional Voice, part 2*, edited by V. L. Laurence, pp. 51–57. The Voice Foundation

McENERY, E. and GAINES, F. (1941) Tongue-tie in infants and children. *Journal of Pediatrics*, **18**, 252–255

McWILLIAMS, B. J. (1983) Multiple speech disorders. In *Paediatric Otolaryngology*, edited by C. D. Bluestone and S. E. Stool, pp. 1508–1520. Philadelphia: W. B. Saunders

McWILLIAMS, B. J., BLUESTONE, C. D. and MUSGRAVE, R. G. (1969) Diagnostic implications of vocal cord nodules in children with cleft palate. *The Laryngoscope*, **79**, 2072–2080

McWILLIAMS, B. J., MORRIS, H. L. and SHELTON, R. L. (1984) *Cleft Palate Speech*. Ontario: B. C. Decker Inc.

MASON, R. M. (1973) Preventing speech disorders following adenoidectomy by preoperative examination. *Clinical Paediatrics*, **12**, 405

MONSEN, R. B. (1983) General effects of deafness on phonation and articulation. In *Speech of the Hearing Impaired*, edited by I. Hochberg, H. Levitt and M. J. Osberger, pp. 23–34. Baltimore: University Park Press

MORREES, C. F., BURSTONE, C. J., CHRISTIANSEN, R. L., HIXON, E. H. and WEINSTEIN, S. (1971) Research related to malocclusion, a state-of-the-art workshop, the oral-facial growth and development programme, NIDR. *American Journal of Orthodontia*, **59**, 1–18

MORRIS, H. L., KRUEGER, L. J. and BUMSTED, R. M (1982) Indications of congenital palatal incompetence (cleft palate) before diagnosis. *Annals of Otology, Rhinology and Laryngology*, **91**, 115

NEEDLEMAN, H. (1977) Effects of hearing loss from early recurrent otitis media on speech and language development. In *Hearing Loss in Children*, edited by B. Jaffe, pp. 640–650. University Park Press

NEIMAN, G. S. and SIMPSON, R. K. (1975) A roentgencephalometric investigation of the effect of adenoid removal upon selected measures of velopharyngeal function. *Cleft Palate Journal*, **12**, 377

NEMEC, J. (1961) The motivation background of hyperkinetic dysphonia in children: a contribution to psychologic research in phoniatry. *Logos*, **4**, 28–31

NICOLOSI, L., HARRYMAN, E. and KRESCHEK, J. (1983) *Terminology of Communication Disorders Speech-Language-Hearing*. Baltimore: Williams and Wilkins

PARADISE, J. L. (1981) Otitis media during early life: how hazardous to development? *Pediatrics*, **68**, 869–873

PENNICEARD, R. (1981) Educational retardation and conductive hearing problems: an overview of the present state of knowledge. *ILEA Edition*, **2**, 3–18

PERKINS, W. H. (1971) *Speech Pathology, an Applied Behavioral Science*. St Louis: The C. V. Mosby Company

PETERSON, S. J. (1975) Nasal emission as a component of misarticulation of sibilant affricates, *Journal of Speech and Hearing Disorders*, **40**, 106–114

PRATER, R. J. and SWIFT, R. W. (1984) *Manual of Voice Therapy*. Boston: Little, Brown and Co

RAZZELL, R. E., ANTHONY, J. F. K. and WATSON, A. C. H. (1983) A UK survey of subjective nasality assessment. In *Proceedings of the 20th Congress of the International Association of Logopaedics and Phoniatrics*, Edinburgh, UK, edited by M. Edwards, pp. 209–214. London: The College of Speech Therapists

RUSTIN, L. and COOK, F. (1983) Intervention procedures for the dysfluent child. In *Approaches to the Treatment of Stuttering*, edited by P. Dalton, pp. 47–75. London: Academic Press

RUTTER, M. and MARTIN, J. A. M. (1972) *The Child with Delayed Speech*. London: William Heinemann Medical Books

SELLEY, W. (1979) Dental and technical aids for the treatment of patient suffering from velopharyngeal disorders. In *Diagnosis and Treatment of Palato Glossal Malfunction*, edited by R. E. Ellis and F. C. Flack. London: The College of Speech Therapists

SHINE, R. E. (1980) Direct management of the beginning stutterer. *Seminars in Speech, Language and Hearing Disorders*, **1**, 339–350

SIMON, B., FOWLER, S. M. and HANDLER, S. D. (1983) Communication development in young children with long-term tracheostomies: preliminary report. *International Journal of Paediatric Otorhinolaryngology*, **6**, 37–50

SIMON, B. and HANDLER, S. D. (1981) The speech pathologist and management of children with tracheostomies. *Journal of Otolaryngology*, **10**, 440–448

TOOHILL, R. J. (1975) The psychosomatic aspects of children with vocal nodules. *Archives of Otolaryngology*, **101**, 591–595

TUCKER, H. M., RUSNOR, M. and COHEN, L. (1982) Speech development in aphonic children. *The Laryngoscope*, **92**, 566–568

VAN DEINSE, J. (1982) *Journal of Research in Singing*, **5**, 33–49

WARREN, D. W. (1964) Velopharyngeal orifice size and upper pharyngeal pressure-flow patterns in normal speech. *Journal of Plastic and Reconstructive Surgery*, **33**, 148–162

WERTZ, R. T. and MEAD, M. D. (1975) Classroom teacher

and speech clinician severity ratings of different speech disorders. *Language Speech and Hearing Survey in Schools*, **6**, 119–124

WILLIAMS, W. N. and WALDRON, C. M. (1985) Assessment of lingual function when ankyloglossia (tongue-tie) is suspected. *Journal of the American Dental Association*, **110**, 353–356

WILSON, D. K. (1979) *Voice Problems of Children*, 2dn edn. Baltimore: Williams and Wilkins

WINITZ, H. (1969) *Articulatory acquisition and behaviour*. Engelwood Cliffs: Prentice Hall

WITZELL, M. A. (1983) Speech problems in craniofacial anomalies. *Communicative Disorders*, **7**, 45–59

WOOD, K. (1971) Terminology and nomenclature. In *Handbood of Speech Pathology*, edited by L. E. Travis, pp. 3–26. New York: Appleton-Century-Crofts

WORLD HEALTH ORGANIZATION (1978) *International Classification of Diseases, 9th revision*. Geneva: WHO

WYNTER, H. (1974) An investigation into the analysis and terminology of voice quality and its correlation with the assessment reliability of speech therapists. *British Journal of Disorders in Communication*, **9**, 102–109

12

Otitis media with effusion (glue ear)

A. Richard Maw

Otitis media with effusion is one of the commonest chronic otological conditions of childhood. It is described by a variety of synonyms. Otitis media with effusion results from alteration of the mucociliary system within the middle ear cleft where serous or mucoid fluid accumulates in association with a negative pressure. The pressure change is almost invariably caused by malfunction of the eustachian tube. Although there are no signs of inflammation, bacteria can be cultured from the effusion in as many as 50% of cases, particularly if special techniques are used.

An effusion frequently remains in the middle ear following acute suppurative otitis media, but usually spontaneous clearance occurs within a few weeks. Chronic otitis media with effusion is especially prevalent in children with cleft palate (Stool and Randall, 1967; Paradise, Bluestone and Felder, 1969). It frequently occurs in association with chronic upper respiratory tract infection and conditions affecting the nose and sinuses. These include allergic rhinitis, fibrocystic disease and ultrastructural cilial abnormalities of the respiratory tract mucosa. It is found very often in children suffering with Down's syndrome (Stome, 1981) or Hurler's syndrome and other craniofacial abnormalities.

The condition occurs in childhood as overt or covert hearing loss presenting as an educational or behavioural problem. In younger children it may present as speech and language delay or as an articulation defect. Often the hearing loss is first detected on routine screening examinations before or at 3.5 years of age, or later at a preschool testing. Sometimes attention is drawn to it by frequent episodes of otalgia which indicate an exacerbation of acute suppurative otitis media superimposed on the middle ear effusion. Occa-

sionally, presentation is with complications such as otorrhoea secondary to perforation of the tympanic membrane.

Treatment varies widely and is naturally dependent on the duration and severity of the condition. It is accepted that mild forms of the disease resolve spontaneously, particularly in the summer months. Unilateral effusions, though not without effect, seem less detrimental to normal childhood development than if the condition is bilateral. As yet, no satisfactory study has demonstrated any long-term benefit from the large variety of medical measures prescribed as treatment. Topical and systemic vasoconstrictor substances, and anti-allergy remedies have their proponents. Antibiotics have been prescribed; systemic steroids have also been tried; but all methods remain unproven.

Surgical treatment is often recommended to the ears in the form of myringotomy and aspiration with or without insertion of a ventilation tube. Surgery may also be recommended to the sinuses as antral lavage and to the postnasal space and pharynx in the form of adenoidectomy and tonsillectomy. It is removal of the adenoids and tonsils which is mainly responsible for the morbidity and mortality in relation to treatment. The main reasons postulated for adenoidectomy as a means of treatment and as a method for prevention of recurrence of the effusion are centred on the size of the adenoids and their possible role as a focus of ascending eustachian tube infection. In addition, they may alter nasopharyngeal pressure relationships. The potential source of infection from the tonsils has been similarly implicated. Tonsillectomy is often additionally advised on grounds which, on their own merit, might not substantiate a need for removal of the tonsils alone. Arguments for

(Bateman, 1959; Gottschalk, 1972; Potsic, 1980; Marshak and Ben Neriah, 1980) and against (Editorial, 1977; Sade, 1979; Roydhouse, 1980; Stool, 1980; Stell, 1981) adenoidectomy and adeno-tonsillectomy for all types of middle ear disease in childhood have been discussed and reported in symposia worldwide (Lim *et al.*, 1976, 1984; Paradise, 1976; Senturia *et al.*, 1980).

Considering the large numbers of these operations performed for this condition, it is interesting that so few studies have been carried out to validate their efficacy. It seems that the belief that adenoidectomy relieves acute suppurative otitis media has been extrapolated, as yet without convincing supportive evidence, as grounds for the management of chronic otitis media with effusion.

This chapter does not address itself to the particular problem of unilateral middle ear effusion arising in association with a postnasal space neoplasm. This situation naturally requires an entirely different clinical approach.

Terminology

Since the original description by Politzer (1869) there has been a vast literature relating to this condition. Over the years the changing nomenclature has indicated current attitudes, often in relation to supposed aetiology (Black, 1984a). It has been variously termed catarrhal, exudative, seromucinous, serous, secretory and non-suppurative otitis media. More recently, middle ear effusion and otitis media with effusion have been current terminology. To many clinicians and lay persons it is known as 'glue ear'. An acceptable classification for otitis media with effusion should allow further subdivision according to the nature of the effusion and the duration of the condition. It may be defined as the presence within the middle ear cleft of an effusion which may be serous or mucoid but not frankly purulent. Although not associated with clinically obvious signs or symptoms of infection, bacteria may be cultured from the effusion in approximately one-third to one-half of the cases.

Incidence and natural history

All forms of otitis media mainly affect infants and young children. It is probably a worldwide problem. Population studies are often unsatisfactory and difficult to compare, some reporting prevalence, and others incidence. It is likely that the first episode of acute suppurative otitis media occurs before the age of one year in 50–60% of cases. Around 70% of children have experienced their first attack before the age of 3 years. Teele,

Klein and Rosner (1980) found that following the first attack of acute otitis media in infants, 40% had no effusion after one month and 90% were effusion free after 3 months. However, unlike acute otitis media, the epidemiology of otitis media with effusion is poorly documented. Reported studies rely on different otoscopic and tympanometric methods for identification.

In the UK, Brooks (1976) reported an incidence of 50% in children aged 5–7 years. Tos and Poulsen in 1979 and Tos, Holm-Vensen and Sorensen (1982) found an incidence of 30% in Danish children aged 2–4 years. Lous and Fiellau Nikolajsen (1981), also from Denmark, reported a 26% incidence in 7-year-old children. Silva *et al.* (1982), in New Zealand, found 17.1% of a sample of 879 5-year-old children had either unilateral or bilateral otitis media with effusion. Suarez Nieto *et al.* (1983) indicated a prevalence of 8.7% in 472 children screened from a population of 5414 Spanish children aged from 2 to 12 years. The prevalence decreased with increasing age from 38.8% at 2 years to 1.1% at 11 years, fitting a logarithmic regression curve. A prospective study of 70 babies followed from birth to one year showed that 54% had one or more episodes of otitis media and 10 developed bilateral middle ear effusions (Marchant *et al.*, 1984). As judged symptomatically and by otoscopic findings, the incidence reached a maximum by about the fifth year in the series studied by Pukander, Sipila and Karma (1984) and thereafter there was a gradual decrease. Recently in the USA, Casselbrant *et al.* (1985) have demonstrated a cumulative incidence in preschool children aged between 2 and 6 years – the incidence was 53% in the first year and 61% in the second year. Findings were based on pneumatic otoscopy and tympanometry. They also showed that 80% of the effusions resolved within 2 months. The prevalence showed a seasonal variation and a strong association with the presence of upper respiratory infection. The incidence was independent of age within the 2–6-year-old age group.

It has been suggested, but not proven, that otitis media with effusion develops as a sequel to the more widespread use of antibiotics. There may also be an inverse relationship with the decreasing incidence in complications of suppurative otitis media in conjunction with the advent of antibiotic treatment (Feigin, 1982). This development is seen either to be a result of incomplete resolution of the acute infection or a reflection of changing virulence of the organisms causing acute suppuration. An alternative postulate has been interference by antibiotics of local IgM production within the middle ear. Finally, there may be altered resistance to infection within the community whose general health has improved.

There appear to be racial differences in incidence of otitis media – Eskimos and American Indians being more frequently affected than American whites, and black children having a lower incidence than white children. Most studies demonstrate a higher incidence of suppurative otitis media and otitis media with effusion in males than in females. The racial variations may be due to genetic and anatomical differences in the skull base and eustachian tube. The male predilection may reflect the overall male predominance for childhood infections. Recently, Tos and Stangerup (1985) have reported reduced pneumatization of the mastoid air cell system in children with a history of otitis media with effusion or tubal dysfunction. Boys had smaller systems than girls and the degree of middle ear pathology was greater in boys. This was thought to relate to the more frequent upper respiratory tract infection in boys. The study supports the environmental, rather than the hereditary theory of mastoid pneumatization. Socio-economic, genetic and environmental factors affect the development of otitis media. Accepted risk factors are: a family history of otitis media in parents or siblings, parental occupation and smoking; and in Scandinavia, the type of nursery care (Klein, 1979).

The distribution of patients within any clinic reflects the method of referral and the facilities and expertise of the referring physicians. At present there seems to be a peak incidence of children aged between 3 and 6 years attending otolaryngology clinics. However, as the diagnosis in infancy is difficult and the condition is often asymptomatic, it is probably more prevalent in this age group than is realized (Marchant *et al.*, 1984). After the age of 10 years it is less frequent and at this stage one experiences the complications rather than the effects of the primary condition.

Studies by Henderson *et al.* (1982) have confirmed that the incidence of acute otitis media with effusion is increased in children with viral respiratory infection ($P<0.001$). Of these infections, respiratory syncytial virus, influenza virus and adenovirus conferred a greater risk than infection with parainfluenza virus, enterovirus or rhinovirus. There is a close seasonal relationship between the incidence of acute suppurative otitis and otitis media with effusion, with a peak in January, February and March and a minimum incidence in August, September and October. This seasonal change correlates with the incidence of respiratory syncytial viral infections (Hinchcliffe, 1976).

Due to the enormous increase in literature in the 1950s, it was thought by some authors that there was a real increase in the incidence of the disease at that time. However, this may have been apparent rather than real. Coincidental improvement of otological services for children with more sophisticated audiological screening tests and the advent of otological microscopy are probably responsible for more accurate and frequent diagnosis. The increase may reflect improved availability of otolaryngological and paediatric services. It may be due to earlier recognition of the condition by general practitioners and an awareness by parents of the effect of hearing difficulties during childhood. The number of therapeutic procedures for the condition has risen dramatically in recent years. A rise has occurred in North America, Scandinavia, Japan and in the UK. It is now said by some to be reaching epidemic proportions and the condition has been termed the 'new dyslexia' (Black, 1985a).

Aetiology

The major underlying factors responsible for the production of otitis media with effusion are a combination of eustachian tube malfunction with superadded infection. It is the wide variety of conditions affecting eustachian tube function which confer the more generalized clinical picture to otitis media with effusion. These may be considered under three main headings:

(1) *eustachian tube malfunction*
　　cleft palate
　　submucous cleft palate
(2) *altered mucociliary system*
　　infection (nose, sinus, postnasal space, tonsils, pharynx)
　　allergy
　　immunological factors
　　surfactant deficiency
　　ultrastructural changes in cilia
　　fibrocystic disease
　　hormonal factors
　　other factors
(3) *nasopharyngeal disproportion*
　　craniofacial abnormalities
　　adenoids and nasopharynx.

Eustachian tube malfunction

The underlying tubal dysfunction may reflect the situation that exists before the normal change occurs from the childhood to the adult configuration of the eustachian tube. This is said to occur at about the age of 7 years (Holborow, 1970). It is after this time that spontaneous resolution of otitis media with effusion occurs. Following the demonstration by Stool and Randall (1967) of otitis media with effusion in children with cleft palate, Paradise, Bluestone and Felder (1969) indicated the universality of effusions in these children in whom the underlying defect causing tubal dysfunction is an abnormal mode of action of the tensor palati muscle. There is also evidence that otitis media with effusion improves following palatal repair.

Tubal dysfunction may result either from skull base abnormalities or where there are anatomical variations in the nasopharynx. These may be defined in relation to differences in the angle subtended by the floor of the anterior cranial fossa and basisphenoid with the level of the hard palate. Consequently otitis media with effusion is more common in acknowledged craniofacial abnormalities such as Down's and Hurler's syndromes.

Bluestone and Cantekin (1979) described otitis media in conjunction with both tubal obstruction and abnormal patency. Functional and mechanical obstruction may occur (Bluestone and Beery, 1976), the former where there is a collapse of the eustachian tube with increased compliance. The situation is found as a result of differences in the structure of tubal cartilages in young children. Mechanical obstruction may be either extrinsic as in the case of postnasal space tumour or adenoid hyperplasia, or may be intrinsic as a result of mucosal disease (Bluestone, 1982). These mechanisms correlate with the previously held *hydrops ex vacuo* theory which suggests that in tubal obstruction, due to gas absorption, a negative pressure develops in the middle ear cleft. As a result, a sterile transudate is formed. This is clearly not the sole mechanism, as it is now realized that bacterial or viral infection with an accompanying inflammatory exudate is a more likely co-factor as a cause for otitis media with effusion in many cases. It has been shown that transudation, exudation and absorption all contribute to middle ear effusion formation, regardless of the effusion type (Lim, 1979).

Altered mucociliary system

Infection

Positive bacterial cultures were demonstrated in 40% of middle ear fluid specimens by Senturia *et al.* (1958) and subsequently other workers have produced positive cultures in 22–52% of effusions. The bacteria found in cases of chronic otitis media with effusion are similar to those cultured in acute suppurative otitis media (Klein, 1980), which in turn are similar to the bacteria found in the nasopharynx. *Streptococcus pneumoniae* and *Haemophilus influenzae* account for the majority of cases. The remainder are caused by group A β-haemolytic streptococcus, *Staphylococcus aureus* and *Branhamella catarrhalis*. Mills, Uttley and McIntyre (1984) have suggested that some cases of

otitis media with effusion result from incomplete resolution of acute suppurative otitis media. Treatment with penicillin of resistant strains of *H. influenzae* and *Staph. aureus* may be a factor in the process. The same authors (Mills, Uttley and McIntyre, 1985) have more recently confirmed, from studies of bacterial flora, that invasion of the middle ear may occur from the nasopharynx in cases with effusion. Experimental evidence from a study by De Maria *et al.* (1984) suggested that a surface endotoxin of *H. influenzae* may be responsible for the induction of otitis media with effusion.

The close relationship between respiratory viral infection, particularly with respiratory syncytial virus and acute suppurative otitis media, has been mentioned and it must be stressed that both show a close seasonal relationship with otitis media with effusion. Ruokonen, Sandelin and Makinen (1979) showed a 50% incidence of *H. influenzae* in adenoid specimens in children with otitis media with effusion or recurrent acute otitis, compared with 14% in non-otitis media cases. Similarly, virus isolates were positive in 28% of otitis cases compared with 3% in the remainder without otitis. However, Maw and Speller (1985) have shown no significant differences in the cultures of bacteriological swabs from the postnasal space of children with otitis media with effusion, compared with age-matched children undergoing surgery for strabismus during the same season of the year. There was only a slight preponderance of *Streptococcus pyogenes* ($P<0.05$) in the patient group.

Allergy

The role of allergy as a causative factor for otitis media with effusion is unproven. Some studies have suggested an increased incidence in otitis media with effusion in allergic patients. This has not yet been supported by accurately controlled studies with total and specific immunoglobulin estimations. It may be that the increased susceptibility to respiratory infections found in patients with respiratory allergy is responsible for their tubal dysfunction (Clemis, 1976). Alteration of immune responses within the middle ear system may occur as a result of immediate hypersensitivity, as a cytotoxic response, as a response by the complement system or due to delayed hypersensitivity via a cellular immune mechanism (Lim and De Maria, 1982). Phillips *et al.* (1974) showed the mean IgE content of the middle ear exudate to be 12 times higher than the mean serum IgE for the same children. However, the IgE, IgM and IgA concentrations were the same both in exudate and serum. By contrast, other studies revealed no abnormalities of IgE (Mogi, Maeda and Yoshida, 1976).

More recently, Borge (1983) has shown that children with otitis media with effusion have a higher positive family history of atopy and a higher incidence of atopic disease compared with the control subjects. However, the selection criteria did not include IgE estimations in both controls and atopic subjects.

Church *et al.* (1981) demonstrated large numbers of mast cells in the adenoids. These are capable of binding IgE and releasing histamine and other inflammatory mediators on antigen challenge. Subsequently, Collins *et al.* (1985) showed that the total amount of histamine in patients with bilateral otitis media with effusion was significantly higher than in patients without the condition. They suggested that adenoidectomy may reduce a potential source of inflammatory mediator from the vicinity of the eustachian tube. However, in a study based on serum IgE levels, Maw (1986) was not able to show any difference of outcome in cases with otitis media with effusion following treatment with adenoidectomy or by insertion of a ventilation tube, whether atopy was present or not. Mills and Brain (1985) have shown a relationship between a previous history of acute otitis media and otitis media with effusion, but no aetiological relationship between the latter and allergy. In a review paper, Clemis (1976) concluded that allergic factors, although not the only cause, are important in the aetiology of otitis media with effusion. However, it seems that a true causal relationship has yet to be proven.

Immunological factors

On the basis of protein and enzyme studies, Palva, Raunio and Nousianen (1974) claimed that the middle ear effusion must result from active secretion rather than transudation. In support of this, middle ear mucosal biopsies from patients with otitis media with effusion have an increased density of mucous glands and goblet cells compared with those suffering from otosclerosis or tympanosclerosis. Whereas in the latter conditions the glands are infrequently active, in cases of effusion, 90% are found to be active. Palva, Lehtinen and Virtanen (1983) postulated that the adenoid or even the lymphoid tissue of the entire oropharynx could act as a source of bacterial antigen. This might maintain an immune complex disease in some patients with otitis media with effusion.

Because of the pathological similarities between rheumatoid arthritis and otitis media with effusion, De Maria, McGhee and Lim (1984) measured rheumatoid factor both in middle ear and serum samples in patients with chronic otitis media with effusion. The factor was present in 85% of effusions but in only 8% of serum samples. Titres were seven times higher in mucoid than in serous effusions. The presence of the factor was unrelated to the patient's age or history; or to the bacterial growth from the effusion.

Surfactant deficiency

It has also been suggested that, perhaps as a result of proteolytic enzyme activity from bacteria, a deficiency develops in the eustachian tube of surfactant, a surface tension lowering substance. Surface active phospholipids which reduce surface tension at the liquid/air interface have been demonstrated in dogs and rabbits by thin layer chromatography (Hills, 1984).

Ultrastructural changes and fibrocystic disease

Otitis media with effusion occurs more commonly with the immotile cilia syndrome and particularly with that form of the condition which constitutes the Kartagener's syndrome. Likewise, an alteration of mucociliary activity from whatever cause will affect middle ear function. It is also responsible for the association of otitis media with effusion and patients suffering from mucoviscidosis or fibrocystic disease.

Hormonal changes

Hormone dysfunction with high oestrogen levels or cases with hypothyroidism may alter tubal function sufficiently to produce an effusion, although this is infrequent in children.

Other factors

Finally, there have been suggestions that otitis media may in some cases result from or coexist with a leak of perilymph. This raises the possibility of an aetiological correlation between conductive and sensorineural hearing loss (Knight and Phillips, 1980).

Whatever the precise infective, immunological or other mechanism involved, the end result of tubal dysfunction is the same.

Nasopharyngeal disproportion

Craniofacial abnormalities

Children with Down's syndrome are known to have a disproportionate increase in the basal angle of the skull in relation to their cranial capacity. This alone, or in combination with the size of the adenoids, may be responsible for the nasopharyngeal disproportion and resultant eustachian tube malfunction found in Down's syndrome. A similar explanation may hold true for other cases with craniofacial abnormalities such as Hunter's or Hurler's syndromes. Indeed, even in normal children the actual size of the adenoids may be less important than their size in relation to the nasopharynx.

Adenoids and nasopharynx

The range in size of normal adenoids at different ages is difficult to ascertain. Almost all studies have been performed using lateral radiographs, often with a lateral cephalometric technique. Physiological variations in the size of the nasopharyngeal airway occur during sleep and during crying. They also relate to the position of the mouth and movement of the soft palate. Jeans *et al.* (1981) have shown that the growth of the soft tissues of the postnasal space representing the adenoids outstrips growth of the nasopharynx from 3 to 5.5 years of age with the resultant reduction in the nasopharyngeal airway. Subsequently, growth of the nasopharynx increases while soft tissues remain relatively unchanged and thus the airway increases. There is a significant difference in the mean area of the nasopharynx between males and females throughout development, although more so from 13 years onwards. The difference between the sexes in the area of the nasopharyngeal soft tissues is only significant at the age of 5 years and the difference in the airway is only significant from 13 years onwards.

Very careful studies were made by Linder-Aronson (1970) in relation to the size of the adenoids and nasopharynx and symptoms of nasal obstruction. He confirmed that enlarged adenoids led to mouth breathing. Furthermore, when obstruction was present, it was associated with a particular type of facial skeleton. There was noted to be reasonable agreement between the clinical assessment of adenoid size and the measurement on radiographs. The nasal airflow was lower for larger than for smaller adenoids and it was increased following adenoidectomy. The study appeared to support the hypothesis that adenoids affect the mode of breathing which then influences the individual's dentition. Hibbert and Whitehouse (1978) reported the correlation of lateral radiographic studies with adenoid size.

Johnson, Murray and Maran (1983) have indicated the errors inherent in this type of technique. Lateral cephalometric radiographs are therefore recommended to assess accurately the size of the adenoids and postnasal space airway. Studies of interobserver variability in clinical and radiological assessments of adenoid size and their correlation with adenoid volume have been made (Maw, Jeans and Fernando, 1981). These confirmed the findings of Hibbert and Tweedie (1977) of an extremely close correlation between adenoid weight and volume ($R = 0.997$; $P<0.001$). Jeans, Fernando and Maw (1981) have reported a radiological study based on interobserver agreement to assess accuracy in the measurement of adenoid enlargement.

Quarnberg (1981) has shown a relationship between large adenoids and the occurrence of acute otitis media in children aged less than 4 years. He also showed a similar relationship with radiological clouding of the maxillary sinuses. It was suggested that both factors might be responsible for the prolongation of acute otitis media. McNicholl (1983) has demonstrated nasal abnormality at the vomeroethmoid suture in children with otitis media with effusion. This he postulated may cause turbulence in the postnasal space. Todd (1984) noted a large eustachian tube calibre in patients with otitis media and in cleft palate patients compared with controls ($P<0.001$). However, the eustachian tube diameter was smaller than in patients with otitis media with effusion and allergic airway disease. ($P<0.05$).

Clinical presentation

As suggested by the definition, in its quiescent phase, otitis media with effusion has none of the signs and symptoms usually attributed to infection of the middle ear cleft. Thus, the most frequent presentation is with latent or overt hearing loss. Whichever is the case, the loss often fluctuates in severity. When latent in infants and young children it may present with impaired speech and language development (Rapin, 1979). There may be behavioural difficulties and scholastic retardation (Silva *et al.*, 1982, 1986; Stewart *et al.*, 1984). Only rarely do younger children complain of hearing difficulty. It is frequently first detected on routine screening tests; either clinically, audiometrically or by impedance studies. Indirect symptoms such as shouting, insularity, increasing the volume of the television and delay in reading development are commonly found.

Otalgia often occurs, frequently in a recurrent form. When present, it usually results from secondary infection of the fluid within the middle ear cleft. Invariably this results from an ascending eustachian tube infection. It is frequently coincident with a cold or minor upper respiratory tract infection, but occasionally follows sinus infection or an episode of allergic rhinitis. It often follows swimming.

It is possible to recognize certain clinical subgroups of otitis media with effusion:

(1) latent or overt hearing impairment without significant postnasal obstruction, otalgia or upper respiratory tract infection

(2) obvious postnasal obstruction with hearing impairment but only occasional upper respiratory tract infection, minimal allergy and, rarely, otalgia

(3) upper and lower respiratory tract disease with generalized nasal obstruction and hearing impairment without otalgia of which there may be three types: non-specific catarrhal conditions; rhinosinusitis; and allergy

(4) recurrent otalgia and hearing impairment with only occasional otorrhoea, few upper respiratory tract infections, occasional mild nasal obstruction and/or mild allergy

(5) acute upper respiratory tract infections which are infrequently tonsillitis, leading to otalgia, with hearing impairment and occasional otorrhoea

(6) cases with chronic irreversible eustachian tube malfunction, for example cleft palate, Down's, Hurler's and other syndromes with craniofacial abnormality, or ultrastructural cilial abnormalities of the respiratory tract mucosa.

Diagnosis and screening

Clinical, audiometric and tympanometric assessment may be used for screening and diagnosis. In most centres, they form the basis by which to judge selection for medical or surgical treatment. They also provide a means of evaluating improvement or otherwise, at follow-up examinations. There is considerable variation in appearance of the tympanic membrane in otitis media with effusion (Malcolmsen, 1969). There is a similar degree of inter- and intraobserver variability in the otoscopic assessment of the tympanic membrane with a pneumatic otoscope. An experienced otoscopist should have a high degree of specificity and rather better sensitivity (Paradise, Smith and Bluestone, 1976b).

The use of magnification with an operating microscope may further improve diagnostic accuracy. The degree of retraction of the pars tensa may be assessed by the extent of splitting and derangement of the light reflex, by the rotation and displacement of the malleus handle, and by the prominence of the lateral process of the malleus. The pars flaccida may be indrawn to a variable degree. Attic retraction and sometimes erosion of the outer attic wall anterior and posterior to the neck of the malleus may occur at a later stage. The degree of retraction of the tympanic membrane reflects the negative middle ear pressure which reduces the mobility of the membrane. Both retraction and mobility should always be assessed with a Siegle's or similar type of pneumatic otoscope. The colour and loss of translucency of the membrane range from pale grey or amber to a black or so-called 'blue drum'. It may be thickened, dull and opalescent, or thin and reflective. With poor illumination, minimal changes may be difficult to distinguish from the normal state. Increased vascularization of radial vessels is very frequent and, in some cases, there is also an increase in the malleolar vessels. Fluid levels and air bubbles may be visible within the middle ear cleft. Atelectatic change of the pars tensa and pars flaccida may be present to a variable degree.

Tuning fork tests may be helpful particularly in children over 4 years of age when a negative Rinne test is said to predict a hearing loss in excess of 15–20 dB (Yung and Morris, 1981). However, the author's own studies refute this suggestion (Capper, Slack and Maw, 1987).

Pure-tone audiometry is only of limited diagnostic value for the identification of otitis media with effusion. It does, however, provide some assessment of the severity of the disease. It can be used as a guide by which to monitor the progress and the effects of treatment. Fiellau Nikolajsen (1983) showed some relationship between the severity of hearing loss and middle ear changes. He confirmed some further relationship between hearing loss and impedance results. Dry ears had a mean hearing threshold of 17 dB. The mean for minimal otitis media with effusion was 23 dB, for moderate 29 dB and for infected middle ears, 34 dB. Overall in 79 out of 88 ears tested, the mean hearing threshold averaged 23 dB. Fria, Cantekin and Eichler (1985) showed the speech awareness threshold in infants aged between 7 and 24 months with otitis media with effusion to be in the order of 24.6 dB hearing level. Older children from 2 to 12 years of age with otitis media with effusion had mean three frequency pure-tone audiometric and speech reception thresholds of 24.5 dB and 22.7 dB respectively. It was found that the hearing acuity was not related to age or the duration of history of otitis media with effusion. There was no relationship between hearing level and the type of impedance curve. Ruben and Math (1978) have shown that the presence of conductive hearing loss due to otitis media with effusion may delay the diagnosis of an underlying sensorineural hearing loss.

Tympanometry was first introduced into Scandinavia (Metz, 1946), then into the UK (Brooks, 1968) and later into the USA. It provides an effective screening test for the detection of negative middle ear pressure, although it will not distinguish between such a pressure change with and without middle ear effusion (Beery *et al.*, 1975; Grimaldi, 1976; Cantekin, Beery and Bluestone, 1977). There are limitations in its use with young children where there is increased compliance of the external auditory meatus (Paradise, Smith and

Bluestone, 1976). Most normal studies show maximum compliance in a range of +200 to −200 mm of water with a rounded or peak curve. The advent of screening programmes led to the development and validation of less expensive automatically recording impedance meters (Fria, Cantekin and Probst, 1980). Diagnostic predictability of 84% may be achieved with a simple peak versus no peak pattern of classification, and compares favourably with 85.8% accuracy with more sophisticated impedance and otoadmittance meters (Cantekin, Beery and Bluestone, 1977). Fiellau Nikolajsen (1983) modified Jerger's (1970) nomenclature subdividing the tympanograms into four types:

> type A with middle ear pressure from +200 to −99 mm of water
> type C_1 with middle ear pressure from −100 to −199 mm of water
> type C_2 with middle ear pressure from −200 to +400 mm of water
> type B had flat curves without a well-defined compliance maximum.

Recently Alhady and Sharnoubi (1984) have demonstrated a very highly significant relationship in mean values of middle ear pressure in patients with adenoidal hyperplasia. They also showed a significant relationship in patients with chronic sinusitis compared with patients suffering with chronic tonsillitis in whom there was no relationship.

Management

It is accepted that there may be numerous forms of treatment for otitis media with effusion and, as yet, a correct management approach remains to be defined (Lim, 1985). As Snow (1980) pointed out, none of the treatment methods available are mutually exclusive and some may be efficacious to a limited extent. Naturally, management of the effect of the effusion on hearing thresholds varies according to the duration and severity of the hearing loss. Many cases resolve spontaneously without treatment. Although these and other milder cases do not require intervention, they need observation and follow-up. Other similar cases may be managed by improved teaching techniques and individual attention in the classroom, until spontaneous resolution has occurred. It is unlikely that thresholds of less than 20 dB across the speech frequencies will require treatment, which may also be witheld in unilateral cases for longer periods of time than if the condition is bilateral.

The variable effect on an individual's hearing acuity is difficult to assess, particularly in young children. Furthermore, the differential effects of intermittent conductive hearing loss as against a continuous problem are unclear. However, there seems little doubt that where the condition is prolonged for more than several months, linguistic and learning abilities are affected and psychosocial changes seem to occur. These are difficult to monitor and evaluate.

The effects of recurrent bouts of otalgia both locally on the ear and more generally on childhood development is not known. Most studies have not demonstrated any long-term benefit from the wide variety of medical treatments so far investigated in properly controlled trials. Few studies have demonstrated whether treatment can prevent the development of later complications within the middle ear.

Medical treatment

Longitudinal studies show that, not only is there seasonal variation in the condition, but relapses and remissions occur several years after treatment has been prescribed. Many reported studies present results only 6 weeks and 3 months after treatment. Fraser, Mehta and Fraser (1977) could not demonstrate any improvement in children with otitis media with effusion either as a result of autoinflation of the eustachian tube or using 0.5% ephedrine hydrochloride nose drops. There was no effect from medication with an antihistamine-sympathomimetic amine mixture. Other similar medical regimens have not proved to be effective in obtaining a cure (Hayden *et al.*, 1984; Hughes, 1984). Stewart *et al.* (1985) showed no effect on otitis media with effusion from a mucolytic agent (bromhexine hydrochloride). There have been preliminary reports of the effect of gaseous ventilation of the middle ear cleft with sulphur hexafluoride. However, long-term studies are unavailable (Andreasson *et al.*, 1983).

Management of nasal allergies with topical steroid preparations such as beclomethasone and flunisolide may reduce eustachian tube malfunction, but trials in relation to otitis media with effusion are awaited. Extrapolation of the management of acute suppurative otitis media has led to the recommendation of similar regimens for the management of otitis media with effusion. However, a study by Van Buchem, Dunk and Van T. Hof (1981) did not demonstrate significant differences in the clinical course of acute otitis media whether or not antibiotics had been prescribed. To date, there have not been any convincing statistically controlled trials indicating a sustained cure rate for otitis media with effusion following antibiotic treatment. Short-term reports of the effectiveness of co-trimoxazole (Marks, Mills and Shaheen, 1981) have been contradicted by longer term follow-up studies (Marks, Mills and Shaheen, 1983). More recently, Thomsen *et al.* (1986) have shown short-term cure rates for otitis media with effusion following long-term treatment with a combination of amoxycillin and clavulanic acid. The effect was only demonstrable for 3 months in children over the age of 5 years. Despite a report by Persico, Podoshin and Fradis (1978) showing improved response rates postoperatively in the treatment of otitis media with effusion with ampicillin and prednisolone, compared with ampicillin alone, there seems little convincing supportive evidence to recommend the use of systemic steroids.

The development of vaccines against *Streptococcus pneumoniae* and certain viruses that seem to be associated with acute otitis media may hold some hope of reducing the incidence of this condition. However, at the present time there does not appear to be any effective medical cure for otitis media with effusion.

Surgical treatment

Myringotomy and ventilation tube insertion

Myringotomy incision for relief of *acute suppurative otitis media* should be made either over the point of maximum bulging of the tympanic membrane or in a curvilinear fashion vertically in the postero-inferior segment. The incision splits the middle fibrous layer of the tympanic membrane and care must be taken to avoid middle ear structures.

For aspiration of *serous or mucoid effusions*, a radial incision is made, separating the fibres of the middle layer. The incision is preferably placed in the anteroinferior or anterosuperior quadrant. To prevent early closure of a simple myringotomy,

thermal incisions have been suggested, but probably offer no significant benefit over use of a sharp, thin myringotome. Care must be taken to avoid excessive damage to the fibrous layer which may lead to thin, triangular scar formation at the site of the incision.

Immediate improvement of the hearing loss can be achieved by this procedure. Unfortunately, in all reported series, there is a significant recurrence rate, with reaccumulation of the fluid and return of the hearing impairment. This situation can be overcome by insertion of a ventilation tube often referred to as a grommet. For insertion of a ventilation tube the wire should be cut short. The tube is held with fine forceps by the flange or by the wire and not by the lumen. The upper edge of the flange is introduced into the incision and the remainder of the tube is pressed into position with a fine needle or with the tip of the myringotome (*Figure 12.1*). It is held in place by the tension of the separated fibres of the middle layer. The lumen should be patent and free from secretions, blood or trauma resulting from serrations of the crocodile forceps. The type of material used for manufacture of the tube and whether or not it is inserted in the anterosuperior or anteroinferior quadrants do not appear to affect the time of extrusion. However, tube design, the experience of the operator and whether or not the tube fits loosely when inserted, all significantly affect extrusion rates (Mackenzie, 1984). Since Armstrong's initial report in 1954 subsequent studies have demonstrated the limitation of ventilation tubes both in the long term for hearing improvement and in the shorter term because of the need for re-insertion. Gundersen and Tonning (1976) confirmed satisfactory improvement in speech reception thresholds to 20 dB or less in the short term. Later however, Gundersen, Tonning and Kveberg (1984) reported longer term follow-up

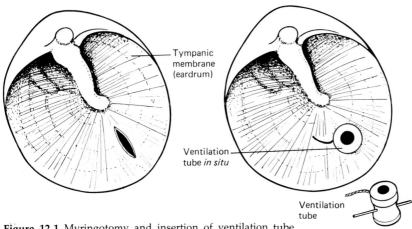

Figure 12.1 Myringotomy and insertion of ventilation tube

with a mean of 12.5 years in 95 out of 100 patients. A total of 179 ears were treated and 28 were found to have permanent hearing loss due to chronic otitis media or adhesions with an average loss of 34 dB. The results led the authors to question the long-term efficacy of ventilation tube insertion.

The mean duration for survival of a functioning tube appears to be about 6–12 months, with no demonstrable benefit of hearing gain after 12 months (Brown, Richards and Ambegaokar, 1978).

Ventilation tubes are associated with more complications than occur with myringotomy alone. There is frequently short-lived otorrhoea. Scarring and tympanosclerosis of the tympanic membrane occur in a significant number of patients. Residual perforation of the tympanic membrane occasionally follows use of a tube. In one-quarter to one-third of cases with established otitis media with effusion, re-insertion is required on one or more occasions until spontaneous resolution of the effusion occurs (Curley, 1986). Richards *et al.* (1971) and Kilby, Richards and Hart (1972) from Cardiff demonstrated that 24 months following myringotomy in one ear and insertion of a Shepard ventilation tube in the other, all of the tubes had been extruded. There was no significant difference in hearing thresholds in either ear and fluid was still present in 30% of ears in each group. Impedance studies showed no significant differences, but thin tympanic membrane scars were more frequent in ears treated with tubes. Brown, Richards and Ambegaokar (1978), also from Cardiff, reported the 5-year follow-up of 55 cases. They showed no difference in the hearing thresholds 6 months following insertion of ventilation tubes compared with myringotomy alone. They also showed a 42% incidence of tympanosclerosis and a 13% incidence of thin scars. There was a recurrence rate of 33% which was the same whether or not a tube had been inserted. Adenoidectomy had been performed in all cases and tonsillectomy in a few.

As time passes, the incidence of tympanosclerosis increases and was shown by Miller, Wilson and Richards (1982) to be as high as 70% after 10 years. In a study from the present author's department, Slack *et al.* (1984) confirmed this figure for at least some degree of tympanosclerosis 21 months after insertion of ventilation tubes. In this study, such tympanic membrane changes were almost never seen in the contralateral unoperated ear. Birck and Mravec (1976) studied 736 children and 2237 ventilation tube insertions. Adenoidectomy with or without tonsillectomy was performed in 44% of patients and of these, 35% required a further tube insertion. There was a failure rate of 27% for adenoidectomy alone. As with other studies, a high incidence of failure was noted in the group of children suffering with

allergic disease in addition to middle ear effusion. Otorrhoea was reported in 15% of cases.

From Copenhagen, Tos and Poulsen (1976) reported the late results of treatment with tubes in 109 patients. Adenoidectomy was usually also performed at the same time, although had previously been carried out in 37%. They showed a 60% total cure rate and a 25% partial cure rate and indicated that re-insertion of tubes was required in 23% of cases. The studies of Miller, Wilson and Richards (1982) have been confirmed by Tos *et al.* (1984) and dispute the suggestion that middle ear ventilation with a tube may prevent serious long-term complications such as atelectasis and attic retraction. In many centres, myringotomy and aspiration alone are practised in the first instance, reserving tube insertion for recurrent cases.

The high complication rate resulting from ventilation tubes has led some authors to suggest a policy of unilateral rather than bilateral insertion, especially in young children (Lildholt, 1979; To, Pahor and Robin, 1984). Lildholt reported 91 children with bilateral otitis media with effusion in which adenoidectomy was performed together with unilateral myringotomy and tube insertion. The contralateral ear was left untreated and no difference was found in the middle ear pressure or hearing level one month after extrusion of the tube. One-quarter of the ears suffered otorrhoea. The study is slightly invalidated, in that certain cases had been submitted to previous adenoidectomy. Such a compromise regimen of unilateral treatment for bilateral cases has also been suggested by Bonding, Tos and Poulsen (1982) and Sade (1979). The former studied the effect in bilateral cases, of unilateral tube insertion compared with myringotomy alone, repeating the work of Kilby, Richards and Hart which had been performed 10 years earlier in 1972. They suggested that, in 75% of cases, resolution of effusions had occurred following adenoidectomy and myringotomy and that part of the improvement was spontaneous and unrelated to treatment. It was suggested that a ventilation tube did not improve long-term eustachian tube function. More recently, Lildholt (1983) repeated his recommendation for elective unilateral tube insertion. Notwithstanding any of these problems, ventilation tube insertion is the most common surgical procedure performed in children in the USA (Vogelsang and Birck, 1984) and is fast reaching similar proportions in the UK (Black, 1984b).

Surgical treatment may be indicated for any obvious underlying condition affecting eustachian tube function. It is accepted that earlier rather than late closure of a cleft palate defect will result in improvement of the aural condition. Occasionally, antral washouts are required and sometimes submucosal diathermy is helpful to reduce the nasal obstruction caused by swollen inferior turbinates.

Adenoidectomy and adenotonsillectomy

Since before the turn of the century, and in particular in the preantibiotic era, adenoidectomy had become the accepted method of treatment for the relief of recurrent suppurative middle ear disease. This rationale was based on the assumption that, in some way, the adenoids affected the eustachian tube function and by the *ex vacuo* theory, produced a transudate within the middle ear cleft. This hypothesis was supported by the frequent finding of a unilateral middle ear effusion in association with postnasal space carcinoma involving the eustachian tube cushion. It would seem more reasonable to recommend adenoidectomy in cases presenting with significant symptoms of nasal obstruction and otitis media with effusion but often these are just the cases which are excluded from randomly allocated studies. Recommendation for surgery in children with small non-obstructive adenoids was based on the premise that they acted as a focus of potential ascending eustachian tube infection. Studies by Maw and Speller (1985) refuted this. Adenoidectomy was frequently combined with tonsillectomy, presumably for those cases where there was coexistent upper respiratory tract infection and tonsillitis. Often, however, the aural condition was used to justify tonsillectomy where it could not be advised on its own merits.

Naturally a very high incidence of these surgical procedures in small children has been a cause for concern. Ultimately in 1958, Sataloff and Menduke, and later, McKee (1963a,b) reported some poorly controlled studies showing a limited efficacy of these operations. Doubt was cast upon these results when subsequent studies demonstrated the presence of middle ear disease in 60% of cases where either adenoids had previously been removed or were not found to be present (Dawes, 1970; Mawson and Fagan, 1972). In that year, there were 917 000 tonsil and adenoid operations in the USA, with a rate of 4.5 per 1000. In 1978, 25 000 Danish children, equivalent to approximately 40% of the total birthrate, had been treated by adenoidectomy partly on account of otitis media with effusion. A survey by Hibbert (1977) showed that in the UK 80% of otolaryngologists advised adenoidectomy as part of the treatment for otitis media with effusion and most surgeons felt it was an enlargement of the adenoids which produced the effusion. This was thought to result from obstruction of the eustachian tube orifice.

Snow (1980) carefully reviewed the literature regarding adenoidectomy, adenotonsillectomy and treatment with various medical measures in cases persisting for more than 6 weeks. Such cases were recommended for myringotomy and ventilation tube insertion. Adenoidectomy was not said to be indicated for the majority of first episodes of otitis media with effusion unless there was nasal obstruction, rhinorrhoea or adenoiditis. He suggested that adenoidectomy is more likely to be recommended in recurrent otitis media with effusion following ventilation tube insertion. The position of tonsillectomy in his view is much less certain and is not usually recommended on the basis of otitis media with effusion by itself. Stell (1981) reviewed research from his own and other departments and reached the conclusion that adenoidectomy might be abandoned with virtually no ill effects except in certain cases of obstructive upper airway disease or cor pulmonale. However, his references were not specifically directed to otitis media with effusion or its treatment.

The number of operative procedures on the tonsils and adenoids has diminished during the last decade, but they still account for 50% of all major surgical operations performed on children, 25% of all hospital admissions and 10% of all hospital bed days in the USA, where 25% of all children will undergo this type of surgery (Bluestone, 1982). Black (1985b) confirmed the steady falling rate for adenotonsillectomy operations in the UK by as much as 46% between 1967 and 1980. The reduction within the Oxford Regional Health Authority in children younger than 9 years, suggests the fall for adenoidectomy alone to be significantly less than for the combined procedure. During the same period there was an increase in the frequency of myringotomy as judged on a national basis. Black demonstrated a significant increase in all surgery for 'glue ear' from 47.2% to 68.1%. He noted a social class gradient for these operations and in particular for myringotomy and adenoidectomy, the highest rate for surgery being in the upper social classes. He revealed a twofold difference between health districts, and his data excluded those children managed in private hospitals.

The arguments for and against adenoidectomy and adenotonsillectomy for otitis media with effusion continue. The few studies directed specifically to the problem are not without their design faults. The numbers are usually small. Inclusion criteria are often unsatisfactory and evaluation of an end point for the middle ear condition has been difficult to define. Not all have been randomly controlled nor even prospective and only more recent investigations have included impedance studies in their assessment. There has been failure to evaluate the adenoids and tonsils separately and in many there is a tendency, for ethical reasons, to exclude the most severely affected children. Seldom has inter- and intraobserver variability been considered. Not all studies account for the obvious variables of age, sex, atopy, seasonal variation and adenoid size. Finally, there is often a failure to identify precisely the type and severity of the middle ear effusion to be assessed.

In an uncontrolled study, Lemon (1962) noted a 40% recurrence rate of secretory otitis media in 100 non-adenoidectomy cases compared with only 3% in 100 children submitted to adenoidectomy. In an initial study of 1413 children, McKee (1963a) confirmed a reduction in the incidence of otitis media following adenotonsillectomy. Subsequently, with 200 further children he demonstrated that the benefit with respect to otitis media was attributable to adenoidectomy alone (McKee, 1963b). Similarly Roydhouse (1970) found a reduction in otitis media following adenotonsillectomy in 251 cases, particularly during the first year postoperatively. Stroyer Andersen *et al.* (1979) showed some beneficial effect of adenoidectomy in cases with secretory otitis.

Bluestone, Cantekin and Beery (1975) demonstrated radiographically, retrograde obstruction of the eustachian tube in relation to otitis media and enlarged adenoids. They found adenoidectomy was more successful in the prevention of otitis media in children where there was retrograde obstruction of the eustachian tube, than in children without evidence of preoperative obstruction. They also showed improved prevention of otitis media following adenoidectomy where there were larger, rather than smaller adenoids, particularly if the child did not suffer from allergic rhinitis. Atopic individuals were more likely to develop otitis media following adenoidectomy. This study was uncontrolled, of short follow-up and with limited numbers.

In a later study, commenced in 1971, and reported by Roydhouse in 1980, it was demonstrated that the cure rate for otitis media with effusion was no better following adenoidectomy and ventilation tubes, compared with tubes alone. The cases were followed from 3.7 to 4.3 years. However, there was a greater relapse rate in the non-adenoidectomy group who required 9% more tubes. In addition, radiographs of the adenoids suggested that the group cured without adenoidectomy tended to have smaller adenoids.

Mawson, Adlington and Evans (1967) studied 400 patients and found a significant reduction in sore throats but no altered incidence of otitis media following adenotonsillectomy. Dawes (1970) demonstrated that in two-thirds of 270 cases of middle ear effusion, the adenoids were either not present or had been previously removed. Mawson and Fagan (1972) subsequently showed

that 65% of 81 children with middle ear effusions had previously been submitted to adenoidectomy.

Rynel Dagoo, Ahlbom and Schiratzki (1978) omitted cases with severe prolonged nasal obstruction in a study of 76 children randomly allocated to control and adenoidectomy groups. They demonstrated in both groups a reduction of colds, suppurative and serous otitis media and of nasal obstruction which was more obviously reduced in the adenoidectomy group in the first year. However, if middle ear fluid was found at the time of adenoidectomy, myringotomies and insertion of ventilation tubes were also performed. There were only 12 cases of serous otitis media in the adenoidectomy group and 18 in the control group with crude criteria for middle ear diagnosis. The validity of this study is therefore considerably reduced.

In a small, very carefully controlled prospective study of 42 cases, Fiellau Nikolajsen, Falbe-Hansen and Knudstrup (1980) could not demonstrate any beneficial effect of adenoidectomy on impedance measurements. However, the 20 children randomly allocated for adenoidectomy and myringotomy, compared with the 22 for myringotomy alone would probably not constitute the type of case normally submitted for adenoidectomy in some other centres. Furthermore, some had previously been submitted to adenoidectomy before the study commenced. With rather inadequate supportive data, Sade (1979) reported no better improvement in otitis media with effusion after adenoidectomy and insertion of a ventilation tube compared with insertion of a tube alone. A recent study by Widemar *et al.* (1985) was reported to show no effect of adenoidectomy on tympanic membrane changes, pure-tone audiometry and impedance findings in cases with otitis media with effusion. However, bilateral myringotomies had been performed in all cases and insertion of tubes in those with mucoid secretions. These additional procedures somewhat invalidate their assumptions, for the study lacks a group treated by adenoidectomy alone. By contrast, a retrospective study by Marshak and Ben Neriah (1980) showed a statistically non-significant improvement rate ($P<0.3$) in otitis media with effusion after adenoidectomy and myringotomy (74%) compared with myringotomy alone (59%), but Birck and Mravec (1976) recorded a 27% failure rate for adenoidectomy alone particularly where allergy was coexistent.

Prospective randomized studies by the author (Maw, 1983; 1985a,b; 1986) showed that adenoidectomy alone produces significant clearance of middle ear effusion in 31.3% of cases at 6 months, and 41.7% at one year, judged by pneumatic otoscopy. It also results in no peak/peak conversion of impedance curves in 22.5% of cases at 6 months and 29.8% at one year. There is an audiometric hearing gain of 12.78 dB at 6 months and 13.52 dB at one year. The effect of adenoidectomy was enhanced in older children – aged more than 5 years – compared with younger children and in those with larger, rather than smaller adenoids, as demonstrated by preoperative lateral cephalometric radiographs. The sex of the child and the presence or absence of atopy had no effect on the outcome. The improvement in relation to adenoid size was short lived and any effect after 6 months may have resulted from age rather than adenoid size.

The combination of tonsillectomy with adenoidectomy provided no additional benefit. Indeed, compared with adenoidectomy alone, although the combined procedure had a more beneficial effect when assessed after 6 months, the effect was reversed after one year. The reduced effectiveness by the addition of tonsillectomy may be due to palatal scarring altering nasopharyngeal anatomy and function. The addition of myringotomy and ventilation tube insertion with adenoidectomy and adenotonsillectomy, resulted in only slightly improved hearing thresholds after 6 months and no significant difference after one year. There was improved otoscopic clearance of effusion and impedance change when a ventilation tube was also used. However, to achieve this slight benefit and maintain adequate hearing thresholds, re-insertion of the tube was required in 26% of the cases in the adenoidectomy group and 34% in the adenotonsillectomy group.

Treatment with a ventilation tube alone, produced much the same hearing thresholds after 6 months and 12 months as those cases treated by adenoidectomy and adenotonsillectomy alone. However, with only a tube, re-insertion was required in 54% of cases to achieve continued and satisfactory overall hearing thresholds.

Bulman, Brook and Berry (1984) have demonstrated significant benefit from adenoidectomy at 3 and 6 months postoperatively as judged by pure tone audiometry. Any further benefit after 6 months was not demonstrable possibly because of removal of the more severely affected cases from the trial. Paradise *et al.* (1986) have recently confirmed significant improvement in recurrent acute otitis media and otitis media with effusion following adenoidectomy. The beneficial effects were seen to persist for at least 2 years postoperatively. Their study was well controlled, prospective and of a very careful design. The correlation between adenoid size radiologically or volumetrically and the presence or absence of middle ear effusion is poor. However, Hibbert (1979) showed reduction of the postnasal space airway ($P<0.05$) in children with middle ear effusions, compared with age-matched controls, and the author's own

studies substantiate this finding (Phillips, Maw and Harvey, 1987). It seems possible therefore that, although the adenoids are no larger in children with middle ear effusion, some aspects of the morphology of the postnasal space may be different.

On the basis of these investigations, it would seem that surgery should not be recommended until bilateral effusions have been confirmed to have had significant effect on hearing thresholds for at least 3 months. Treatment of unilateral cases may be further deferred, but naturally other factors such as speech, language and learning require consideration. Adenoidectomy should probably be recommended selectively in those cases with larger than average adenoids as demonstrated on a lateral cephalometric radiograph. Improved results may be expected in children more than 5 years of age. However, younger children with obstructive adenoids would also be expected to benefit by adenoidectomy. In addition, myringotomies should be performed bilaterally.

Insertion of a single ventilation tube provides immediate restoration of hearing acuity. It would be expected that after approximately 6–12 months, extrusion will occur and the child's parents should be advised of the likely need for repeat insertion in at least 25% of cases. By limiting tube insertion to only one ear, any complications would be significantly reduced. Naturally, the state of the tympanic membrane with respect to the degree of atelectasis may indicate a need for bilateral tube insertion and perhaps even prolonged ventilation with a long-term type of tympanostomy tube. Recommendation for adenoidectomy can be made in the knowledge that overall, regardless of adenoid size, there is at least a 40% rate of clearance of effusion after one year. Careful selection of cases with regard to age and adenoid size may significantly improve this figure. Unless there are very specific indications for tonsillectomy in children with otitis media with effusion, the operation should not be additionally recommended. Obviously, some children with combined aural and obstructive upper airway disease due to their tonsillar enlargement may require tonsillar surgery.

Sequelae

The linguistic and learning effects of untreated otitis media with effusion, especially if bilateral, are well recognized and documented (Silva *et al.*, 1986). In severe cases, without treatment it seems likely that tympanic membrane retraction, particularly in the attic region will occur.

Tympanosclerosis frequently develops following ventilation tube insertion and this is not often an accompaniment of simple myringotomy and aspiration (Tos, Bonding and Poulsen, 1983). Brown, Richards and Ambegaokar (1978) reported a 42% incidence at 5 years and a 13% incidence of thin scars in the ears with tubes, compared with a zero incidence of either condition in the control ear. A 10-year follow-up rate of 67% was obtained for 34 of these patients. Miller, Wilson and Richards (1982) noted a most significant finding of increased pars flaccida pathology which was of similar incidence in the tubed and untubed control ear. Barfoed and Rosberg (1980) demonstrated tympanosclerosis in 61% of cases 4.5–7.5 years following tube insertion and also noted more marked pseudomembrane formation, cicatrization and atrophy. These occurred particularly at the site where the tympanic membrane had been disrupted by placement of the tube. Slack *et al.* (1984) have confirmed that the incidence of tympanosclerosis progresses rapidly, so that even after one year, slightly less than 40% of cases have some degree of the condition and after 21 months, the incidence is 70%. Furthermore, there is a gradual increase in the distribution of the sclerotic process throughout the drum. It appears that there is a predisposition for its development to commence in the posteroinferior quadrant in cases where the ventilation tube is inserted anteroinferiorly. There is some equivocal relationship between tympanosclerosis development and mucoid rather than serous effusions.

The development of attic retraction sacs in relation to otitis media with effusion was reported by Tos and Poulsen (1980). More recently, Tos *et al.* (1984) have confirmed the data reported by Miller, Wilson and Richards (1982). In a sample of healthy, non-selected children, they showed attic retraction, atrophy or tympanosclerosis in 24% of 5-year olds, 37% of 6-year olds and 39% of 7-year olds. There was a correlation between the tympanometric profile, the frequency of otitis media and the eardrum abnormality which did not seem to be corrected by treatment with ventilation tubes.

Suppuration after tube insertion has been reported in as many as 34% in the series by Barfoed and Rosberg (1980); 41% of cases by Kokko (1974) and 30% of cases in Lildholt's series (1983). Persistent perforation develops more frequently where there is otorrhoea and all series of any size, document the development of a small number of cholesteatomata in the operated ears.

In view of the findings by Miller, Wilson and Richards (1982) and Tos *et al.* (1984) one must question further the ability of ventilation tubes to forestall the progression of tympanic membrane changes due to negative middle ear pressure. This is particularly related to those changes which occur in the attic. All otologists have witnessed the steady progression of tympanic membrane changes which occur in some cases of otitis media with effusion as a result of chronic negative middle ear pressure. Ultimately a state of severe atelectasis develops which is extremely difficult both to arrest or correct. A thin two-layered membrane becomes indrawn onto the medial wall of the middle ear. It is draped over the ossicles and indrawn towards the eustachian tube and attic regions. Often some degree of ossicular erosion occurs particularly of the long process of the incus. Outer attic wall erosion also occurs revealing the neck of the malleus and body of the incus over which the thin retracted membrane is applied. At this stage, middle ear ventilation is invariably impossible to achieve. These patients, especially if bilateral disease is present, require a hearing aid. Attempts at reconstructive surgery in these instances are demanding and often unrewarding.

References

ALHADY, R. A. and SHARNOUBI, M. E. (1984) Tympanometric findings in patients with adenoid hyperplasia, chronic sinusitis and tonsillitis. *Journal of Laryngology and Otology*, **98**, 671–676

ANDREASSON, L., BYLANDER, A., IVARSSON, A. and TJERNSTROM, O. (1983) Treatment with sulfur hexafluoride in children with serous otitis media. *Archives of Otolaryngology*, **109**, 358–359

ARMSTRONG, B. W. (1954) A new treatment for chronic secretory otitis media. *Archives of Otolaryngology*, **59**, 653–654

BARFOED, C. and ROSBERG, J. (1980) Secretory otitis media. *Archives of Otolaryngology*, **106**, 553–556

BATEMAN, G. H. (1959) Secretory otitis media. *Journal of Laryngology and Otolaryngology*, **71**, 261–276

BEERY, Q. C., ANDRUS, W. S., BLUESTONE, C. D. and CANTEKIN, E. I. (1975) Tympanometric pattern of classification in relation to middle ear effusions. *The Laryngoscope*, **85**, 56–64

BIRCK, H. D. and MRAVEC, J. J. (1976) Myringotomy for middle ear effusions. Results of a two-year study. *Annals of Otology, Rhinology and Laryngology, 85*, (suppl. 25), 263–267

BLACK, N. (1984a) Is glue ear a modern phenomenon? A historical review of the medical literature. *Clinical Otolaryngology*, **9**, 155–163

BLACK, N. (1984b) Surgery for glue ear – a modern epidemic. *The Lancet*, **1**, 835–837

BLACK, N. (1985a) Glue ear: the new dyslexia? *British Medical Journal*, **290**, 1963–1965

BLACK, N. (1985b) Geographical variations in the use of surgery for glue ear. *Journal of the Royal Society of Medicine*, **78**, 641–648

BLUESTONE, C. D. (1982) Current concepts in otolaryngology. Otitis media in children: to treat or not to treat. *New England Journal of Medicine*, **306**, 1399–1404

BLUESTONE, C. D. and BEERY, Q. C. (1976) Concepts on the pathogenesis of middle ear effusion. *Annals of Otology, Rhinology and Laryngology*, **85**, (suppl. 25), 182–186

BLUESTONE, C. D. and CANTEKIN, E. I. (1979) Eustachian tube dysfunction. In *Otolaryngology* (revised edn), edited by G. English, pp. 1–40. Hagerstown, Md: Harper and Row

BLUESTONE, C. D., CANTEKIN, E. I. and BEERY, Q. C. (1975) Certain effects of adenoidectomy on eustachian tube ventilatory function. *The Laryngoscope*, **85**, 113–127

BONDING, P., TOS, M. and POULSEN, G. (1982) Unilateral insertion of grommets in bilateral secretory otitis media. Tympanometric findings after 1–3 years. *Acta Oto-Laryngologica Supplementum*, **286**, 161–162

BORGE, P. (1983) Atopy and secretory otitis media. Immunological studies and responses to topical corticosteroid therapy. *Journal of Laryngology and Otology*, **97**, 117–129

BROOKS, D. (1976) School screening for middle ear effusion. *Annals of Otology, Rhinology and Laryngology*, **85**, (suppl. 25), 223–229

BROOKS, D. N. (1968) An objective method of detecting fluid in the middle ear. *International Audiology*, **7**, 280–286

BROWN, M. J. K. M., RICHARDS, S. H. and AMBEGAOKAR, A. G. (1978) Grommets and glue ear: a five-year follow-up of a controlled trial. *Proceedings of the Royal Society of Medicine*, **71**, 353–356

BULMAN, C. H., BROOK, S. J. and BERRY, M. G. (1984) A prospective randomised trial of adenoidectomy vs grommet insertion in the treatment of glue ear. *Clinical Otolaryngology*, **9**, 67–75

CANTEKIN, E. I., BEERY, Q. C. and BLUESTONE, C. D. (1977) Tympanometric patterns found in middle ear effusions. *Annals of Otology, Rhinology and Laryngology*, **86**, (suppl. 41), 16–20

CAPPER, J. W. R., SLACK, R. W. T. and MAW, A. R. (1987) Tuning fork tests in children – an evaluation of their usefulness. *Journal of Laryngology and Otology* (in press)

CASSELBRANT, M. L., BROSTOFF, L. M., CANTEKIN, E. I., FLAHERTY, M. R., DOYLE, W. J., BLUESTONE, C. D. *et al.* (1985) Otitis media with effusion in pre-school children. *The Laryngoscope*, **95**, 428–436

CHURCH, M. K., COLEMAN, J. W., HOLGATE, S. T., PAO, G. J. K. and WELCH, M. T. (1981) The effect of polyamine, 48/80 and calcium ionophone on histamine release from human dispersed lung and adenoid mast cells. *British Journal of Pharmacology*, **74**, 979–980

CLEMIS, J. D. (1976) Identification of allergic factors in middle ear effusions. *Annals of Otology, Rhinology and Laryngology*, Suppl. 25, 234–237

COLLINS, M. P., CHURCH, M. K., BAKSHI, K. N. and OSBORNE, J. (1985) Adenoid histamine and its possible relationship to secretory otitis media. *Journal of Laryngology and Otology*, **99**, 685–691

CURLEY, J. W. A. (1986) Grommet insertion: some basic questions answered. *Clinical Otolaryngology*, **11**, 1–4

DAWES, J. D. K. (1970) The aetiology and sequelae of exudative otitis media. *Journal of Laryngology and Otology*, **84**, 583–610

De MARIA, T. F., BRIGGS, B. R., LIM, D. J. and OKAZAKI, N. (1984) Experimental otitis media with effusion following inoculation of non-viable *H. influenzae*. *Annals of Otology, Rhinology and Laryngology*, **93**, 52–56

De MARIA, T. F., McGHEE, R. B. and LIM, D. J. (1984) Rheumatoid factor in otitis media with effusion. *Archives of Otolaryngology*, **110**, 279–280

FEIGIN, R. D. (1982) Otitis media: closing the information gap. *New England Journal of Medicine*, **306**, 1417–1418

FIELLAU NIKOLAJSEN, M. (1983) Tympanometry and secretory otitis media. *Acta Oto-Laryngologica Supplementum*, **394**, 1–73

FIELLAU NIKOLAJSEN, M., FALBE-HANSEN, J. and KNUDSTRUP, P. (1980) Adenoidectomy for middle ear disorders: a randomized controlled study. *Clinical Otolaryngology*, **5**, 323–377

FRASER, J. G., MEHTA, M. and FRASER, P. M. (1977) The medical treatment of secretory otitis media. Clinical trial of three commonly used regimes. *Journal of Laryngology and Otology*, **91**, 707–765

FRIA, T. J., CANTEKIN, E. I. and EICHLER, J. A. (1985) Hearing acuity in children with otitis media with effusion. *Archives of Otolaryngology*, **111**, 10–16

FRIA, T. J., CANTEKIN, E. I. and PROBST, G. (1980) Validation of an automatic otoadmittance middle ear analyzer. *Annals of Otology, Rhinology and Laryngology*, **89**, 253–256

GOTTSCHALK, G. H. (1972) Serous otitis. A conservation approach to treatment. *Archives of Otolaryngology*, **96**, 110–112

GRIMALDI, P. M. E. B. (1976) The value of impedance testing in diagnosis of middle ear effusion. *Journal of Laryngology and Otology*, **90**, 141–152

GUNDERSEN, T. and TONNING, F. M. (1976) Ventilation tubes in the middle ear; long term observations. *Archives of Otolaryngology*, **102**, 198–199

GUNDERSEN, T., TONNING, F. M. and KVEBERG, K. H. (1984) Ventilating tubes in the middle ear. Long-term observations. *Archives of Otolaryngology*, **110**, 783–784

HAYDEN, G. F., RANDALL, J. E., RANDALL, J. C. and HENDLEY, J. O. (1984) Topical phenylephrine for the treatment of middle ear effusion. *Archives of Otolaryngology*, **110**, 1512–1514

HENDERSON, F. W., COLLIER, A. M., SANYAL, M. A., WATKINS, J. M., FAIRCLOUGH, D. L., CLYDE, W. A. *et al.* (1982) A longitudinal study of respiratory viruses and bacteria in the aetiology of acute otitis media with effusion. *New England Journal of Medicine*, **306**, 1377–1383

HIBBERT, J. (1977) The current status of adenoidectomy: a survey among otolaryngologists. *Clinical Otolaryngology*, **2**, 239–247

HIBBERT, J. (1979) Some aspects of adenoidectomy. *ChM Thesis*, University of Liverpool, Liverpool

HIBBERT, J. and TWEEDIE, M. C. K. (1977) The value of signs and symptoms in the diagnosis of enlarged adenoids. *Clinical Otolaryngology*, **2**, 297–304

HIBBERT, J. and WHITEHOUSE, G. H. (1978) The assessment of adenoidal size by radiological means. *Clinical Otolaryngology*, **3**, 43–47

HILLS, B. A. (1984) Analysis of eustachian surfactant and its function as a release agent. *Archives of Otolaryngology*, **110**, 3–9

HINCHCLIFFE, R. (1976) Epidemiology and otolaryngology. In *Scientific Foundations in Otolaryngology*, edited by R. Hinchcliffe and D. Harrison, pp. 133–150. London: Heinemann

HOLBOROW, C. A. (1970) Eustachian tubal function. Changes in anatomy and function with age and the relationship of these changes to aural pathology. *Archives of Otolaryngology*, **92**, 624–626

HUGHES, K. B. (1984) Management of middle ear effusions in children. *Journal of Laryngology and Otology*, **98**, 677–684

JEANS, W. D., FERNANDO, D. C. J. and MAW, A. R. (1981) How should adenoid enlargement be measured? A radiological study based on inter-observer agreement. *Clinical Radiology*, **32**, 337–340

JEANS, W. D., FERNANDO, D. C. J., MAW, A. R. and LEIGHTON, B. C. (1981) A longitudinal study of the growth of the nasopharynx and its contents in normal children. *British Journal of Radiology*, **54**, 117–121

JERGER, J. (1970) Clinical experience with impedance audiometry. *Archives of Otolaryngology*, **92**, 311

JOHNSON, A. P., MURRAY, J. A. M. and MARAN, A. G. D. (1983) Errors in the assessment of nasopharyngeal airway by radiograph. *Journal of Laryngology and Otolaryngology*, **97**, 1017–1026

KILBY, D., RICHARDS, S. H. and HART, G. (1972) Grommets and glue ear: two year results. *Journal of Laryngology and Otology*, **86**, 881–888

KLEIN, J. O. (1979) Epidemiology of otitis media. *Proceedings of the 2nd National Conference of Otitis Media*, held in Colombus, Ohio, edited by R. J. Wiet and S. W. Coulthard, pp. 18–20. Columbus, Ohio: Ross Laboratories

KLEIN, J. O. (1980) Microbiology of otitis media. *Annals of Otology, Rhinology and Laryngology*, Suppl. 68, 98

KNIGHT, N. J. and PHILLIPS, M. J. (1980) Round window rupture and acquired sensorineural loss in children. *Clinical Otolaryngology*, **5**, 117–128

KOKKO, E. (1974) Chronic secretory otitis media in children. *Acta Oto-Laryngologica Supplementum*, **327**, 1–44

LEMON, A. N. (1962) Serous otitis media in children. *The Laryngoscope*, **72**, 32–44

LILDHOLT, T. (1979) Unilateral grommet insertion and adenoidectomy in bilateral secretory otitis media; preliminary report of the results in 91 children. *Clinical Otolaryngology*, **4**, 87–93

LILDHOLT, T. (1983) Ventilation tubes in secretory otitis media. *Acta Oto-Laryngologica Supplementum*, **398**, 1–70

LIM, D. J. (1979) Normal and pathological mucosa of the middle ear and Eustachian tube. *Clinical Otolaryngology*, **4**, 213–234

LIM, D. J. (1985) Recent advances in otitis media with effusion. Report of research conference. *Annals of Otology, Rhinology and Laryngology*, **94**, (suppl. 116), 1–32

LIM, D. J., BLUESTONE, C. D., KLEIN, J. O. and NELSON, J. D. (1984) *Recent Advances in Otitis Media with Effusion*. Philadelphia: B. J. Decker Inc.

LIM, D. J., BLUESTONE, C. D., SAUNDERS, W. H. and SENTURIA, B. H. (1976) Recent advances in middle ear effusions. *Annals of Otology, Rhinology and Laryngology*, **85**, (suppl. 1), 1–299

LIM, D. J. and De MARIA, T. F. (1982) Pathogenesis of otitis media bacteriology and immunology. *The Laryngoscope*, **92**, 278–286

LINDER-ARONSON, S. (1970) Adenoids. Their effect on mode of breathing and nasal airflow and their relationship to characteristics of the facial skeleton and dentition. *Acta Oto-Laryngologica Supplementum*, **265**, 1–132

LOUS, J. and FIELLAU NIKOLAJSEN, M. (1981) Epidemiology of middle ear effusion and tubal dysfunction. A one year prospective study comparing monthly tympanometry in 387 non-selected seven-year-old children. *International Journal of Paediatric Otorhinolaryngology*, **3**, 303–317

McKEE, W. J. E. (1963a) A controlled study of the effects of tonsillectomy and adenoidectomy in children. *British Journal of Preventative and Social Medicine*, **17**, 49–69

McKEE, W. J. E. (1963b) The part played by adenoidectomy in the combined operation of tonsillectomy with adenoidectomy. *British Journal of Preventative and Social Medicine*, **17**, 133–140

MACKENZIE, I. J. (1984) Factors affecting the extrusion rates of ventilation tubes. *Journal of the Royal Society of Medicine*, **77**, 751–753

McNICHOLL, W. D. (1983) Otitis media with effusion in children and its association with deformation of the vomeroethmoid suture, *Journal of Laryngology and Otology*, **97**, 203–212

MALCOLMSEN, K. G. (1969) Long term follow-up of chronic exudative otitis media. *Proceedings of the Royal Society of Medicine*, **62**, 43–46

MARCHANT, C. D., SHURIN, P. A., TURCZYK, V. A., WASIKOWSKI, D. E., TUTIHASI, M. A. and KINNEY, S. E. (1984) Course and outcome of otitis media in early infancy: a prospective study. *Journal of Pediatrics*, **104**, 826–831

MARKS, N. J., MILLS, R. F. and SHAHEEN, O. H. (1981) A controlled trial of cotrimoxazole therapy in serous otitis media. *Journal of Laryngology and Otology*, **95**, 1003–1009

MARKS, N. J., MILLS, R. P. and SHAHEEN, O. H. (1983) Cotrimoxazole in the treatment of serous otitis media. A follow-up report. *Journal of Laryngology and Otology*, **97**, 213–215

MARSHAK, G. and BEN NERIAH, Z. (1980) Adenoidectomy versus tympanotomy in chronic secretory otitis media. *Annals of Otology, Rhinology and Laryngology*, **89**, (suppl. 68), 316–318

MAW, A. R. (1983) Chronic otitis media with effusion (glue ear) and adenotonsillectomy: prospective randomized controlled study. *British Medical Journal*, **287**, 1586–1588

MAW, A. R. (1985a) Age and adenoid size in relation to adenoidectomy in otitis media with effusion. *American Journal of Otolaryngology*, **6**, 245–248

MAW, A. R. (1985b) Factors affecting adenoidectomy for otitis media with effusion (glue ear). *Journal of the Royal Society of Medicine*, **78**, 1014–1018

MAW, A. R. (1986) Adenoidectomy and adenotonsillectomy for otitis media with effusion (glue ear) in children: a prospective randomized controlled study. MS Thesis, University of London, London

MAW, A. R. and HEROD, F. (1986) Otoscopic, impedance and audiometric findings in glue ear treated by adenoidectomy and tonsillectomy. A prospective randomized study. *The Lancet*, **1**, 1399–1402

MAW, A. R., JEANS, W. D. and FERNANDO, D. C. J. (1981) Inter-observer variability in the clinical and radiological assessment of adenoid size and the correlation with adenoid volume. *Clinical Otolaryngology*, **6**, 317–322

MAW, A. R. and SPELLER, D. C. E. (1985) Are the tonsils and adenoids a reservoir in otitis media with effusion (glue ear). *Clinical Otolaryngology*, **10**, 265–269

MAWSON, S. R., ADLINGTON, P. and EVANS, M. (1967) A controlled study. Evaluation of adenotonsillectomy in children. *Journal of Laryngology and Otology*, **81**, 777–790

MAWSON, S. R. and FAGAN, P. (1972) Tympanic effusions in children. *Journal of Laryngology and Otology*, **86**, 105–119

METZ, O. (1946) The acoustic impedance measured on normal and pathological ears. *Acta Oto-Laryngologica Supplementum*, **63**, 1–254

MILLER, J. J., WILSON, F. and RICHARDS, S. H. (1982) Grommets and glue ear; a 10-year follow-up of a controlled trial. *Clinical Otolaryngology*, **7**, 135

MILLS, R. and BRAIN, C. (1985) A history of acute suppurative otitis media and allergic symptomatology in children with chronic secretory otitis media and controls. *Clinical Otolaryngology*, **10**, 303–306

MILLS, R., UTTLEY, A. and McINTYRE, M. (1984) Relationship between acute suppurative otitis media and chronic secretory otitis media: role of antibiotics. *Journal of the Royal Society of Medicine*, **77**, 754–757

MILLS, R., UTTLEY, A. H. C. and McINTYRE, M. F. (1985) A bacteriological study of the middle ear and upper respiratory tract in children with chronic secretory otitis media. *Clinical Otolaryngology*, **10**, 335–341

MOGI, G., MAEDA, S. and YOSHIDA, T. (1976) Immunochemistry of otitis media with effusion. *Journal of Infectious Diseases*, **133**, 126–236

PALVA, T., LEHTINEN, H. and VIRTANEN, H. (1983) Immune complexes in the middle ear fluid and adenoid tissue in chronic secretory otitis media. *Acta Oto-Laryngologica Supplementum*, **95**, 539–543

PALVA, T., RAUNIO, V. and NOUSIANEN, R. (1974) Secretory otitis media. Protein and enzyme analysis. *Annals of Otology, Rhinology and Laryngology*, **83**, (suppl. 11), 35–43

PARADISE, J. L. (1976) Paediatricians' view of middle ear effusions; more questions than answers. *Annals of Otology, Rhinology and Laryngology*, **85**, (suppl. 25), 20–24

PARADISE, J. L., BLUESTONE, C. D. and FELDER, H. (1969) The universality of otitis media in 50 infants with cleft palate. *Paediatrics*, **44**, 35–42

PARADISE, J. L., BLUESTONE, C. D., ROGERS, K. D. *et al.* (1986) Efficacy of adenoidectomy for recurrent otitis media: results from parallel randomised and non randomised clinical trials. *Proceedings of the International Symposium on Acute and Secretory Otitis Media*, Part 1, Jerusalem, Israel, 17–22 November, 1985, edited by J. Sade. Amsterdam: Kugler Publications

PARADISE, J. L., SMITH, C. G. and BLUESTONE, C. D. (1976) Tympanometric detection of middle ear effusion in infants and young children. *Paediatrics*, **58**, 198–210

PERSICO, M., PODOSHIN, L. and FRADIS, M. (1978) Otitis media. A steroid and antibiotic therapeutic trial before surgery. *Annals of Otology, Rhinology and Laryngology*, **87**, 191–196

PHILLIPS, M. J., KNIGHT, N. J., MANNING, H., ABBOTT, A. L. and TRIPP, W. G. (1974) IgE and secretory otitis media. *The Lancet*, **2**, 1176–1178

PHILLIPS, D. E., MAW, A. R. and HARVEY, K. (1987) The nasopharynx and adenoid in children with glue ear compared with normal controls. *Clinical Otolaryngology* (in press)

POLITZER, A. (1869) *Diseases of the Ear*, 5th edn, translated by M. J. Ballin and C. J. Heller. Philadelphia: Lee and Febiger

POTSIC, W. P. (1980) The role of adenoidectomy in secretory otitis media. In *Controversy in Otolaryngology* edited by J. B. Snow, pp. 154–159. Philadelphia: W. B. Saunders

PUKANDER, J., SIPILA, M. and KARMA, P. (1984) Occurrence of and risk factors in acute otitis media. In *Recent Advances in Otitis Media with Effusion*, edited by D. J. Lim *et al.*, pp. 9–13. Philadelphia: B.C. Decker Inc

QUARNBERG, Y. (1981) Acute otitis media. A prospective clinical study of myringotomy and antimicrobial treatment. *Acta Oto-Laryngologica Supplementum*, **375**, 1–157

RAPIN, J. (1979) Conductive hearing loss effects on children's language development and scholastic skills. *Annals of Otology, Rhinology and Laryngology*, **88**, (suppl. 60), 3–12

RICHARDS, S. H., KILBY, D., SHAW, J. D. and CAMPBELL, H. (1971) Grommets and glue ear: a clinical trial. *Journal of Laryngology and Otology*, **85**, 27–32

ROYDHOUSE, N. (1970) A controlled study of adenotonsillectomy. *Archives of Otolaryngology*, **92**, 611–616

ROYDHOUSE, N. (1980) Adenoidectomy for otitis media with mucoid effusion. *Annals of Otology, Rhinology and Laryngology*, **89**, (suppl. 68), 312–315

RUBEN, R. J. and MATH, R. (1978) Serous otitis media associated with sensorineural loss in children. *The Laryngoscope*, **88**, 1139–1154

RUOKONEN, J., SANDELIN, K. and MAKINEN, J. (1979) Adenoids and otitis media with effusion. *Annals of Otology, Rhinology and Laryngology*, **88**, 166–171

RYNEL DAGOO, B., AHLBOM, A. and SCHIRATZKI, H. (1978) Effects of adenoidectomy: a controlled two year follow-up. *Annals of Otology, Rhinology and Laryngology*, **87**, 272–278

SADE, J. (1979) *Secretory Otitis Media and its Sequelae.* New York: Churchill Livingstone

SATALOFF, J. and MENDUKE, H. (1958) Adenoids and hearing loss in children. *American Journal of Diseases in Children*, **95**, 529–533

SENTURIA, B. H., BLUESTONE, C. D., LIM, D. J. and SAUNDERS, W. H. (1980) Recent advances in otitis media with effusion. *Annals of Otology, Rhinology and Laryngology*, **89**, (suppl. 68), 1–362

SENTURIA, B. H., GESSERT, C. F., CAR, C. D. and BAUMANN, H. S. (1958) Studies concerned with tubo-tympanitis. *Annals of Otology, Rhinology and Laryngology*, **67**, 440–467

SILVA, P. A., CHALMERS, D., STEWART, I. A. and WILLIAMS, S. M. (1986) Some audiological, psychological, educational and behavioural characteristics of children with bilateral otitis media with effusion: a longitudinal study. In *Proceedings of International Symposium on Acute Secretory Otitis Media*, Part 1, Jerusalem, Israel, 17–22 November, 1985, edited by J. Sade. Amsterdam: Kugler Publications

SILVA, P. A., KIRKLAND, C., SIMPSON, A., STEWART, I. A. and WILLIAMS, S. M. (1982) Some developmental and behavioural characteristics associated with bilateral secretory otitis media. *Journal of Learning Disabilities*, **15**, 417–425

SLACK, R. W. T., MAW, A. R., CAPPER, J. W. R. and KELLY, S. (1984) A prospective study of tympanosclerosis developing after grommet insertion. *Journal of Laryngology and Otology*, **98**, 771–774

SNOW, J. B. (1980) Role of tonsillectomy and adenoidectomy in the management of children with middle ear effusion. *Annals of Otology, Rhinology and Laryngology*, **89**, 43–46

STELL, P. M. (1981) Adenoidectomy (editorial). *Clinical Otolaryngology*, **6**, 1–3

STEWART, I., KIRKLAND, C., SIMPSON, A., SILVA, P. and WILLIAMS, S. (1984) Some developmental characteristics associated with otitis media with effusion. In *Recent Advances in Otitis Media with Effusion*, edited by D. J. Lim *et al.*, pp. 329–331. Philadelphia: B.C. Decker Inc

STEWART, I. A., GUY, A. M., ALLISON, R. S. and THOMSON, N. J. (1985) Bromhexine in the treatment of otitis media with effusion. *Clinical Otolaryngology*, **10**, 145–149

STOME, M. (1981) Down's syndrome: a modern otorhino-laryngological perspective. *The Laryngoscope*, **91**, 1581–1594

STOOL, S. E. (1980) Myringotomies and tympanostomy tubes are sufficient. In *Controversy in Otolaryngology*, edited by J. B. Snow, p. 150. Philadelphia: W. B. Saunders

STOOL, S. E. and RANDALL, P. (1967) Unexpected ear disease in infants with cleft palate. *Cleft Palate Journal*, **4**, 99–103

STROYER-ANDERSEN, M., MEISTRUP LARSEN, U., MEISTRUP LARSEN, K. I. and PETERSEN, E. (1979) *Acta Oto-Laryngologica Supplementum*, **360**, 195–197

SUAREZ NIETO, C., MALLAGUIZA CALVO, R. and BARTHE GARCIA, P. (1983) Aetiological factors in chronic secretory otitis media in relation to age. *Clinical Otolaryngology*, **8**, 171–174

TEELE, D., KLEIN, J. and ROSNER, B. (1980) Epidemiology of otitis media in children. *Annals of Otology, Rhinology and Laryngology*, **89**, (suppl. 68), 5–6

THOMSEN, J., SEDERBERG-OLSEN, J., BALLE, V., BOMHOLT, A., STANGERUP, S. E., TOS, M. *et al.* (1986) Long term antibiotic treatment of patients with secretory otitis media. A double blind placebo controlled study. Proceedings of the *International Symposium on Acute and Secretory Otitis Media*, Part 1, Jerusalem, Israel, 17–22 November, 1985, edited by J. Sade. Amsterdam: Kugler Publications

TO, S., PAHOR, A. L. and ROBIN, P. E. (1984) A prospective trial of unilateral grommets for bilateral secretory otitis media in children. *Clinical Otolaryngology*, **9**, 115–117

TODD, N. W. (1984) Otitis media and eustachian tube calibre. *Acta Oto-Laryngologica Supplementum*, **404**, 1–17

TOS, M., BONDING, P. and POULSEN, G. (1983) Tympano-sclerosis of the drum in secretory otitis after insertion of grommets. A prospective comparative study. *Journal of Laryngology and Otology*, **97**, 489–496

TOS, M., HOLM-VENSEN, S. and SORENSEN, C. H. (1982) Spontaneous course and frequency of secretory otitis in 4-year-old children. *Archives of Otolaryngology*, **108**, 4–10

TOS, M. and POULSEN, G. (1976) Secretory otitis media. Late results of treatment with grommets. *Archives of Otolaryngology*, **102**, 672, 675

TOS, M. and POULSEN, G. (1979) Tympanometry in 2-year-old children. Seasonal influence on secretory otitis media and tubal dysfunction. *Annals of Otology, Rhinology and Laryngology*, **41**, 1–10

TOS, M. and POULSEN, G. (1980) Attic retractions following secretory otitis media. *Acta Oto-Laryngologica*, **89**, 479–486

TOS, M. and STANGERUP, S. E. (1985) Secretory otitis and pneumatisation of the mastoid process: sexual differences in the size of the mastoid air cell system. *American Journal of Otolaryngology*, **6**, 199–205

TOS, M., STANGERUP, S. E., HOLM-JENSEN, S. and SORENSEN, C. H. (1984) Spontaneous course of secretory otitis and changes of the ear drum. *Archives of Otolaryngology*, **110**, 281–289

VAN BUCHEM, F. L., DUNK, J. H. M. and VAN T. HOF, M. A. (1981) Therapy of acute otitis media. Myringotomy, antibiotics or neither? *The Lancet*, **2**, 883–887

VOGELSANG, M. W. and BIRCK, H. G. (1984) Ventilation tubes in the paediatric population. In *Recent Advances in Otitis Media with Effusion*, edited by D. J. Lim *et al.*, pp. 306–308. Philadelphia: BC Decker Inc

WIDEMAR, L., SVENSSON, C., RYNEL-DAGOO, B. and SCHIRATZKI, H. (1985) The effect of adenoidectomy on secretory otitis media. A 2-year controlled prospective study. *Clinical Otolaryngology*, **10**, 345–350

YUNG, M. W. and MORRIS, T. M. O. (1981) Tuning fork tests in diagnosis for serous otitis media. *British Medical Journal*, **283**, 1576

13

Acute suppurative otitis media and acute mastoiditis

Joselen Ransome

Acute suppurative otitis media is one of the most common diseases in childhood: this is because the middle ear cleft is readily infected from the nose and nasopharynx by way of the eustachian tube, and the incidence of such infections peaks in early childhood before maturation of the immune system. It does however occur at any age.

Definition

Acute suppurative otitis media

Acute suppurative otitis media is inflammation of the mucous membrane lining of the middle ear cleft (consisting of the eustachian tube, tympanic cavity, mastoid antrum and mastoid air cells) produced by pus-forming organisms.

Acute mastoiditis

Acute mastoiditis, formerly a common complication of acute suppurative otitis media, is now rare in countries with well-developed primary medical care. While some degree of mastoiditis inevitably occurs early in the course of acute suppurative otitis media, since the middle ear and mastoid mucosa are in continuity, the clinical entity of acute mastoiditis consists of persistence of pain in and behind the ear despite adequate antibiotic therapy or time for natural resolution, together usually with persistence of otorrhoea, fever, and tenderness over the mastoid antrum.

Anatomy of the middle ear cleft

This is described in detail in Volume 1, Chapter 1. Here the reader's attention is drawn to the important ways in which the child's anatomy differs from that of the adult.

The eustachian tube

The eustachian tube is relatively shorter, wider and straighter in the infant and young child than in the adult. Hence infected material from the nose, adenoids and sinuses more readily passes along the eustachian tube to the tympanic cavity, particularly during feeding (especially in the supine position), coughing, sneezing and vomiting. Furthermore, the period when the tube is wider and straighter coincides with the period when children are particularly prone to upper respiratory infections and when they are also more likely to have a large mass of adenoid tissue. In older children and adults, forcible nose-blowing may propel infected mucus into the tympanic cavity.

The mastoid process

The mastoid process has not developed at birth and thus the stylomastoid foramen with the emerging facial nerve is relatively superficial in infancy and, therefore, the nerve is more easily cut by a postauricular incision. The mastoid process begins to develop during the second year of life, by a downward growth of bone. When complete, at puberty, the stylomastoid foramen and facial nerve are then much more deeply placed on the inferior aspect of the skull deep to, and just anterior to, the mastoid process.

The mastoid antrum

The mastoid antrum is fully formed at birth but, as the mastoid process has not developed, it is very superficial, about 2 mm deep to the bony surface. It reaches the adult depth of about 15 mm at puberty. Thus, between infancy and puberty the antrum acquires an increased bony covering at the rate of approximately 1 mm per annum.

The mastoid air cells

Pneumatization of the mastoid bone occurs at the same time as the development of the mastoid process. Resorption of haemopoietic marrow occurs and, at the same time, mucous membrane from the antrum grows into the bony spaces so formed to line them, forming a complex system of interlinked air cells. Persistent infection of the bony framework of these air spaces constitutes the clinical entity of acute mastoiditis. In a small percentage of individuals, pneumatization does not take place, so although the mastoid antrum is always present, the mastoid bone is acellular and of 'ivory' type, and these patients do not develop acute mastoiditis. Intermediate types also occur, either as normal variants, or due to arrest of pneumatization by childhood ear infections.

The tympanic membrane

The tympanic membrane is fully formed at birth but is more horizontally placed, making access for myringotomy difficult. Along with the developments outlined above, it gradually assumes a more vertical plane.

Acute suppurative otitis media

Aetiology

Route of infection

By way of the eustachian tube

The relative incompetence of the eustachian tube in younger children is referred to above. The vast majority of infecting organisms reach the middle ear by way of the eustachian tube in both children and adults, most commonly from an ordinary head cold. Even after the eustachian tube reaches its adult, more protective, form, infection still reaches the middle ear by direct spread along the mucosa, or infected mucus can be propelled into the middle ear by forcible nose-blowing, sneezing, pressure changes as in flying, and forcing water up the nose as in jumping into swimming pools.

By way of the tympanic membrane

The route can be by way of the tympanic membrane, either due to a pre-existing perforation, when infected material may enter the middle ear during hair-washing, face-washing and swimming; due to a traumatic perforation by an unsterile object; or due to operative trauma, for example myringotomy, tympanotomy, or through a ventilation tube.

Blood-borne infection

It is thought that some viral infections of the middle ear, including the acute specific fevers and influenza, may be blood-borne. While this chapter is concerned with acute suppurative otitis media and hence with pyogenic infections, pyococci frequently follow and invade tissues already affected by viruses.

Age

Acute suppurative otitis media is a common disease of childhood, with about five children in every 100 having at least one attack in their first 10 years (Lewis *et al.*, 1967). The peak incidence is sometimes stated to be from 5 to 7 years, after which it declines rapidly. However, several studies have shown that the incidence is highest among preschool children, especially before the second birthday. In one such study of a population of 146 822 of all ages living in various parts of Finland, about 50% of all cases of acute suppurative otitis media were found in infants under 2 years old (Pukander *et al.*, 1982). The annual incidence in this study was 4.4%.

Sex

According to Bordley, Brookhouser and Tucker (1986) 60–65% of otitis media cases in children are males. The Finnish study referred to above showed that the annual attack rate was 4.84% in males and 4.07% in females. No rationale for this apparent inequality has been identified.

Socio-economic factors

The incidence is highest in low hygiene populations, and under conditions of overcrowding and malnutrition.

Climate

A higher incidence of acute suppurative otitis media is seen in cold climates, especially in winter. The incidence is also higher in urban areas than in the country.

Racial factors

Studies in the USA (Bordley, Brookhouser and Tucker, 1986) have shown a higher incidence of acute suppurative otitis media in white children compared with black; a particularly high incidence is seen in Eskimos and American Indians.

Nasopharyngeal tissue masses

Adenoids

Adenoids tend to block the eustachian tubes and also to act as a focus of infection from which organisms pass up the tube. However, controversy continues as to the exact role of the adenoids in acute suppurative otitis media as well as in non-suppurative middle ear effusions. Maw (1985) has shown that adenoidectomy is beneficial in resolving middle ear effusions, although the age of the child might be more significant, as children over 6 years showed better clearance than children under 6. It can be argued that the presence of adenoids, in impeding eustachian tube function, would play a similar role in acute suppurative otitis media. McKee, as long ago as 1963 (1963a,b) in two careful studies showed evidence of the effectiveness of adenoidectomy in significantly reducing the incidence of acute suppurative otitis media. Interestingly, he also showed that adenoidectomy alone was as effective in reducing acute suppurative otitis media as adenoidotonsillectomy, suggesting that tonsils rarely play any part in the aetiology. McKee also commented on the importance of age, the worst results having been achieved in children over 8, in whom the number of attacks would be declining anyway. However, it is well known that both children and adults with no adenoids can suffer frequent otitis media due to the many other factors involved. Careful assessment of the possible role of adenoids, as compared with other aetiological factors, in each individual case, is therefore mandatory.

Other nasopharyngeal masses

These act in a similar way to adenoids and include polyps, teratoma, angiofibroma, lymphoma and, in adults, carcinoma (*see* Volume 4, Chapter 19).

Respiratory disease

Chronic rhinitis and sinusitis produce a constant flow of infected mucus which may enter the eustachian tubes, while the infected sputum of bronchitis, bronchiectasis and pneumonia may also be coughed into the nasopharynx and enter the tubes.

Allergy

The importance of allergy as an aetiological factor in acute suppurative otitis media is still debatable. While allergic oedema of the eustachian tube undoubtedly occurs and might provide a rationale for recurrent acute suppurative otitis media in some cases, many atopic subjects have no ear problems.

Pre-existing middle ear effusion

A pre-existing middle ear effusion may act as a ready culture medium for invading pyococci.

Immunodeficiency syndromes

Immunodeficiency syndromes, including hypogammaglobulinaemias, are rare but important causes of recurrent upper respiratory infections including acute suppurative otitis media, and should always be excluded when recurrences are very frequent.

Chronic systemic disorders

Chronic systemic disorders undoubtedly predispose to acute suppurative otitis media as they do to other infective disease. Examples occurring in both children and adults are diabetes, leukaemias, anaemias, cystic fibrosis and nephritis.

Cleft palate

Children with cleft palate have a high incidence of middle ear disease, either acute suppurative otitis media or otitis media with effusion, due to eustachian tube dysfunction secondary to the tensor palati anomaly.

Primary ciliary dyskinesia

Primary ciliary dyskinesia, although excessively rare and more usually associated with otitis media with effusion, can also contribute to recurrent acute suppurative otitis media.

Pathology

Microbiology

While acute suppurative otitis media is appropriately considered as a bacterial disease, viruses undoubtedly play a role in many cases, paving the way for pyococcal invasion. Attempting to culture viruses from the middle ear in acute suppurative otitis media has a low yield of about 5% – possibly they are inactivated or absent by the time the full clinical picture has developed. At the present time, the most commonly isolated pathogens are *Streptococcus pneumoniae* and *Haemophilus influenzae;* the next most common are group A beta-haemolytic streptococcus, *Staphylococcus aureus,* and *Neisseria catarrhalis.* Gram-negative bacilli such as *Pseudomonas aeruginosa,* various *Proteus* species and *Klebsiella pneumoniae* have also been reported.

Middle ear inflammatory process

This can proceed quite rapidly, and consists of a stage of mucosal oedema with increased secretion, followed by hyperaemia, white cell infiltration and pus formation. This process clearly cannot be limited to the tympanum since the air spaces and mucosa of the entire middle ear cleft are in continuity; hence, tubal occlusion occurs due to mucosal swelling, preventing drainage, and involvement of the mastoid air cells also occurs. If pus accumulates under pressure and there is tubal occlusion, the tympanic membrane may rupture. Destruction of cilia, normally present in the anterior part of the tympanum and in the tube, contributes to the poor drainage of thick secretions through the tube.

Spread of infection

Spread of infection can occur due to retrograde thrombophlebitis, bone necrosis, congenital dehiscences and fracture lines, as follows:

(1) intracranially, giving rise to extradural abscess, subdural abscess, meningitis, brain abscess, lateral sinus thrombosis, and otitic hydrocephalus
(2) to the labyrinth causing suppurative labyrinthitis
(3) to the facial nerve canal, causing facial paralysis
(4) to the neck, by breaking through the mastoid tip, producing Bezold's or Citelli's abscess
(5) to the petrous apex.

Details of (1) and (2) can be found in Volume 3, Chapter 12.

Symptoms

The variation in the clinical picture in any infection is due to the varying virulence of the invading microorganism, varying host defence, and effectiveness of and compliance in treatment.

Acute suppurative otitis media can vary from a relatively minor attack of earache with tympanic membrane hyperaemia lasting a few hours, to a fulminating febrile illness perhaps with complications requiring surgery.

By far the most common presenting symptom of acute suppurative otitis media is *pain* in the affected ear or ears which is accurately described and well located by older children and adults, who point to the ear canal and say the pain is 'deep inside', and frequently severe and throbbing. Children too young to describe their pain tend to pull at the ear lobe, or repeatedly push the ear into their pillow. The child may already be irritable, restless, off his food and seem feverish, or these symptoms may develop some hours after the onset of pain. Usually the attack will have been preceded by an upper respiratory infection, and symptoms and signs of this may be present. *Deafness* in the affected ear or ears will soon be noticed by older children and adults; the disease is often bilateral in children and the parents of young children would notice deafness in these cases, but in unilateral cases it may not be apparent.

At this stage the disease may not progress and will gradually resolve, with the pain subsiding and the hearing gradually recovering.

In many cases, however, it proceeds to a stage of intense pain, followed by rupture of the tympanic membrane and a complaint of *aural discharge*. A small percentage of both children and adults also complain of giddiness.

There may be a history of one or more of the predisposing factors described under aetiology.

Signs

Before describing these it is important to consider the method of examining young children. It is of the utmost importance to gain their confidence as there may be only one chance to examine them – an abortive or clumsy attempt at otoscopy may result in a distraught and terrified child who will not submit to examination a second time. Children can be thought of as miniature adults with their own name and distinctive personality, and their own (sometimes inappropriate) views as to how the consultation should be conducted. They fear pain and the unknown, and should therefore be examined with the utmost gentleness, speaking to the child by name and reassuring him that by keeping still the examination will not be painful. The best position for examination is on the mother's lap: she holds the child's head against her chest with one hand on his forehead, and with her other hand restrains his arms. If possible the child's legs should be held firmly by the mother between her thighs.

Ears

In the early stages of acute suppurative otitis media the tympanic membrane will be injected along the handle of the malleus, around the periphery, and sometimes over the pars flaccida. Later the whole tympanic membrane becomes hyperaemic and opaque. If infection continues and pus begins to accumulate under pressure, the pars tensa starts to bulge, mainly posteriorly, and acquires a yellowish colour (*see Plate 1a*). Finally the tympanic membrane ruptures and discharge will be seen in the external canal, which may be serous, serosanguineous, mucopurulent or frankly purulent. It is important to note whether the discharge has the shiny, glossy appearance of mucus – if the discharge contains mucus it can *only* come from the middle ear. The presence or absence of an offensive odour from the discharge should also be noted – if present it suggests underlying chronic otitis media. (*See also* Differential diagnosis *below*.) At this time the pain usually subsides. After mopping or aspirating discharge it is usually possible to see a small central perforation, commonly in the posterior segment of the pars tensa. Sometimes, however, the perforation may be difficult to see as the oedematous edges of the middle ear mucosa tend to obscure it. It may be located by applying a negative pressure with a Siegle's speculum, or aspirating under the operating microscope, when a blob of discharge may be seen emerging from the perforation. The perforation may also be anterior, but is only marginal or in the pars flaccida in acute-on-chronic middle ear disease. If the infection has followed trauma to the tympanic membrane a jagged perforation may be seen. If a ventilation tube is *in situ*, pus may be seen pulsating through the lumen.

Mastoid tenderness, elicited by pressure over McEwen's triangle, may be present early in the course of acute suppurative otitis media. It assumes significance as a sign of mastoiditis if it persists or increases despite adequate treatment.

During resolution the hyperaemia fades and the perforation heals, often leaving no trace but sometimes leaving a scar.

In older children and adults the Rinne and Weber tests will indicate conductive deafness. In younger children the hearing for a whispered voice will be impaired.

Nose and throat

As stated, the commonest cause of acute suppurative otitis media is the common cold, and examination of the nose and throat may show inflammation of the mucosa and nasal mucoid discharge. If there is bacterial rhinitis and/or sinusitis, mucopurulent or purulent nasal and postnasal discharge may be seen. Sometimes there is also acute adenoiditis with yellow patches of purulent exudate similar to tonsillitis.

General signs

Children are frequently febrile, but adults rarely so. A temperature of 40°C is not unusual in children. The disease may present in neonates as a pyrexia of 'unknown' origin, occasionally even with meningitis. Other general signs would be those of any underlying general or predisposing condition.

Signs of complications

Acute suppurative otitis media may be a serious illness. Complications may develop rapidly and it is necessary to be alert to the signs of these.

Tenderness and oedema over the mastoid process with protuberance of the pinna (*see Plate 1b*) indicate mastoiditis, as do *sagging of the posterosuperior canal wall*, and *granulation tissue* pouting through the perforation, with *discharge persisting* for 3–4 weeks from the onset. (*See also below*, Differential diagnosis and Acute mastoiditis.)

Sick children should always be tested for *neck stiffness*, and in severe cases a thorough examination of the central nervous system should be carried out to exclude intracranial complications. *Nystagmus* must be looked for in patients complaining of vertigo, and the *fistula test* carried out.

Investigations

Microbiology

In all cases when otorrhoea is present, an *ear swab* should be taken for culture and sensitivity of organisms. It is not necessary routinely to culture for viruses, since these are seldom found and there is no specific treatment anyway. If the ear is not discharging it is often useful to take *nose and throat swabs*, since the ear will usually contain the same organisms.

Blood studies

A full blood count including differential white cell count is helpful in patients with acute suppurative otitis media. In very ill patients, or those in whom complications, particularly intracranial ones, are suspected, a rising leucocyte count may be the only indication that pus is accumulating *somewhere* as other symptoms and signs may be diminished by antibiotic treatment. The full blood count will also exclude or identify leukaemias, anaemias and neutropenia.

Quantitative immunoglobulin electrophoresis to detect varying degrees and types of hypogammaglobulinaemia should also be carried out in patients with frequent attacks of acute suppurative otitis media.

Audiometry

Pure tone audiometry needs to be performed fairly early in the course of acute suppurative otitis media, but need not be done when the patient is in severe pain and febrile. It will obviously show conductive deafness, but its value lies in establishing a baseline and monitoring the resolution of the disease.

Tympanometry should not be carried out in the acute stage as it is painful and adds no useful information, but again when improvement begins it can be undertaken to establish a baseline as, not infrequently, acute suppurative otitis media leaves an unresolved middle ear effusion.

Mastoid X-rays

X-rays are only required if mastoiditis is diagnosed. Clouding of the mastoid air cells is always present in acute suppurative otitis media, but when there is doubt as to whether mastoid surgery is needed, X-rays are useful as evidence of breaking down of air cells (coalescent mastoiditis, *Figure 13.1*) will strengthen the indications (*see* Volume 1, Chapter 17.)

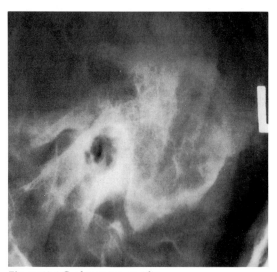

Figure 13.1 Coalescent mastoiditis

Urine examination

Urine examination is carried out in recurrent cases to exclude diabetes.

Diagnosis

This is usually straightforward and is based on the history of earache, deafness, and perhaps otorrhoea, probably preceded by a respiratory infection, together with the inflammatory changes found on examination which have been described above. However, there are some pitfalls and these are discussed later.

Differential diagnosis

This is considered later under Acute mastoiditis.

Prognosis

In this antibiotic era complete resolution of acute otitis media is the rule, with absence of complications, healing of the tympanic membrane, and restoration of normal hearing. In a few, a sterile middle ear effusion or a perforation persists. Only a very small percentage proceed to acute mastoiditis. The life-threatening intracranial complications are very rare, and are more often associated with a pre-existing chronic otitis media.

Complications

Mastoiditis

Mastoiditis may also lead to postauricular abscess or Bezold's and Citelli's abscess.

Facial paralysis

This subject is discussed in Volume 3, Chapter 24. Here it can be stated that facial paralysis occurring in the course of acute suppurative otitis media or acute mastoiditis almost invariably recovers completely with medical or surgical treatment of the primary condition; surgery of the nerve trunk is not required.

Intracranial complications

Extradural abscess, subdural abscess, meningitis, brain abscess, lateral sinus thrombosis and otitic hydrocephalus may occur.

Labyrinthitis

Labyrinthitis can also occur.

Petrositis

Petrositis and Gradenigo's syndrome are both complications.

Mastoiditis and petrositis are described below. Intracranial complications and labyrinthitis are rare nowadays but when they do occur it is more commonly in association with chronic otitis media. These conditions are described in Volume 3, Chapter 12.

Sequelae

(1) Persistence of a sterile middle ear effusion after resolution of the acute inflammatory stage, causing persistence of hearing impairment.
(2) High-tone sensorineural deafness, usually mild, presumably due to the inflammatory process involving the deep surface of the round window membrane.

(3) Persistent perforation of the tympanic membrane can occur, more particularly in debilitated patients who have suffered a fulminating attack of acute suppurative otitis media leading to more widespread necrosis of the tympanic membrane; discharge may also persist, and the disease may evolve into *chronic suppurative otitis media.*

(4) Extensive scarring of the tympanic membrane, middle ear adhesions and resorption of ossicles may occur in recurrent cases (adhesive otitis). Hyalinized collagen deposits in the middle ear and tympanic membrane (tympanosclerosis) may also occur.

Treatment of acute suppurative otitis media

Treatment of acute suppurative otitis media is considered under the following headings:

(1) curative
    medical
        general
        analgesics
        topical
        antibiotics
        [decongestants]
    surgical – myringotomy
(2) [prophylactic]
(3) treatment of associated conditions
(4) treatment of complications.

The square brackets indicate treatment modes not generally considered to be appropriate.

Curative

Medical treatment

General

Both children and adults are best managed in bed in the acute phase, in a warm room, of adequate humidity to maintain ciliary function. Febrile and toxic children will need no persuasion to stay in bed; afebrile children can be allowed up but kept indoors. As in any infective illness, nourishment and fluid intake must be adequate, and supplementary vitamins, especially C, can be added if the patient's normal diet is thought to be inadequate. Some patients, both children and adults, are better managed in hospital, depending on the severity, length of history, response to previous treatment, and other factors such as association with diabetes or other illness. Hospitalization provides the opportunity for frequent observation of the general and local condition, and for investigations, if complications are suspected or surgery is considered.

Analgesics

These must be given in adequate dosage and with sufficient frequency to control pain.

Topical

When otorrhoea is present the discharge should be gently mopped with dry sterile cotton wool or sucked from the canal, as often as it recurs. A piece of cotton wool can be placed at the orifice of the ear canal to prevent the discharge running down and excoriating the skin of the ear lobe.

Antibiotics

Most otologists and primary care physicians in the UK would favour early administration of antibiotics in all but the most minor cases, despite the fact that some cases may be viral, and notwithstanding the need to avoid overprescribing. Van Buchem, Peeters and Van't Hof (1985) disagree with this and advocate witholding antibiotics for 3–4 days, asserting that the vast majority of cases recover with symptomatic treatment only. However, the widely observed and rapid decline, since the advent of antibiotics, of acute mastoiditis, formerly an extremely common complication of acute suppurative otitis media, supports the concept that antibiotics limit the disease and minimize its consequences. Minor cases in which the pain lasts for only a few hours do not require treatment, nor those in whom pain is very slight. In practice a 'trial' of *no* treatment is usually inevitable as it may be 12–24 hours before the patient can obtain medical care.

Route of administration Oral administration is the route of choice except in very severe cases. In these one or more antibiotics may be given intravenously.

Duration Antibiotics should usually be given for 5–10 days, depending on the severity of the case. If a patient is treated at home the importance of treatment compliance should be emphasized.

Choice of antibiotic Administration should not be begun before an ear swab is taken (or nose and throat swabs if the ear is not discharging), but after this there is no need to wait for the result. Amoxycillin is a useful first-line treatment as it is well tolerated and the common bacteria of acute suppurative otitis media are usually sensitive to it. Other useful antibiotics are erythromycin, trimethoprim, trimethoprim with sulphamethoxazole (co-trimoxazole), and cefaclor. Severe and fulminating cases can be given a combination of ampicillin, flucloxacillin and metronidazole intravenously.

The response to the chosen regimen should be monitored carefully and, if ineffective, it should be altered according to the results of the swab cultures and organism sensitivities.

Decongestants

Both systemic and topical decongestants are often prescribed in the hope that they will improve the patency of the eustachian tube and thus improve middle ear drainage. The use of *systemic decongestants* has a logical basis as pseudoephedrine and phenylephrine have been shown to increase tubal patency in dogs (Jackson, 1971); unfortunately, however, many trials have now shown that systemic decongestants are no better than a placebo in the management of middle ear disease. Admittedly, some trials were more concerned with secretory otitis media but Olson *et al.* (1978) studied 169 children with acute suppurative otitis media and treated all with antibiotics plus either pseudoephedrine or placebo; the outcome was the same in both groups. Possibly the doses commonly used do not produce effective vasoconstriction, or vasoconstriction may occur, only to be followed by the rebound phenomenon observed in the nose after the use of some nasal sprays. Since systemic administration of pseudoephedrine and similar compounds may sometimes cause sleep disturbance, irritability and, occasionally, psychotic symptoms, especially in children, the conclusion is inescapable that their *use is unwise.*

Topical decongestants are also widely prescribed but the passage of drops or nebulized particles through the nose and nasopharynx seems hardly likely to produce a useful effect on the eustachian tube. Lilholdt *et al.* (1982) did not find any improvement in eustachian tube function in 40 children with proved severe tubal dysfunction after their noses were sprayed with either oxymetazoline hydrochloride or placebo. The use of topical decongestants in acute suppurative otitis media is *not* recommended as they are unlikely to produce a useful effect on the eustachian tube.

Surgical treatment

While the vast majority of ears with acute suppurative otitis media will respond to the above regimen of appropriate antibiotics, bed-rest and analgesia, and while some tympanic membranes will rupture spontaneously with or without treatment, in a very small minority there is persistence of pain and temperature with a red bulging tympanic membrane despite adequate medical management. *Myringotomy* should then be undertaken with a view to releasing pus accumulating under pressure.

The operation is carried out under general anaesthesia using an operating microscope, and with full aseptic procedures. The patient is placed supine on the operating table with the head turned to one side. Using an aural speculum and angled myringotome, a radial incision is made in

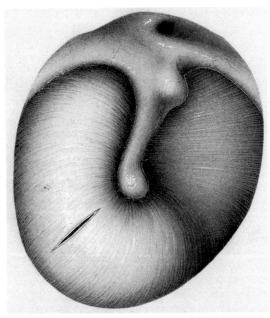

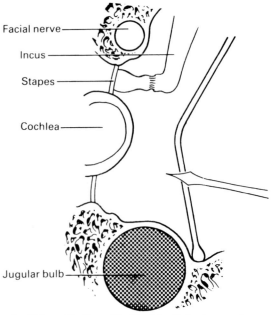

Figure 13.2 Position of myringotomy incision in acute suppurative otitis media. (Reproduced from 'Myringotomy', J. Ransome, in *Operative Surgery*, 4th edn, Volume *The Ear*, edited by John Ballantyne and Andrew Morrison, pp. 27–37. London: Butterworths)

the posteroinferior segment; the maximum bulging is posterior in acute suppurative otitis media, and the inferior incision avoids the risk of damaging the ossicular chain, chorda tympani and facial nerve (*Figure 13.2*). Pus then gushes out under pressure, and a swab is taken and sent for culture and sensitivities. Residual pus is gently sucked out. The incision should be about 3–4 mm in length; tiny incisions tend to heal too quickly and allow pus to reaccumulate in the middle ear cleft. Ventilation tubes should *not* be inserted in acute suppurative otitis media.

Postoperatively, on recovering from anaesthesia the patient will usually say that the earache has disappeared, and generally the temperature quickly returns to normal. Antibiotic treatment is continued until resolution is virtually complete, but the regimen is changed if necessary as soon as the results of the swab taken at operation are known.

Prophylactic treatment

Long-term daily treatment with antibiotics or sulphamethoxazole has been shown to be effective in reducing the number of episodes in patients prone to acute suppurative otitis media. However, all antibiotics are potentially toxic and long-term prophylaxis with oral antibiotics is not generally recommended as the risks may be greater than the risk of another attack of acute suppurative otitis media. (Note that this statement applies *only* to recurrent acute suppurative otitis media and it is recognized that there may be a place for such prophylaxis in other conditions.) Occasionally acute suppurative otitis media occurs so frequently and with such severity that a trial of continuous antibiotic treatment, especially in the winter, is justified.

Treatment of associated conditions

The treatment of acute suppurative otitis media, especially when recurrent, should include a search for and management of treatable associated disease. The role of the *adenoids* has been considered under Aetiology above, and many otologists would consider it necessary to remove the adenoids in some cases of recurrent acute suppurative otitis media. Adenoidectomy should be carefully and thoroughly performed with special attention to removal of adenoid tissue from the fossae of Rosenmüller. *Rhinitis and sinusitis* should also be looked for and treated vigorously. The presence of *lower respiratory infection* requires treatment with the help of a paediatrician or respiratory physician. *Other conditions* referred to under Aetiology must receive the appropriate management, for example early repair of cleft palate.

Treatment of complications and sequelae

Persistence of middle ear effusion

This is a common sequel to an attack of acute suppurative otitis media and therefore there must be careful follow-up of each case, with otoscopy supplemented by tympanometry and pure tone audiometry as necessary, until complete resolution occurs or persistence of fluid is found. The management is described in Chapter 12.

Persistent perforation of the tympanic membrane

See Volume 3, Chapter 10.

Labyrinthitis and intracranial complications

These are described in Volume 3, Chapter 12.

Facial paralysis

Facial paralysis occurring in the course of middle ear cleft infection is usually due to a dehiscent facial nerve canal – when the infection is controlled in most cases the facial nerve recovers.

Mastoiditis and petrositis

Mastoiditis and petrositis are described below.

Acute mastoiditis
Aetiology and pathology

In developed countries with effective primary and secondary health care, acute mastoiditis is nowadays rare, largely due to the widespread use of antibiotics for acute suppurative otitis media. However, if the preceding attack is untreated, or fails to respond, the inflammatory process will persist and increase in the mastoid air cells. The accumulation of pus in the air cells leads to necrosis of the bony walls of the cells producing the so-called 'coalescent mastoiditis'. For a time the disease may remain walled off within the mastoid bone, but eventually it will spread:

(1) laterally through the lateral outer table of the mastoid bone to give a *subperiosteal abscess* and, if pus ruptures through the periosteum, a *subcutaneous abscess*
(2) superiorly and posteriorly, giving rise to:
  (i) extradural abscess
  (ii) subdural abscess
  (iii) meningitis
  (iv) brain abscess of (*a*) the temporal lobe or (*b*) the cerebellum
  (v) lateral sinus thrombosis
  (vi) otitic hydrocephalus

(3) medially causing *labyrinthitis* or *petrositis* and *Gradenigo's syndrome*

(4) inferiorly through the mastoid process tip or medial wall causing *Bezold's abscess*, caused by pus tracking along the sternomastoid muscle or *Citelli's abscess* caused by pus tracking along the posterior belly of the digastric muscle

(5) anteriorly to the facial nerve canal causing facial paralysis, and also to the postero-superior external auditory canal wall, causing the appearance of sagging of the meatal skin in that area.

Predisposing factors

These are the same as described above for acute suppurative otitis media. The disease can occur at any age, but is far more common in children.

History

The patient will have had an attack of acute suppurative otitis media, with the characteristic symptoms and signs described above, anything from a few days up to 3 or 4 weeks previously. The attack of acute suppurative otitis media will probably have been preceded by a head cold or other upper respiratory infection or, in children, by an acute specific fever, such as measles or scarlet fever.

Symptoms

General

Mastoiditis is frequently a serious illness with pyrexia and general malaise. Fever, restlessness and refusal of food may be the only symptoms in very young children.

Local

Commonly there is persistence of earache, otorrhoea and increasing hearing impairment, from the time of onset of the preceding acute suppurative otitis media. Sometimes the original symptoms abate, especially if antibiotic treatment has been given, only to recur, together with fever, some 2–4 weeks later. Occasionally the only symptom is persistent profuse otorrhoea. The patient may complain of nasal obstruction or nasal discharge. The presence of unilateral headache is a danger sign suggesting the onset of intracranial complications. Similarly a complaint of giddiness is a warning that labyrinthitis is imminent, or developing.

Signs

General

The patient will frequently appear pale, ill and restless. There may be pyrexia of 40°C or more in children, though in adults pyrexia may be low or absent.

Local

External auditory canal

On examination of the external auditory canal, there may be discharge, either mucopurulent or purulent, but seldom offensive, unless acute disease has occurred on previously chronic otitis media; the discharge may be seen to pulsate through a perforation. Sagging of the postero-superior canal wall may be present.

Tympanic membrane

Perforation of the tympanic membrane is almost invariably present, and is nearly always postero-central – occasionally, however, mastoiditis can develop behind an intact tympanic membrane, which will appear red and full or bulging.

Granulations or a polyp, bright red in colour, may be seen pouting through the perforation when disease has been present for weeks rather than days.

Signs of complications such as severe headache, drowsiness, vomiting, and neck stiffness are serious indications of intracranial complications and must prompt an immediate and thorough examination of the central nervous system. Vertigo with nystagmus suggests labyrinthitis.

Postauricular area

Mastoid tenderness elicited by pressure over McEwen's triangle, will invariably be present. It will proabably have persisted from the onset of the preceding acute suppurative otitis media attack, and may increase.

Swelling over the mastoid bone may be present, and if so either the postauricular groove is accentuated indicating that the pus is still sub-periosteal, or the postauricular groove is absent, because either the periosteum has given way and the pus is subcutaneous, or there is simple inflammatory oedema over the mastoid.

The presence of fluctuation will distinguish the later abscess formation from the earlier simple inflammatory oedema.

Protuberance of the pinna can occur either due to simple inflammatory oedema over the mastoid, or to subcutaneous abscess; subperiosteal abscess with retention of the postauricular groove does not push the pinna forwards unless the abscess is very large.

Investigations

These are the same as for acute suppurative otitis media but the points below should be remembered.

Microbiology

It is particularly important to obtain an ear swab and an early report on the culture and sensitivities in case the organisms are not sensitive to the first treatment. Patients, particularly children, may have a serious illness which in turn may lead to further complications such as meningitis, and valuable time will be lost in treating this potentially lethal condition if culture is not performed. In more severe cases initial blood cultures are also indicated.

Blood studies

A full blood count should be carried out promptly, and repeated during the course of the disease. A rising leucocyte count invariably indicates pus accumulating and unless there is an obvious cause such as a fluctuant postauricular abscess, signs of intracranial spread must be looked for.

Audiometry

A pure tone audiogram may show as much as 40–50 dB of conductive hearing loss; comparison with an audiogram performed during the preceding acute suppurative otitis media attack may show that the hearing loss has increased. If the patient is ill, or the mastoid is very tender, only Rinne and Weber tests are called for.

Mastoid X-rays

While seldom required in simple acute suppurative otitis media, X-rays will show not only clouding of cells, which is always present in acute suppurative otitis media but also breaking down of bony air cell walls, indicating progressive disease, or coalescent mastoiditis. The films are also a useful guide, if surgery is required, as to the extent of pneumatization, which varies greatly (*see* Chapter 2).

Diagnosis

Diagnosis is made on the history, symptoms and signs, supported by X-rays, as already described. The principal features can be summarized as follows: an attack of acute suppurative otitis media fails to resolve and is followed by persistent or recurrent earache, pyrexia and otorrhoea, increasing deafness, together with mastoid tenderness and sometimes a protuberant pinna.

Differential diagnosis of acute suppurative otitis media and acute mastoiditis from other conditions

Acute suppurative otitis media

Acute suppurative otitis media may sometimes have to be distinguished from the following conditions.

Otitis externa

Otitis externa may also give earache and otorrhoea, and the tympanic membrane may appear red as the outer layer is in continuity with the canal epithelium and is frequently involved in the inflammatory process. The discharge is frequently watery, but if purulent it never has the shiny, glossy appearance of middle ear discharge due to the presence of mucus. The hearing in otitis externa is normal or only slightly impaired (except when the canal is blocked by discharge), whereas in acute suppurative otitis media the hearing loss is usually more marked. Itching is a very common feature of otitis externa, but does not occur in acute suppurative otitis media. Very severe otitis externa may mimic acute mastoiditis (*see below*).

Tympanic membrane hyperaemia

The whole tympanic membrane can become quite diffusely red in a child who is crying. Since he may be crying because he has earache, time must be allowed for him to settle down and then the examination is repeated. The insertion of an aural speculum may cause slight flushing down the handle of the malleus and round the periphery of the pars tensa, so examination should be very gentle to avoid confusion with this early sign of developing acute suppurative otitis media.

Otitis media with effusion

The tympanic membrane may sometimes look pinkish and opaque, but is never as intensely red as in acute suppurative otitis media.

Myringitis haemorrhagica bullosa

This condition frequently occurs during epidemics of respiratory viruses such as influenza, and is characterized by excruciating earache followed by a small quantity of serosanguineous discharge. Inspection of the tympanic membrane shows either the presence of haemorrhagic blebs, or the outlines of ruptured blebs. When uncomplicated the hearing is usually normal. Secondary bacterial invasion of the middle ear may occur, so the two conditions may coexist.

Other causes of otalgia

There are many causes of otalgia remote from the ear itself, and these are discussed in Volume 3, Chapter 13. The diagnostic point here is that the patient with pain *referred* to the ear from some other structure will have a perfectly normal tympanic membrane and hearing.

Acute mastoiditis

This may have to be distinguished from the following conditions.

Acute severe otitis externa

Acute severe otitis externa is usually localized in the form of a furuncle. This may lead to really marked postauricular oedema and protuberance of the pinna and this, together with severe earache and some purulent otorrhoea, produces the resemblance to acute mastoiditis. However, in furunculosis there is severe pain on pushing the tragus gently in and on pulling gently on the pinna; this does not occur in acute mastoiditis. There will be no history of a preceding attack of acute suppurative otitis media. The hearing is usually normal or only slightly impaired (unlike mastoiditis) unless the canal is completely occluded by swelling or discharge. If the postauricular groove is accentuated, this is a sign of subperiosteal pus which has spread from the mastoid. X-rays of the mastoids will show apparent cloudiness of the air cells in either condition (due in external otitis to the overlying oedema), but if breaking down of the bony mastoid air cell walls is shown, this indicates that mastoiditis is present.

Postauricular lymphadenitis

Very rarely, suppuration in a postauricular lymph node, due to infection in the skin or scalp, may cause confusion. However the tympanic membrane, external auditory canal and hearing will be found to be normal.

Erysipelas

Erysipelas may occasionally affect the skin of the postauricular area, and resemble mastoiditis because of pain, fever and red oedematous skin. However, careful examination will reveal a raised, red spreading edge of the lesion, contrasting sharply with the normal pale adjacent skin. The external canal skin, tympanic membrane, and the hearing will all be normal.

Complications of acute mastoiditis

These have been referred to under Pathology and will not be described here, except petrositis. The reader is reminded that labyrinthitis and the intracranial complications are discussed in the chapter on complications of otitis media (Volume 3, Chapter 12).

Acute petrositis

The degree of pneumatization of the temporal bone is extremely variable, but may extend right through the petrous bone to its apex. If so, when there is mastoiditis, there is nothing except host defence and timely treatment to prevent infection spreading right to the petrous apex. However, acute petrositis is now excessively rare, and even in the preantibiotic era it was not common.

Clinical picture

The clinical picture is that of the preceding acute suppurative otitis media and acute mastoiditis which fails to respond to treatment, sometimes even if this included cortical mastoidectomy. There is persistence of earache and temperature, then pain is felt in the distribution of the ipsilateral trigeminal (fifth cranial) nerve. Finally, involvement of the ipsilateral abducent (sixth cranial) nerve gives rise to diplopia, and examination of the eye movements will show paralysis of the external rectus muscle of the eyeball on the affected side (sixth nerve paralysis).

Gradenigo's syndrome

The features of this are acute infection of the middle ear cleft, associated with discharge of pus from the ear, pain in the distribution of the trigeminal nerve and sixth nerve paralysis. The syndrome is due to the close anatomical relationship of the fifth and sixth nerves with the petrous apex. But, besides acute petrositis, it may also be due to an extradural abscess or a patch of meningitis overlying the petrous apex.

Diagnosis

Diagnosis depends on the foregoing clinical picture, assisted by polytomography and/or computerized tomographic scanning of the temporal bone.

Treatment

Intensive antibiotic treatment is begun immediately and, in a previously untreated case with a short history, this may well be all that is required. However if the patient fails to respond in 24–48 hours, or if cortical mastoidectomy has already been performed but the disease nevertheless progresses to petrositis, further surgical exploration will be required. This is considered below following surgical treatment of acute mastoiditis.

Treatment of acute mastoiditis

Medical

Even when a child or adult presents with an advanced case of acute mastoiditis with postauricular oedema and protuberant pinna, the treatment is initially medical in hospital, and the majority of these cases will resolve completely. Exceptions are cases with postauricular fluctuation, previous adequate medical management, or suspected intracranial complications.

The patient should be admitted to hospital so that he can be monitored carefully to ensure resolution or to detect lack of progress or early signs of complications. The treatment regimen is as described for acute suppurative otitis media, with a preference for intravenous antibiotic therapy in advanced cases.

Surgical

Cortical mastoidectomy

Cortical mastoidectomy is indicated:

(1) if subperiosteal fluctuation, suspected intracranial complications, or a neck abscess are present when the case presents
(2) if there is persistence of pain, temperature, and otorrhoea, or even profuse otorrhoea on its own, after 2–4 weeks of adequate medical management including use of the correct antibiotic based on culture results, and known compliance in the antibiotic regimen.

The aim of the operation is to exenterate the mastoid air-cell system as completely as possible; the ossicular chain is not disturbed.

Preoperative investigations

Besides those previously mentioned, the patient's fitness for general anaesthesia should be assessed, when possible an immediate preoperative audiogram should be performed, and the central nervous system examined to exclude or assess intracranial complications (with particular reference to facial movements to exclude a preoperative facial paralysis or nystagmus). Mastoid X-rays not only help to confirm the indications for surgery, but also give guidance to the surgeon on the extent of pneumatization and the positions of the dura of the middle and posterior cranial fossae.

Preparation

A postauricular incision is used and as it is fairly close to the hair-line, the hair should be taped out of the way with Sellotape or other adhesive tape. It is not usually necessary to shave the hair.

Anaesthesia

Premedication will always be required as for any other operation requiring general anaesthesia. A general anaesthetic with endotracheal intubation is given.

The operation

This is performed under general anaesthesia. A curved incision is made through the skin of the postauricular region a few millimetres behind and parallel to the postauricular groove.

Care must be taken in the lower half of the incision in infants, in whom the mastoid process is undeveloped, and the facial nerve, as it leaves the stylomastoid foramen is therefore superficial; in the upper half of the incision the lower border of the temporalis muscle should be identified and retracted superiorly. If it is necessary to incise it to obtain adequate exposure, the vessels running at its lower border are first ligated or diathermized (*Figure 13.3*).

In older children and adults, the tendon of the sternomastoid muscle has a wide attachment to the superficial aspect of the mastoid process; the fibres are scraped off with a periosteal elevator. Between the temporalis muscle and the sternomastoid the soft tissues, including the postauricular muscles and periosteum, are incised down to the bone.

The periosteum is elevated forwards as far as the lateral end of the posterior bony meatal wall, backwards for a few millimetres, and upwards to the level of the upper attachment of the pinna. All bleeding points are secured and a self-retaining retractor is inserted.

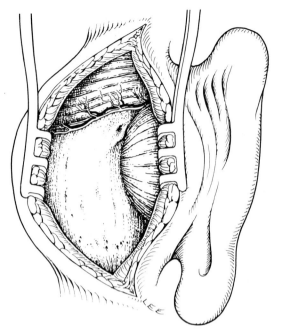

Figure 13.3 Cortical mastoidectomy incision and exposure of mastoid bone. (Reproduced from 'Cortical mastoidectomy', J. Ransome, in *Operative Surgery*, 4th edn, Volume *The Ear*, edited by John Ballantyne and Andrew Morrison, pp. 67–71. London: Butterworths)

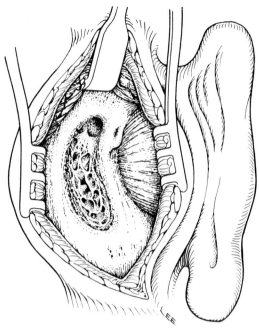

Figure 13.4 Exposure of mastoid antrum. (Reproduced from 'Cortical mastoidectomy', J. Ransome, in *Operative Surgery*, 4th edn, Volume *The Ear*, edited by John Ballantyne and Andrew Morrison, pp. 67–71. London: Butterworths)

In exenterating part of the mastoid bone to uncover the antrum it must be remembered that the antrum is at a depth of 15 mm in the adult, but only a few millimetres in the infant; the surface marking of the antrum is McEwen's triangle; and the position of the middle and posterior fossa dura can be judged by examining the lateral oblique X-ray of the mastoid.

Bearing in mind these landmarks, bone is gradually removed with the drill until the antrum is exposed (*Figure 13.4*).

If pus is encountered a further swab is taken and sent for culture. To confirm that the antrum – rather than merely a large cell – has been entered, a small Dundas Grant probe is passed into the aditus. This should be performed gently to avoid dislodging the short process of the incus. At the same time the size of the aditus can be judged; if it is very small it may be enlarged slightly with a fine bone curette to ensure adequate drainage of the middle ear. (Note that the bony posterior meatal wall must be preserved, and the skin is not dissected from it.)

The air cells are now followed and removed in every direction. It is particularly important to clear all the cells from the sinodural angle. The smooth bone covering the middle fossa dura above and the lateral sinus posteriorly is usually easily recognized (*Figure 13.5*).

There is frequently a group of cells in relation to the vertical part of the facial nerve which are best removed under the operating microscope. In a well-pneumatized skull, cells may extend anteriorly into the root of the zygoma and posteriorly into

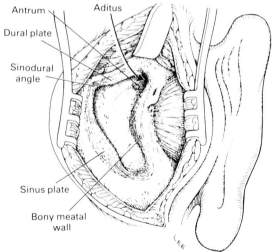

Figure 13.5 Completion of air cell exenteration. (Reproduced from 'Cortical mastoidectomy', J. Ransome, in *Operative Surgery*, 4th edn, Volume *The Ear*, edited by John Ballantyne and Andrew Morrison, pp. 67–71. London: Butterworths)

the occipital bone; these too must be followed as far as is practicable.

It is not necessary to remove the whole tip of the mastoid process unless it is necrotic, but the lateral wall and all cells up to the tip should be removed.

The bony cavity thus created has the antrum as its deepest point, and is bounded above by the dural plate, posteriorly by the sinus plate and anteriorly by the bony meatal wall and aditus. In patients with intracranial complications, a small area of both middle fossa dura and lateral sinus should be exposed; if this reveals granulations or an extradural abscess, exposure of dura is continued until healthy dura is found.

A small drain is inserted into the antrum and led out near the mastoid tip. The skin is closed with interrupted sutures, and a dressing pad and bandage should be applied firmly to prevent a subcutaneous haematoma.

Postoperative care

As soon as the patient is conscious, the facial movements are examined to exclude operative damage to the facial nerve. Antibiotic therapy is continued.

The patient's temperature should be taken every 4 hours. It usually falls dramatically within the first 24 hours, when the patient can be allowed to get out of bed.

The drain should be removed when there is no further discharge either through the wound or through the external meatus. In practice this is usually after 2–3 days, but the drain should be left longer if necessary.

The sutures can be removed on the fifth to seventh day.

A postoperative audiogram is obtained as soon as the ear is dry. At this stage there should be some improvement, although normal hearing may not be regained until 2–3 weeks after the operation.

Complications

Complications of the operation are few and due mainly to errors of technique.

Persistent deafness This may be due to incus dislocation or removal. This should be suspected when the ear becomes dry and the tympanic membrane heals but conductive deafness persists. Impedance audiometry will confirm disruption of the ossicular chain. Tympanotomy and reconstruction of the ossicular chain may then be indicated.

Persistent infection due to residual disease may cause a conductive deafness. This should resolve with proper medical treatment and good drainage.

However, if it persists, reopening of the mastoid and exenteration of the remaining cells is required.

Complete facial nerve paralysis If present immediately postoperatively, but not preoperatively, the facial nerve has been damaged at operation, and the mastoid must be reopened and the facial nerve explored.

Meatal stenosis This may occur if the bony meatal wall is taken down and the skin dissected off the bony wall. It requires excision of the stenosed area and firm packing of the canal until re-epithelialization occurs.

Simple incision and drainage of a postauricular abscess

This condition occurs when pus spreads beyond the confines of the middle ear cleft and ruptures through the lateral surface of the mastoid process into the subperiosteal space. (This then would normally be an indication for cortical mastoidectomy since incision and drainage alone may not be sufficient to enable the mastoiditis to resolve.) However in two circumstances simple incision of the abscess (*Figure 13.6*) is indicated:

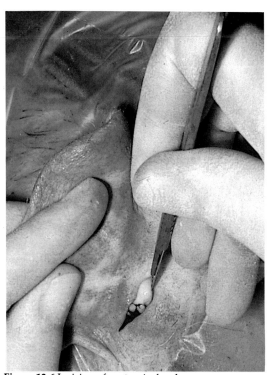

Figure 13.6 Incision of postauricular abscess. (Reproduced by kind permission of Mr J. B. Booth)

(1) In infants, who may occasionally develop a postauricular abscess from a middle ear infection, but in whom the mastoid is not pneumatized nor the mastoid process developed. Particular care must be taken with the incision because of the superficial placing of the facial nerve (*see* Anatomy at the beginning of this chapter).

(2) In any patient, of any age, judged too ill to sustain even the not very long procedure of cortical mastoidectomy, in whom time is of the essence and rapid evacuation of at least some pus is thought to be adequate for the time being. For such cases an even simpler alternative is needle aspiration.

The procedure consists of a simple postauricular incision over the point of maximum fluctuation. When the pus is found a swab is taken, then as much pus as possible is sucked out. A small drainage tube is stitched in and the incision closed.

Myringotomy

Myringotomy alone is obviously not a sufficient form of surgery for acute mastoiditis, but in those few patients who require surgery, but in whom there has been no spontaneous perforation of the tympanic membrane, a myringotomy should be performed as well as other appropriate procedures.

Surgical treatment of acute petrositis

The indication is the presence of acute petrositis, perhaps with Gradenigo's syndrome, and failure to respond rapidly to medical treatment.

The following account of the various approaches to the petrous cells used in the past, has been given by Mawson (1979). It is emphasized that such surgery would be exceptionally rare nowadays; it is difficult and hazardous, and should only be performed by those with very considerable familiarity with the field.

Extrapetrosal drainage

A cortical mastoidectomy operation is performed or reopened. Any fistulous tracks found must be followed. If necessary surgery must proceed to radical mastoidectomy. Tracks may then be found which lead towards the apex from the hypotympanum or attic.

Various routes for a deep exploration are as follows, and are illustrated in *Figure 13.7*.

Eagleton's operation

A wide exposure of the dura of the middle fossa is made by removal of the tegmen, the base of the zygoma and part of the squamous temporal bone. The dura of the middle fossa is gently elevated towards the petrous apex.

Almoor's operation

The petrous apex is approached through a triangle bounded by the tegmen tympani above, the carotid artery anteriorly and the cochlea posteriorly.

Ramadier's operation

Here the petrous apex is approached more widely. The tympanic plate of the external auditory canal, posterior to the base of the glenoid fossa suture line, is removed. The carotid artery is lifted forward by a gauze sling. The petrous apex may then be explored through the posterior wall of the bony carotid canal.

Frenckner's operation

Sometimes a group of cells runs under the arch of the superior semicircular canal. This is a good approach to the petrous apex, but it would have to be combined with an approach to the hypotympanum.

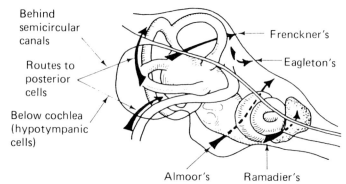

Figure 13.7 Routes to the petrous apex. (After S. Mawson, 1979)

References

BORDLEY, J. E., BROOKHOUSER, P. E. and TUCKER, G. F. Editors. (1986) Otitis media and mastoid disease. In *Ear, Nose and Throat Disorders in Children*, p. 68. New York: Raven Press

JACKSON, R. T. (1971) Pharmacological mechanisms in the eustachian tube. *Annals of Otology, Rhinology and Laryngology*, (St Louis), **80**, 313–318

LEWIS, R. S., MAWSON, S. R., EDWARDS, W. G. and LUDMAN, H. (1967) Acute suppurative otitis media. In *Essentials of Otolaryngology*, p. 82. London: W Heinemann

LILHOLDT, T., CANTEKIN, E. I., BLUESTONE, C. D. and ROCKETTE, H. E. (1982) Effect of a topical nasal decongestant on eustachian tube function in children with tympanostomy tubes. *Acta Oto-Laryngologica*, **94**, 93–97

McKEE, W. J. E. (1963a) A controlled study of the effects of tonsillectomy and adenoidectomy in children. *British Journal of Preventive and Social Medicine*, **17**, 49–69

McKEE, W. J. E. (1963b) The part played by adenoidectomy in the combined operation of tonsillectomy with adenoidectomy. *British Journal of Preventive and Social Medicine*, **17**, 133–140

MAW, A. R. (1985) Factors affecting adenoidectomy for otitis media with effusion (glue ear). *Journal of the Royal Society of Medicine*, **78**, 1014–1018

MAWSON, S. R. (1979) Acute inflammation of the middle ear cleft. In *Scott-Brown's Diseases of the Ear, Nose and Throat*, 4th edn. edited by J. Ballantyne and J. Groves, Vol. 2, pp. 189–190. London: Butterworths

OLSON, A. L., KLEIN, S. W., CHARNEY, E., MacWHINNEY, J. B., McINERNEY, T. K., MILLER, R. L. *et al.* (1978) Prevention and therapy of serous otitis media by oral decongestant. *Pediatrics*, **61**, 679–684

PUKANDER, J., LUOTONEN, J., SIPILÄ, M., TIMONEN, M. and KARMA, P. (1982) Incidence of acute otitis media. *Acta Oto-Laryngologica*, **93**, 447–453

VAN BUCHEM, F. L., PEETERS, M. F. and VAN'T HOF, M. A. (1985) Acute otitis media: a new treatment strategy. *British Medical Journal*, **290**, 1033–1037

14

Vestibular disorders

Susan Snashall

Embryology

The membranous labyrinth of the inner ear develops from the otic capsule between the fourth and twelfth weeks of intrauterine life. The cartilage around the capsule differentiates into the osseous labyrinth at 6–7 weeks' gestation and, at that time, is separated from the membranous portion by the perilymphatic space (Dayal, Far-kushidy and Kokshanian, 1973). As the vestibular system is older phylogenetically, each stage in the development of this system is in advance of that of the auditory system, and is therefore less vulnerable to environmental insult.

The semicircular canals arise from the utricular portion of the otic vesicle and have attained gross morphology at the 30 mm stage. The cochlear duct extends from the saccular portion and has two and a half coils at the 50 mm stage (Anniko, 1983). The neuroepithelium is differentiated in the utricle at 7 weeks and the semicircular canals at 8 weeks, being complete in all cristae and maculae at 12–14 weeks. By comparison, the basal turn of the cochlea is not fully differentiated until mid-term (Dayal, Farkushidy and Kokshanian, 1973; Anniko, 1983).

The vestibular nerve is among the first of the central nervous system tracts to myelinate at around 16 weeks, coinciding with the myelination of the intersegmental tract systems of the cervical spinal cord (Hamilton and Mossman, 1972). The auditory nerve is not myelinated until 20–24 weeks (Eisenberg, 1983). The vestibular system is functional well before birth with a feeble Moro reflex present as early as the ninth to tenth weeks (Holt, 1975) and the vestibulo-ocular reflex is present at 24 weeks (Hamilton and Mossman, 1972).

The different types of congenital dysplasia of the inner ear reflect this sequence of events. Vestibular dysplasia is usually confined to the less common and more severe anomalies. As these arise early in fetal life they may be associated with other morphological abnormalities (Chandra Sekhar and Sachs, 1975).

Four types of inner ear dysplasia are recognized:

(1) Michel aplasia: total aplasia of the osseous labyrinth
(2) Mondini dysplasia: dysplasia of the osseous labyrinth
(3) Bing-Siebenman dysplasia: normal osseous, abnormal membranous labyrinth
(4) Scheibe dysplasia: cochleosaccular dysgenesis.

Scheibe dysplasia is the most common type. In children with this congenital anomaly the deafness is often not accompanied by vestibular dysfunction and there may be no associated abnormalities in other systems. X-ray studies of the petrous temporal bone will also be normal. Some environmental hazards will cause only microscopic abnormalities of the neuroepithelium. Hultcrantz and Anniko (1984) demonstrated changes in the crista ampularis after gamma irradiation on the twelfth gestational day in mice. Wright *et al.* (1982) demonstrated otoconial abnormalities after administration of prostaglandin inhibitors in pregnancy.

Development of vestibular-based functions

The function of the vestibular system can be divided into two categories: the maintenance of posture and stability of vision. In both capacities it integrates with other sensory and motor systems and cannot be considered in isolation. Assessment of vestibular function depends upon the integrity of systems such as the oculomotor tracts and close control of variables related to these systems.

Maintenance of posture

The primary archaic responses (disappearing by the age of 6 months) such as the Moro response, and the secondary inherent responses (persisting into childhood), for example the parachute reaction, are elicited as part of the neurological examination of the infant. They are not performed specifically to assess vestibular function. In the presence of otherwise normal development some of these may be used in this context and therefore deserve description.

The primary archaic responses

The Moro response

Sudden bilateral extension of the upper limbs followed by flexion is evoked by sudden jarring of the cot or by suddenly dropping the head backwards by 2 cm. To limit the stimulus to movement of the head in space, the infant is held on the examiner's forearms with hands supporting the infant's head. The examiner drops from the standing position (*Figure 14.1a*) to the crouching position (*Figure 14.1b*) by bending the knees. The baby is thus suddenly lowered and the reflex obtained (Eviatar and Eviatar, 1978). This response is always present at birth in normal children and disappears by the sixth month.

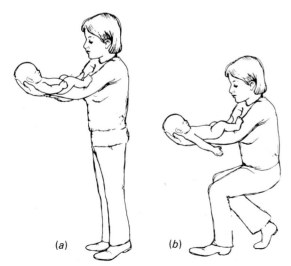

Figure 14.1 The Moro response. (*a*) starting position; (*b*) finishing position

Tonic labyrinthine response

'An increase in extensor tone when supine and flexor tone when prone is not always demonstrable in normal infants but is sometimes found in infants with cerebral palsy' (MacKeith and Robson, 1970).

The secondary inherent responses

Righting responses

These reflexes maintain the head in the upright position and arise at the level of the red nucleus by integration of visual, proprioceptive and vestibular stimuli. To test for vestibular function these reflexes should be elicited with the baby blindfolded.
(a) The earliest righting reflex appears at 10 weeks and consists of extension of the head when the baby is held in ventral suspension.
(b) Later head righting reflexes can be obtained by changing the infant's position rapidly from upright to prone or supine. The head will be lifted to restore it to the vertical position.

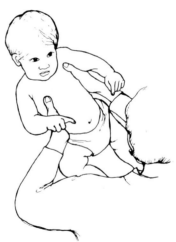

Figure 14.2 Righting responses–oblique suspension

(c) From 4 months the infant will tilt the head to maintain it vertical (*Figure 14.2*) if the trunk is tilted through 30° (oblique suspension). At 5 months this manoeuvre is accompanied by the lower limbs moving away from the side to which the infant has been tilted (MacKeith and Robson, 1970).
(d) The propping reaction (*Figure 14.3*) is elicited in the same manner with the baby in the sitting position. The head should remain vertical. The upper limb on the side to which the trunk has been tilted abducts as does the contralateral lower limb.

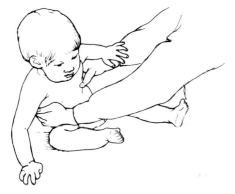

Figure 14.3 Righting responses–propping reaction

Protective reactions

Parachute reaction
(a) Downward parachute: the baby is held in vertical suspension and moved suddenly downwards. Up to the age of 5 months this elicits the Moro response, but above this age the lower limbs extend and abduct.
(b) Forward parachute: held in ventral suspension and moved forward and down the upper limbs abduct and extend and the fingers splay. This reflex can also be elicited by holding the baby in vertical suspension and moving rapidly to ventral suspension. For vestibular testing this should be performed with the infant blindfolded (Eviatar and Eviatar, 1978).

Motor milestones

The ages of sitting unsupported, crawling and walking unaided bear some relation to vestibular function (Kaga *et al.*, 1981), but are also dependent upon the neurodevelopmental state of the infant. Those who bottom shuffle instead of crawling are known to walk later than other normal children (MacKeith and Robson, 1970). In the neurological examination of children the abnormalities found are more often due to failure to develop function than to its loss (MacKeith and Robson, 1970). The importance of vision for postural control, in particular low contrast vision in the peripheral field, cannot be overemphasized (Marron and Bailey, 1982). Attempts have been made to separate those aspects of motor control due to the vestibular system from other measurements of neurodevelopment, but the results were disappointing (DeGangi, Berk and Larsen, 1980; Bundy and Fisher, 1981). One measure of postural status that can be quantified is body sway using the vestibulospinal stability test (Black *et al.*, 1977). Postural sway decreases during the first decade and then remains stable until it increases again in old age. However, it is not related to vestibular function alone. The development of motor and perceptual skills over a 3-year period in normal children and those with minimum brain dysfunction, perceptual and attention deficit, showed that many of the differences seen at the age of 7 years had disappeared 3 years later (Rasmussen *et al.*, 1983; Gillberg, 1985). The development of motor milestones cannot be considered in isolation from the overall development of the child.

Stability of vision

The vestibulo-ocular reflex can be evoked by rotational or caloric stimuli, and enables clear vision to be maintained while the head is in motion. It consists either of nystagmus or of deviation of the eyes equal and opposite to the movement of the head. The fast phase of vestibular nystagmus is central in origin and is affected by maturational changes within the reticular formation. Visual-vestibular interaction has a complex effect upon the vestibulo-ocular reflex and is responsible for many of the changes that take place with increasing maturity.

Response to rotation

In the neonatal period, rotation is most conveniently achieved by holding the infant at arms length in vertical suspension while the examiner rotates about his own axis (*Figure 14.4a* and *b*). As the infant is on the circumference of the circle, looking inwards, the eyes will open and deviate in the direction of rotation (*Figure 14.4c*).

For the first few weeks of life there is deviation of the eyes alone. Between the fourth and sixth week nystagmus is superimposed upon this deviation. Both optokinetic and vestibular nystagmus will be in the same direction so that once nystagmus intervenes the test cannot be used to assess vestibular function. After this age the alert baby will usually fix his eyes on the examiner's face (Farmer, 1964; Eviatar and Eviatar, 1978).

In the laboratory, rotation testing is undertaken with the subject seated in a chair capable of impulse, ramp or sinusoidal acceleration. Infants are held supported on an adult's lap and tolerate sinusoidal acceleration particularly well. To maintain the lateral semicircular canal in the plane of rotation, the head should be flexed 30°. This position cannot be maintained for long periods in infants (Kaga *et al.*, 1981).

The position of the head during recording of rotation or caloric responses affects the quality of induced nystagmus (Schrader, Koenig and Dichgans, 1985). Care must therefore be taken to

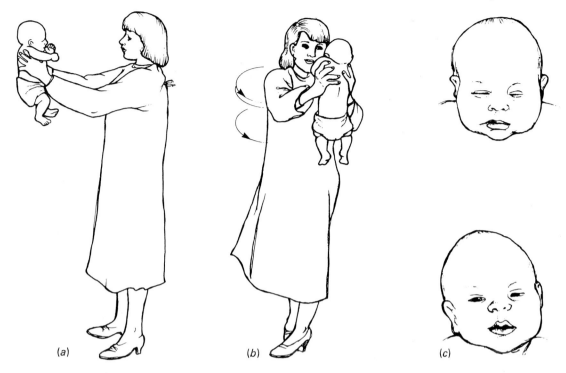

Figure 14.4 Neonatal rotation test. (*a*) starting position; (*b*) finishing position; (*c*) eyes closed at beginning of rotation, open and deviated at end of rotation

ensure that the infant's head is maintained in the vertical plane throughout the test procedure.

Perrotatory nystagmus was recorded in 182 infants in the first year of life by Eviatar and Eviatar (1979). The percentage of babies with perrotatory nystagmus in the first 90 days of life was greatest in full-term infants. By 180 days of age all except the preterm infants exhibited nystagmus. These latter findings were thought to be due to immaturity of the central nervous system at birth.

Postrotatory nystagmus was found to be replaced by tonic deviation of the eyes in two earlier studies of rotation responses in neonates (Groen, 1963; Mitchell and Cambon, 1969). Testing in complete darkness gives better results than using a blindfold (Cyr, 1980; Ornitz, 1983). Absence of nystagmus may be due to lack of alertness in the young or preterm infant (Ornitz, 1983). This factor was illustrated by Reding and Fernandez (1968) who demonstrated absence of nystagmus and presence of tonic deviation to rotation during non-REM sleep in children aged 6–9 years.

The frequency of perrotatory nystagmus is low at birth and increases uniformly during the first 6 years of life, although it does not reach adult values until 10–15 years of age (Tibbling, 1969; Kaga *et al.*, 1981). In parallel with frequency of

beat, the amplitude of the nystagmus is large in infants, gradually decreasing as frequency increases. The duration of perrotatory nystagmus increases rapidly during the first year of life, and more slowly in the following 6 years (Tibbling, 1969; Kaga *et al.*, 1981). The standard deviation in older children was greater than for adults. Theoretically the maximum velocity of the slow phase of vestibular nystagmus is a better indicator of vestibular function than is frequency or duration, but the validity of this measurement depends upon accurate calibration which may be difficult in the very young child. In spite of this, the maximum velocity of the slow phase of both primary (perrotatory) and secondary (postrotatory) nystagmus has been recorded. The maximum velocity of the slow phase of primary nystagmus can be considered as representative of vestibular responsiveness. Tibbling (1969) found that young infants exhibited a high slow component velocity which decreased with age. This was supported by Ornitz *et al.* (1979) for responses measured in total darkness. Eviatar and Eviatar (1979), testing with the infant blindfolded, found that the slow phase velocity increased up to the sixth month and then remained stable. Herman, Maulucci and Stuyck (1982) reported a higher gain of vestibulo-ocular reflex in children. Secondary nystagmus which reflects vestibular adaptation was also found to be of higher velocity in infants (Ornitz *et al.*, 1979) and the secondary nystagmus: primary nystagmus ratio was significantly greater in early infancy. It was postulated that strong adaptation was protective when the infant was subjected to unpredictable passive motion.

Caloric responses

Studies of ice water calorics in the neonatal period include those of Mitchell and Cambon (1969), Eviatar and Eviatar (1979), Pignataro *et al.* (1979) and Donat, Donat and Lay (1980). Caloric nystagmus was found to be absent in some very young infants but Eviatar and Eviatar (1979) reported that it was present in 90% of infants at the age of 9 months. Frequency, velocity, amplitude and latency showed age-related changes similar to those for rotation. Donat, Donat and Lay (1980) described caloric-evoked tonic deviation of the abducting eye with disconjugate deviation of the adducting eye. This internuclear ophthalmoplegia was thought to be due to lack of myelination of the medial longitudinal fasciculus. Iced water is a painful, albeit alerting, caloric stimulus.

The bithermal caloric test was shown to give uniform and reproducible results in children aged 2–7 years (Koenigsberger *et al.*, 1970), measuring duration with eyes fixed on a target. Values for duration and left/right difference are quoted. Michishita (1967) recorded frequency, duration and slow phase velocity of caloric nystagmus from birth to 15 years of age with very similar results to those for rotation reported by Tibbling (1969). Calculations for canal paresis and directional preponderance indicated that differences would have to exceed 25% and 35% respectively to be indicative of pathology.

The variance for these calculated values is similar to that found in rotation testing (Kaga *et al.*, 1981) in normal children but, to some extent, arises from technique. It is difficult to maintain the child in a constant state of alertness. Also the external meatus is small so that inequalities of irrigation can easily occur. Ornitz (1983) has stressed the requirement for total darkness when testing children, as even small sources of light can be sufficient for visual inhibition of nystagmus.

Eye movement control

Adventitious eye movements

Both drift and microsaccades (Carpenter, 1977) are common in the dark, and are particularly prevalent in children. The 'Bell's phenomenon' in which the eyes deviate upwards upon closure is universal and will inhibit nystagmus. Bell's phenomenon

is reversed during a mental alerting task with the eyes closed (Goebel *et al.*, 1983). When testing children care is needed to maintain eye opening and mental alertness. Recording electronystagmography by DC rather than AC helps to distinguish adventitious movements from nystagmus and makes possible the recording of tonic deviation. Eviatar and Eviatar (1981) were, however, able to document the absence of spontaneous and positional nystagmus in normal infants under the age of one year using AC recording.

Smooth pursuit

At birth smooth pursuit is only possible at low velocities. This is thought to reflect foveal immaturity (Kremenitzer *et al.*, 1979). At greater velocities catching up saccades are required (Herman, Maulucci and Stuyck, 1982). At 8 weeks an infant will follow a continuously moving target and at 20 weeks a target with intermittent motion (Bower, Broughton and Moore, 1971). Atkinson and Braddick (1979) felt that tracking was probably fully developed by the age of 3 years, but Gilligan *et al.* (1981) demonstrated improvement up to the age of 10 years. Conjugate eye movements were complete at the age of 3 years. Herman, Maulucci and Stuyck (1982) demonstrated maturation of visual motor skills up to the age of 18 years.

Saccadic movements

These are present at birth but are not accurate until much later. Infants require more than one saccade to reach a target or may overshoot (Bower, Broughton and Moore, 1971).

Optokinetic nystagmus

This is present at birth when it may be utilized to test vision (Gorman, Cogan and Gellis, 1957). It is, however, only present at low velocities and is accompanied by tonic deviation of the eyes in the direction of the slow phase, instead of the fast phase as in adults (Kremenitzer *et al.*, 1979).

Visual–vestibular interaction

This is concerned with the effect of visual stimuli upon vestibular evoked eye movements. As visual motor and pursuit skills mature this effect will increase. Herman, Maulucci and Stuyck (1982) found that, in children, the vestibular stimulus dominates the retinal stimulus so that visual suppression of the rotation-induced vestibuloocular reflex was found to be less in children than adults. Visual suppression is due to low contrast peripheral field sensitivity rather than foveal vision so that immaturity of the retinal stimulus does not account for this immaturity. The development of coupling between the visual and vestibular systems in childhood is an extremely complex area which has been largely neglected by physiological research (Ornitz, 1983).

Physiological vertigo syndromes

Physiological vertigo will occur when there is a mismatch of input from different sensory systems. The multisensory vertigo syndromes were comprehensively reviewed by Brandt and Daroff (1980). Height vertigo, visual vertigo, somatosensory vertigo, auditory vertigo, head extension vertigo, and bending over vertigo receive scant attention in children but differ very little from their presentation in adults. Motion sickness, however, presents a quite different problem as it is much more prevalent in childhood.

Motion sickness

The incidence of this complaint depends upon the parameters used (Money, 1970), but by any criterion the disorder is far more common in children than adults. Surprisingly, there have been very few studies of motion sickness in this age group. Sharma (1980) found 16.6% of male and 29.2% of female children to be affected. Motion sickness is believed to result from conflicting kinetic input from visual, vestibular and non-vestibular proprioceptive systems, in the presence of an intact vestibular system. It results in the same symptoms as those produced by excessive vestibular stimulation (Money, 1970).

An intact visual system is not required and blind children frequently experience motion sickness. During childhood an individual progresses from field dependency (relying on visual clues for orientation in space) to one of field independence (relying on internal clues). Deich and Hodges (1973) related field dependence to motion sickness in fifth, seventh and college grade students (10–18 years). Both field dependence and motion sickness decreased with age but there was no relation of field dependence to motion sickness, nor sex to field dependence. Girls are more susceptible to motion sickness than boys, and this is thought to be cultural as their vestibular experience is often less than that of boys (Deich and Hodges, 1973; Lentz and Collins, 1977; Sharma, 1980).

Infants below the age of 2 years are usually resistant to motion sickness, either because they travel supine (Money, 1970) or because of lack of visual input (Brandt and Daroff, 1980). Children are most susceptible to motion sickness from 2 to 12 years of age with a subsequent gradual decrease

in symptoms (Lentz and Collins, 1977; Brandt and Daroff, 1980; Sharma, 1980; Kuritzky, Ziegler and Hassanien, 1981). Decrease in motion sickness with age is attributed to experience moderating the vestibular response and to the development of central inhibition (Groen, 1963) with improvement in vestibulo-ocular reflex suppression (Hood, 1980; Fluur, 1983). Motion sickness is more prevalent in children who suffer from migraine (Toglia, Thomas and Kuritzky, 1981; Del Bene, 1982). In addition, visual vertigo and vestibular dysfunction contribute to motion sickness in this group.

Vestibular stimulation

Repetitive vestibular stimulation is pleasurable and calming to infants whether from self-stimulation or by those caring for the child. Self-stimulation in the form of body rocking or head banging or rolling begins at about 6 months of age when the gain of the vestibulo-ocular reflex is at its highest (Ornitz, 1983). It does not usually last beyond the age of 2 years. Self-stimulation has been found to accelerate motor milestones (Sallustro and Atwell, 1978). Applied vestibular stimulation has been demonstrated to improve the development of ocular-motor skills and the integrative functions of the cerebellum (Clark, Kreutzberg and Chee, 1977; Weeks, 1979). In an older age group, vestibular stimulation affected the duration of postrotational nystagmus in three children with learning disability (Ottenbacher, 1982). It follows therefore that vestibular hypofunction is sometimes related to delay in motor milestones (Rapin, 1974; Eviatar and Eviatar, 1981), and is implicated in children suffering from cognitive, perceptual and attentional problems. This is discussed in more detail at the end of this chapter.

Symptomatology and history taking

Vestibular disorders may present with dysequilibrium or be asymptomatic (Brookhouser, Cyr and Beauchaine, 1982). In the young child vertigo frequently goes unrecognized. It should be suspected if the child lies face down wedged against the side of the cot with the eyes closed, not wanting to be moved (Farmer, 1964). Sudden falling or tipping over, with crying, pallor, and sweating are also indicative of vertigo (Basser, 1964). In older children vertigo should be suspected if they are unwilling to get out of bed after the acute phase of an illness has passed. Lack of vestibular function is usually symptomless as children have such good compensation for loss of vestibular input (Dix, 1948). It should, however, be suspected if there is inexplicable delay in the acquisition of motor milestones, learning to skate or cycle, or spatial disorientation in a darkened environment. Such children may be fearful of any situation in which the lights are turned out, as in a film show.

History

Acute episodic vertigo

Attacks of vertigo can begin in the second year of life before the child is able to describe the symptom, objective observations being all that is available. The infant may suddenly cry out in fear and drop to a crawling position, cling for support to any available object, or be observed to be ataxic. Nystagmus is sometimes reported, and the child is pale. If the attack lasts long enough, sweating or vomiting may occur. Once the child is a little older descriptions such as 'the skies are falling' or 'the world is going round' are given. Headache with the attack should be suspected if it is accompanied by screaming.

In children around the age of one year vestibular dysfunction can present as torticollis with abnormal tilting or twisting of the head. It is important to establish whether there is any loss of consciousness, however brief, during the attack or subsequent amnesia, or bizarre movements. The speed with which the attack comes on, its duration, and the manner in which the child returns to normal are often pathognomonic.

In addition to the description of the acute attack the following details must be established: accompanying symptoms, precedency, precipitating or aggravating events, frequency or periodicity of attacks, age of onset and sequelae. Accompanying symptoms to be explored are hearing loss, tinnitus, headache, visual obscuration, lassitude, photophobia, and neurological deficit such as ocular palsies, hemiparesis or paraesthesia.

Preceding and precipitating events to be elicited are as follows: exertion, barotrauma or head injury; changes in position; infections, especially otitis media, meningitis and viral illnesses. As pyrexial illness is so common in children, care must be taken to establish a causal relationship. For example, labyrinthitis occurs with, or immediately after, a viral illness whereas cerebellar ataxia is delayed by 7–10 days.

For recurrent attacks of vertigo the chronology of symptoms and their periodicity must be established as some vertiginous disorders of childhood are strikingly periodic. The vertigo syndromes of childhood tend to be different according to the age of the child. For example, paroxysmal torticollis is a disorder of the first 3 years of life; benign paroxysmal vertigo is usually confined to the second to tenth years, and basilar artery migraine begins in the first year of life and subsequently changes to common migraine. When confronted with one form of vertigo the presence of any pre-existing forms should be explored. The acute attack of vertigo must be distinguished from other recurrent paroxysmal epileptic and non-epileptic disorders (Collins, 1983/84) which are presented in detail in the section on differential diagnosis.

Persistent vertigo, imbalance or motor delay

Dysequilibrium due to primary vestibular deficit must be distinguished from ataxia due to central nervous system disease (Harrison, 1962a; Beddoe, 1977; Busis, 1983). Whereas delay in the acquisition of motor milestones or balancing skills can result either from poor sensory input or central nervous system immaturity, deteriorating function is more likely to be due to posterior fossa disease (Curless, 1980). The distinction must therefore be made between delay, arrest or deterioration in motor and postural performance. The presence of any concomitant ocular-motor, visual or neurological deficit is ascertained. If there is no imbalance in daylight, specific enquiry should be made regarding the child's performance in the dark. A history of fear of the dark or of being blindfolded can be helpful. Some children with vestibular disorders will be afraid of swings and roundabouts and of rough play.

Small children frequently fall, but children with vestibular disorders may be noticed to be more clumsy and fall more frequently than their peers. Distinction is made between unsteadiness on rapid movement and ataxia of gait. The presence or absence of motion sickness is relevant. As bilateral vestibular weakness is usually symptomless a high index of suspicion is required.

General health

The development, visual, and hearing status of the child is ascertained. The presence of any middle ear, renal or endocrine disease, serious medical disorder or any physical deformity is established. The child's personality is relevant to migrainous disorders and also to hyperventilation. Problems with interpersonal relationships and school performance can lead to anxiety.

The frequency, location and duration of headache or vomiting is recorded in the same manner as for the attack of vertigo. Repeated physical trauma or exposure to toxic chemicals could cause dizziness. A detailed drug history, including commonly prescribed drugs for minor disorders, for example piperazine for infestation, is mandatory.

Past history

The health of the mother during pregnancy with regard to viral illness and also to systemic illness requiring the administration of ototoxic antibiotics (McCracken, 1976; Wright *et al.*, 1982) is explored. In the perinatal period prolonged or repeated anoxia will result in brain damage rather than vestibular destruction. The administration of aminoglycoside antibiotics in association with loop-inhibiting diuretics is associated with vestibular and cochlear ototoxicity (Finitzo-Hieber *et al.*, 1979; Camarda *et al.*, 1981; Davis *et al.*, 1982; Finitzo-Hieber, McCracken, and Brown, 1985). In childhood a history of trauma, surgery, infectious diseases, viral illness, meningitis or the administration of ototoxic antibiotics is noted.

Developmental history

Motor milestones, social and speech development are all relevant to vestibular function. School performance and learning ability are ascertained.

Family history

Enquiry should be made after the following familial disorders: migraine, seizures, deafness, endocrine disease, renal disease, motion sickness, and syndromes with aural manifestations or ataxia. Infections which cross the placental barrier, such as syphilis, may affect a number of siblings. The general state of health of the family is important as other members of the family will have been exposed to the same environment. The possibility of consanguinity is explored.

Physical examination

The examination of the child suspected of vestibular deficit or dysfunction must include complete otolaryngological, neurological and neurodevelopmental investigation. Particular attention is required in the following areas:

The ear: the tympanic membrane, which should preferably be examined under the operating microscope, noting any congenital abnormality of the external ear, however minor.

The nose and throat: infection, congenital abnormality, the state of the airway.

Hearing and speech: an objective assessment using distraction or toy tests of hearing and listening to the child's expressive language. For details the reader is referred to other chapters in this volume. The parents' subjective report is insufficient.

Tuning fork tests

Eye movements: the cover test for latent strabismus, in addition to pursuit, convergence and nystagmus.

Postural control: righting reflexes, positional nystagmus, hopping, heel-toe walking, kicking a ball, gait and stance with eyes open and closed, head tilt, asymmetry of movement, removal of proprioceptive input.

Neurological: hand-eye coordination, cranial nerves, tendon reflexes, tone, developmental abnormalities, congenital defects and syndromes, abnormal movements.

Vision: visual acuity, ophthalmoscopy, heterochromia.

General examination: congenital defects, pigmentary disorders, musculoskeletal defects and disorders, heart sounds.

Investigation

In many instances it is possible to reach a diagnosis on the basis of careful history and detailed examination. Most of the causes of vertigo in childhood are not associated with any abnormality on investigation, which can be unproductive if not used selectively. Audiovestibular and electroencephalographic investigation frequently provide useful information and, in some instances, X-ray and laboratory tests are required. Referral for a paediatric opinion is often advisable.

Auditory tests

Pure-tone audiometry is essential in all children capable of giving reliable responses and is supported by speech discrimination tests. Impedance testing should also be routine.

Electrophysiological tests

An EEG should be performed whenever there is any possibility of altered consciousness associated with vertigo. It is also helpful in cases of persistent or progressive dysequilibrium. Evoked response audiometry may be required to assess hearing, but also provides information on neurological status.

Vestibular tests

Electronystagmography allows evaluation of vestibular function without the influence of visual and proprioceptive input. Providing the following precautions are taken to allow for the differences encountered when testing children, electronystagmography and the bithermal caloric test can be undertaken even in very young children.

(1) To overcome vestibulo-ocular reflex suppression by visual fixation, caloric or rotation responses should be measured in total darkness with mental alerting. An infra-red viewer is required to ensure that the eyes remain open and the child alert.

Compared with adults the caloric nystagmus of children is of lower frequency and greater amplitude. Although the mean maximum velocity of the slow phase is similar, the variance is higher and the response is often dysrhythmic. Calculations for canal paresis and directional preponderance should take this wide range of normal values into account. Published data for caloric responses in children are anomalous as illumination and recording conditions are not uniform. Each laboratory should therefore define its own normal data for the bithermal caloric test. Although convenient, the iced water caloric test is not recommended for children as it is distressing and is less accurate. As a small ear canal can cause inequality of irrigation, the volume should be measured after each caloric test.

(2) If electronystagmography is used to record the response, a DC machine will minimize the likelihood of adventitious eye movements masquerading as nystagmus (as may occur with AC equipment).

(3) Acceptance of the test is helped by the display of a photograph of a child wearing electrodes. Throughout the procedure the child should be included in the conversation as any sense of isolation produces anxiety.

(4) Stability of gaze for recording spontaneous nystagmus is improved by proprioceptive clues.

(5) Attention for smooth pursuit tracking is maintained by the use of an intermittent light source.

(6) Optokinetic tracking can be recorded from birth provided a full field stimulus is used. Attention for the small optokinetic drum is so difficult that results are poor even in children 5–15 years old.

(7) Rotation responses either to sinusoidal harmonic rotation or to ramp acceleration and deceleration are of greater gain in children than adults, with rather less fixation suppression. The test is well tolerated and gives invaluable information on the overall vestibular status of the child.

Vestibulospinal stability test: this new technique of quantifying body sway gives a rapid objective recording of stability and has a place in the screening of children where more demanding investigations are not tolerated.

Radiology

Plain skull films and mastoid X-rays are performed if indicated. Inner ear abnormalities which are detectable on petrous bone tomography are likely to be associated with vestibular abnormality, if not total lack of function. Tomography is therefore more rewarding than in the investigation of straightforward genetic cochlear deafness. Computerized tomographic scanning is obligatory where there is any suspicion of central nervous system disorder causing unsteadiness, particularly if it is progressive.

Urinalysis

This is indicated for estimation of protein and red blood cells in children with sensorineural deafness and vestibular disorder. It should be repeated at yearly intervals as renal involvement can be progressive.

Blood tests

Serology: screening for congenital syphilis is mandatory in all children with progressive cochlear and vestibular dysfunction in the first or second decade. In young children a viral screen is advisable if congenital deafness is present.

Blood chemistry: sugar, creatinine, calcium phosphate, electrolytes, T3 and T4 are advocated.

Haematology: full blood count, erythrocyte sedimentation rate (ESR), and autoimmune profile are indicated when vertigo is accompanied by fluctuating deafness.

Electrocardiography is indicated in congenital deafness and vestibular deficit of unknown aetiology to detect those syndromes with cardiac and labyrinthine dysgenesis.

Pathological vertigo syndromes
Vestibular disorders with auditory symptoms
External meatus

Impacted cerumen may cause dysequilibrium.

Middle ear cleft
Otitis media with effusion

This condition usually gives rise to no more than mild positional vertigo or occasional slight dizziness. There are, however, reports of balance disturbance and episodic rotational vertigo which respond to the insertion of tympanostomy tubes (*Clinical Otolaryngology,* 1978; Fried, 1980; Blaney, 1983).

Blaney reported serous otitis as the cause for five out of 25 children presenting to the clinic with rotational vertigo. Busis (1983) regarded eustachian tube dysfunction as the commonest cause of vestibular disturbance in children. Markedly negative middle ear pressure in association with thick mucus in the middle ear cleft may cause dramatic attacks of transient rotational vertigo accompanied by pallor and nausea, which are not precipitated by movement and with little change in hearing.

Alternatively, parents of preschool children with serous otitis not infrequently notice that the child 'walks clumsily', 'falls all over the place' or 'walks into things'. They may query whether he or she has adequate vision to account for this. These symptoms of imbalance respond immediately to correction of middle ear pressure. In the author's experience 50% of children with serous otitis may have some balance disturbance. This responds to correction of the underlying condition in one-half of those affected. The presence of balance disturbance should weight the scales in favour of surgical intervention for serous otitis even if the hearing is relatively unaffected.

Suppurative otitis media

Either acute or chronic suppuration may serve as an irritative or invasive focus involving the labyrinth. Some of the topical antibiotics used for this condition are also vestibulotoxic. In spite of this, suppuration relatively rarely causes vertigo.

Cholesteatoma

Both congenital (Schwartz *et al.*, 1984; Wang *et al.*, 1984) and acquired cholesteatoma may invade the labyrinth and give rise to vertigo. In any child with a discharging ear or attic disease in association with vertigo the fistula test should be performed.

Labyrinthine

Congenital vestibular deficit

Of all the congenital sensory deficits this is the most silent. It is usually associated with congenital deafness, but vestibular hypofunction may also contribute to the handicap of other disorders such as Down's syndrome (Zarnoch, 1980). When congenital deafness is accompanied by episodic vertigo or abnormal vestibular responses, polytomography may reveal an enlarged vestibule with dilatation of the ampullated portions of the horizontal and superior semicircular canals, in addition to an abnormal cochlea (Hill, Freint and Mafee, 1984; Brama, 1985). Congenital vestibular

deficit with deafness is more often symptomless and only detected by examination.

There have been a number of studies of vestibular function in deaf school children (Arnvig, 1955; Sandberg and Terkildsen, 1965; Swisher and Gannon, 1968; Brookhouser, Cyr and Beauchaine, 1982). In an unselected population in schools for the deaf the incidence of reduced or absent caloric or rotation responses varies from 10 to 36% depending on the technique used. Brookhouser, Cyr and Beauchaine (1982) demonstrated that caloric responses are sometimes suppressed in children. They recommend that results be recorded with eyes open in the dark and with a mental alerting task, using sign language where required. In this manner they found 22% to have caloric abnormalities. These were correlated with results of the tandem Romberg test in the Jendrassik position.

Although not correlated with the severity of the deafness the presence of caloric weakness is useful for the determination of aetiology and therefore prognosis. Arnvig (1955) found caloric reduction most prevalent in those with deafness due to meningitis (91%) and those with retinitis pigmentosa, who accounted for one-half of the children with reduced vestibular function. Kumar, Fishman and Torok (1984) reported that vestibular deficit in Usher's syndrome is found in that variety of the disease that has the worst prognosis for visual deficit. Karjalainen *et al.* (1985) postulated that vestibular tests may facilitate the detection of heterozygote carriers of Usher's syndrome with central vestibular abnormalities.

Waardenburg's syndrome accounts for 2% of all congenital deafness and 30% of these patients will also have congenital vestibular failure (Schweitzer and Clack, 1984). Patients with Waardenburg's syndrome and vestibular disorder experience dizziness or episodic vertigo rather than delayed milestones or imbalance. In Hurler's syndrome there is disruption of the statoacoustic nerve by deposits of Hurler cells between the nerve fibres (Friedman *et al.*, 1985). This disruption may cause a retrocochlear auditory and vestibular deficit in addition to the degeneration of the organ of Corti.

A congenital vestibular disorder may therefore be anticipated in those cases of congenital deafness which are associated with other defects particularly of the head and neck, vision, or petrous temporal bone.

Apart from prognosis and diagnosis vestibular assessment allows better rehabilitation. Harris *et al.* (1984) linked vestibular weakness in congenital deafness due to cytomegalovirus with delayed motor milestones and imbalance. Brookhouser, Cyr and Beauchaine (1982) recommended that all deaf children have vestibular assessment for recreational and occupational counselling. They suggested that this be performed early in those with deafness greater than 110dB as vestibular weakness is more likely in this group.

There is no advantage in caloric assessment for the purposes of aural rehabilitation using 'vestibular hearing' (Swisher and Gannon, 1968) as the caloric test stimulates the lateral semicircular canal. It is the saccule that is responsible for vestibular hearing (Lenhardt, 1985). This is one explanation of the better hearing in those with normal vestibular function.

Trauma

Head injury produces vertigo by perilymph fistula (*see below*), or by labyrinthine concussion with or without fracture of the temporal bone. Vertigo may be short-lived even if destruction of the labyrinth is complete as children adapt quickly to altered vestibular function. Recording nystagmus in the absence of visual fixation soon after the injury is important for medico-legal reasons as vestibular responses may remain abnormal permanently.

It is possible to lose vestibular function without deafness in a longitudinal fracture. Vartiainen, Karjalainen and Karja (1985) reported one such case of vertigo in 61 children following acute blunt head injury. This child had vertigo due to a traumatic perilymph fistula. The incidence of sensorineural deafness was 7%. Perilymph fistula may follow even minor trauma to the head.

Infection

Bacterial infection is transmitted to the labyrinth from the middle ear (*see above*) or via the cochlear aqueduct from meningeal infection. Deafness due to meningitis is accompanied by loss of vestibular function in 66% (Arnvig, 1955). Infection with congenital syphilis presents with deafness, tinnitus and vertigo in a pattern not dissimilar from endolymphatic hydrops (Wilson and Zoller, 1981). Viral labyrinthitis is more usual, the pathogenesis being the same as in adults via the modiolus with the difference that it is easily overlooked (Tieri *et al.*, 1984). Cochlear function may be affected. The child is often too young to describe the symptoms and the lack of mobility is ascribed to the causative illness. The vertigo subsides in a few days without recognition of labyrinthine involvement (Hyden, Odkvist and Kyle, 1979). Subsequent caloric weakness may be demonstrated even in the absence of vertigo. The viruses most often associated with labyrinthitis in adults and children are mumps, measles, varicella zoster and cytomegalovirus (Davis and Straus, 1973; Straus and Davis, 1973; Ronson and Hinchcliffe, 1976; Karmody, 1983). Epidemic labyrinthitis does not involve the cochlea.

Menière's disease

Menière's disease is uncommon in children, accounting for only 2% of Harrison and Naftalin's (1968) series of 423 cases with this condition. Earlier reports of childhood Menière's disease include those of Brain (1938), Crowe (1938), Simonton (1940), Ombredanne and Aubry (1941), Ford (1944), Cawthorne (1954), and Golding-Wood (1960). Some of these were traced by Meyerhoff, Paparella and Shea (1978) when they presented a series of eight cases. Parving (1976), Beddoe (1977) and Sade and Yaniv (1984) documented an additional seven cases. Filipo and Barabara (1985) reported that 7% of referrals for Menière's disease are under the age of 20 years.

From these published data (*Table 14.1*), Menière's disease would appear to be almost twice

Table 14.1 Age of onset of Menière's disorder

Author	Brain	Crowe	Simonton	Ombredanne and Aubry	Ford	Cawthorne	Golding-Wood	
Date	1938	1938	1940	1941	1944	1954	1960	
Total no. cases	41	1	1	1	1*	424	314	
Onset 0–9 years	0	1	1	0	1	0	0	
Onset 10–19 years	1	0	0	1	1	6	3	
Author	Harrison and Naftalin	Parving	Beddoe	Meyerhoff, Paparella and Sade	Sade and Yaniv	Filipo and Barabara		Total
Date	1968	1976	1977	1978	1984	1985		
Total no. cases	423	2	2	8	5	5		1228
Onset 0–9 years	5	1*	1	3	5*	1		19
Onset 10–19 years	6	1	1	5*	0	4		29

* Series in which some or all of the cases were bilateral

as common after the age of 10 years than it is in the younger children as mentioned by Gates (1980). Children presenting with deafness, tinnitus and vertigo merit a comprehensive search for aetiological factors. Adrenal, pituitary and thyroid gland insufficiency, allergy, autoimmune disease, syphilis, trauma, perilymph fistula, acoustic neuroma and congenital abnormalities of the inner ear, petrous temporal bone and base of skull should be considered (Meyerhoff, Paparella and Shea, 1978; Filipo and Barabara, 1985).

A large vestibular aqueduct has been associated with congenital sensorineural deafness and vertigo (Valvassori and Clemis, 1978; Hill, Freint and Mafee, 1984) but Rizvi and Elliott Smith (1981) found no significant correlation between a large vestibular aqueduct and endolymphatic hydrops when comparing this population with a control group.

The criterion for diagnosing Menière's disease in childhood is no different from that in adults; namely a predominantly low tone cochlear deafness with tinnitus and episodic rotational vertigo. Between attacks vestibular function may return to normal (Busis, 1983). Some children with Menière's disease in infancy have progressive sensorineural deafness (Sade and Yaniv, 1984), but others go into spontaneous remission with no residual cochlear or vestibular deficit. Harrison and Naftalin (1968) regarded this group as being 'pseudo-Menière's', but it is possible that this is remission rather than recovery. Although Meyerhoff, Paparella and Shea (1973) regarded saccus decompression more successful than medical therapy in children, Filipo and Barabara (1984) reported a good response to diuretics in three out of five children. Other forms of medical therapy have not proved beneficial, with the exception of steroids for autoimmune and inflammatory endolymphatic hydrops (Bachynski and Wise, 1984; Hughes *et al.*, 1984).

Of the 15 children with Menière's disease under the age of 10 years reported in the literature (*see Table 14.1*) five are known to have bilateral disease; a much higher proportion than in the older children (2/21). This reported high proportion of bilateral disease in the very young is in agreement with the author's own experience.

Perilymph fistula

Perilymph fistula is an important cause of sudden, fluctuating or progressive hearing loss associated with tinnitus, vertigo or imbalance. Unfortunately, it is extremely difficult to diagnose without surgical exploration of the ear (Halvey and Sade, 1983). A high index of suspicion for this disorder is required if surgical closure of the leak is to stabilize the hearing, abolish vertigo and prevent recurrent

meningitis (Grundfast and Bluestone, 1978; Healy, Friedman and Ditroia, 1978; Althaus, 1981).

In children fistula is often associated with congenital abnormalities of the head and neck, for example craniosynostosis, Pendred's syndrome, Klippel-Feil syndrome, a large cochlear aqueduct, Mondini defect, or lateral dilatation of the internal acoustic meatus. It may be precipitated by such events as barotrauma, exertion or a Valsalva manoeuvre (Althaus, 1981; Milner *et al.*, 1983; Supance and Bluestone, 1983; Weider and Musiek, 1984; Cremers *et al.*, 1985). Malformation of the round window niche associated with perilymph leak can be present without any radiological evidence of labyrinthine deformity (Pashley, 1982) and on tympanotomy the round window is often obscured by mucosal folds (Flood *et al.*, 1985).

In the absence of a clear history of trauma, exertion or surgery, this condition may be confused with other causes of progressive or sudden deafness. Halvey and Sade (1983) were unable to identify any significant preoperative differences between those with and without fistula at operation. A number of tests have been advocated to aid diagnosis. A unilateral sensorineural hearing loss with poor speech discrimination and a change in hearing thresholds in the recumbent position should alert the clinician (Busis, 1983; Flood *et al.*, 1985). Very small changes in threshold are, however, difficult to establish in children and transtympanic electrocochleography may be required for diagnosis.

Vestibular function is often deranged in perilymph fistula. This can be documented by recording spontaneous or positional nystagmus, posturography, and the fistula test. The latter was thought to be more specific for perilymph leak than more general evidence of peripheral vestibular disorder when recorded with the eyes closed (Daspit, Churchill and Linthicum, 1980). Results have, however, been disappointing as the fistula test recorded by electronystagmography can activate a latent spontaneous nystagmus that is not necessarily due to a perilymph leak. Supance and Bluestone (1983), in a large study of perilymph fistulae in children, confirmed by tympanotomy, found that the fistula test did not correlate with the operative findings. Exploratory tympanotomy was carried out in 33 infants and children (44 ears) identifying a perilymph leak in 29 ears. Middle ear anomalies were found in 20 ears. Preoperative factors determined to be highly suggestive of perilymph fistula were sudden onset of sensorineural hearing loss, congenital deformities of the head, and abnormal findings on tomography of the temporal bones, especially Mondini-like inner ear dysplasias.

The vestibular abnormalities most frequently associated with perilymph fistula were positional nystagmus and abnormal platform posturography. Vertigo was present in 10 of the 33 children explored, of whom four were found to have a fistula. Perilymph gushers during surgery for congenital stapes fixation may be anticipated in X-linked progressive mixed deafness; abnormal vestibular symptoms and signs and abnormalities on polytomography of the temporal bones may be found (Cremers *et al.*, 1985).

In summary the features suggestive of a perilymph fistula are:

History

Head injury, barotrauma, sneezing, Valsava manoeuvre, laughing, blowing a wind instrument
Sudden or fluctuating sensorineural deafness
A sensation of 'pop' in the ear followed by deafness or vertigo
Tullio phenomenon
Continuous dizziness increased by postural change
A past history of recurrent meningitis.

Findings

Spontaneous or positional nystagmus
Positive Romberg test, including posturography
Unilateral sensorineural hearing loss, change of hearing with position
Congenital abnormalities of the head and neck including minor abnormalities of the pinna
Abnormal petrous bone tomography, especially Mondini dysplasia, dilatation of the distal end of the internal auditory canal or an abnormally large vestibule.

Ototoxic drugs

Whether or not the aminoglycoside antibiotics used in the neonatal period cause significant ototoxicity is a debate which remains to be fully resolved. Animal studies suggest that young animals are more susceptible to vestibular and cochlear toxicity than are adults of the same species (Prieve and Yanz, 1984). Prospective, long-term studies of infants who received aminoglycoside antibiotics in the neonatal period have failed to provide convincing evidence that, in those children subsequently proved to be deaf or partially hearing, ototixicity was the sole factor (Finitzo-Hieber *et al.*, 1979; Finitzo-Hieber, McCracken and Brown, 1985). McCracken (1976) and Elfving, Pettay and Raivio (1973) similarly found it difficult to evaluate a cause–effect relationship with regard to vestibular deficit in two out of 13 infants treated with gentamicin.

As the incidence of vestibular ototoxicity is only of the order of 1% (Noone, 1982) large numbers of subjects are required if statistically significant differences are to be shown between groups. In spite of this difficulty Eviatar and Eviatar (1981, 1982), in a prospective study of 43 infants treated with aminoglycosides compared with 250 control preterm infants, found abnormal vestibular test results only in the treated infants. Head control was delayed in two of 26 treated with kanamycin, eight of 17 treated with gentamicin and only one untreated control. All except the one control baby and one of the gentamicin group had positional nystagmus with additional abnormalities of rotation of caloric responses. The caloric abnormality was unilateral in six of the infants. Only two of the infants with vestibular dysfunction had an associated hearing loss. Delayed head control usually arises from cerebral palsy and it is therefore important to know whether vestibular function is normal so that a realistic prognosis can be given.

These recommendations were in agreement with those of Camarda *et al.* (1981), demonstrating vestibular deficit in 52 subjects aged 2–26 years with ototoxic hearing loss and delayed motor control. The new antibiotic, netilmicin, would appear to have a far lower incidence of ototoxicity as only one case was found out of 804 neonates, infants and children treated (Chiu *et al.*, 1983). The 572 neonates in this study were evaluated for ototoxicity by brainstem evoked responses in the neonatal period only and it is therefore possible that vestibular toxicity was missed in this age group. The only case of toxicity reported was a 14-year-old girl with vertigo, tinnitus and deafness.

Perinatal risk factors

Perinatal risk factors in the aetiology of vestibular loss parallel those for hearing loss and contribute to the disability in this age group. Thiringer *et al.* (1984) redefined those risk factors correlated with sensorineural deafness in 146 deaf preschool children.

Six factors were identified:

(1) hereditary tendency to deafness
(2) rubella or other virus infection in pregnancy
(3) malformations of the ear, face, syndrome-like appearance, chromosome defects and alcohol fetopathia
(4) asphyxia requiring more than 10 minutes resuscitation and/or intensive care treatment
(5) very low birthweight infants
(6) neonatal sepsis/meningitis.

All these factors will predispose the infant to ototoxicity, both vestibular and cochlear, making cause–effect difficult to disentangle. Ototoxicity is related more to total dose, and slow clearing from perilymph than it is to peak levels of drug concentration (Ohtani *et al.*, 1982).

In older children there are a number of conditions in which treatment with an ototoxic antibiotic with or without loop inhibitor diuretics is likely (Davis *et al.*, 1982), for example cystic fibrosis, severe burns, renal failure. Monitoring of patients receiving aminoglycoside antibiotics is usually achieved by pure-tone audiometry and measurement of blood levels. Although, ideally, caloric testing should be performed, the condition of the patient may make this impractical. There is the additional problem that patients become adapted to the caloric stimulus if it is performed frequently. Longridge and Mallinson (1984) have described a method by which the vestibulo-ocular reflex can be used as a screening test which correlates with caloric responses in those patients capable of discriminating the letter 'E'.

Neurotoxic chemicals such as solvents should also be considered in the aetiology of vestibulo-oculomotor dysfunction (Odkvist *et al.*, 1982).

Retrolabyrinthine

Lesions of the eighth cranial nerve give rise to progressive deafness, tinnitus and imbalance. In childhood and adolescence these symptoms are more likely to be due to progressive, genetic, infective, or hydropic disorders of the labyrinth. Meningitis can give rise to audiovestibular deficit by infection around the statoacoustic nerve within the internal auditory meatus (Keane *et al.*, 1983). Benign cerebellopontine angle tumours do occasionally occur in children, particularly those with a family history of von Recklinghausen's disease (*see below*). Each case of asymmetrical progressive sensorineural deafness or imbalance should therefore be investigated on its merits if these rare conditions are not to be overlooked.

Vestibular disorders without other ear symptoms

Referral of children with vertigo to an otologist is relatively rare. In a recent survey of 175 children aged 10–20 years seen in an otolaryngology clinic over a 33-month period, Ruben (1985) reported that none presented with vestibular symptoms. Blaney (1983), also reporting referrals to an otolaryngology clinic, listed 27 children presenting with dizziness in a period of 18 months. Children may not complain of vertigo or imbalance, either because they are too young or because they do not realize that it is an abnormal symptom (Gates, 1980). The recognition that the child's symptoms are due to vertigo often depends upon correct interpretation of the parent's description of the child's behaviour. Children with vertigo are therefore usually referred to paediatric clinics rather than an otolaryngology clinic. The disorders described in this section are not thought to arise

primarily in the labyrinth but, nevertheless, cause rotational, episodic vertigo. Both benign paroxysmal vertigo of childhood and benign paroxysmal torticollis are regarded as migraine equivalents by many authors (Sanner and Bergstrom, 1979; Eeg-Olofsson *et al.*, 1980; Koehler, 1980).

Benign paroxysmal vertigo of childhood

First described by Basser in 1964, this disorder is characterized by brief, sudden and severe episodes of spontaneous vertigo in otherwise healthy children. There are concomitant autonomic symptoms such as pallor, sweating, and occasionally vomiting. The onset is abrupt, causing confusion with seizures, but there is no loss or alteration of consciousness. Typically the child suddenly cries out with fear, drops to all fours or clings for support, and remains acutely unsteady for 30–60 seconds. He/she rapidly returns to complete normality within at most a few minutes and resumes whatever he/she was previously doing. Nystagmus may be observed during the attack, and the children, who are frequently articulate for their age, describe 'the world going round' or 'the walls falling down'. The attacks are recurrent, of variable frequency, and there are no precipitating factors or sequelae. Attacks typically commence before the age of 4 years (Fried, 1980) and disappear spontaneously in a matter of months or years. The paroxysms can occasionally occur in older children or the young teenager (Busis, 1983).

Almost one-half of the affected children go on to develop migraine in adolescence (Koenigsberger *et al.*, 1970; Chutorian, 1972; Koehler, 1980). Most children have a family history of migraine (Koenigsberger *et al.*, 1970; Eeg-Olofsson *et al.*, 1980; Koehler, 1980; Mira *et al.*, 1984). Sometimes the attacks are associated with headache and photophobia (Mira *et al.*, 1984). Early studies of caloric tests in children with benign paroxysmal vertigo were performed with the eyes open and fixed on a target. Caloric abnormalities were common compared to a control group (Koenigsberger *et al.*, 1970; Koehler, 1980). Studies of caloric responses in the absence of fixation using electronystagmographic (ENG) recording gave normal results between attacks (Eeg-Olofsson *et al.*, 1980; Mira *et al.*, 1984).

The paroxysms are distinguished from other causes of episodic vertigo by the absence of auditory symptoms, and the complete absence of abnormal findings between attacks, especially the EEG and X-ray studies. Although Beddoe (1977) and Busis (1983) recommend that the diagnosis of benign paroxysmal vertigo of childhood should not be made unless there is evidence of residual vestibular disturbance on the caloric test, this is not necessarily the case. As some reports found normal caloric responses in patients with this condition the presence of persistent vestibular disorder should alert the clinician to the possibility of recurrent perilymphatic fistula, Menière's disorder, or posterior fossa pathology.

Benign paroxysmal torticollis

First described by Snyder in 1969 this condition commences before the first birthday and recovers spontaneously by the age of 5 years. The paroxysms are characterized by head tilting to one side which persists for hours or days. The symptom is worse in the upright position and attempts to right the head are met with resistance. Usually the child is not distressed but the attacks may be accompanied by pallor, agitation or vomiting. Ataxia may accompany the attack which may be preceded by rolling of the eyes. There is spontaneous and sudden recovery. Of 10 children described by Dunn and Snyder (1976), one progressed to develop migraine. Food allergies to milk or chocolate are also reported in this group. Both Dunn and Snyder (1976) and Sanner and Bergstrom (1979) believed this condition to be a variant of benign paroxysmal vertigo of childhood and to be related to migraine. Once again the children tend to be articulate and, once they are old enough, will describe 'the house turning'.

Migraine: classical and basilar artery

Migraine is a hereditary disorder affecting 5% of schoolchildren (Fried, 1980). In a study of 386 children with this condition, Watson and Steel (1974) found 43 to have vertigo of whom 23 did not have an associated headache. A diagnosis of migraine without headache is tenable if the patient has transient neurological disturbances as well (Busis, 1983). In childhood, the manifestations of migraine are more protean than in adults, and it is only as they mature that the symptoms change to include paroxysmal headache (Watson and Steel, 1974).

Classical migraine typically begins in the 5–15 year range (Watson and Steele, 1974), but in basilar artery migraine the onset of symptoms can be in the first 3 years of life (Golden and French, 1975; Eviatar, 1981). At this age the child is too young to complain of either vertigo or headache and the diagnosis must be made on the parents' observations. Typically the attacks last 1–3 days during which time the infant becomes progressively lethargic, anorexic and photophobic. Initially unsteady, the infant eventually prefers to lie undisturbed, wedged against the side of the cot with the eyes tightly closed. Picking up the child may induce vomiting. Having had disturbed nights the child finally awakes screaming with pain, clutching at the head or pulling his hair. The attack then subsides over the next 24 hours and the child returns to normal. Symptoms may last only a matter of hours, but in some cases neurological sequelae can last for weeks. The attacks are characterized by transient neurological disturbance and visual obscuration. Ataxia, ocular palsies, hemiparesis, facial palsy, drop attacks and blindness are likely to be present.

In basilar artery migraine there may be bilateral weakness or paraesthesia of the limbs, tinnitus and occasionally transient deafness. The attacks are separated by symptom-free intervals and may be remarkably periodic (Ouvrier and Hopkins, 1970; Watson and Steel, 1974; Golden and French, 1975; Eviatar, 1981).

Children at risk for migraine have a strong family history of the condition (Watson and Steel, 1974; Eviatar, 1981; Busis, 1983). Children with a previous history of motion sickness, vertigo, dizziness, visual vertigo, vomiting attacks, and periodic abdominal pain are at risk of developing classical migraine with headache (Papatheophilou, Jeavons and Disney, 1972; Kuritzky, Zeigler and Hassanein, 1981; Del Bene, 1982). Caloric abnormalities are present in a proportion of children with basilar artery migraine and adults with classical migraine (Eviatar, 1981; Toglia, Thomas and Kuritzky, 1981). Watson and Steel (1974) found no EEG abnormality in children with migraine, but Eviatar reported a significant number of children with vertigo and EEG abnormalities.

The abrupt onset of both headache and vertigo in migraine are similar to the onset of these symptoms in epileptic disorders. Seizure headaches may be distinguished on the EEG evidence but also on the family history. Children with this condition have a family history of seizures rather than migraine (Swaiman and Frank, 1978).

Vestibular neuronitis

First described by Dix and Hallpike in 1952, vestibular neuronitis consists of an episode of vestibular failure characterized by rotational vertigo, vomiting and autonomic disturbance in association with an upper respiratory infection. The acute symptoms last days to weeks and then gradually subside. Approximately 50% of those affected have only one attack. Over the ensuing months to years the remaining 50% experience gradually decreasing episodes of vertigo precipitated by movement or lightheadedness. Children recover more quickly from this disorder than do adults (Gates, 1980).

Vestibular neuronitis is a disease of young adults, but may affect any age group. Harrison

(1962b) reported three cases under the age of 20 years out of a total of 67. In a series of 50 children referred with vertigo Eviatar and Eviatar (1977) found vestibular neuronitis in five children. In a similar series of 27 children Blaney (1983) was unable to make this diagnosis in any child. Out of a total of 28 children presenting with vertigo to the present author over a period of 2 years, one case was thought to be due to this condition. Beddoe (1977) regarded vestibular neuronitis as common over the age of 10 years.

Cervical vertigo and odontogenic vertigo

Cervical vertigo is thought to arise from disordered input from the cervical nerves to the vestibular nuclei and is extremely uncommon in childhood. The mechanism of odontogenic vertigo arising from irritative foci in the maxilla, mandible or temporomandibular joint is less clear, but impacted wisdom teeth should be considered as a cause of dizziness in young people (Eidelman, 1980).

Benign paroxysmal positional vertigo

In contrast to benign paroxysmal vertigo of childhood, benign positional vertigo is a purely peripheral labyrinthine phenomenon. It may be caused by head or whiplash injury, or arise spontaneously. In children it is usually caused by trauma. If positional vertigo arises spontaneously in a child it is often of the central type rather than the benign paroxysmal peripheral type (Curless, 1980). Eadie (1967) found that out of 115 cases with benign positional vertigo 9% were in the age group 11–12 years.

Metabolic causes of imbalance

Hyperlipidosis

Cochlear vessels involute from fetal life onwards (Johnsson and Hawkins, 1972). Hyperlipoproteinaemia is thought to accelerate presbyacusis, but this is not a significant factor in children except in familial forms of this condition. Type II hyperlipoproteinaemia develops in infancy and is heralded by xanthomata in the tendons of the hands and feet. Hyperlipoproteinaemia can cause inner ear dysfunction characterized by the symptoms of Ménière's disease which improve on appropriate management (Pillsbury, 1981).

Hypothyroidism

Although this is an important cause of imbalance in the elderly, it is unlikely to give rise to symptomatic unsteadiness in children. Vestibular function may be found to be abnormal in cases of congenital deafness and myxoedema (Pendred's syndrome).

Central vestibular disorders

Congenital anomalies of the skull base

Structural anomalies of the upper cervical vertebrae and foramen magnum may present with ataxia or vertigo resulting from pressure on, and stretching of, the cerebellum, brainstem and lower cranial nerves. Platybasia is a familial disorder that produces upward displacement of the floor of the posterior fossa and narrowing of the foramen magnum. Neurological symptoms do not appear until the second or third decade and include progressive spasticity, incoordination, nystagmus and weakness of the lower cranial nerves. It may be associated with other malformations of the central nervous system including the Chiari malformations.

The Chiari malformations are characterized by cerebellar elongation and protrusion through the foramen magnum into the cervical spinal cord. In *type I* malformation the cerebellar herniation exists alone or with malformations of the base of the skull such as platybasia, basilar impression, or Klippel-Feil syndrome. Type I is often asymptomatic in childhood but may become clinically apparent in adolescence with hydrocephalus, signs of cervical cord compression, suboccipital headache, vertigo, laryngeal paralysis and progressive cerebellar signs. Downbeating vertical nystagmus has been reported to be associated with this condition. Other central vestibular signs found on electronystagmographic recording such as saccadic smooth pursuit, optokinetic disruption, ocular dysmetria and failure of fixation suppression are present, but are not as diagnostic of Chiari malformation (Chait and Barber, 1979).

Type II Chiari malformation is the most common form of this condition, comprising type I malformation together with non-communicating hydrocephalus and lumbosacral spina bifida.

Type III may have any of the features of types I and II with occipital cranial bifidum or cervical spinal bifida.

Types II and III present early in childhood with widespread neurological abnormalities, whereas type I may present with vertigo or ataxia in adolescence, or simply a failure to learn to cycle or skate. Diagnosis is by computerized tomographic (CT) scanning of the skull base, or preferably by magnetic resonance scanning (Longridge and Mallison, 1984).

Klippel-Feil syndrome, characterized by fusion and reduction in number of the cervical vertebrae, causes variable neurological symptoms. It is commonly associated with other malformations including congenital deafness.

Hereditary cerebellar ataxias

Heredodegenerative diseases that involve the cerebellum and begin in childhood are uncommon. They present with slowly progressive ataxia, and posterior fossa tumours must be excluded before making this diagnosis. The more common familial cerebellar degenerations are ataxia telangiectasia, Friedreich's ataxia and Ramsay Hunt syndrome, of which Friedreich's ataxia is associated with congenital deafness. Refsum's disease is of more relevance to the otologist as it presents with cerebellar ataxia, deafness, retinitis pigmentosa and polyneuritis. The combination of night blindness, cerebellar ataxia and vestibular deficit causes progressive difficulty in walking. The onset of symptoms is usually between the ages of 4 and 7 years. It is due to an underlying disorder of lipid metabolism and is detected by the presence of lipiduria and raised serum phytanic acid. A phytol-free diet lowers the serum phytanic acid with improvement in neurological signs (Menkes, 1985). Inheritance is autosomal recessive.

In contrast to the heredodegenerative diseases, acute intermittent familial cerebellar ataxia is a self-limiting disease inherited by a dominant trait with variable penetrance. This disorder gives rise to acute episodes of ataxia beginning in the first 2 years of life, and disappearing around the age of 15 years. The attacks are characterized by sudden onset of gait and truncal ataxia with upper limb ataxia, intention tremor and dysarthria. Headache, vomiting, nystagmus and sometimes seizures may occur. In childhood the attacks last about 4 weeks, decreasing in duration with increasing maturity. Eventually the attacks are mild and last only days at a time. Afflicted members of the family are symptom-free between attacks. There are no skin or biochemical disturbances during the attack. It is postulated that the attacks result from toxic effects upon the immature cerebellum from infections including ascariasis (Hill and Sherman, 1968).

Hereditary disease of the peripheral and cranial nerves

The most common heredodegenerative condition is Charcot-Marie-Tooth disease. Peroneal muscular atrophy is the usual presentation of this disease (Menkes, 1985) but congenital sensorineural deafness is present in a proportion of cases (Cornell, Sellars and Beighton, 1984). As the deafness is retrocochlear it is likely to be accompanied by vestibular weakness. Neurofibromatosis affects both peripheral and cranial nerves. The optic nerve is the most common and earliest site of involvement; bilateral acoustic neuromata are less common. The presence of seizures in early childhood associated with café-au-lait spots and with or without subcutaneous neurofibromata, should alert the clinician to the possibility of intracranial tumours (Menkes, 1985). Congenital nystagmus is a recessive trait in which there is fine and rapid nystagmus, usually pendular, which is asymptomatic but may be associated with vertigo and ataxia (White, 1969).

Infection

Bacterial meningitis may present with ataxia or this symptom may develop during the course of the illness. Ataxia at the time of meningitis is not necessarily associated with deafness. In a study of six such children only one was left with sensorineural deafness (Schwartz, 1972). Infection from the meninges to the labyrinth takes place via the internal auditory canal causing a purulent labyrinthitis with residual deafness and dysequilibrium (Eavey *et al.*, 1985). The imbalance resolves although the vestibular weakness will persist together with the hearing loss. In these patients, the labyrinth usually becomes ossified (Becker *et al.*, 1984). Symptomatic dizziness can persist in the absence of deafness and be associated with central manifestations. Eviatar and Eviatar (1977) identified post-meningitis dizziness in three of a series of 50 children presenting with vertigo.

Brainstem encephalitis gives rise to either vertigo or ataxia. The symptom is persistent and is accompanied by fever and neurological signs such as supranuclear or internuclear ophthalmoplegia, vertical nystagmus and directional preponderance of induced nystagmus (Ellison and Hanson, 1977; Curless, 1980; Fried, 1980).

Cerebellar encephalitis may present a similar picture and is distinguished from acute cerebellar ataxia by the identification of a causative organism (Menkes, 1985). Acute cerebellar ataxia is prevalent in the first 3 years of life and follows 7–21 days after a non-specific infectious illness. There is sudden truncal ataxia with other neurological symptoms and signs. In the very young child it may be difficult to distinguish from acute labyrinthitis. Symptoms may persist for several months and, although it is a self-limiting condition, there are sometimes permanent sequelae.

Trauma

Dizziness and vertigo in the post-concussion syndrome are less common in children than in adults as the vestibular system is more plastic, but Eviatar and Eviatar (1977) reported four cases and Toglia, Rosenberg and Ronis (1970) 43 individuals under the age of 25 years in a series of 235 whiplash patients with closed head injuries. The numbers are small considering the frequency of closed head injury in the paediatric population. The possibility of a contrecoup injury to the temporal lobe vestibular cortex as it strikes the sphenoid ridge should be considered if vertigo develops days or weeks after a closed head injury (Busis, 1983).

Neoplasia

Persistent, progressive ataxia or vertigo in the absence of pyrexial illness is likely to be due to posterior fossa neoplasia. The presence of other neurological symptoms and signs, particularly disorders of eye movement control point to a central rather than peripheral aetiology (Curless, 1980; Hood, 1980).

Demyelination

The clinical picture of multiple sclerosis as it occurs in children differs little from that seen in adults. The diagnosis is difficult to make in this age group as it depends upon long observation. The first attack is more likely to occur after, rather than before, puberty. Molteni (1977) reported vertigo as the presenting symptom in four out of 14 cases of childhood multiple sclerosis. Menkes (1985) found six with vertigo and 10 with dizziness and vomiting as presenting symptoms in 36 children with this condition. Both authors felt that this incidence was similar to that in adults.

Seizure disorders

Seizures give rise to vertigo in three ways: as an aura of a grand mal fit (de Jesus, 1980), as vertiginous epilepsy (Alpers, 1960), or as vestibulogenic epilepsy (Behrman and Wyke, 1958). Vertigo as an aura of a grand mal fit is the most common, and is easy to distinguish from other causes.

Vertiginous seizures are a variety of temporal lobe epilepsy which can be confused with other causes of acute episodic vertigo. Vertiginous seizures may be distinguished from benign paroxysmal vertigo as the attacks last seconds rather than minutes, there is a transient 'absence' or loss of consciousness, and they are followed by lethargy, postictal depression, or brief amnesia. The child does not describe the sensation of movement with the clarity of a child with paroxysmal vertigo. Concomitant nystagmus does not occur.

There is a high incidence of associated visceral complaints and sensory symptoms such as visual and auditory hallucinations. There may also be motor or emotional components. Vertiginous seizures should be distinguished from minor motor seizures in which balance may be lost as a result of muscle contraction and from myoclonic-astatic epilepsy of early childhood (Bower, 1981). A family history of seizures is common and attacks of vertiginous epilepsy usually change to focal fits in the second decade. The EEG is diffusely abnormal and the attacks respond to anticonvulsants. The incidence of vertiginous epilepsy is much higher in some series (Eviatar and Eviatar, 1977) than in others (Blaney, 1983). This is largely due to differing patient populations in different clinics, but has caution should be exercised against the assumption that vertigo with an abnormal EEG is vertiginous epilepsy.

Vestibulogenic epilepsy originates in the reticular formation of the brainstem and is precipitated by vestibular stimulation. Unlike vertiginous epilepsy which arises in the vestibular cortex there is concomitant nystagmus. Vestibulogenic epilepsy is a rare disorder that is not specifically a phenomenon of childhood.

Differential diagnosis

Paroxysmal disorders

Peripheral and central disorders of vestibular function must be differentiated from other recurrent paroxysmal disorders. In the young child unable to describe the symptom of vertigo, great care is required in history taking. Breath holding spells and seizures are most likely to be confused with vertigo. Breath holding spells have a peak incidence between 2 and 3 years. The attack consists of a precipitating event, for example sudden fear, frustration or trauma, followed by crying, exhalation, cyanosis and limpness. The child regains consciousness, is transiently confused and then fully recovers. The mechanism is the Valsalva manoeuvre. The attack lasts 2–20 seconds.

In the second, less common, form of breath holding an unexpected painful stimulus precipitates sudden limpness, pallor, loss of consciousness and apnoea. The child may quickly regain consciousness or progress to opisthotonos and seizures. Diagnosis is by the ocular compression test which induces cardiac asystole for more than 2 seconds in 35% of cases. There is a positive family history in 30% and the EEG between attacks is normal (Rabe, 1974).

Recurrent syncope is seen in infants and adolescents. Usually it is a reaction to emotional stress, mild hypoglycaemia and environmental factors, but the possibility of cardiac syncope should be considered. This is particularly the case with children with congenital deafness who may be expected to have episodic vertigo. The surdo-cardiac syndrome is familial and produces congenital deafness, a prolonged Q-T interval, fainting and sudden death. The attacks begin in late infancy (Rabe, 1974).

Infantile spasms occuring in mentally handicapped infants are associated with an abnormal EEG which is diagnostic. Myoclonic-astatic epilepsy of early childhood is similar to infantile spasms but occurs in children over the age of 2 years. In such a 'drop attack' the child is suddenly flung forwards or backwards as if pushed violently (the myoclonic attack) or suddenly collapses due to loss of muscle tone (the astatic attack). Consciousness may be lost momentarily (Bower, 1981).

Night terrors may be confused with positional vertigo or basilar artery migraine occurring at night. Night terrors occur in the first 3 hours of deep, non-REM sleep. The child suddenly sits bolt upright, screaming with terror, and remains unaware of the surroundings for 10–20 minutes before dropping back into quiet sleep (Rabe, 1974).

In slightly older children hypoglycaemia may give rise to faintness or dizziness which usually arises in relation to a fixed interval after a meal, typically during the morning.

Psychosomatic dizziness and hyperventilation

These disturbances may present as vestibular disorders and must be distinguished from organic disease. The older the child at the onset of symptoms the more likely it is to be psychogenic (Beddoe, 1977). Two groups are most at risk: those under excessive social pressure to achieve (Fried, 1980), and adolescent females. Hyperventilation may be accompanied by nausea, vertigo, headache, palpitations, faintness and visual disturbance. Diagnosis is facilitated by reproducing the symptoms with hyperventilation (Pincus, 1978). Functional dizziness may be distinguished from vertigo by turning the child on an office chair to see whether rotation induced vertigo mimics the complaint (Drachman and Hart, 1972; Kerr, 1983).

Vestibular disorders associated with abnormal development, behaviour and learning ability

Vestibular stimulation has already been noted to enhance the development of eye movement control and coordination. Poor vestibular function should therefore be regarded as an additional handicap where it exists in a multihandicapped child (Zarnoch, 1980). Studies have been reported of vestibular disorders in motor delay (Rapin,

1974), learning disorders (Ayres, 1978) and autism (Tjernstrom, 1973). Studies in learning-disabled children in particular have largely failed to isolate vestibular function from other influences upon induced nystagmus. The abnormalities found can be ascribed to differences in visual-vestibular interaction in both the learning-disabled (Ornitz, 1983) and the autistic (Tjernstrom, 1973) groups. Learning disability is multifactorial and is associated with minor, widespread, pathology in the central nervous system (Fuller, Guthrie and Alvord, 1983; Gillberg, 1985). Scattered lesions within the brainstem and higher centres may give rise to central signs on electronystagmography which may be confused with immaturity of eye movement control seen in some normal children.

Disorders of eye movement control and vestibular sensitivity do occur in children with developmental, learning and behaviour problems but, in any study of such children, comparison with age-matched controls and careful control of variables such as illumination and mental alerting, are advisable (Ornitz, 1983; Snashall, 1983). Assessment of vestibular function and eye movements will provide information that is helpful in planning realistic management goals for these children.

Management of vertigo
Medical

The treatment of vertigo in children is the same in principle as that in adults with some minor differences. The management of motion sickness has received little attention. Many children require vestibular sedatives such as dimenhydrinate, but most can be managed by positioning the child in the vehicle so that there is not a mismatch of visual and vestibular information (Jay, Jay and Hoyt, 1980).

Benign paroxysmal vertigo usually requires no more than reassurance of the parents, but dimenhydrinate may be helpful. The migrainous disorders respond to reassurance, antihistamines or beta blockers and dietary measures. Exclusion diets of known precipitants of migraine such as chocolate, cheese, oranges and tomato derivatives along with the 'E' factors often produce dramatic results.

The various seizure disorders respond to anticonvulsants to a greater or lesser degree.

Ménière's disorder is more difficult to manage in children than in adults as routine medication has poor compliance. The fluctuation in hearing is such that assessment of response to therapy is difficult. Low salt diet, diuretics and betahistine may be used in conjunction with antihistamines, but many children with this condition do just as well without treatment.

Psychological

Although most children have very little difficulty coping with vertigo once the initial fear has passed they can occasionally become psychologically disabled by this symptom. This is particularly likely in adolescent girls who experience recurrent positional or movement-induced vertigo. Strong reassurance may be required to persuade these patients to resume normal mobility.

Surgical

If secretory otitis is present it should be corrected surgically as this will provide the fastest and most consistent response. If there is suspicion of a perilymphatic fistula, surgical exploration should be considered especially if there is any bony abnormality of the temporal bone. If there is unremitting vertigo due to endolymphatic hydrops with or without distension of the vestibule, endolymphatic sac surgery may be appropriate.

References

ALPERS, B. J. (1960) Vertiginous epilepsy. The *Laryngoscope*, **70**, 631–637

ALTHAUS, S. R. (1981) Perilymph fistulas. The *Laryngoscope*, **91**, 538–562

ANNIKO, M. (1983) Embryonic development of the vestibular sense organs and their innovation. In *Development of Auditory and Vestibular Systems*, edited by R. Romand, pp. 378–385, pp. 375–423. London: Academic Press

ARNVIG, J. (1955) Vestibular function in deafness and severe hardness of hearing. *Acta Oto-Laryngologica*, **4**, 283–288

ATKINSON, J. and BRADDICK, O. (1979) New techniques for assessing vision in infants and young children. *Child: Care, Health and Development*, **5**, 389–398

AYRES, A. J. (1978) Learning disabilities and the vestibular system. *Journal of Learning Disability*, **11**, 18–29

BACHYNSKI, B. and WISE, J. (1984) Cogan's syndrome: a treatable cause of neurosensory deafness. *Canadian Journal of Ophthalmology*, **19**, 145–147

BASSER, L. S. (1964) Benign paroxysmal vertigo of childhood. *Brain*, **87**, 141–152

BECKER, T. S., EISENBERG, L. S., LUXFORD, W. M. and HOUSE, W. F. (1984) Labyrinthine ossification secondary to childhood bacterial meningitis: implications for cochlear implant surgery. *American Journal of Neuroradiology*, **5**, 739–741

BEDDOE, G. M. (1977) Vertigo in childhood. *Otolaryngologic Clinics of North America*, **10**, 139–144

BEHRMAN, S. and WYKE, B. D. (1958) Vestibulogenic seizures. *Brain*, **81**, 529–541

BLACK, F. O., O'LEARY, D. P., WALL, C. and FURMAN, J. (1977) The vestibulo-spinal stability test: normal limits. *Transactions of American Academy of Ophthalmology and Otolaryngology*, **84**, 549–560

BLANEY, A. W. (1983) The dizzy child. *Proceedings of the Irish Otolaryngological Society*, pp. 55–61

BOWER, T. G., BROUGHTON, J. and MOORE, M. K. (1971) Development of the object concept as manifested in changes in the tracking behaviour of infants between 7 and 20 weeks of age. *Journal of Experimental Child Psychology*, **11**, 182–193

BOWER, B. (1981) Fits and other frightening or funny turns in young children. *The Practitioner*, **225**, 297–304

BRAIN, W. R. (1938) Vertigo: neurologic, otologic, circulatory and surgical aspects. *British Medical Journal*, **2**, 605–608

BRAMA, I. (1985) Congenital neural hearing loss due to inner ear malformation. *Journal of Laryngology and Otology*, **99**, 293–295

BRANDT, T. and DAROFF, R. B. (1980) The multisensory physiological and pathological vertigo syndromes. *Annals of Neurology*, **7**, 195–203

BROOKHOUSER, P. E., CYR, D. G. and BEAUCHAINE, K. A. (1982) Vestibular findings in the deaf and hard of hearing. *Otolaryngology – Head and Neck Surgery*, **90**, 773–777

BUNDY, A. C. and FISHER, A. G. (1981) The relationship of prone extension to other vestibular functions. *American Journal of Occupational Therapy*, **35**, 782–787

BUSIS, S. N. (1983) Vertigo. In *Pediatric Otolaryngology*, edited by C. D. Bluestone and S. E. Stool, pp. 261–270. Philadelphia: W. B. Saunders

CAMARDA, V., MORENO, A. M., BOSCHI, V., DI CARLO, A., SPAZIANI, G. and SAPONARA, M. (1981) Vestibular otoxicity in children: a retrospective study of 52 cases. *International Journal of Pediatric Otorhinolaryngology*, **3**, 195–198

CARPENTER, R. H. S. (1977) *Movement of the Eyes*, p. 96. London: Pion Ltd

CAWTHORNE, T. (1954) Aural vertigo. In *Modern Trends in Diseases of the Ear, Nose and Throat*, edited by Maxwell Ellis, p. 13. London: Butterworths

CHAIT, G. C. and BARBER, H. O. (1979) Arnold-Chiari malformation – some neurological features. *Journal of Otolaryngology*, **8**, 65–79

CHANDRA SEKHAR, H. K. and SACHS, M. (1975) Mondini defect in association with multiple congenital anomalies. *The Laryngoscope*, **85**, 117–125

CHIU, T. A., AYOUB, E. M., LORBER, R. R., DANZIG, M. R. and NORRED, S. (1983) Evaluation of a new aminoglycoside antibiotic in the treatment of infections in neonates, infants and children. *Clinical Therapeutics*, **6**, 954–1102

CHUTORIAN, A. (1972) Benign paroxysmal vertigo in childhood. *Developmental Medicine and Child Neurology*, **14**, 513–515

CLARK, D. L., KREUTZBERG, J. R. and CHEE, F. K. W. (1977) Vestibular stimulation influence on motor development in infants. *Science*, **196**, 1228–1229

COLLINS, K. J. (1983/1984) Vertigo and dizziness in childhood: clinical aspects of diagnosis. *Journal of the Otolaryngological Society of Australia*, **5**, 209–211

CORNELL, J., SELLARS, S. and BEIGHTON, P. (1984) Autosomal recessive inheritance of Charcot-Marie-Tooth disease associated with sensorineural deafness. *Clinical Genetics*, **25**, 163–165

CREMERS, C. W. R. J., HOMBERGEN, G. C. H. J., SCAF, J. J., HUYGEN, P. L. M., VOLKERS, W. S. and PINCKERS, A. J. L. G. (1985) X-linked progressive mixed deafness with perilymphatic gusher during stapes surgery. *Archives of Otolaryngology*, **111**, 249–254

CROWE, S. J. (1938) Menière's disease: study based on examinations made before and after divisions of vestibular nerve. *Medicine*, **17**, 1

CURLESS, R. G. (1980) Acute vestibular dysfunction in childhood, central versus peripheral. *Child's Brain*, **6**, 39–44

CYR, D. G. (1980) Vestibular testing in children. *Annals of Otology, Rhinology and Laryngology*, **74**, (suppl.), 63–68

DASPIT, C. P., CHURCHILL, D. and LINTHICUM, F. H. (1980) Diagnosis of perilymph fistula using ENG and impedance. *The Laryngoscope*, **90**, 217–223

DAVIS, A. J. and STRAUS, M. (1973) Viral disease of the labyrinth. *Annals of Otology, Rhinology and Laryngology*, **82**, 584–594

DAVIS, R. R., BRUMMETT, R. E., BENDRICK, T. W. and HIMES, D. L. (1982) The otoxic interaction of viomycin, capromycin and polymycin B with ethacrynic acid. *Acta Oto-Laryngologica*, **93**, 211–217

DAYAL, V. S., FARKUSHIDY, J. and KOKSHANIAN, A. (1973) Embryology of the ear. *Journal of Otolaryngology*, **2**, 136–142

DeGANGI, G. A., BERK, R. A. and LARSEN, L. A. (1980) The measurement of vestibular based functions in preschool children. *American Journal of Occupational Therapy*, **34**, 452–459

DEICH, R. F. and HODGES, P. M. (1973) Motion sickness, field dependence and levels of development. *Perceptual and Motor Skills*, **36**, 1115–1120

de JESUS, C. P. V. (1980) Neurologic aspects of vertigo. *Ear, Nose and Throat Journal*, **59**, 366–376

DEL BENE, E. (1982) Multiple aspects of headache risk in childhood. *Advances in Neurology*, **33**, 187–198

DIX, M. R. (1948) The effect of streptomycin on the eighth nerve system. *Journal of Laryngology and Otology*, **62**, 735–745

DIX, M. R. and HALLPIKE, C. S. (1952) The pathology, symptomatology and diagnosis of certain common disorders of the vestibular system. *Proceedings of the Royal Society of Medicine*, **45**, 341–354

DONAT, J. F. G., DONAT, J. R. and LAY, K. S. (1980) Changing response to caloric stimulation with gestational age in infants. *Neurology*, **30**, 776–778

DRACHMAN, D. A. and HART, C. W. (1972) An approach to the dizzy patient. *Neurology*, **22**, 324–334

DUNN, D. W. and SNYDER, C. H. (1976) Benign paroxysmal vertigo of childhood. *American Journal of Diseases of Childhood*, **130**, 1099–1100

EADIE, M. J. (1967) Paroxysmal positional giddiness. *Medical Journal of Australia*, **1**, 1169–1173

EAVEY, R. D., GAO, Y. Z., SCHUKNECHT, H. F. and GONZALEZ-PINEDA, M. (1985) Otologic features of bacterial meningitis of childhood. *Journal of Pediatrics*, **106**, 402–407

EDITORIAL (1978) Vertigo and glue ear in children. *Clinical Otolaryngology*, **3**, 198–200

EEG-OLOFSSON, O., ODKVIST, L., LINDSKOG, U. and ANDERSON, B. (1980) Paroxysmal vertigo in childhood. *Acta Otolaryngologica*, **93**, 283–289

EIDELMAN, D. (1981) Vertigo of dental origin: case reports. *Aviation, Space and Environmental Medicine*, February 1, 22–124

EISENBERG, R. B. (1983) Development of hearing in children. In *Development of Auditory and Vestibular Systems*, edited by R. Romand. London: Academic Press

ELFVING, J., PETTAY, O. and RAIVIO, M. (1973) A follow up study on the cochlear, vestibular and renal function in children treated with gentamycin in the newborn period. *Chemotherapy*, **18**, 141–153

ELLISON, P. H. and HANSON, P. A. (1977) Herpes simplex: a possible cause of brainstem encephalitis. *Pediatrics*, **59**, 240–243

EVIATAR, L. (1981) Vestibular testing in basilar artery migraine. *Annals of Neurology*, **9**, 126–130

EVIATAR, L. and EVIATAR, A. (1977) Vertigo in children: differential diagnosis and treatment. *Pediatrics*, **59**, 833–838

EVIATAR, L. and EVIATAR, A. (1978) Neurovestibular examination of infants and children. *Advances in Oto-Rhino-Laryngology*, **23**, 169–191

EVIATAR L. and EVIATAR, A. (1979) The normal nystagmic response of infants to caloric and perrotatory stimulation. *The Laryngoscope*, **89**, 1036–1045

EVIATAR, L. and EVIATAR, A. (1981) Aminoglycoside ototoxicity in the neonatal period: possible aetiological factor in delayed postural control. *Otolaryngology – Head and Neck Surgery*, **89**, 818–821

EVIATAR, L. and EVIATAR, A. (1982) Development of head control and vestibular responses in infants treated with aminoglycosides. *Developmental Medicine and Child Neurology*, **24**, 372–379

FARMER, T. W. (1964) *Pediatric Neurology*. New York: Harper and Row Inc

FILIPO. R. and BARABARA, M. (1985) Juvenile Menière's disease. *Journal of Laryngology and Otology*, **99**, 193–196

FINITZO-HEIBER, T., McCRACKEN, G. H. and BROWN, K. C. (1985) Prospective controlled evaluation of auditory function in neonates given netilmicin or amikacin. *Journal of Pediatrics*, **106**, 129–136

FINITZO-HEIBER, T., McCRACKEN, G. H., ROESER, R. J., ALLEN, D. A., CHRANE, D. F. and MORROW, J. (1979) Otoxicity in neonates treated with gentamycin and kanamycin: results of a 4-year controlled follow up study. *Pediatrics*, **63**, 443–450

FLOOD, L. M., FRASER, G., HAZELL, J. W. P. and ROTHERA, M. P. (1985) Perilymph fistula. Four years experience with a new audiometric test. *Journal of Laryngology and Otology*, **99**, 671–676

FLUUR, E. (1983) Clinical investigation of the efferent inhibition of the vestibular function. *Advances in Oto-Rhino-Laryngology*, **29**, 89–101

FORD, F. R. (1944) *Diseases of the Nervous System in Infancy, Childhood and Adolescence*, p. 401. Springfield, Illinois. Charles C. Thomas

FRIED, M. D. (1980) The evaluation of dizziness in children. *The Laryngoscope*, **90**, 1548–1560

FRIEDMAN, I., SPELLACY, E., CROW, J. and WATTS, R. W. E. (1985) Histopathological studies of the temporal bones in Hurler's disease (mucopolysaccharidosis IH). *Journal of Laryngology and Otology*, **99**, 29–41

FULLER, P. W., GUTHRIE, R. D. and ALVORD, E. C. (1983) A proposed neuropathological basis for learning disabilities in children born prematurely. *Developmental Medicine and Child Neurology*, **25**, 214–231

GATES, G. A. (1980) Vertigo in children. *Ear, Nose and Throat Journal*, **59**, 358–365

GILLBERG, I. C. (1985) Children with minor neurodevelopmental disorders. III: neurological and neurodevelopmental problems at age 10. *Developmental Medicine and Child Neurology*, **27**, 3–16

GILLIGAN, M. B., MAYBERRY, W., STEWART, L., KENYON, P. and GAEBLER, C. (1981) Measurement of ocular pursuits in normal children. *American Journal of Occupational Therapy*, **35**, 249–255

GOEBEL, J. A., STROUD, M. H., LEVINE, L. A. and MUNTZ, H. R. (1983) Vertical eye deviation and nystagmus inhibition during mental alerting. *The Laryngoscope*, **93**, 1127–1132

GOLDEN, G. S. and FRENCH, J. H. (1975) Basilar artery migraine in young children. *Pediatrics*, **56**, 722–726

GOLDING-WOOD, P. H. (1960) Ménière's disease and its pathological mechanism. *Journal of Laryngology and Otology*, **74**, 804–828

GORMAN, J. J., COGAN, D. C. and GELLIS, S. S. (1957) An apparatus for grading the visual acuity of infants on the basis of optokinetic nystagmus. *Pediatrics*, **19**, 1088–1092

GROEN, J. J. (1963) Postnatal changes in vestibular reactions. *Acta Oto-Laryngologica*, **56**, 390–397

GRUNDFAST, K. M. and BLUESTONE, C. D. (1978) Sudden or fluctuating hearing loss and vertigo in children due to perilymph fistula. *Annals of Otology, Rhinology and Laryngology*, **87**, 761–770

HALVEY, A. and SADE, J. (1983) The perilymph fistula. *American Journal of Otology*, **5**, 109–112

HAMILTON, W. J. and MOSSMAN, H. W. (1972) *Human Embryology: Prenatal Development of Form and Function*, 4th edn. Cambridge: Hoffer

HARRIS, S., AHIFORS, K., IVARSSON, S., LERNMARK, B. and SVANBERG, L. (1984) Congenital cytomegalovirus infection and sensorineural hearing loss. *Ear and Hearing*, **5**, 352–355

HARRISON, M. S. (1962a) Vertigo in childhood. *Journal of Laryngology and Otology*, **76**, 601–616

HARRISON, M. S. (1962b) Epidemic vertigo: vestibular neuronitis. *Brain*, **85**, 613–619

HARRISON, M. S. and NAFTALIN, L. (1968) *Ménière's Disease.* Springfield, Illinois: Charles C. Thomas

HEALEY, G. B., FRIEDMAN, J. M. and DITROIA, J. (1978) Ataxia and hearing loss secondary to perilymph fistula. *Pediatrics*, **61**, 238–241

HERMAN, R., MAULUCCI, R. and STUYCK, J. (1982) Development and plasticity of visual and vestibular generated eye movements. *Experimental Brain Research*, **47**, 69–78

HILL, J. H., FREINT, A. J. and MAFEE, M. F. (1984) Enlargement of the vestibular aqueduct. *American Journal of Otolaryngology*, **5**, 411–414

HILL, W. and SHERMAN, H. (1968) Acute intermittent familial cerebellar ataxia. *Archives of Neurology*, **18**, 350–357

HOLT, K. (1975) Movement and child development. *Clinics in Developmental Medicine*, **55**. Philadelphia: Lippincott

HOOD, D. (1980) Unsteadiness of cerebellar origin: investigation into its cause. *Journal of Laryngology and Otology*, **94**, 865–876

HUGHES, G. B., KINNEY, S. E., BARNE, B. P., CALABRESE, L. H. (1984) Practical versus theoretical management of autoimmune inner ear disease. *The Laryngoscope*, **94**, 758–767

HULTCRANTZ, M. and ANNIKO, M. (1984) Malformation of the vestibular organs following low dose gamma irradiation during embryonic development. *Acta Oto-Laryngologica*, **97**, 7–17

HYDEN, D., ODKVIST, L. and KYLE, P. (1979) Vestibular symptoms in mumps and deafness. *Acta Oto-Laryngologica Supplementum*, **360**, 182–183

JAY, W. M., JAY, M. S. and HOYT, C. S. (1980) Visual suppression of motion sickness. Letter. *New England Journal of Medicine*, **302**, 1091

JOHNSSON, L. and HAWKINS, J. (1972) Vascular changes in the human inner ear associated with ageing. *Annals of Otology, Rhinology and Laryngology*, **81**, 364–376

KAGA, K., SUSUKI, J-I., MARSH, R. R. and TANAKA, Y. (1981) Influence of labyrinthine hypoactivity on gross motor development of infants. *Annals of the New York Academy of Science*, **374**, 412–420

KARJALAINEN, S., TERASVIRTA, M., KARJA, J. and KAARAINEN, H. (1985) Usher's syndrome type III: ENG findings in four affected and six unaffected siblings. *Journal of Laryngology and Otology*, **99**, 43–48

KARMODY, C. S. (1983) Viral labyrinthitis: early pathology in the human. *The Laryngoscope*, **93**, 1527–1533

KEANE, W. M., POTSIC, W. P., ROWE, L. E., KONKLE, D. F. and EVE, I. L. (1983) Meningitis and hearing loss in children. *The Hearing Journal*, February, 24–27

KERR, A. G. (1983) A symptomatic approach to vertigo. *Journal of Laryngology and Otology*, **97**, 813–815

KOEHLER, B. (1980) Benign paroxysmal vertigo of childhood: a migraine equivalent. *European Journal of Pediatrics*, **134**, 149–151

KOENIGSBERGER, M. R., CHUTORIAN, A. M., GOLD, A. P. and SCHVEY, M. S. (1970) Benign paroxysmal vertigo of childhood. *Neurology*, **20**, 1108–1113

KREMENITZER, J. P., VAUGHAN, H. G., KURTZBERG, D. and DOWLING, K. (1979) Smooth pursuit eye movements in the newborn infant. *Child Development*, **50**, 442–448

KUMAR, A., FISHMAN, G. and TOROK, N. (1984) Vestibular and auditory function in Usher's syndrome. *Annals of Otology, Rhinology and Laryngology*, **93**, 600–608

KURITZKY, A., ZIEGLER, D. K. and HASSANIEN, R. (1981) Vertigo, motion sickness and migraine. *Headache*, **21**, 227–231

LENHARDT, M. (1985) Vestibular hearing. *Journal of the Speech and Hearing Association of Virginia*, **26**, 47–50

LENTZ, J. M. and COLLINS, W. E. (1977) Motion sickness and susceptibility and related behavioural characteristics in men and women. *Aviation, Space and Environmental Medicine*, **48**, 316–322

LONGRIDGE, N. S. and MALLINSON, A. I. (1984) A discussion of the dynamic illegible 'E' test: a new method of screening for aminoglycoside vestibulotoxicity. *Oto-laryngology – Head and Neck Surgery*, **92**, 671–677

McCRACKEN, G. H. (1976) Clinical pharmacology of antimicrobial agents. In *Infectious Diseases of the Fetus and Newborn Infant*, edited by J. S. Renington and J. O. Klein, pp. 1020–1067. Philadelphia: W. B. Saunders and Company

MacKEITH, R. C. and ROBSON, P. (1970) Postural reactions in the first year of life. *Update*, **2**, 1275–1282

MARRON, J. A. and BAILEY, I. L. (1982) Visual factors and orientation-mobility performance. *American Journal of Optometry and Physiological Optics*, **59**, 413–426

MENKES, J. H. (1985) *Textbook of Child Neurology*. Philadelphia: Lea and Febiger

MEYERHOFF, W. L., PAPARELLA, M. M. and SHEA, D. (1978) Ménière's disease in children. *The Laryngoscope*, **88**, 1504–1511

MICHISHITA, K. (1967) Studies of normal vestibular reaction in children. *Journal of Otorhinological Society of Japan*, **70**, 37–60

MILNER, L. S., DAVIDGE-PITTS, K. J., ROSEN, E. U. and ANDERSON, M. G. (1983) Recurrent meningitis due to round window fistula in Klippel Feil syndrome. *South African Medical Journal*, **64**, 413–414

MIRA, E., PIACENTINO, G., LANZI, G., BALOTTIN, U. and FAZZI, E. (1984) Benign paroxysmal vertigo in childhood: a migraine equivalent. ORL; *Journal of Otolaryngology and its related specialities*, **46**, 97–104

MITCHELL, T. and CAMBON, K. (1969) Vestibular response in the neonate and infant. *Archives of Otolaryngology*, **90**, 40–41

MOLTENI, R. A. (1977) Vertigo as a presenting feature of multiple sclerosis in childhood. *American Journal of Diseases of Children*, **131**, 553–554

MONEY, K. E. (1970) Motion sickness. *Physiological Reviews*, **50**, 1–39

NOONE, P. (1982) Clinical application of aminoglycosides. *British Journal of Audiology*, **16**, 141–146

ODKVIST, L. M., LARSBY, B., THAM, R., AHLFELDT, H., ANDERSON, B., ERIKSSON, B. and LIEDGREN, S. R. C. (1982) Vestibulo-oculomotor disturbances in humans exposed to Styrene. *Acta Oto-Laryngologica*, **94**, 487–493

OHTANI, I., OHTUSUKI, K., AIKAWA, T., OMATA, T., OUCHI, J. and SAITO, T. (1982) Otoxicity of aminoglycoside antibiotics by rapid intravenous injection. *Journal of Oto-Rhino-Laryngology*, **44**, 156–169

OMBREDANNE, M. and AUBRY, M. (1941) Syndrome de Menière chez un enfant de 13 ans. Section intracranienne du nerf auditif. Guerison depuis 3 ans. *Bulletin de la Société de Pediatrie de Paris*, **38**, 193

ORNITZ, E. M. (1983) Normal and pathological maturation of vestibular function in the human child. In *Development of Auditory and Vestibular Systems*, edited by R. Romand, New York: Academic Press, Inc

ORNITZ, E. M., ATWELL, C. W., WALTER, D. O., HARTMANN, E. E. and KAPLAN, A. R. (1979) The maturation of vestibular nystagmus in infancy and childhood. *Acta Oto-Laryngologica*, **88**, 244–256

OTTENBACHER, K. (1982) Patterns of postrotatory nystagmus in three learning disabled children. *American Journal of Occupational Therapy*, **36**, 657–663

OUVRIER, R. and HOPKINS, I. (1970) Occlusive disease of the vertebro-basilar arterial system in childhood. *Developmental Medicine and Child Neurology*, **12**, 186–192

PAPATHEOPHILOU, R., JEAVONS, P. M. and DISNEY, M. E. (1972) Recurrent abdominal pain: a clinical and electroencephalographic study. *Developmental Medicine and Child Neurology*, **14**, 31–44

PARVING, A. (1976) Menière's disease in childhood. *Journal of Laryngology and Otology*, **90**, 817–821

PASHLEY, N. R. T. (1982) Simultaneous round and oval window fistulae in a child. *Annals of Otology, Rhinology and Laryngology*, **91**, 332–335

PIGNATARO, O., ROSSI, L., GAINI, R., OLDINI, C., SAMBATARO, G. AND NINO, L. (1979) The evolution of the vestibular apparatus according to the age of the infant. *International Journal of Pediatric Otolaryngology*, **1**, 165–170

PILLSBURY, H. C. (1981) Metabolic causes of hearing loss and vertigo. *Otolaryngologic Clinics of North America*, **14**, 347–354

PINCUS, J. H. (1978) Hyperventilation syndrome. *British Journal of Hospital Medicine*, **19**, 312–313

PRIEVE, B. A. and YANZ, (1984) Age-dependent changes in susceptibility to ototoxic hearing loss. *Acta Oto-Laryngologica*, **98**, 428–438

RABE, E. F. (1974) Recurrent paroxysmal nonepileptic disorders. *Current Problems in Paediatrics*, **4**, no. 8

RAPIN, I. (1974) Hypoactive labyrinth and motor development. *Clinical Paediatrics*, **13**, 922–936

RASMUSSEN, P., GILLBERG, C., WALDENSTROM, E. and SVENSON, B. (1983) Perceptual, motor and attentional deficits in seven-year-old children: neurological and neurodevelopmental aspects. *Developmental Medicine and Child Neurology*, **25**, 315–333

REDING, G. R. and FERNANDEZ, C. (1968) Effects of vestibular stimulation during sleep. *Electroencephalographic and Clinical Neurophysiology*, **24**, 75–79

RIZVI, S. and ELLIOTT SMITH, L. (1981) Idiopathic endolymphatic hydrops and the vestibular aqueduct. *Annals of Otology, Rhinology and Laryngology*, **90**, 77–79

RONSON, K. and HINCHCLIFFE, R. (1976) Sudden deafness: the role of viruses in acute auditory failure. *British Journal of Audiology*, **10**, 107–109

RUBEN, R. J. (1985) Otorhinolaryngologic disorders of adolescents: a review. *International Journal of Pediatric Otorhinlaryngology*, **9**, 1–30

SADE, J. and YANIV, E. (1984) Menière's disease in infants. *Acta Oto-Laryngologica*, **97**, 33–37

SALLUSTRO, F. and ATWELL, C. W. (1978) Body rocking, head banging and head rolling in normal children. *Journal of Pediatrics*, **93**, 704–708

SANDBERG, L. E. and TERKILDSEN, K. (1965) Caloric tests in deaf children. *Archives of Otolaryngology*, **81**, 350–355

SANNER, G. and BERGSTROM, B. (1979) Benign paroxysmal torticollis in infancy. *Acta Pediatrica Scandinavica*, **68**, 219–223

SCHRADER, V., KOENIG, E. and DICHGANS, J. (1985) The effect of lateral head tilt on horizontal postrotatory nystagmus I and II and the Purkinje effect. *Acta Oto-Laryngologica* **100**, 98–105

SCHWARTZ, J. F. (1972) Ataxia in bacterial meningitis. *Neurology*, **22**, 1071–1074

SCHWARTZ, R. H., GRUNDFAST, K. M., FELDMAN, B., LINDE, R. E. and HERMANSEN, K. L. (1984) Cholesteatoma medial to an intact tympanic membrane in 34 young children. *Pediatrics*, **74**, 236–240

SCHWEITZER, V. G. and CLACK, T. D. (1984) Waardenberg's syndrome: a case report with CT scanning and cochleovestibular evaluation. *International Journal of Pediatric Otorhinolaryngology*, **7**, 311–322

SHARMA, K. (1980) Susceptibility to motion sickness. *Acta Geneticae Medicae et Gemellologiae (Roma)*, **29**, 157–162

SIMONTON, K. M. (1940) Menière's symptom complex: review of the literature. *Annals of Otology, Rhinology and Laryngology*, **49**, 80

SNASHALL, S. E. (1983) Vestibular function tests in children. *Journal of the Royal Society of Medicine*, **76**, 555–559

SNYDER, C. H. (1969) Paroxysmal vertigo in infancy. *American Journal of Diseases of Children*, **117**, 458–460

STRAUS, M. and DAVIS, G. L. (1973) Viral disease of the labyrinth. *Annals of Otology, Rhinology and Laryngology*, **82**, 577–583

SUPANCE, J. S. and BLUESTONE, C. D. (1983) Perilymph fistulas in infants and children. *Otolaryngology – Head and Neck Surgery*, **91**, 663–671

SWAIMAN, K. F. and FRANK, Y. (1978) Seizure headaches in children. *Developmental Medicine and Child Neurology*, **20**, 580–585

SWISHER, L. P. and GANNON, R. P. (1968) A comparison of auditory and vestibular responses in hearing impaired children. *Acta Oto-Laryngologica*, **66**, 89–96

THIRINGER, K., KANKKUNEN, A., LIDEN, G. and NIKLASSON, A. (1984) Perinatal risk factors in the aetiology of hearing loss in preschool children. *Developmental Medicine and Child Neurology*, **26**, 799–807

TIERI, L., MASI, R., MARSELLA, P. and PINELLI, V. (1984) Sudden deafness in children. *International Journal of Pediatric Otorhinolaryngology*, **7**, 257–264

TIBBLING, L. (1969) The rotatory nystagmus response in children. *Acta Oto-Laryngologica*, **68**, 459–467

TJERNSTROM, O. (1973) Nystagmus inhibition as an effect of eye closure. *Acta Oto-Laryngologica*, **75**, 408–418

TOGLIA, J. U., ROSENBERG, P. E. and RONIS, M. L. (1970) Post-traumatic dizziness. *Archives of Otolaryngology*, **92**, 485–492

TOGLIA, J. U., THOMAS, D. and KURITZKY, A. (1981) Common migraine and vestibular function. Electronystagmographic study and pathogenesis. *Annals of Otology, Rhinology and Laryngology*, **90**, 267–271

VALVASSORI, G. E. and CLEMIS, J. D. (1978) The large vestibular aqueduct syndrome. *The Laryngoscope*, **88**, 723–728

VARTIAINEN, E., KARJALAINEN, S. and KARJA, J. (1985) Auditory disorders following head injury in children. *Acta Oto-Laryngologica*, **99**, 529–536

WANG, R., ZUBICK, H. H., VERNICK, D. M. and STROME, M. (1984) Bilateral congenital middle ear cholesteatomas. *The Laryngoscope*, **94**, 1461–1463

WATSON, P. and STEEL, J. C. (1974) Paroxysmal dysequilibrium in the migraine syndrome of childhood. *Archives Otolaryngology*, **99**, 177–179

WEEKS, Z. R. (1979) Effects of the vestibular system on human development, part 1. Overview and effects of stimulation. *American Journal of Occupational Therapy*, **33**, 376–381

WEIDER, D. J. and MUSIEK, F. E. (1984) Bilateral congenital oval window microfistulae in a mother and son. *The Laryngoscope*, **94**, 1455–1458

WHITE, J. C. (1969) Familial periodic nystagmus, vertigo and ataxia. *Archives of Neurology*, **20**, 276–280

WILSON, W. R. and ZOLLER, M. (1981) Syphilitic otitis. *Annals of Otology, Rhinology and Laryngology*, **90**, 21–24

WRIGHT, C. G., HOUSE, R. C., JOHNSSON, L. G., WEINBERG, A. G. and HUBBARD, D. G. (1982) Vaterite otoconia in two cases of otoconial membrane dysplasia. *Annals of Otology, Rhinology and Laryngology*, **91**, 193–199

ZARNOCH, J. M. (1980) Vestibular characteristics of the Down's population. *Seminars in Speech, Language and Hearing*, **1**, 87–97

15

Congenital anomalies of the nose

Michael J. Cinnamond

Despite its complicated embryological development, most significant congenital anomalies of the nose are rare. While a precise explanation for this infrequency is lacking, it may well be that, owing to the intimate association between development of the face and brain, severe structural abnormalities of this region are largely incompatible with continued fetal existence.

There is much to be said for entrusting the long-term management of children with congenital nasal defects to a few large centres, where the necessary radiological, maxillofacial, neurosurgical and other skills are readily available. Few otolaryngologists will gain significant experience, during their working lifetime, in the care of such children and, moreover, many of these patients have additional congenital abnormalities, especially of the face and central nervous system.

Development of the nose

In order that the reader may understand more fully the teratogenesis of those anomalies which do occur, a brief summary of the embryology of the nose will be given here. For a fuller description Volume 1, Chapter 5 should be consulted.

At about the third week of fetal life, paired thickenings (the olfactory or nasal placodes) appear in the cranial ectoderm, near the embryonic anterior neuropore.

Invagination of the placodes, consequent on growth of the surrounding mesoderm, results in the formation of the nasal pits which, as they deepen, serve to delineate medial and lateral prominences of the frontonasal process. The medial prominences fuse to form the central portion of the upper lip, the premaxilla and the primitive nasal septum (*Figure 15.1*).

The floor of the nose is, at first, formed by medial growth of the maxillary processes of the mandibular arch. As the nasal pits deepen, they become slit-like; progressive thinning of the mesoderm, dorsally and caudally, results in the formation of the bucconasal membrane, separating the lumen of the nose from the buccal cavity.

The bucconasal membrane eventually breaks down, forming the primitive posterior nasal apertures which, thus, lie horizontally in the roof of the buccal cavity or stomatodaeum (*Figure 15.2*). The lower, free border of the developing nasal septum, at this stage, lies in contact with the dorsum of the tongue.

Meanwhile, paired lateral palatal processes are formed, one on each side of the tongue (*Figure 15.3*). Fusion of these with each other, with an unpaired, ventrally sited, median process and with the caudal border of the septum, gives rise to the definitive palate, finally separating the nasal and nasopharyngeal cavities from the mouth (*Figure 15.4*).

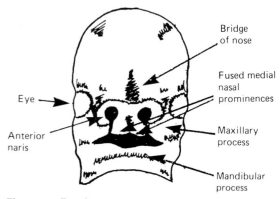

Eye

Anterior naris

Bridge of nose

Fused medial nasal prominences

Maxillary process

Mandibular process

Figure 15.1 Development of the face and nasal pyramid

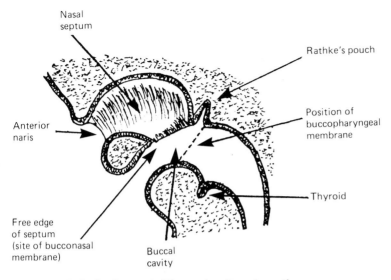

Figure 15.2 Early development of the nasal cavity and mouth

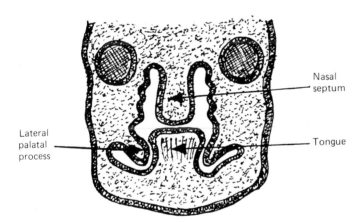

Figure 15.3 Lateral palatal processes

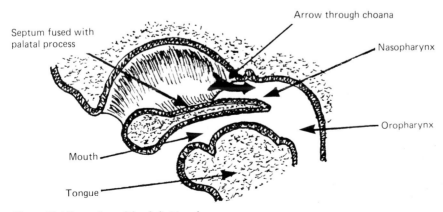

Figure 15.4 Formation of the definitive choana

Choanal atresia

Choana is derived from a Greek word, Χοανη, meaning a funnel. The choanae are, by definition, the posterior apertures of the nose (Friel, 1974); the use of the term 'posterior choanae' is, therefore, tautology.

Atresia of the choanae was first described by Roederer in 1775 (Devgan and Harkins, 1977). It is one of the more commonly observed congenital abnormalities of the nose, although its true incidence is uncertain. The most consistently quoted figure is one per 8000 live births, but this is probably an underestimate; bilateral choanal atresia is likely to have been, and may still be, a frequently unrecognized cause of death in the neonatal period. Females appear to be affected about twice as often as males and the condition may be unilateral or bilateral in the proportion 3:2 (Kaplan, 1985).

Embryology

Much confusion exists about which embryological structure is actually involved in choanal atresia. Some authors (Sprinkle and Sporck, 1983; Kaplan, 1985) subscribe to the theory that the anomaly may arise as a result of persistence of the buccopharyngeal membrane. It is difficult to reconcile this view with the embryology of the region, however, as the buccopharyngeal membrane, in the developing fetus, lies posterior to the site of Rathke's pouch, which in turn lies posterior to the nasal septum (*see Figure 15.2*).

It has also been suggested that the aberration is due to a failure of the bucconasal membrane to undergo involution (Sprinkle and Sporck, 1983). The primitive posterior nasal apertures, produced by breakdown of the bucconasal membrane are, however, considerably more anteriorly placed than the definitive choanae. While this mechanism may explain some instances of choanal atresia, it is the author's view that the majority of cases are due to persistence of the epithelial cells which proliferate within the nasal cavities during the sixth to eighth weeks of intrauterine development.

Pathology

Choanal atresia may be bony (90%) or membranous (10%) and is generally sited just in front of the posterior end of the nasal septum. In most instances where the atretic plate is of the bony type, it is thin and easily perforated; occasionally a much more substantial atresia occurs, a considerable proportion of the posterior nasal cavity being obliterated by dense bone. In this latter form, it is

frequently observed that the nasal cavity is funnel shaped (Pracy, 1979; Pirsig, 1986).

Asymmetry of the facial skeleton is common, especially in those with unilateral atresia, and most patients will have a high arched palate. Other orthodontic abnormalities, such as transverse maxillary compression, have been described and there may be deformed or absent teeth, especially those of the second dentition. Pirsig (1986) is of the opinion that congenital choanal atresia should not be considered as an isolated plate of bone but, rather, as one component of a skull base anomaly developing between the fourth and twelfth weeks of gestation.

Computerized tomography (CT) has demonstrated thickening of the vomer, bowing of the lateral wall of the nasal cavity and fusion of bony elements in the choanal region (Wetmore and Mahboubi, 1986). Maurizi *et al.* (1985) have observed various changes in the cell morphology of the nasal ciliated columnar mucous membrane. They described unevenness of the mucosal surface, thickening of the basal membrane and the presence of ciliary abnormalities including compound cilia, cilia with excessive cytoplasm and ciliary structures with loss of the peripheral membrane.

Incomplete obstruction of the posterior nasal aperture may also occur, usually taking the form of bony stenosis; if severe, this may mimic true atresia, necessitating similar management. Congenital atresia of the anterior nares has been described but is excessively rare (McNab Jones, 1971).

Clinical features

Unilateral choanal atresia, unless specifically sought at birth, may not become apparent until later childhood or even adulthood. Feeding difficulties may occur, especially during breast feeding when the non-affected side of the nose is occluded by contact with the breast. More commonly, however, it presents as a unilateral nasal discharge.

Bilateral atresia, on the other hand, almost always presents as a respiratory emergency, and is, thus, apparent at birth. Newborn infants are, by instinct, nose breathers. The reflexes, which in the older child or adult will result in breathing through the mouth in response to nasal obstruction, do not develop until some weeks or months after birth. If, however, the mouth is held open, either by insertion of an artificial airway or during crying, then mouth breathing will occur. Thus, neonates with bilateral choanal atresia, or other cause of severe nasal obstruction, will sometimes demonstrate a cyclical change in oxygenation, becoming cyanosed during quiet periods, normal colour returning when the child cries.

While choanal atresia may be found as an isolated anomaly, about 60% of cases are associated with one or more supplementary congenital defect (Kaplan, 1985). In addition to random affiliations, however, choanal atresia has, recently, been linked with a limited number of specific defects – the so-called CHARGE association (Pagon *et al.*, 1981):

C colobomatous blindness
H heart disease
A atresia of the choanae
R retarded growth or development, including the central nervous system
G genital hypoplasia in males
E ear deformities, including deafness.

Diagnosis

The time-honoured method of determining patency of the nose in the newborn infant, is the visualized ability to pass a soft red-rubber catheter through each side of the nose into the oropharynx. Failure to pass the catheter, however, is not conclusive evidence for the presence of atresia of the posterior nares; the tip may become impacted in the adenoid or may be deflected by minor abnormalities of the turbinates, causing the tube to curl up inside the nasal cavity. In consequence, the author prefers to use a stethoscope, from which the bell has been removed, the open end of the tube being held over each nostril in turn and the presence or absence of an air-blast noted.

There are, however, causes of total nasal obstruction in the neonate other than choanal atresia: these include massive congenital hypertrophy of the turbinates or adenoid. Radiographic demonstration that contrast medium is held up at the choanae (choanography), has been the traditional method of confirming the diagnosis of atresia. Recently, it has been suggested that computerized tomography gives rather more information, especially with regard to whether the obstruction is membranous or bony and, in the latter case, the actual structures involved and their thickness (Brown *et al.*, 1986).

Management

The essential aim of treatment of choanal atresia is the creation of patent nasal airways. In the case of unilateral atresia, there is seldom any urgency in the presentation and surgery can be undertaken as a planned or 'cold' procedure. Bilateral atresia, however, always presents as a respiratory emergency and management must, therefore, be considered under two headings:

(1) primary, or emergency, treatment
(2) secondary, or definitive, surgery.

Emergency management

In most cases, and especially where it is planned to proceed to definitive surgery within 24 hours or so, it will suffice to insert a standard neonatal Waters airway, taping it securely into position. The child may, if necessary, be fed through an indwelling nasogastric tube. In a few cases, where the child's general condition is precarious, perhaps because of additional pathology, it will be found necessary to delay surgery. In these circumstances, it is probably wiser to intubate the larynx or, if this is not possible, to perform a tracheostomy.

Definitive management

This is best carried out as soon as possible. Four approaches to the posterior end of the nasal cavity have been described:

(1) transnasal
(2) transpalatal
(3) trans-septal
(4) transantral.

Of these, only the first two are in common use today. In all surgery of this region, use of the operating microscope not only provides much better illumination but makes the operation easier and safer. General anaesthesia with orotracheal intubation is employed.

The transnasal route is valid only in membranous atresia or where the bony plate is thin. The simplest procedure is perforation of the atretic lamina followed by dilatation. Although Lichtwitz's trocar and cannula is often used to achieve the primary puncture, there is an inherent risk in this method of causing serious damage to the cervical spine and spinal cord. Instead, the author recommends the use of female urethral dilators which, being curved, direct the perforating force safely downwards, into the lumen of the nasopharynx.

The atretic plate is, almost always, thinnest and weakest at the junction of the floor of the nose and posterior end of the septum. It is, therefore, towards this point that the tip of the instrument should be directed. If gentle pressure does not succeed in perforating the atresia, it is probably too thick and some other method should be employed instead. Once puncture has been achieved, the opening may be widened, using progressively larger dilators, up to about 5 mm (14–16 FG).

Many surgeons recommend the insertion of Portex or Silastic tubes to prevent re-stenosis of the choanae, but the author feels that these do not help and prefers, instead, to dilate serially the choanae once a week for 4–6 weeks.

Other transnasal methods which have been advocated are drilling out the bony atresia with diamond paste burrs or vaporizing the obstruction using the CO_2 gas laser. In either case, it is imperative that an aural speculum is used to protect the skin of the nasal vestibule as it is very easy, otherwise, to cause circumferential damage, resulting in stenosis of the anterior naris.

Where the atresia is thick, it is preferable to employ the transpalatal approach. The most comfortable operating approach is similar to that used in cleft palate surgery, the child's head overhanging the end of the table and resting on the surgeon's lap. The Denis Browne mouth gag gives rather better exposure of the hard palate and is to be preferred to the more usual Boyle–Davis instrument.

An incision is made around the summit of the alveolar ridge or at the gingivopalatal margin if teeth are present. The mucous membrane of the hard palate is elevated, using McKenty or Cottle septal elevators and the flap is developed posteriorly, until the edge of the hard palate is reached. Care must be taken to avoid damage to the greater and lesser palatine vessels and nerves as they traverse the bony palate on either side, close to its posterior edge. The nasopharynx is entered by separation of muscle fibres from the posterior edge of the hard palate and incision of the superior mucosal layer of the soft palate.

Using diamond paste or cutting burrs of suitable size, the posterior end of the hard palate is removed to expose the bony atresia. Much has been written about preservation of mucosal flaps, intended to re-line the new choanae, but in the author's experience, this is almost always impossible to achieve. Continuity of the nasal cavity can now be restored by drilling away the obstructing bone, the posterior end of the vomer being removed at the same time. Care is needed, at this stage, to avoid damage to the vessels and nerves which run in the lateral nasal wall.

Before replacing and suturing the palatal flap, soft Silastic tubes may be inserted and anchored in position with an anterior septal transfixion suture; the tubes should be removed 4–6 weeks later. As in the transnasal approach, the author does not believe that such tubes are necessary.

Pirsig (1986), in a very comprehensive review of the surgery of choanal atresia, has drawn attention to the possibility of subsequent maldevelopment of the upper dental arch in patients who have undergone the transpalatal operation. There is also risk of palatal perforation if the palatal flap is too short.

Septal deviation

Some degree of nasal septal deviation is found in 58% of all newborn babies, and in 4% of births there is also an associated external nasal deformity (Gray, 1985). Two mechanisms have been proposed to explain how such deformities may arise:

(1) differences in the rate of growth of the septum as compared to other midfacial structures, resulting in a septum which is too big for the space it has to occupy
(2) trauma to the nose, either as the result of prolonged contact with the uterine wall or during parturition, especially when this is protracted.

It should be noted that septal deviation is a frequent concomitant of clefting of the upper lip and palate.

The resulting nasal obstruction, which may affect one or both sides, usually presents, in the neonate, as difficult or slow feeding, often accompanied by colic due to air swallowing. If, as frequently happens, nasal infection supervenes, the child will become snuffly and in some cases the nasal blockage is so severe as to mimic choanal atresia.

Inspection of the nose may reveal displacement of the quadrilateral cartilage, but more posteriorly sited deformities of the perpendicular plate of the ethmoid or vomer, are not always visible. Gray (1985) described specially shaped nasal struts which he used to determine the septal configuration. A good estimate of nasal patency may be made by comparing the air-blast heard over each nostril, as described in the section on choanal atresia.

Both external pyramidal and internal septal deformities may be corrected, within the first few days of life, using specially designed, neonatal nasal septum forceps (Gray, 1985; Alpini *et al.*, 1986). By about 6 years of age, the nose is large enough to allow septoplasty to be performed, but it is recommended that tissue removal be kept to an absolute minimum, otherwise subsequent growth and development of the nose may be jeopardized.

Congenital nasal masses

Congenital nasal masses are rare, occurring once in every 20000–40000 live births. All intranasal masses in children, and especially if unilateral, should be treated with the gravest suspicion and circumspection. Failure to differentiate between a simple nasal polyp and a communicating meningoencephalocoele may lead to cerebrospinal fluid rhinorrhoea, with resultant risk of meningitis. The differential diagnosis of nasal swellings in a child is given in *Table 15.1*.

Table 15.1 Causes of nasal swellings in childhood

Cystic	*Solid*
Congenital	Congenital
meningoencephalocoele	glioma
meningocoele	haemangioma
dermoid cyst	lymphangioma
epidermoid cyst	neurofibroma
Acquired	neuroblastoma
sebaceous cyst	rhabdomyosarcoma
lacrimal duct cyst	chordoma
mucocoele	craniopharyngioma
	Acquired
	lipoma
	papilloma
	lymphoma
	nasopharyngeal carcinoma
	angiofibroma
	ethmoidal polyp
	antrochoanal polyp
	abscess

Nasal dermoids

These are cysts or sinuses occurring anywhere in the midline of the nose from the glabella to the columella, whose walls contain skin adnexae (Bradley, 1981). They are formed as the result of sequestration of epithelial elements during fusion of the median nasal processes. The diagnosis is often delayed until adolescence or adulthood and may only become manifest if infection ensues (*see Plate 2b*).

Dermoid sinuses, recognized by a dimple or minute opening sometimes containing a single hair, may extend deeply into the nasal septum, occasionally reaching as far as the cribriform plate. Contrast sinography will assist in determining both the extent and configuration of the sinus tract.

Complete excision is usually difficult to achieve, but may be facilitated by prior cannulation of the external punctum and instillation of methylene blue.

Nasal gliomata

These account for approximately 5% of all congenital nasal swellings. They are said to be more common in males and may occur entirely outside the nasal cavity (60%), entirely within the nasal cavity (30%) or in a combination of both sites (10%).

Although the exact embryological details are uncertain, it seems likely that gliomata and meningoencephalocoeles share a common origin, resulting from faulty closure of the anterior neuropore. However, while meningoencephalocoeles retain their communication with the subarachnoid space, gliomata become detached from the intracranial cavity by closure of the skull sutures, although in some cases a fibrous tract may remain, connecting the glioma to the skull base (*Figure 15.5*).

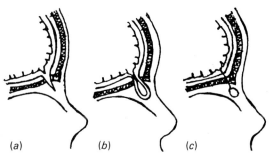

Figure 15.5 Embryogenesis of meningoencephalocoeles and gliomata. (*a*) Normal development – dura projecting into prenasal space; (*b*) meningoencephalocoele – herniation of intracranial tissue; (*c*) nasal glioma – neural tissue trapped by skull closure. (Modified from Swift and Singh (1985) by courtesy of the authors and publisher)

Macroscopically, gliomata are smooth and rubbery with a grey, yellow or purple surface. On histological examination, there are aggregates of mature glial cells, predominantly astrocytes, interspersed with fibrous tissue (Swift and Singh, 1985).

Most cases are diagnosed at or soon after birth, presenting as either a subcutaneous lump, to one side of the nasal bridge, or as an obstructing intranasal mass. Unlike a meningoencephalocoele, a glioma does not increase in size with straining or crying. Tomography or CT scanning of the anterior skull base is usually carried out, although it should be noted that absence of a bony defect does not rule out an intracranial communication. Generally, the diagnosis is not in doubt but should always be confirmed by biopsy, having first checked for the presence of cerebrospinal fluid by needle aspiration.

Nasal gliomata tend to enlarge slowly with age although, occasionally, rapid expansion may occur. Treatment is by excision. Intranasal masses may require a lateral rhinotomy approach although laser excision is also effective. Incomplete removal may lead to recurrence. In those few cases where a dural connection can be demonstrated, anterior craniotomy will be necessary to prevent cerebrospinal fluid leak.

Nasal meningoencephalocoeles

Meningoencephalocoeles, sometimes incorrectly referred to as encephalocoeles, are local herniations of glial tissue and meninges, through a defect in the skull. While these may occur at any site, they are commonly classified into five main groups, depending upon the size and site of herniation (*Table 15.2*). Cranioschisis, it should be noted, refers to very large bony defects in the skull. Most of the meningoencephalocoeles seen by otorhinolaryngologists are of the frontoethmoidal or basal types.

Table 15.2 Classification of meningoencephalocoeles

Occipital	Basal
Cranial vault	transethmoidal
interfrontal	sphenoethmoidal
anterior fontanelle	trans-sphenoidal
interparietal	frontosphenoidal or
posterior fontanelle	spheno-orbital
temporal	Cranioschisis
Frontoethmoid	cranial upper facial cleft
nasofrontal	basal lower facial cleft
nasoethmoidal	occipitocervical cleft
naso-orbital	acrania and anencephaly

Modified from Sprinkle and Sporck (1983) by courtesy of the authors and publisher

Frontoethmoidal meningoencephalocoeles probably share a common origin with nasal gliomata, as described in the previous section; the origin of other groups will depend on local developmental abnormalities. The sac-like protrusion of meninges contains brain tissue and the subarachnoid space, which is filled with cerebrospinal fluid, communicates freely with the cranial cavity. Injury to a meningoencephalocoele is, therefore, likely to cause cerebrospinal fluid rhinorrhoea and meningitis.

A meningoencephalocoele usually presents as either a soft cystic mass overlying the root of the nose (frontoethmoidal type) or as a pedunculated intranasal swelling (basal type). Crying or straining is said to increase the size and tension of the mass, although, in the case of intranasal swellings, this may not be easy to detect. All such swellings must be subject to rigorous radiological examination, including plain films, tomography and CT scanning, to determine the exact site and size of the cranial defect.

In those few cases where the skull defect is small and readily accessible, local external excision with careful plugging of the cranial opening, may suffice. Most cases, however, will require the assistance of a neurosurgeon. Craniotomy is performed, with removal of the herniated brain tissue, followed by closure of the bony defect using tantalum mesh and repair of the meninges with fascia or homologous dura.

Other malformations
Haemangioma

Haemangiomata, which most authorities regard as vascular hamartomata, rather than true neoplasms, are common in childhood (Walter and Israel, 1970). Although the majority of these tumours are found in the head and neck region, primary involvement of the nose is relatively rare. Histologically, haemangiomata have been identified as capillary, cavernous, mixed or hypertrophic, although the usefulness of this classification for either prognosis or typing has been questioned (Batsakis, 1974).

Despite being unsightly and disfiguring, almost all of these lesions will regress spontaneously, with little or no residual deformity (Thomson and Lanigan, 1979). Those few tumours which do not involute are said to be associated with increasing numbers of arteriovenous fistulae, the development of which can be monitored by serial Doppler examinations. In the majority of cases, therefore, masterly inactivity is the treatment of choice, active intervention being restricted to those instances where tumour growth continues.

Agenesis of the nose

Total agenesis of the nose is an exceptionally rare abnormality with fewer than a dozen cases having been reported in the literature (Sprinkle and Sporck, 1983). In two cases reported by Gifford and McCollum (1979), there was an associated absence of the nasopharynx and no evidence of any nasal development. The child may learn to mouth breathe, or surgery may be undertaken in a bid to establish a nasal airway. A nasal prosthesis is probably more cosmetically acceptable than the results of surgical reconstruction.

Partial agenesis with failed development of one nasal cavity has also been reported.

Cleft nose

This deformity is also very rare. The actual degree of clefting which occurs varies considerably, from minor notching of the nasal tip to total midline division of the nose into widely separated nasal cavities. There may be associated median clefting of the upper lip and palate or notching of the alar margins (*see Plate 2a*). Most cases exhibit hypertelorism and it has been suggested that there are strong associations between separation of the eyes, cephalic anomalies and the probability of mental deficiency (DeMyer, Zeman and Palmer, 1963).

Surgical repair of these anomalies is likely to require the assistance of a maxillofacial surgeon and, perhaps, a neurosurgeon. In the more severe cases, multiple procedures will be necessary and, where bony elements are involved, it may be advantageous to delay repair until growth of the nose and face have ceased.

Proboscis lateralis

This unusual deformity consists of a tube of skin and soft tissue, arising at the inner canthus of the eye. The nasal cavity, on the affected side, may be completely normal or there may be maldevelopment, of varying degree, up to and including total agenesis.

The embryological defect would appear to result from imperfect fusion of the lateral nasal and maxillary processes. As a consequence, there is also failure in development of the nasolacrimal duct.

Where there is maldevelopment of the nasal cavity, repair will be facilitated by incorporation of some of the extraneous tissue of the tube in reconstruction of the nose. Some form of dacryocystorrhinostomy will also be required.

References

ALPINI, D., CORTI, A., BRUSA, E. and BINI, A. (1986) Septal deviation in newborn infants. *International Journal of Pediatric Otorhinolaryngology*, **11**, 103–107

BATSAKIS, J. (1974) *Tumours of the Head and Neck*, p. 250. Baltimore: Williams and Wilkins Co

BRADLEY, P. J. (1981) Nasal dermoids in children. *International Journal of Pediatric Otorhinolaryngology*, **3**, 63–70

BROWN, O. E., SMITH, T., ARMSTRONG, E. and GRUNDFAST, K. (1986) The evaluation of choanal atresia by computed tomography. *International Journal of Pediatric Otorhinolaryngology*, **12**, 85–98

DeMYER, W., ZEMAN, W. and PALMER, C. G. (1963) Familiar alobar holoprosencephaly (arrhinencephaly) with median cleft lip and palate. *Neurology*, **13**, 913–918

DEVGAN, B. K. and HARKINS, W. B. (1977) Congenital choanal atresia – twenty years experience. *International Surgery*, **62**, 397–399

FRIEL, J. P. (1974) Editor. *Dorland's Illustrated Medical Dictionary*, 25th edn, p. 305. Philadelphia: W. B. Saunders

GIFFORD, G. H. and McCOLLUM, D. W. (1972) Congenital malformations. In *Pediatric Otolaryngology*, edited by C. F. Ferguson and E. L. Kendig Jr. Philadelphia: W. B. Saunders

GRAY, L. (1985) Septal manipulation in the neonate: method and results. *International Journal of Pediatric Otorhinolaryngology*, **8**, 195–209

KAPLAN, L. C. (1985) Choanal atresia and its associated anomalies. Further support for the CHARGE association. *International Journal of Pediatric Otorhinolaryngology*, **8**, 237–242

McNAB JONES, R. (1971) Affections of the external nose and nasal cavities. In *Scott-Brown's Diseases of the Ear, Nose and Throat*, edited by J. Ballantyne and J. Groves, 3rd edn, pp. 15–48. London: Butterworths

MAURIZI, M., OTTAVIANI, F., PALUDETTI, G., SPRECA, A. and ALMADORI, G. (1985) Choanal atresia: a surface and ultrastructural study of the nasal mucous membranes. *International Journal of Pediatric Otorhinolaryngology*, **10**, 53–66

PAGON, R. A., GRAHAM, J. M. JR, ZONANA, J. and YONG, S.-L. (1981) Coloboma, congenital heart disease and choanal atresia with multiple anomalies: CHARGE association. *Journal of Pediatrics*, **99**, 223–227

PIRSIG, W. (1986) Surgery of choanal atresia in infants and children: historical notes and updated review. *International Journal of Pediatric Otorhinolaryngology*, **11**, 153–170

PRACY, R. (1979) Congenital diseases of the nose. In *Scott-Brown's Diseases of the Ear, Nose and Throat*, edited by J. Ballantyne and J. Groves, 4th edn, pp. 73–81. London: Butterworths

SPRINKLE, P. M. and SPORCK, F. T. (1983) Congenital malformations of the nose and paranasal sinuses. In *Pediatric Otolaryngology*, edited by C. H. Bluestone and S. E. Stool, pp. 769–780. Philadelphia: W. B. Saunders

SWIFT, A. C. and SINGH, S. D. (1985) The presentation and management of the nasal glioma. *International Journal of Pediatric Otorhinolaryngology*, **10**, 253–261

THOMSON, H. G. and LANIGAN, M. (1979) The Cyrano nose: a clinical review of hemangiomas of the nasal tip. *Plastic and Reconstructive Surgery*, **63**, 155–160

WALTER, J. B. and ISRAEL, M. S. (1970) *General Pathology*, 3rd edn, pp. 578–582. London: J. & A. Churchill

WETMORE, R. F. and MAHBOUBI, S. (1986) Computed tomography in the evaluation of choanal atresia. *International Journal of Pediatric Otorhinolaryngology*, **11**, 265–274

16

Craniofacial anomalies

David R. James

The term *craniofacial anomalies* literally encompasses all congenital deformities of the cranium and face. More specifically, however, the term has come to imply congenital deformities of the head that interfere with physical and mental well-being (Marsh and Vannier, 1985). There are practically no epidemiological studies of craniofacial malformations as such. Myrianthopoulos (1982) reviewed data gleaned from epidemiological studies of malformations that were selected 'because of their careful design, large number of observations and high degree of ascertainment'. On this basis, there appear to be of the order of 175 major craniofacial malformations per 10 000 births, and the proportion of craniofacial malformations out of all malformations is about 21%.

The initial attempts at surgical correction of facial deformity were directed at the mandible. Osteotomies of the mandible have been described at every part of the bone in order to achieve forward, backward, or rotational repositioning of the constituent parts. These techniques have been comprehensively reviewed by Rowe (1960). The most universally useful technique has proved to be the *sagittal splitting* osteotomy introduced by Trauner and Obwegeser (1957), with later modifications by Dal Pont (1961) and Hunsuck (1968).

The first maxillary osteotomies used to correct facial deformity were at the Le Fort I level, and the development of this procedure has recently been reviewed by Drommer (1986). Gillies performed the first craniofacial dysjunction at the Le Fort III level in 1942 (Gillies and Harrison, 1950). Obwegeser explored the techniques of subcranial facial osteotomy during the 1950s and 1960s, laying the foundations for the routine surgical correction of the great majority of cases of facial deformity (Obwegeser, 1969).

During the 1960s, Tessier devised advanced techniques for the surgical correction of the craniofacial deformity which afflicted patients suffering from the craniosynostoses (Tessier, 1967). These patients, while comparatively few in number, suffer particularly severe forms of craniofacial deformity. Both Obwegeser and Tessier exploited subcranial osteotomies, but Tessier also addressed the problem of orbital hypertelorism. Segmental orbital rim movements had been used by a number of surgeons, but the results were unsatisfactory. Tessier reasoned that successful surgical correction required mobilization of the orbit posterior to the equator of the globe of the eye, and that this required a combined intracranial and extracranial approach. Tessier and his neurosurgical colleague Guiot, were the first surgeons to reposition the bony orbits by a courageous craniofacial approach (Tessier *et al.*, 1967). Surgeons from all parts of the world subsequently journeyed to Paris to learn from Tessier before returning home to help develop the discipline of craniofacial surgery, of which he is the undisputed father.

Classification of craniofacial anomalies

Developments in craniofacial surgery in turn stimulated interest in the classification of craniofacial anomalies. Hitherto, descriptions of patients with such deformities were reported as individual cases, as groups of patients having similar collections of clinical signs (malformation syndromes), and as part of voluminous textbooks containing extensive lists of various types of facial dysmorphology.

Craniofacial anomalies can be broadly divided into three main subgroups:

the craniosynostoses
craniofacial clefts
miscellaneous craniofacial anomalies.

The craniosynostoses

At birth the cranial sutures are non-ossified zones between the bony plates of the cranial vault and the various small bones of the cranial base which appear as radiolucencies on routine skull radiographs. The sutures were originally considered to be the primary site of growth of the bony cranium, but they are now thought to be tension-responsive zones that deposit bone in response to intracranial expansion. The sutures remain biologically active for variable periods of time postnatally before fusing on a predictable schedule. *Craniosynostosis* is the term used to describe premature fusion of one or more cranial sutures *in utero*.

The incidence of craniosynostosis is not precisely known. In a World Health Organization study, several participating centres reported this condition with an incidence ranging from one in 4500 to one in 30 000 births; yet another study quoted an incidence of one in 2000 births (Myrianthopoulos, 1982).

Three types of craniosynostosis are described.

Primary craniosynostosis

This may be found as an idiopathic developmental error occurring in otherwise normal individuals. It also occurs as part of complex syndromes involving other developmental aberrations; such syndromes often show Mendelian inheritance. It should be noted, however, that there is no familial incidence in the large majority of cases of primary craniosynostosis.

Secondary craniosynostosis

A failure of brain growth as in microcephaly or an encephaloclastic process occurring during the first years of life will result in premature fusion of the cranial sutures. A similar process may also be seen when severe hydrocephalus has been treated with a low-pressure shunt.

Metabolic craniosynostosis

Metabolic craniosynostosis results from premature sutural fusion determined by obvious biochemical disorders such as the mucopolysaccharidoses, rickets, hypophosphatasia or hypercalcaemia.

Pathology of craniosynostosis

From a pathologist's point of view, craniosynostosis can be regarded as a normal developmental process occurring at an abnormally young age. There is little or nothing in the suture pathology to suggest that the process differs fundamentally from normal suture closure. Histological studies of the sutures have concentrated mainly on those of the cranial vault, but it has become increasingly evident that, in many cases of craniosynostosis, the basal sutures are also involved.

The cranial deformities which are seen in the craniosynostoses represent the secondary pathology of the condition. The volumetric capacity of the skull is unlikely to be reduced by the premature fusion of one or two sutures, but when multiple sutures are involved, the cranial volume is affected. In this latter case, the skull shows pathological changes indicative of raised intracranial pressure. These include convolutional impressions (circular or oval areas of thinning of the cranial vault seen on skull radiographs as 'hammer or copper beating') and the formation of small cerebral herniae in areas of even more defective cranial development. The variations in skull shape consequent upon the premature fusion of specific sutures will be discussed below.

Changes in the brain, the organs of special sense and the facial viscera may be regarded as the tertiary pathology of craniosynostosis. Much concern over the condition relates to possible detrimental effects on the brain. There are few convincing reports of cerebral damage directly related to the distorted shape of the cranium, but minor degrees of cerebral damage would escape detection at post-mortem. Serious cerebral anomalies are most often found in association with the genetically determined craniosynostoses, especially Apert syndrome. The chief secondary neuropathological complication is hydrocephalus, which may be severe enough to demand treatment. Vision may be affected and perhaps mentality. When the cranial capacity is reduced, the term *craniostenosis* is applied.

Symptomatology

Where medical and nursing scrutiny is routine and effective in the neonatal period, the majority of cases of craniosynostosis are diagnosed early. In a minority of patients, usually where the deformities are mild, the diagnosis may be delayed. A variety of signs and symptoms are associated with craniosynostosis.

Raised intracranial pressure

This is an important but relatively uncommon feature of craniosynostosis, with the associated symptoms of *headache, failing vision* and *mental deterioration*. Papilloedema is a very serious clinical finding, and is most likely to develop early in life, when there is maximum disproportion between the volume of the growing brain and the capacity of the stenosed skull. Mental changes occur in less than 20% of cases, and there is poor correlation between mental status and the severity of the craniosynostosis.

Exorbitism and orbitostenosis

Exorbitism, or the protrusion of the orbital contents anterior to the bony orbit, is a feature of some cases of the complex craniosynostosis syndromes (*Figure 16.1*). The magnitude of the exorbitism

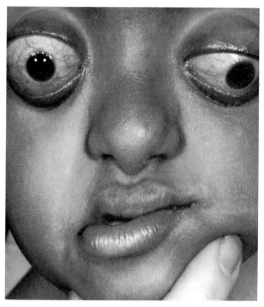

Figure 16.1 Patient with Pfeiffer syndrome exhibiting severe exorbitism and a divergent squint. He experienced occasional dislocation of the globes with retraction of the eyelids behind them

varies between specific diagnoses as well as between individuals with the same syndrome. The orbital volume is reduced by encroachment of the roof, lateral and medial walls, reflecting disturbed bony development within the anterior and middle cranial fossae secondary to craniosynostosis; this reduction in orbital capacity is sometimes termed *orbitostenosis*. In addition, the orbital floor is hypoplastic as a result of the severe maxillary retrusion often seen in these syndromes.

Exorbitism, apart from being unsightly, may interfere with function. The extrinsic ocular muscles, especially the medial recti, work at a disadvantage; there is a strong tendency to divergent squinting (*Figure 16.1*) and binocular

vision is frequently impossible. Exorbitism may be sufficiently marked to prevent lid closure during sleep, leading to keratitis and the danger of blindness (*Figure 16.2*). Thus sight may be in danger from both corneal damage and optic atrophy secondary to raised intracranial pressure. In some patients the globe is so proptosed that it may become dislocated through the palpebral fissure, when manual reduction may be necessary.

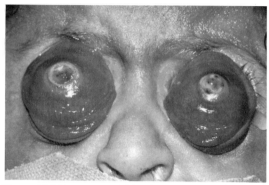

Figure 16.2 Extreme exorbitism in a neonate with Kleeblattschädel (clover-leaf skull) resulting in gross keratitis and loss of vision. (Courtesy of Mr Richard Hayward, FRCS)

Orbital hypertelorism

Greig (1924) coined the term *hypertelorism* to describe what he thought was a discrete syndrome consisting of excessive separation between the eyes. Greig's nomenclature of *ocular* hypertelorism has now been replaced by the term *orbital* hypertelorism in order to exclude excessive interpupillary distances secondary to exotropias. It should be distinguished from *telecanthus*, an increased distance between the medial canthi, which is frequently encountered in severe nasoethmoidal trauma. Orbital hypertelorism is not a primary anomaly *per se*, but is found in a number and variety of diseases and malformation syndromes, most notably the craniosynostoses and craniofacial clefting syndromes (*see Figure 16.23*). There is some evidence to suggest that the severity of hypertelorism progresses in craniosynostosis, whereas it remains constant with growth in patients with clefting. Not only is orbital hypertelorism unsightly, but there may be functional impairment of binocular vision and convergence.

The diagnosis depends on defining deviation from normality, usually two or three standard deviations from the mean. Various measurements such as intercanthal distance and interpupillary distance, standardized for age and sex, are used to measure such deviation. The distribution of these differs in various ethnic groups. For example, intercanthal and interpupillary values for Negroes significantly exceeds those for Caucasians. On this basis, Myrianthopoulos (1982) suggested an incidence of one per 1000 births.

Hypertelorism has been classified according to the degree of separation of the medial orbital walls measured at the anterior lacrimal crests on standard radiographic projections. In first degree hypertelorism the interorbital distance is 30–34 mm which is clinically insignificant. In second degree hypertelorism the interorbital distance is 34–40 mm which is clinically obvious, while a distance of greater than 40 mm signifies third degree hypertelorism which is unusual in craniosynostosis, but is seen in association with frontonasal dysplasia (*see below*). In this extreme state the orbits may appear to face laterally as well as forward, in which case the ocular movements are impaired.

Orbital hypotelorism

An interorbital distance below the normal range (22–30 mm in the adult) is likely to give the eyes a close-set appearance known as *hypotelorism* (*see Figure 16.25*). It results from excessive medial migration of the orbits due to inadequate development of the frontal cribriform area as a result of either metopic craniosynostosis or neural hypoplasia. Vision is not affected.

Orbital dystopia

The term *dystopia* literally refers to an aberrant position of the globe. Orbital dystopia implies a displacement of the bony orbit in one or a combination of the axial (transverse), coronal (mediolateral) and sagittal (anteroposterior) planes; the malposition is usually associated with a degree of rotation (*Figure 16.3*). Dystopia may be a feature of the craniosynostoses or of the clefting syndromes such as Treacher Collins syndrome and craniofacial microsomia.

Midface hypoplasia

Craniosynostosis and midface retrusion are common features of a number of specific syndromes, most of which also include deformities of the hands and feet (*see Figures 16.12* and *16.14*). The membranous components of the facial skeleton fail to grow normally, while the cartilaginous components are largely unaffected. Consequently, relative overgrowth of the nasal septum may produce a prominent, often deviated nose with obstruction of the nasal airway. Delaire *et al.* (1963) have applied the term *faciostenosis* to describe these states of midface hypoplasia. While it is not yet

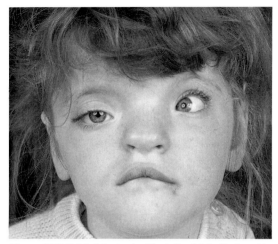

Figure 16.3 Orbital dystopia. The left orbit is displaced in all three planes of space, and demonstrates a degree of rotation

certain that this hypoplasia results from premature fusion of the facial sutures, the concept of faciostenosis is useful, as it emphasizes that affected patients suffer from disorders of visceral function analogous to those seen in *craniostenosis* and *orbitostenosis*.

Airway restriction

Maxillary hypoplasia is a three-dimensional phenomenon. The maxilla is narrow transversely, resulting in a narrow and frequently high-arched palate. The retruded position of the maxilla reduces the postnasal space, while diminished vertical height lowers the capacity of the nasal cavity and paranasal air sinuses; in addition, choanal atresia may occur in cases of Crouzon syndrome. Some of the severely affected children may experience sleep apnoea, while older patients are often mouth breathers who snore unduly. It is possible that respiratory distress may cause some infant deaths, especially in Apert syndrome, which carries a high infant mortality rate.

Speech

Severe midface retrusion can have marked effects on speech. Adequate accommodation of the tongue is precluded by the narrow palate, especially if there is an accompanying palatal cleft – a not uncommon association. Velopharyngeal incompetence is not usually a feature, but may occur in association with a cleft or after large surgical advancements of the maxilla. Crowding of the nasopharyngeal airway and varying degrees of nasal obstruction are common in Crouzon syndrome, and this can result in hyponasal speech.

Hypoplastic paranasal sinuses may reduce vocal resonance, while severe dental malocclusions add to the articulation problems caused by the abnormal tongue position. Impaired hearing is a common finding in Apert and Crouzon syndromes, and this can adversely affect the acquisition of normal speech, as may mental retardation.

Mastication

The skeletal disproportion between maxilla and mandible, and the accompanying dental malocclusion, can seriously impair normal mastication (*see Figure 16.7*). It should be noted that, although there is an apparent mandibular prognathism, the mandible is usually abnormally small in patients with craniosynostosis syndromes. This has important implications for surgical reconstruction, as it is frequently necessary to advance both maxilla and mandible to produce a satisfactory facial harmony (*see Figure 16.21*).

Simple calvarial deformities

There is considerable variation in the shape and size of heads, and when these variations are extreme, they are considered to be deformities. Such a judgement is essentially intuitive, and obviously varies in different ethnic groups and in different cultures. The *cephalic index* (more strictly the horizontal cephalic index), defined as (maximum breadth/maximum length) × 100 offers a useful means of quantitating a visual impression; the dimensions may be measured clinically or from skull radiographs. It will be obvious that it is very difficult to quantitate cranial asymmetry.

All cranial vault sutures and fontanelles are patent in the normal neonatal skull. They ossify and become radiopaque in an orderly, but variable sequence, as follows:

Sutures – metopic (childhood); sagittal, coronal and lambdoid (adulthood); squamosal, occipitomastoid and sphenotemporal (may be patent in the elderly).
Fontanelles – posterior and anterolateral (infancy); posterolateral (during first year of life); anterior (during second year of life).

The shape of the skull may be significantly deformed by premature fusion of the cranial sutures. One must be careful to exclude cranial moulding which usually improves with time, while craniosynostosis becomes progressively more obvious.

The various types of calvarial deformity are summarized in *Table 16.1*. Sagittal synostosis is the most common (*Figure 16.4*), representing about 55–60%, with coronal synostosis being the next most common (20–30%). Metopic, lambdoidal and combinations of premature sutural fusions are far less frequent. While these cranial deformities are found in isolation, they frequently form part of one of the craniosynostosis syndromes described below.

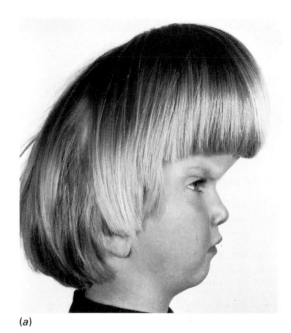

(a)

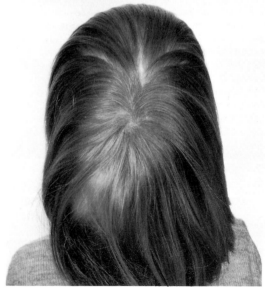

(b)

Figure 16.4 Scaphocephaly. In this child the sagittal suture is completely fused, while the remaining sutures of the cranial vault are normal

Table 16.1 The various types of calvarial deformity

Affected suture	Traditional name	Literal translation	Skull length	Skull width	Skull height
Sagittal	Scaphocephaly	Boat skull	Increased	Decreased	Normal or increased
Metopic	Trigonocephaly	Triangle skull	Normal or increased	Increased	Normal
Unicoronal	Plagiocephaly	Oblique skull	Decreased or normal	Increased	Normal or increased
Bicoronal	Brachycephaly	Short skull	Decreased	Increased	Increased
Multiple sutures	Turricephaly (acrocephaly)	Tower skull	Decreased	Increased	Increased
	Oxycephaly	Sharp skull	Decreased	Increased	Increased
	Kleeblattschädel	Clover-leaf skull	Decreased	Increased	Increased

Note: plagiocephaly is not necessarily synonymous with unilateral coronal synostosis

Craniosynostosis syndromes

Cohen (1979) listed 57 craniosynostosis syndromes, as well as 22 combinations with secondary or occasional craniosynostosis. Simple calvarial deformities may be accompanied by unusual facial appearances, but they are primarily dysplasias of the cranium. Cases of identifiable craniofacial syndrome may present with deformities of the skull vault and minimal facial disturbance.

The commonest of the craniofacial syndromes is Crouzon syndrome which primarily affects the craniofacial region. There are a number of craniofacial syndromes in which craniosynostosis occurs together with syndactyly, the most important of these being Apert syndrome. A significant proportion of the cases of craniofacial syndromes are familial, usually exhibiting autosomal dominant transmission.

Only the commoner syndromes will be described. For an overall perspective of the various craniosynostosis syndromes the reader is referred to the excellent review article by Cohen (1979). A fuller account of the craniosynostoses is provided by David, Poswillo and Simpson (1982).

Crouzon syndrome

Although Friedenwald reported a case of *steeple head* with prominent eyes in 1893, Crouzon, in 1912, was the first to delineate the triad of calvarial deformity, midface hypoplasia and exorbitism. Crouzon syndrome, also called *craniofacial dysostosis*, has autosomal dominant transmission, but up to 50% of cases occur sporadically, representing fresh mutations.

Clinical features

Cranium

Patients may exhibit any of the forms of calvarial deformity, depending on which sutures are involved, the chronological order in which they fuse and the extent of their involvement. The brachycephalic deformities predominate, but it is important to remember that many cases of the syndrome show no obvious calvarial deformity, even when there are marked radiological abnormalities.

Premature and progressive craniosynostosis is variable in onset, but frequently commences during the first year of life and is usually complete

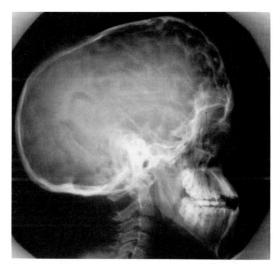

Figure 16.5 Crouzon syndrome. Lateral skull radiograph which demonstrates scaphocephaly due to premature fusion of the sagittal suture, obvious digital markings, basilar kyphosis and widening of the pituitary fossa

by 2–3 years of age. Radiographically, the coronal and sagittal sutures are nearly always involved, while the lambdoidal suture is affected in 80% of cases; other findings include digital markings (90%), basilar kyphosis and widening of the pituitary fossa (*Figure 16.5*). The basal sutures may also fuse prematurely. While this is hard to demonstrate radiographically, post-mortem studies have revealed premature fusion of the sphenofrontal sutures (Kreiborg and Bjork, 1982), a finding which has been confirmed during surgery. Such sphenofrontal craniosynostosis is an important feature of orbitostenosis, since failure of growth across this suture results in reduced anteroposterior depth of the orbit. Cephalometric studies frequently indicate short calvaria, a steep forehead and flattened occiput; often there is protrusion in the area of the anterior fontanelle (the clown's cap deformity) which exaggerates the oxycephalic head shape. The cranial base is commonly short and narrow with the clivus especially shortened.

The signs of raised intracranial pressure may be evident, with headaches noted in 30% and epilepsy in 10%. While some cases of mental impairment result from this increased pressure, the extent to which mental deficiency exists *de novo* is uncertain.

Face

Midface hypoplasia with relative mandibular prognathism, drooping lower lip and short upper lip are typical features (*Figure 16.6*). The nasal bridge is often flattened, and the tip of the nose may appear beak-like. There is deviation of the nasal septum in 35% and obstruction of the nasopharynx in 30% of cases.

Oral findings

These include a narrow high-arched palate, crowding of the dental arches and an anterior open bite (*Figure 16.7*). Ectopic eruption of the maxillary first molar teeth occurs in about half of the patients, and 35% are obligate mouth breathers. Some 3% of patients exhibit a cleft palate and 10% have a bifid uvula.

Eyes

Proptosis is a constant finding, being secondary to the shallow orbits. Divergent strabismus, nystagmus and hypertelorism are frequently found. Exposure conjunctivitis (50%), keratitis (10%), poor vision (45%) and optic atrophy (25%) are reported; rarely there is luxation of the globes.

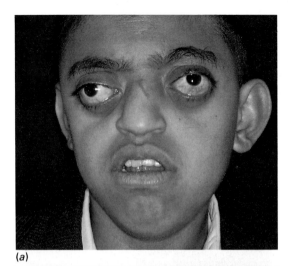

(a)

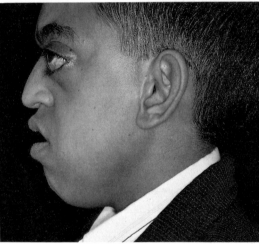

(b)

Figure 16.6 Crouzon syndrome. This 13-year-old boy exhibits the classical features of maxillary hypoplasia with relative mandibular prognathism, exorbitism, short upper lip and drooping lower lip. He also has a divergent strabismus, flattened nasal bridge and beak-like nasal tip

Ears

More than 50% of patients have a conductive hearing loss associated with malformed auditory ossicles, and some 15% patients have atresia of the auditory canals.

Other anomalies

Stiffness of the joints, especially the elbows, has been reported. Cervical spine anomalies occur in 30% of patients, and 85% exhibit calcification of the stylohyoid ligament.

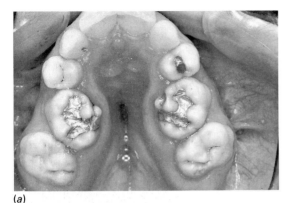

(a)

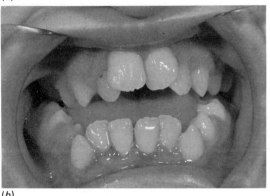

(b)

Figure 16.7 Crouzon syndrome. (*a*) Typical narrow high-arched palate; (*b*) a degree of dental crowding and anterior open bite is also very common

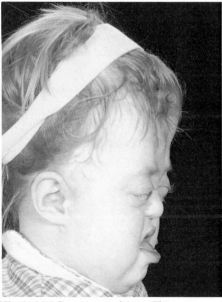

Figure 16.8 Crouzon syndrome. This young patient has a turribrachycephalic skull with a high forehead; she also has severe midface hypoplasia and exorbitism. A similar appearance is frequently seen in Apert syndrome

Differential diagnosis

Having no abnormalities of hands or feet, Crouzon syndrome is easily distinguished from Apert or Pfeiffer syndromes. It may be confused with Saethre–Chotzen syndrome in which the hand and feet anomalies may be minimal or absent. It should also be distinguished from simple craniosynostosis.

Apert syndrome

In 1896 Apert observed an infant with a very brachycephalic head and severe syndactyly affecting all four limbs; by the time he described the case 10 years later (Apert, 1906), eight similar cases had been reported. Apert called the condition *acrocéphalosyndactylie*. The anglicized form *acrocephalosyndactyly* is now usually used to embrace all those syndromes which have the common features of craniosynostosis and digital anomalies. Apert syndrome is distinguished from other acrocephalosyndactylies by the severity of the syndactyly, which involves fusion of the phalanges of at least the index, middle and ring fingers. An incidence of about one in 160 000 has been suggested, but due to high infant mortality, there is probably a significantly lower incidence in the general population. Most cases are sporadic, but there is autosomal dominant inheritance in some cases, and increased paternal age at the time of conception has been found. Prenatal diagnosis has been made by fetoscopy, when hand and foot anomalies have been noted.

Clinical features

Cranium

In typical cases the head is turribrachycephalic, with a high forehead and flattened occiput; the apex of the cranium is located near or anterior to the bregma (*Figure 16.8*). There is often a congenital bone defect in the metopic region, and consequently there may be a soft tissue bulge extending from the fontanelle to the roof of the nose (*Figure 16.9*). There is invariably premature synostosis of the coronal sutures, and there may be additional premature fusion of the squamosal and sagittal sutures, but these are less obvious and usually appear later. The clivus is disproportionately small, and there is an associated shortening of the posterior fossa, but this may become less evident with growth. Post-mortem studies appear to indicate that the cranial malformation is determined before the sutures begin

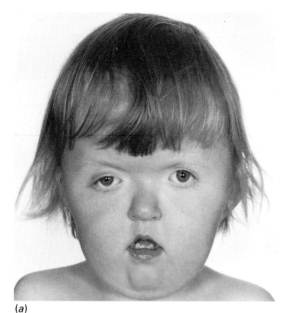

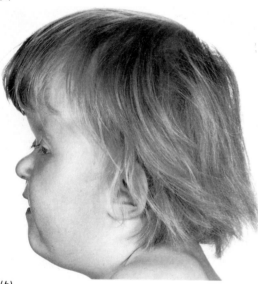

(a)

(b)

Figure 16.9 Apert syndrome. Often a congenital bone defect in the metopic region permits bulging from the fontanelle to the root of the nose

to fuse, and there are various patterns of synostosis in the chondrocranial components of the skull base. David, Poswillo and Simpson (1982) have suggested that in Apert syndrome there is some more fundamental perversion of skull growth than is seen in other forms of craniosynostosis, perhaps due to an underlying biochemical defect in chondrogenesis.

Some degree of mental retardation is found in most patients, although normal intelligence has been observed in some cases. It appears doubtful that cerebral damage results purely as a result of compression by the unyielding skull, and the basis of the mental retardation in Apert syndrome remains unclear.

Face

The facial dysplasia is severe, especially in older patients. The maxilla is grossly hypoplastic, while the nose and mandible are relatively prominent. Facial asymmetry is sometimes present, and can be very pronounced.

Oral findings

The palate is usually highly arched, constricted and may have a median furrow. The soft palate is cleft in about one-third of cases (*Figure 16.10a*), and a bifid uvula is occasionally seen. The

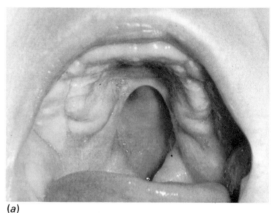

(a)

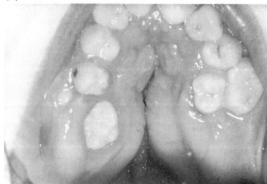

(b)

Figure 16.10 Apert syndrome. (*a*) Cleft of the secondary palate; (*b*) maxillary dental arch exhibiting dental crowding, bulging alveolar ridges and a tendency towards a gothic shape

maxillary dental arch may be V-shaped, with severe dental crowding and bulging alveolar ridges (*Figure 16.10b*). A skeletal class III malocclusion is almost invariable, and an anterior open bite is often seen. Retarded dental eruption is common. All these deformities, together with mental impairment, frequently combine to impair speech.

Eyes

Hypertelorism is common, and there is usually some degree of proptosis. All degrees of orbitostenosis are seen in Apert syndrome, but it is not generally as severe as in Crouzon syndrome. The palpebral fissures may show an antimongoloid slant (*Figure 16.11*).

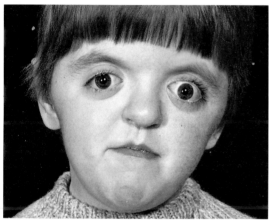

Figure 16.11 Apert syndrome. Mild orbital hypertelorism with an antimongoloid slant of the palpebral fissures and some proptosis

Skeletal system

Deformities of the hands and feet are symmetrical. A mid-digital hand mass with bony and soft-tissue syndactyly of digits two, three and four is always found (*Figure 16.12a*); in addition, digits one and five may be joined to digits two and four respectively (*Figure 16.12b*). The interphalangeal joints of the fingers are stiff, while fingernails of the mid-digital hand mass may be continuous or partly continuous. In the feet, toes two, three and four are joined by soft-tissue syndactyly; toes one and five may either be joined by soft-tissue syndactyly to the second and fourth toes respectively (*Figure 16.12c*). Toenails may be partially continuous with some segmentation.

The upper extremities are shortened, and there may be aplasia or ankylosis of several joints, especially the elbow, shoulder and hip. Progressive synostosis of the bones of the hands, feet and cervical spine have been reported. The epiphyses of the long bones are frequently dysplastic.

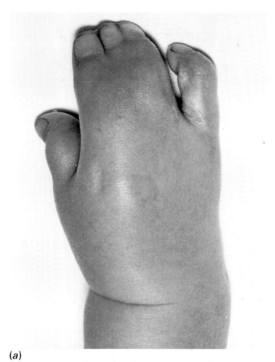

(a)

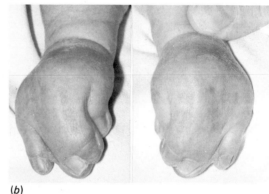

(b)

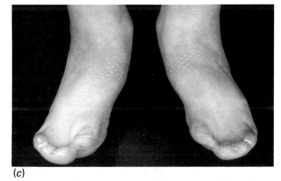

(c)

Figure 16.12 Apert syndrome. Deformities of the hands and feet: (*a*) typical mid-digital hand mass with bony and soft tissue syndactyly of digits two, three and four; (*b*) fusion of all five digits; (*c*) syndactyly of all five digits of the feet

Other findings

Acne vulgaris commonly occurs, with extension to the forearm. Fixation of the stapes is frequently seen, and a variety of cardiovascular and other internal anomalies have been reported.

Differential diagnosis

The syndactyly of Apert syndrome is much more severe and consistent than in other craniosynostosis-syndactyly syndromes such as Pfeiffer, Saethre–Chotzen and Carpenter syndromes. The hands and feet are normal in Crouzon syndrome.

Pfeiffer syndrome

In 1964, Pfeiffer described a syndrome consisting of craniosynostosis with turribrachycephaly, broad thumbs and great toes, and partial soft-tissue syndactyly of the hands and feet as a variable feature. Pfeiffer's report described eight affected individuals in three generations, with two instances of male-to-male transmission. The pedigree indicated autosomal dominant inheritance. It has since become clear that this relatively rare syndrome exhibits complete penetrance and variable expressivity. Sporadic cases have been reported, but no increased paternal age effect has been noted. Since Pfeiffer's original description, a variety of additional craniofacial features have been added.

Clinical features

Cranium

Turricephaly is the commonest deformity, being associated with premature fusion of the coronal sutures (*Figure 16.13a*). Other sutures may be involved, and cases with trigonocephaly and clover-leaf skull have been recorded.

Intelligence is usually normal, but mental retardation does occur, being most severe in those cases associated with clover-leaf skull.

Face

Maxillary hypoplasia with relative mandibular prognathism is common, and the ears are frequently low-set (*Figure 16.13b*). Facial asymmetry, orbital hypertelorism, antimongoloid palpebral fissures, proptosis and strabismus (*see Figure 16.1*) have all been reported.

Oral findings include a high-arched palate, dental malocclusion and, rarely, a bifid uvula.

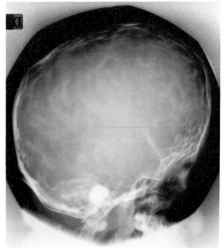

(a)

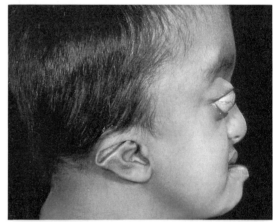

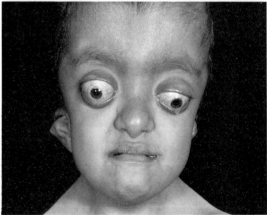

(b)

Figure 16.13 Pfeiffer syndrome. (*a*) Radiograph of the skull of a 9-year-old child demonstrating turricephaly due to premature fusion of the coronal sutures; (*b*) facial photographs of the same patient revealing severe maxillary hypoplasia with relative mandibular prognathism, low set ears, exorbitism and strabismus

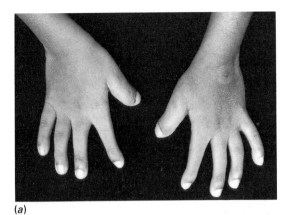

(a)

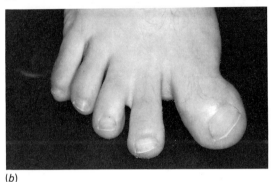

(b)

Figure 16.14 Pfeiffer syndrome. Hands and feet displaying a broad first digit with a varus deformity

Hands and feet

The thumbs and great toes are broad, and usually show varus deformity (*Figure 16.14*). In some patients the great toes may be shortened, but without varus deformity. Cutaneous syndactyly is usually present, involving digits two and three, and at times three and four, of both hands and feet. Clinodactyly and symphalangism of both hands and feet have been reported. Other skeletal anomalies described include fused cervical vertebrae, radiohumeral and radioulnar synostoses (*Figure 16.15*).

Other anomalies

Other features occasionally seen are pyloric stenosis, bicuspid aortic valve, hypoplasia of the gallbladder, single umbilical artery, umbilical hernia, preauricular tags, choanal atresia and hearing loss.

Differential diagnosis

Pfeiffer syndrome should be distinguished from other craniosynostosis – syndactyly syndromes, notably Apert and Saethre–Chotzen syndromes. Facially it is similar to Apert syndrome, but in the latter, the degree of syndactyly is extreme and characteristic. The facial findings of asymmetry, low hairline and beaking of the nose in the Saethre–Chotzen syndrome are not typical of Pfeiffer syndrome. In Crouzon syndrome the hands are normal, while in Pfeiffer syndrome the thumbs and great toes are typical.

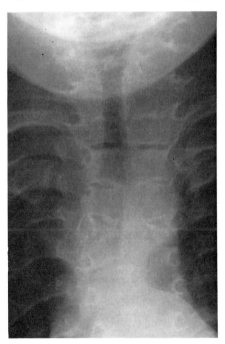

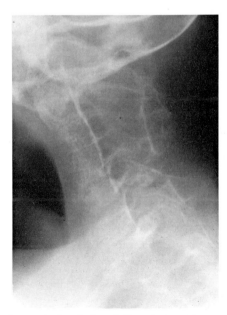

(a)

Figure 16.15 Pfeiffer syndrome. (*a*) Cervical spine radiographs demonstrating fusion of all cervical vertebrae;

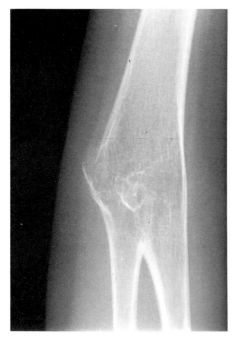
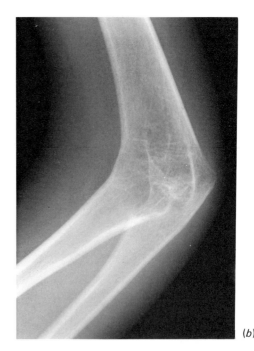

(b)

(b) radiographs of the elbows demonstrating radiohumeral and radioulnar synostosis with the left arm fully extended and the right arm semiflexed

Treatment of the craniosynostoses

The most contentious debate in craniofacial surgery remains that concerning the timing of the various forms of surgery available. Regrettably, despite the fact that such surgery has now been practised for more than 20 years, there are no good objective and scientific studies indicating the long-term results in respect of the obvious parameters of brain and cranial growth, facial growth, eyesight and mental ability. Surgery has been performed at all ages from the neonatal period to adulthood, and the results presented have been largely anecdotal.

There is general agreement that the two conditions which make early surgery mandatory are raised intracranial pressure and the danger of visual impairment due to gross exorbitism. The aims of early craniofacial surgery for craniosynostosis are:

(1) to allow the brain to expand normally
(2) to provide a normal shape to the forehead and skull
(3) to provide eye protection by reducing the exorbitism
(4) to prevent or minimize the problem of impaired facial growth in faciostenosis.

Marchac and Renier (1981) reported the results of early surgery (preferably within the first 6 months), claiming good morphological and functional results that appeared to be maintained over periods up to 8 years (their longest follow-up period). Surgery involved frontal bone advancement by their 'floating forehead' technique and reshaping of the cranium. The photographs appear impressive, but no objective measurement of either morphology or function was made. They also claimed that 'there is a definite improvement in affected facial structures when early surgery has been performed', but no evidence is produced. The severe midface retrusion seen in the craniosynostosis syndromes is almost certainly due to involvement of the sutures of the cranial base, and it is difficult to see how surgery which corrects the cranial vault can have any effect on the growth of the midface.

Examples of early craniofacial surgery are shown in *Figures 16.16* and *16.17*).

Patients with hypertelorism lack stereoscopic vision. Tessier (1967) originally suggested that, if the hypertelorism could be corrected by early surgery, this may result in the acquisition of stereoscopic vision; unfortunately, this does not appear to be the case. Seventy per cent of the adult interorbital distance is reached by the age of 2 years in the normal person, and it is thus assumed that surgical correction of hypertelorism is best delayed until after this age. The results of surgery for hypertelorism depend on the anatomy of the specific deformity and the skill of the surgeon.

Figure 16.18 illustrates correction of hypertelorism in an adolescent.

Faciostenosis or midface retrusion, apart from producing severe facial deformity, may result in the functional problems of corneal exposure,

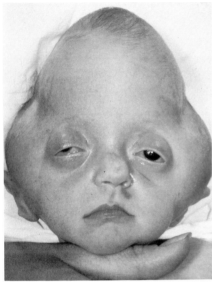

(a)

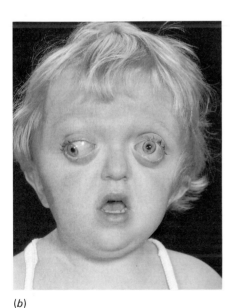

(b)

Figure 16.16 (a)Clover-leaf skull deformity in an infant with Apert syndrome; (b) the patient at 3 years following surgical correction by means of frontal advancement and reshaping of the cranial vault. (Courtesy of Mr Richard Hayward, FRCS)

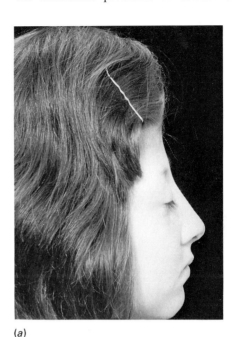

(a)

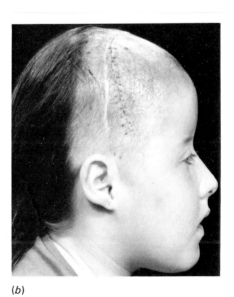

(b)

Figure 16.17 (a) An 8-year-old patient with Crouzon syndrome exhibiting turricephaly and recession of the frontal bone; (b) appearance following frontal advancement and reshaping of the cranial vault. (Courtesy of Mr Richard Hayward, FRCS)

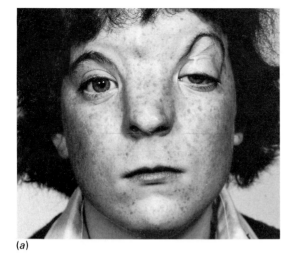

(a)

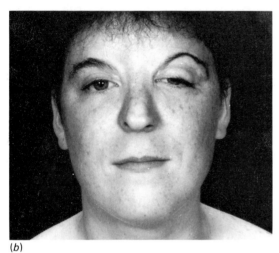

(b)

Figure 16.18 (*a*) A 13-year-old girl with hypertelorism; (*b*) the same patient at the age of 17, 4 years after transcranial correction of her hypertelorism and subsequent soft-tissue adjustment of the left upper eyelid

Details of surgical technique are outside the scope of this chapter, and have therefore not been included. Readers are directed to some of the texts included in the list of references at the end of the chapter. Henderson (1985) covers the subcranial osteotomies comprehensively, and Caronni (1985) is a good source for information about cranial and orbital techniques.

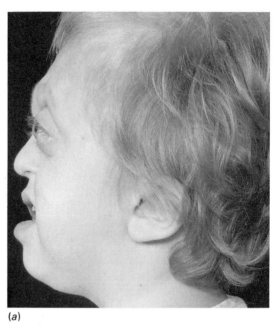

(a)

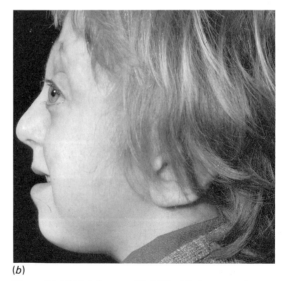

(b)

Figure 16.19 (*a*) A 3-year-old child with Apert syndrome who has had previous cranial vault surgery; (*b*) appearance after a Le Fort III subcranial advancement

impairment of breathing and poor mastication. There are obvious advantages to correcting the deformity early, both from a cosmetic and functional point of view. However, this presents some technical problems, and it is almost certain that further correction will be necessary at a later date. Provided that everybody involved in the decision is aware of these constraints, it appears reasonable to agree to early surgery in appropriate cases (*Figure 16.19*). Undoubtedly better results are obtained in those cases in which surgery is delayed until after puberty (*Figures 16.20* and *16.21*).

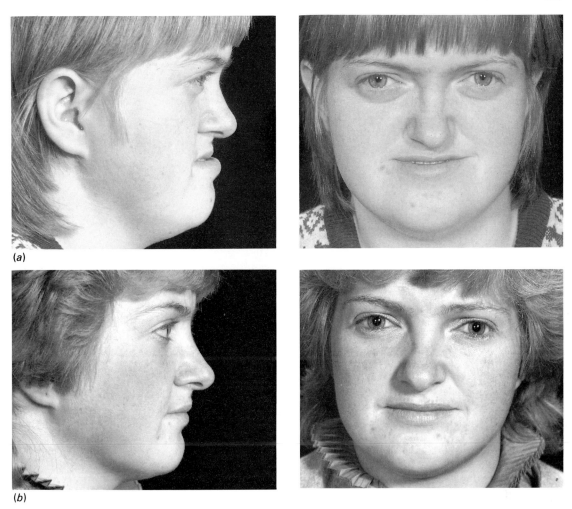

Figure 16.20 (*a*) Crouzon syndrome in 16-year-old girl; (*b*) appearance 4 years after a subcranial Le Fort III advancement

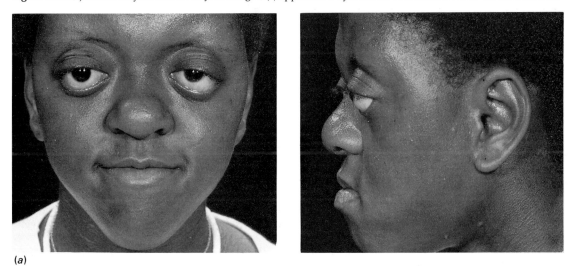

Figure 16.21 (*a*) A 15-year-old girl with Apert syndrome;

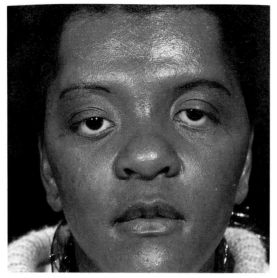 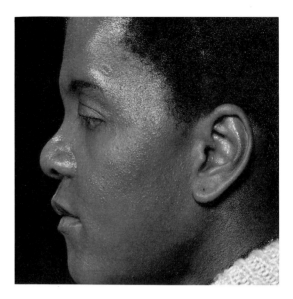

(b)

(b) same patient 2 years after simultaneous transcranial frontal advancement, Le Fort III maxillary advancement, mandibular advancement and genioplasty

Craniofacial clefts

Cleft is a useful word for conveying the mechanism of a malformation, or the resultant features of the deformity. While clefts of the lip and palate are relatively common, there are a number of other clefts occurring in the craniofacial region which are rare. For many years the terminology for these conditions was confusing, and often misleading. Terms such as nasomaxillary hypoplasia and frontonasal dysplasia were used, and adjectives such as orofacial, oronasal and otomandibular employed. Some malformations may bear many names, while others are subjected to eponymous terminology such as Treacher Collins and Goldenhar syndromes.

Numerous attempts have been made to classify craniofacial defects, but none has proved entirely satisfactory. Tessier (1976) devised a descriptive, clinical classification that is unrelated to the embryology of the malformation. It is based on his personal observation of 336 cases of craniofacial clefts. His analysis of this vast and unique collection of rare conditions included clinical and radiographic examination; in 254 cases he carried out an anatomical dissection at the time of surgery. As a result of this work Tessier found that true bony clefts were present where 'hypoplasia' had previously been described, this being the case in both Treacher Collins syndrome and craniofacial microsomia. Bone and soft tissues were rarely involved to the same extent; between the midline and infraorbital foramen soft tissue defects were the more destructive, while lateral to this (with the notable exception of the auricle) bony defects were more severe. Clefts were located along some very definite axes; due to the constancy of most skeletal points, clefts are more easily described with reference to the skeleton than to the soft tissues.

Tessier classification

Tessier utilizes the eyelids and orbits as a reference when describing clefts, as this enables both cranium and face to be included. His original diagrams present a graphic representation of the classification (*Figure 16.22*).

For the purpose of orientation, the orbit is divided into two hemispheres. The lower lid with the cheek and lip constitutes the southern hemisphere, and clefts through it are facial. The upper lid is in the northern hemisphere, and clefts through it are cranial. Using the number zero as the mid-sagittal plane, each site of malformation has been assigned a respective number determined by its axis in relationship to the zero line. Fifteen locations for clefts (0–14) have been described, using the orbit as the point of reference. They are distributed according to eight 'time

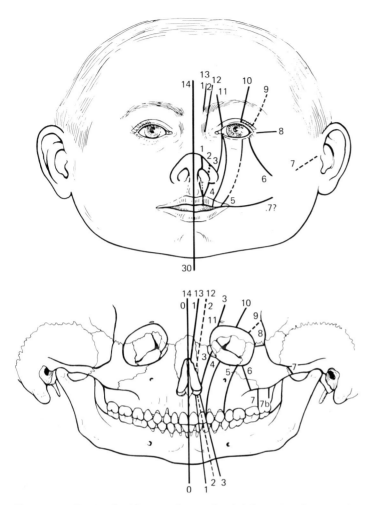

Figure 16.22 Tessier classification of craniofacial clefts. (*a*) Localization of soft-tissue clefts; (*b*) localization of skeletal (bony) clefts. Dotted lines represent either uncertain sites or uncertain clefts

zones', cleft number seven being the most lateral. Cleft lip is not specifically described, but is encountered in most instances of clefts 1, 2 or 3. For specific details of the classification, readers are referred to Tessier's original paper.

It should be remembered that the spectrum of prevalence of the anomalies encompassed within the above classification varies from very uncommon to extremely rare. Selection has therefore been exercised, and only the 'commoner' conditions seen in a craniofacial unit have been included.

Frontonasal dysplasia

This condition, also known as *median cleft face syndrome*, is an ill-defined syndrome. It is a

non-specific developmental alteration, in which the defect occurs with a host of low-frequency anomalies (Goodman and Gorlin, 1983). Frontonasal dysplasia corresponds to clefts 0 and 14 in Tessier's classification. The main features are orbital hypertelorism, broad nasal root, lack of formation of the nasal tip, widow's peak hair anomaly and anterior cranium bifidum occultum. Sedano *et al.* (1970) published a comprehensive review of the condition, and applied the term *frontonasal dysplasia*.

The basic defect is unknown. Embryologically, if the nasal capsule fails to develop, the primitive brain vesicle fills the space normally occupied by the capsule; this produces anterior cranium bifidum occultum, a morphokinetic arrest in the positioning of the eyes and lack of formation of the nasal tip. Most cases of this condition are sporadic.

Both autosomal inheritance and multifactorial transmission have been proposed, but the genetic mode of inheritance remains unclear. It is not known why twinning is commoner in families with frontonasal dysplasia than in the general population.

Clinical features

The facial malformation presents variable clinical combinations, and varies from mild to severe. Orbital hypertelorism is a constant finding, and secondary telecanthus or narrowing of the palpebral fissures occurs in severe cases (*Figure 16.23*).

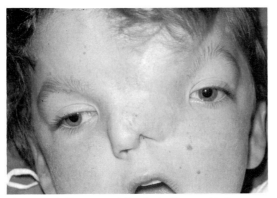

Figure 16.23 Frontonasal dysplasia. Gross orbital hypertelorism with secondary narrowing of the palpebral fissures and a widow's peak hair anomaly

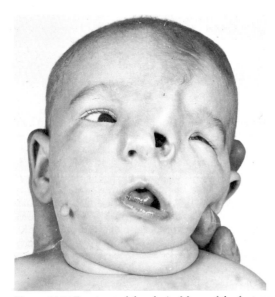

Figure 16.24 Frontonasal dysplasia. Many of the features of this condition are demonstrated; hypertelorism, broad nasal root with coloboma of the nostril, widow's peak hair anomaly, and a preauricular skin tag. This infant also has microphthalmia on the left side

Epibulbar dermoids are common, while anophthalmia, microphthalmia, upper eyelid colobomas and congenital cataracts occur rarely. The anterior hairline may extend in a V shape onto the centre of the forehead (widow's peak). Nasal deformities vary from colobomata of the nostrils to nasal flattening, with widely spaced nares and a broad nasal root (*Figure 16.24*). Other findings include median cleft of the upper lip (cleft palate is rare), preauricular tags, low set ears, absent tragus and conductive deafness.

Mental deficiency is present in some cases, being more likely when the hypertelorism is severe or when extracephalic anomalies are present. Anterior cranium bifidum may be seen radiographically. A large anterior meningo-encephalocoele, and rarely lipoma or teratoma, is sometimes associated with frontonasal dysplasia. Craniosynostosis and brachycephaly have been reported, together with a variety of cerebral anomalies.

Outside the craniofacial region occasional findings include polydactyly, syndactyly, clinodactyly, umbilical hernia and cryptorchidism.

Differential diagnosis

Orbital hypertelorism should be regarded as a non-specific malformation that may occur in a variety of different syndromes. Peterson *et al.* (1971) have listed a variety of disorders in which orbital hypertelorism is a feature. Bifid nose can occur with hypertelorism, several familial cases having been reported. When epibulbar dermoids, eyelid colobomas and preauricular tags are present, frontonasal dysplasia should be distinguished from craniofacial microsomia.

Treatment

Seventy per cent of the adult interorbital distance is reached by the age of 2 years in the normal person. It is thus generally assumed that surgical correction of hypertelorism should be delayed until after this age. In the majority of cases the optic canals are the normal distance apart. Occasionally they are wider apart, and this is usually associated with an increase in width of the cribriform plate. Before any surgery is contemplated it is thus important that a precise assessment of the orbital anatomy is made. For a resumé of imaging techniques the reader should consult Marsh and Vannier (1985). The place of magnetic resonance imaging has not yet been fully determined.

For details of the surgical technique for the correction of orbital hypertelorism the reader is directed to a text on craniofacial surgery, for example, Caronni (1985).

Median cleft lip with orbital hypotelorism

This rare syndrome is also known as *holoprosencephaly, arhinencephaly* and *median facial dysgenesis*. It results from impaired sagittal cleavage of the forebrain into cerebral hemispheres. There exists a whole spectrum of midline face–brain anomalies ranging from the extreme *cyclopia* (one central eye), through *cebocephaly* (orbital hypotelorism and a single blind-ended nostril nose) and *premaxillary agenesis* (hypotelorism, a flat boneless nose and a medial cleft lip) to the less severe forms of *midline facial dysmorphia*. In all forms the incidence is about one in 15 000 births, and the frequency may be as high as one in 250 conceptuses from spontaneous abortion. Chromosomal anomalies are common in this group of disorders, and the majority of cases are sporadic. Some mild examples have exhibited Mendelian inheritance. The more severe forms do not survive long enough to reproduce.

Clinical features

The characteristic features of the syndrome are:

(1) complete median cleft lip with absent premaxilla and prolabium
(2) flat nose with absent columella, septal cartilage and nasal bones
(3) orbital hypotelorism
(4) mongoloid slant of the eyes
(5) fusion of eyebrows in midline, and sparse frontal hair
(6) forebrain formed by a single large ventricle with little cerebral cortex
(7) a cleft palate may be present.

Almost all these features are illustrated in *Figure 16.25*.

Treatment

Severe cases do not survive infancy, and many do not live past childhood. Most exhibit a moderate to severe degree of mental retardation. The degree of facial involvement usually, but not always, predicts the extent of brain malformation. It will thus be obvious that extensive treatment is unrealistic. Where appropriate, lip closure may be helpful.

Lateral and oblique facial clefts

Lateral facial cleft

This relatively rare cleft runs from the angle of the mouth towards the tragus of the ear, although its course is variable. It results from failure of fusion of the maxillary and mandibular processes of the first branchial arch. It may be present as a shallow furrow throughout, or extend as a complete cleft into the oral cavity as far as the anterior border of the masseter muscle. There may be hypoplasia of the muscles of mastication, as well as of the maxilla, zygoma and auricle. Both Treacher Collins syndrome and craniofacial microsomia are forms of lateral facial clefting (Tessier no.7); the macrostomia seen in the Goldenhar variant of craniofacial microsomia is an obvious manifestation of this cleft (*Figure 16.26*).

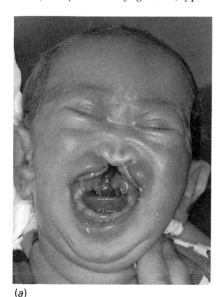

(a)

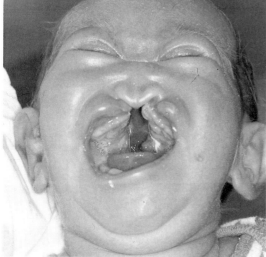

(b)

Figure 16.25 Median cleft lip with orbital hypotelorism. This baby exhibits virtually all the features of this syndrome

Oblique facial cleft

Boo-Chai (1970) has subdivided these extremely rare clefts into:

(1) *naso-ocular cleft*, extending from the nostril to the lower eyelid border with possible extension to the temporal region (along the line of closure of the nasolacrimal groove)
(2) *oro-ocular cleft*, extending from eye to lip. There may be a further subdivision into medial and lateral types, depending on the relationship to the infraorbital foramen.

About 25% of these rare clefts are bilateral, an example being illustrated in *Figure 16.27*.

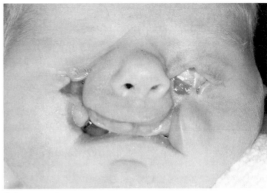

(a)

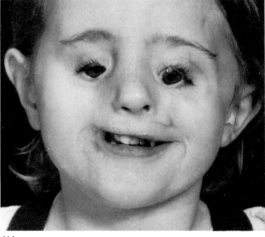

(b)

Figure 16.27 Bilateral oblique facial clefts. These oro-ocular clefts represent the medial variety on the left (Tessier no. 4) and the lateral variety on the right (Tessier no. 5). Such clefts present extremely difficult reconstructive problems. (Courtesy of Mr Eric Gustavson, FRCS)

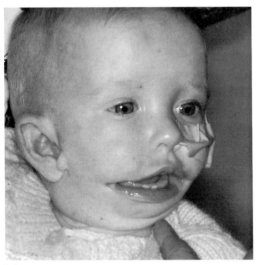

(a)

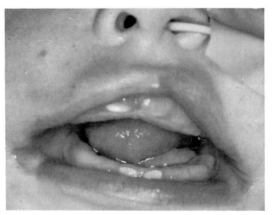

(b)

Figure 16.26 Macrostomia in craniofacial microsomia, an example of cleft No. 7 in the Tessier classification

Treatment

Treatment usually consists of one or more Z-plasties to bring tissue into the cleft. Eyelid colobomas are treated in the usual way by excision of the edges and closure of the defect.

Amniotic band disruption complex

The amniotic band disruption complex occurs in various forms. The most common involves the limbs only, but the complex embraces a spectrum ranging from a ring constriction of the finger to major craniofacial and visceral defects. The most severe combination of anomalies in this disorder includes limb and craniofacial abnormalities acronymically termed the ADAM (*a*mniotic *d*eformity, *a*dhesions, *m*utilations) complex. The incidence is estimated between one in 5000 and one in 10 000 for all forms of the complex, and craniofacial examples are obviously much rarer. There is no evidence that a genetic factor is involved.

The most common hypothesis concerning the complex is that the fetal deformities result from primary amnion rupture without chorionic sac damage at various stages of gestation. The placenta and membranes are often abnormal; fibrous strands attached to the amnion or chorion have been observed, and rarely, a band is attached to the infant (*Figure 16.28*). The earlier the amniotic rupture, the more severe the anomalies.

Facial anomalies include cleft lip (usually bilateral), bizarre midfacial clefts (*Figure 16.29*), hydrocephalus, microcephalus, multiple anterior encephalocoeles and meningocoeles. Eye abnormalities include distorted or colobomatous palpebral fissures, microphthalmia, anophthalmia and corneal opacity. There may be complex nasal malformations, and major visceral anomalies comprise omphalocoele and gastroschisis.

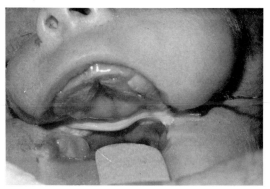

Figure 16.28 Amniotic band disruption complex. Amniotic band producing a most unusual cleft transversely across the palate

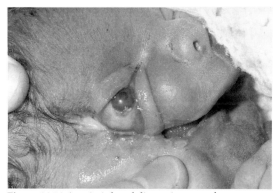

Figure 16.29 Amniotic band disruption complex. Another view of the patient shown in *Figure 16.28*. The facial part of the cleft appears to mimic a Tessier no. 5 oblique facial cleft

Treatment

The prognosis depends on the severity of the deformities. Many of those with the ADAM complex die, and mental retardation is common with central nervous system involvement. Due to the wide variety of clinical features, treatment plans have to be applied on an individual basis.

Craniofacial microsomia

This condition is also known as hemifacial microsomia, first arch syndrome, first and second branchial arch syndrome, otomandibular dysostosis, oculoauriculovertebral dysplasia, Goldenhar syndrome and lateral facial dysplasia. Most of these terms convey the erroneous impression that involvement is limited to facial structures, whereas cardiac, renal and skeletal anomalies may occur in addition. The condition was first reported by von Arlt in 1881. Gorlin *et al.* (1963) used the term hemifacial microsomia to refer to patients with unilateral microtia, macrostomia and failure of formation of the mandibular ramus and condyle; they suggested that oculoauriculovertebral dysplasia (Goldenhar syndrome) was a variant, characterized by vertebral anomalies and epibulbar dermoids. From a craniofacial viewpoint, the most recent appellation of craniofacial microsomia proposed by Converse *et al.* (1977) has the merit of avoiding the implication that the condition is unilateral (it is frequently bilateral), and it emphasizes that the cranium may be involved.

Regardless of the preferred name, this diagnostic group includes a wide spectrum of phenotypes (*Figures 16.30–16.34*). Although craniofacial microsomia is usually sporadic, familial cases are known, with a variety of transmission patterns. The incidence is reported as between one in 5000 births with a 1:1 sex ratio. In about 70% of cases the anomaly is unilateral. When it is bilateral it is always asymmetrical, a notable difference from Treacher Collins syndrome.

Poswillo (1973, 1974), using an animal model, demonstrated that destruction of differentiating tissues in the region of the developing ear and jaws by a teratogenically induced, expanding haematoma produced a branchial arch dysplasia. The severity of the dysplasia was related to the degree of local destruction. Thus craniofacial microsomia should probably be regarded as a non-specific symptom complex, the pathogenesis of which has several different aetiologies. When cardiac, renal or skeletal anomalies coexist, there appears to be an increased chance of genetic involvement.

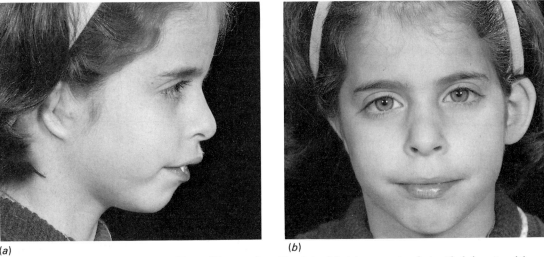

(a)   (b)

Figure 16.30 Craniofacial microsomia. Very mild example, with minimal facial asymmetry, but with deformity of the right auricle

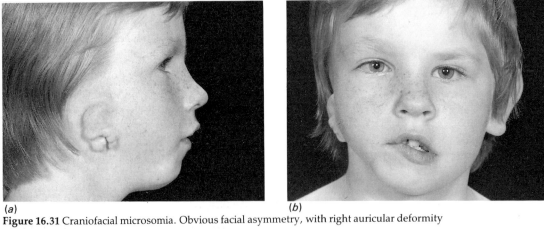

(a)   (b)

Figure 16.31 Craniofacial microsomia. Obvious facial asymmetry, with right auricular deformity

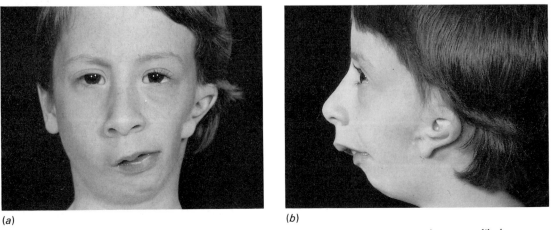

(a)   (b)

Figure 16.32 Craniofacial microsomia. Fairly severe example, with marked facial asymmetry due to mandibular, maxillary and zygomatic hypoplasia. Although abnormal, the left auricle is far less affected than the less severe cases shown in *Figures 16.31* and *16.32*

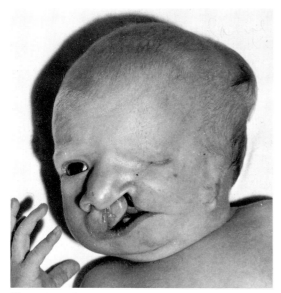

Figure 16.33 Craniofacial microsomia. Severe case of this syndrome, accompanied by a cleft of the lip and palate on the ipsilateral side. The microphthalmia resulted in enucleation of the affected eye

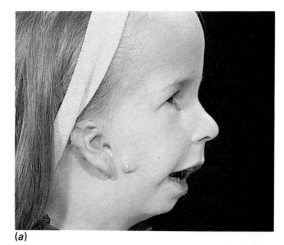

Clinical features

Not uncommonly the infants are small-for-dates, and there may be feeding difficulties which, on occasions, can necessitate tube feeding. In rare cases, nocturnal sleep apnoea may be severe enough to require tracheostomy (*see Figure 16.38*).

Facies

The facies may be striking because of the asymmetry. This may be partly due to hypoplasia and/or displacement of the pinna, but the degree of involvement varies markedly. The maxilla, zygoma and temporal bones on the affected side are reduced and flattened (*Figure 16.35*). Frontal bossing is common, and the ipsilateral eye may be set lower than its neighbour. The chin point is frequently deviated to the affected side due to mandibular hypoplasia, and the asymmetry can be further enhanced by hypoplasia of the parotid gland. Macrostomia, when it occurs, is usually mild (*see Figure 16.26*). Some 30% of patients with craniofacial microsomia have bilateral involvement, but the disorder is always more severe on one side (*see Figure 16.36e*).

Oral findings

Patients may exhibit all degrees of hypoplasia of the mandible, from a minimal decrease in size to complete agenesis of the ascending ramus and

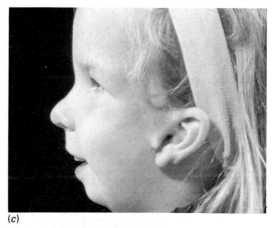

Figure 16.34 Craniofacial microsomia. Bilateral involvement; although there is reasonable symmetry with an absence of cant of the occlusal plane, the external ears are affected to varying degrees. The normal obliquity of the palpebral fissures and lack of zygomatic hypoplasia excludes a diagnosis of Treacher Collins syndrome

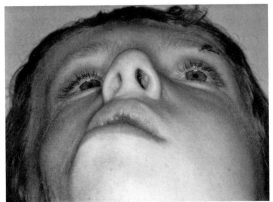

Figure 16.35 Craniofacial microsomia. This view of the face reveals hypoplasia of the mandible, maxilla, zygoma and temporal bones

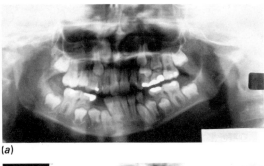

(a)

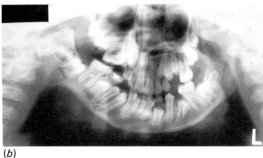

(b)

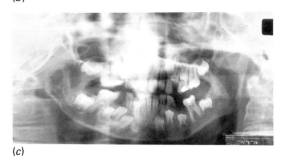

(c)

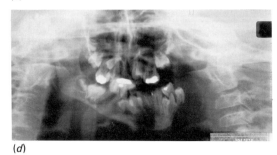

(d)

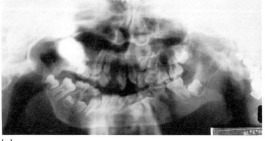

(e)

portion of the body on the affected side (*Figure 16.36*). When the condyle is absent, there is concomitant absence of the glenoid fossa. The gonial angle is often flattened, and this is a reflection of the decreased activity of the masticatory muscles. Moss and James (1984) have shown that there is a significant correlation between muscle activity and the morphology of the ascending ramus. The dental occlusal plane is frequently canted (*Figure 16.37*), and the degree of cant is a direct reflection of the severity of the mandibular and maxillary hypoplasia. Moss and James also found that the angle of the occlusal plane was negatively correlated with muscle activity, and that, in unilateral cases, the deficiency of growth on the affected side was compensated by overgrowth of the other side. In bilateral cases, the occlusal plane is usually normal or only mildly canted, but in such cases the chin is often severely retruded (*see Figure 16.34*). In infants, when severe micrognathia is present, there is a risk of obstructive sleep apnoea (*Figure 16.38*). This risk is enhanced when the pharynx is hypoplastic.

Figure 16.36 Craniofacial microsomia. Orthopantomograms demonstrating varying degrees of mandibular involvement. (*a*) Mild left-sided mandibular hypoplasia; the lack of a well-defined angle reflects reduced activity of the medial pterygoid and masseter muscles; (*b*) mild right-sided hypoplasia; the pronounced antegonial notch indicates good pterygomasseteric activity, and hence a good prognosis for successful bony reconstruction; (*c*) more severe right-sided mandibular hypoplasia with a trivial ascending ramus and right temporomandibular joint; (*d*) complete agenesis of the left ascending ramus; this is the radiograph of the patient shown in *Figure 16.44*; (*e*) bilateral case with coincident right unilateral complete cleft of lip and palate; the right ascending ramus is absent, and the left condyle is hypoplastic

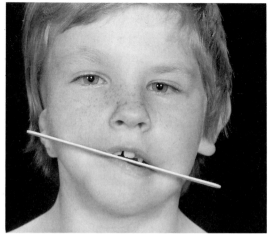

Figure 16.37 Craniofacial microsomia. A wooden spatula placed between the teeth reveals a marked cant of the occlusion. This is a reflection of the degree of mandibular and maxillary hypoplasia

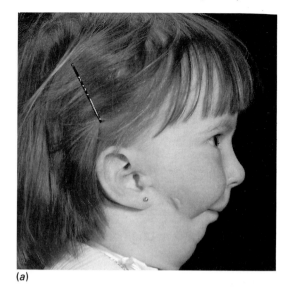

(a)

As well as hypoplasia and/or paresis of the palatal muscles, the tongue may be similarly affected, resulting in some degree of collapse of the dental arches. The incidence of cleft lip and palate is usually quoted as less than 10%, but at the Hospitals for Sick Children, Great Ormond Street, London the incidence is 18% in a group of some 60 patients.

Neuromuscular system

Hypoplasia of the masticatory muscles is present in all but the mildest cases, the masseter, temporalis and medial pterygoid being the most frequently involved, though to a variable degree. Facial weakness, usually affecting the lower face (*Figure 16.39*) occurs in 10% of patients; palatal and tongue musculature are less commonly affected. The incidence of mental retardation is reported as 10%, and occasional cases of occipital encephalocoele are recorded.

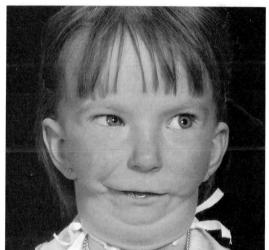

(b)

Figure 16.38 Craniofacial microsomia. This little girl with bilateral involvement has severe mandibular hypoplasia; this resulted in nocturnal sleep apnoea, severe enough to warrant a tracheostomy

Ear

Malformations of the external ear may vary from complete aplasia to a crumpled, distorted pinna displaced anteriorly and inferiorly. Supernumerary ear tags can be found anywhere from the tragus to the angle of the mouth; ear tags may be bilateral, especially when epibulbar dermoids are present. Conductive hearing loss due to middle ear abnormalities and/or absence or deficiency of the external auditory meatus is found in some 40% of patients.

Eye

The palpebral fissure is often somewhat lowered on the affected side. Epibulbar dermoid and/or lipodermoid is a variable finding. It is milky-white to yellow in colour, flattened, ellipsoidal and usually solid rather than cystic. The dermoid is frequently located at the limbus or corneal margin in the *lower* and outer quadrant (*Figure 16.40*); by contrast, the lipodermoid is usually located in the *upper* and outer quadrant. In some patients both

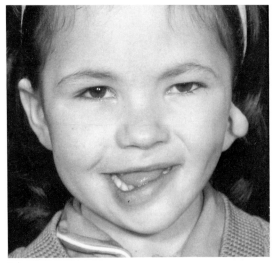

(a)

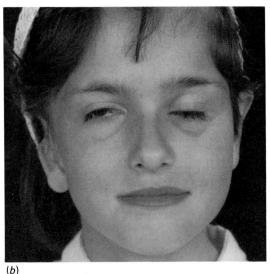

(b)

Figure 16.39 Craniofacial microsomia. (a) When facial weakness occurs in this syndrome, it more frequently affects the lower face as in this child with left-sided involvement; (b) upper facial weakness is occasionally a feature; this girl has trivial involvement of the hard and soft tissues of the face, but nevertheless has a right-sided weakness of the upper branches of the facial nerve

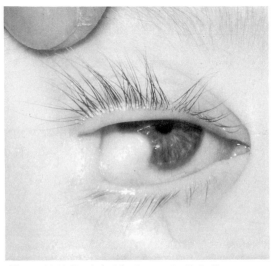

Figure 16.40 Craniofacial microsomia. Epibulbar dermoid affecting the lower and outer quadrant of the right eye

Skeletal anomalies

Vertebral anomalies are found in about half the patients, and include occipitalization of the atlas, cuneiform vertebrae, complete or partial synostosis of two or more vertebrae, supernumerary vertebrae, hemivertebrae and spina bifida. Anomalous ribs, talipes equinovarus and other skeletal defects have been reported.

Other anomalies

Some 50% of affected patients have various forms of congenital heart disease (Gorlin, Pindborg and Cohen, 1976). This can be severe enough to preclude corrective facial surgery. Pulmonary agenesis or hypoplasia has been noted on the affected side. A variety of renal abnormalities can be associated with the condition, including absent kidney, double ureter and anomalous blood supply.

Differential diagnosis

This disorder should be distinguished from Pierre Robin anomaly and Moebius syndrome. Bilateral cases of craniofacial microsomia are frequently confused with Treacher Collins syndrome; such confusion may be avoided if it is remembered that the former condition is asymmetrical, while the latter is symmetrical. Colobomas occur in the upper eyelid in craniofacial microsomia and the lower lid in Treacher Collins syndrome. Epibulbar dermoids may also be observed in frontonasal dysplasia.

lesions are seen in the same eye. Unilateral coloboma of the upper lid is common in patients with epibulbar dermoids (it will be remembered that in Treacher Collins syndrome colobomata occur in the *lower* lid). Choroidal or iridial coloboma and congenital cystic eye can occur in this disorder. Microphthalmia (*see Figure 16.33*) and anophthalmia are associated with severely affected individuals in whom mental retardation is more common.

Treatment

Three main problems have to be faced when considering surgical correction of craniofacial microsomia:

(1) No general agreement exists regarding the best time to carry out reconstructive surgery. At one extreme are those who maintain that all treatment for these patients should be deferred until growth is complete, the argument being that the shortage of investing soft tissues will inevitably cause relapse during the growing stages. Others maintain that enlargement of the deficient mandibular ramus during growth (usually by serial bone grafting) will help stimulate any growth potential that may be present in the soft tissue.
(2) The hypoplasia seen in craniofacial microsomia affects all tissues, both hard and soft. Thus any bony reconstruction has to be planned within the constraints of limited soft tissue (functional) matrix.
(3) Facial asymmetries in general are more difficult to correct than horizontal or vertical disproportions. The fact that the hypoplasia of craniofacial microsomia affects all tissues presents one of the most difficult problems facing the maxillofacial surgeon.

The following observations reflect the author's view about the management of this difficult problem.

(1) In moderate to severe unilateral cases, complete symmetry can never be achieved.
(2) Early surgery is indicated in those patients who demonstrate activity in the masticatory muscles. Ideally, electromyography should be carried out. If this investigation is not available, the presence of certain indicators favours early surgery; these indicators are the presence of a condyle (however rudimentary), a reasonably sized coronoid process, a masseteric process at the angle of the mandible and a degree of antegonial notching, however slight (Towers, 1976). Very early surgery to the midface is better delayed due to the danger of damage to the developing tooth buds filling the maxilla, and the lack of patient cooperation for postoperative orthodontics. Mandibular surgery, however, can be performed at any time, but is better delayed until cooperation for functional orthodontic treatment is possible. If possible, the start of a 'growth spurt' is a useful time for surgical intervention.
(3) In unilateral cases of craniofacial microsomia the unaffected side is not 'normal'. It undergoes hyperplasia in order to compensate for underdevelopment of the affected side (Moss and James, 1984). In reconstruction it is important not to try to make the involved side the same length as the 'normal' side; some reduction in height of the longer side is advisable.
(4) The constraints of the restrictive soft-tissue envelope may be managed by redistributing the bones within it, and not trying to introduce too much increase in bony volume. The reduction in lower face height referred to in (3) will assist this process. If the above process is not possible, it will be mandatory to introduce soft tissue into the area.
(5) The bulk of a bone graft, whether it is vascularized or not, will only survive if subjected to the stimulus of muscle activity. Thus the quality of the masticatory muscles on

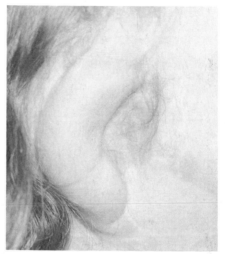

(a)

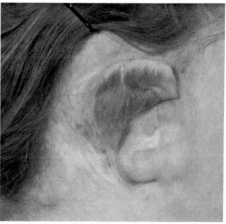

(b)

Figure 16.41 Craniofacial microsomia. Two examples of ear reconstruction which hardly justify the inconvenience and discomfort of the patient and the use of expensive resources

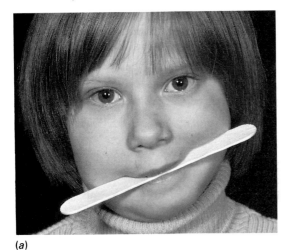

(a)

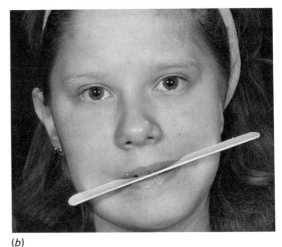

(b)

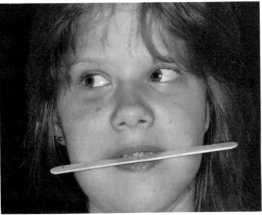

(c)

Figure 16.42 Craniofacial microsomia. Two-stage correction of a moderately affected patient. (*a*) Prior to surgery; (*b*) appearance four years after mandibular osteotomy and bone grafting at 11 years of age; (*c*) patient aged 15 years following maxillary and mandibular osteotomies

the affected side is an important index of the prognosis for bone graft survival. When onlay bone grafts are used, cranial bone survives better than either rib or iliac crest – the two usual sources of bone for reconstruction (Zins and Whitaker, 1983).

(6) The concept of the transfer of vascularized composite flaps containing both bone and soft tissue has received much attention recently. Vascularization of a bone graft in the absence of muscle activity will not ensure its survival.

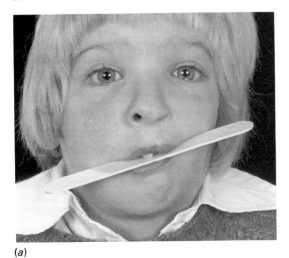

(a)

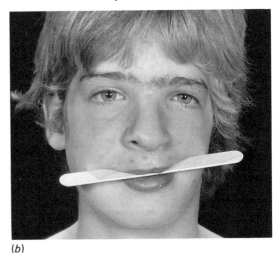

(b)

Figure 16.43 Craniofacial microsomia. A more severe case, complicated by a complete left unilateral cleft of lip and palate. This 13-year-old boy underwent a two-stage reconstruction; a left malar osteotomy and temporal fossa reconstruction was followed by maxillary and mandibular osteotomies (*b*). Further surgery, including a rhinoplasty and soft-tissue augmentation will be necessary

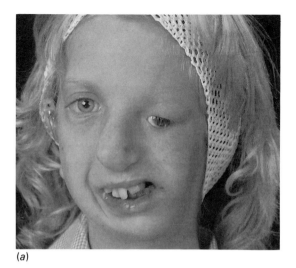

(a)

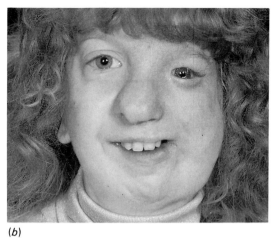

(b)

Figure 16.44 Craniofacial microsomia. (*a*) Patient very severely affected with gross soft-tissue and bony hypoplasia of the left side of the face, including microphthalmia; (*b*) multistaged reconstruction including a microvascular osteocutaneous groin flap has produced only a modest result in this girl at 19 years of age

Similarly, muscles will atrophy and become fibrotic when they lack a nerve supply. The definitive assessment of a series of these flaps is awaited with interest, but the optimism of some enthusiasts appears to ignore proven physiological concepts. Despite the above reservations, the microvascular transfer of soft tissue appears to offer definite advantages over other techniques when surface cover or soft-tissue bulk is required.

(7) Much time and effort is devoted to ear reconstruction. In the author's experience the results are usually disappointing and sometimes frankly mutilating (*Figure 16.41*). When the time comes for correction of the major part of the deformity, both parents and child are sometimes disillusioned and resentful. It is time that the allocation of so much surgical time and effort in pursuit of such disappointing results should be questioned.

For details of the surgical techniques currently employed in the treatment of craniofacial microsomia, the reader is referred to texts by Caronni (1985) and Henderson (1985). The

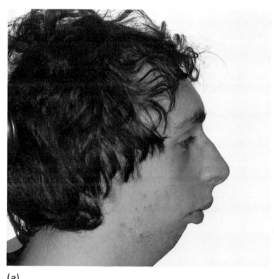

(a)

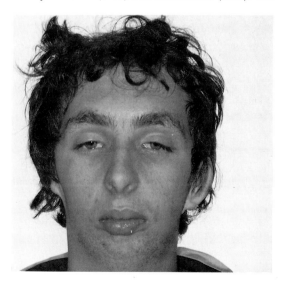

Figure 16.45 Craniofacial microsomia. (*a*) This patient with bilateral involvement exhibits very little asymmetry but gross micrognathia;

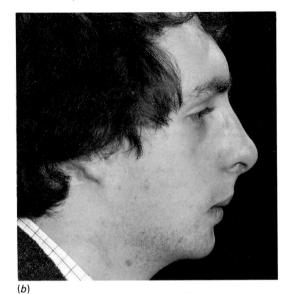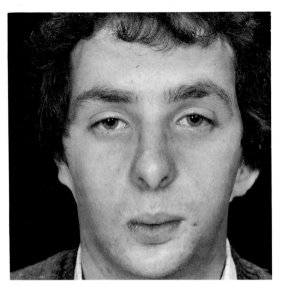

(b)

(b) the appearance at the age of 18 years following a two-staged correction involving bilateral mandibular osteotomies with bone-grafting followed by genioplasty and rhinoplasty

results of such surgery are shown in *Figures 16.42–16.45*.

Treacher Collins syndrome

Synonyms for this condition include mandibulofacial dysostosis, Berry syndrome, Franceschetti–Zwahlen–Klein syndrome and bilateral facial agenesis. Although the syndrome was probably first described by Thomson in 1846 (Gorlin, Pindborg and Cohen, 1976), credit for its discovery is usually given to Berry or, more commonly, to Treacher Collins, who described the essential features of the syndrome in 1900. Franceschetti and Klein (1949) coined the term *mandibulofacial dysostosis*.

The syndrome is inherited as an autosomal dominant trait with high penetrance and marked variability in expressivity. More than half the cases arise as fresh mutations, but before being so assigned, careful examination of family members should be performed, looking for minimal signs of the syndrome. The abnormal gene may have a lethal effect, since miscarriage or early postnatal death is common. Poswillo (1974) used an experimental animal model to formulate an explanation for the causal mechanism of Treacher Collins syndrome. He found that there was early destruction of the neural crest cells of the facial and auditory primordia which migrate to the first and second branchial arches. This destruction, before migration is well under way, leads to the formation of a 'vacuum' in the area of the otic cup into which the surrounding tissues flow. The developing otic pit thus moves upwards into the first arch region and relocates over the angle of the mandible. Additionally, there is a symmetrical, overall hypoplasia of many of the derivatives of the first and second branchial arch mesenchyme.

Clinical features

Facies

The facial appearance is characteristic (*Figure 16.46*). The obliquely slanting palpebral fissures, depressed cheekbones, deformed pinnas, receding chin and large, fish-like mouth present an unforgettable picture. One-quarter of affected patients have a tongue-shaped process of hair that extends towards the cheek (*Figure 16.47*). The body of the malar bones may be totally absent, but more often is grossly and symmetrically underdeveloped, with discontinuity of the zygomatic arches (*Figure 16.48*). The paranasal air sinuses are usually small, and may be absent. The lower orbital rim is sometimes defective, giving support to Tessier's assertion that Treacher Collins syndrome is a clefting syndrome. The nasofrontal angle is usually obliterated, with a high nasal bridgeline. The nose appears large due to the lack of malar development, while the nares may be narrow and the alar cartilages hypoplastic.

Oral manifestations

The mandible is almost always hypoplastic, with the deficiency mainly in the ascending ramus; the gonial angle is high, and antegonial notching is seen. There is a downward curve in the body of

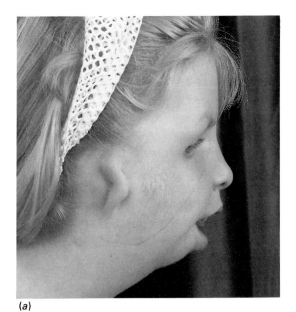

(a)

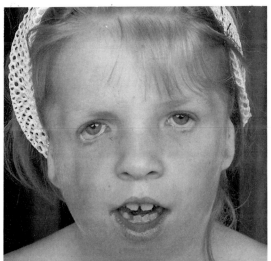

(b)

Figure 16.46 Treacher Collins syndrome. Characteristic facies of an 8-year-old patient with the condition

the mandible and, together with the short ramus, this results in gross retrusion of the chin (*Figure 16.49*). There is usually a high-arched palate, 30% of which are cleft. Macrostomia, seen in 15% of cases, may be unilateral or bilateral. Dental malocclusion is common; the teeth may be widely separated, hypoplastic, displaced or associated with an anterior open bite.

Eyes

There is an antimongoloid obliquity of the palpebral fissures, and a coloboma is present in the outer third of the lower lid in 75% of patients, half of whom also have a deficiency of eyelashes medial to the coloboma. Iridial coloboma may also occur. The lower lacrimal points, Meibomian glands and intermarginal strip may be absent. Microphthalmia has been reported.

Ears

The external ear is frequently deformed, crumpled forward or misplaced. Some patients exhibit an absence of the external auditory canal or ossicular defects resulting in conductive deafness. Anomalies of the ossicles include a fixed malleus, fusion of malformed malleus and incus, monopodal

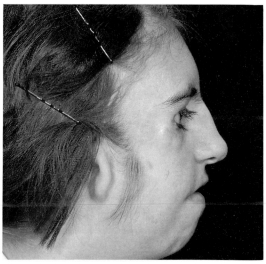

Figure 16.47 Treacher Collins syndrome. Tongue-shaped process of hair present in one-quarter of affected individuals

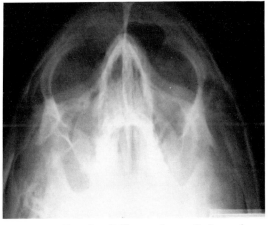

Figure 16.48 Treacher Collins syndrome. Radiograph demonstrating hypoplasia of the malar bones with absence of both zygomatic arches

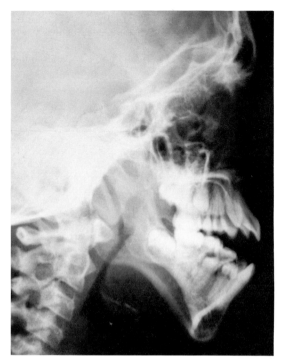

Figure 16.49 Treacher Collins syndrome. Radiograph showing the short ascending ramus of the mandible resulting in marked retrusion of the chin and anterior open bite

stapes, absence of stapes and oval window; there may be complete absence of the middle ear and epitympanic space. Extra ear tags and blind pits may be found anywhere between the tragus and angle of the mouth.

Other anomalies

Those other abnormalities reported include absence of the parotid gland, congenital heart disease, malformed cervical vertebrae, defects of the extremities, cryptorchidism and renal abnormalities. Mental retardation does occur, but in some cases this may be secondary to a severe hearing deficit.

Differential diagnosis

The most important distinction is from bilateral craniofacial microsomia. Treacher Collins syndrome is a symmetrical facial deformity, while craniofacial microsomia is never symmetrical. Other isolated and rare syndromes may exhibit some of the facial features seen in Treacher Collins syndrome, and the 'commonest' of these is acrofacial dysostosis (Nager syndrome).

Treatment

Poswillo (1974) argued persuasively that the early reconstruction of the hypoplastic facial skeleton in Treacher Collins syndrome will permit expansion of the modified functional matrix. While the skeletal structures of the mid and lower face are morphologically deficient, their design is such that in the presence of a system of masticatory muscles there exists a reasonable functional matrix capable of growth and development after surgical reconstruction. Occasionally very early surgery is mandatory when obstructive sleep apnoea is precipitated by the severe micrognathia (*Figure 16.50*).

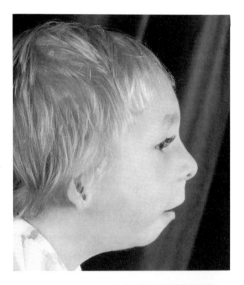

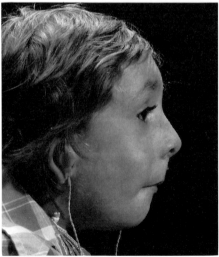

Figure 16.50 Treacher Collins syndrome. This 4-year-old boy experienced obstructive sleep apnoea which was relieved by mandibular advancement and bone-grafting

Surgery is directed at three main areas:

(1) the eyes, with antimongoloid slant of the palpebral fissues and lower lid colobomas
(2) the malar hypoplasia
(3) the mandibular hypoplasia with the marked retrognathia and anterior open bite.

For details of the techniques involved, readers should consult an appropriate craniofacial text such as that by Caronni (1985).

Miscellaneous craniofacial anomalies

Some craniofacial anomalies cannot be classified as one of the craniosynostoses or a clefting syndrome. These disorders include dysplasias, hamartomata, certain benign neoplasms and a miscellany of specific syndromes. The conditions described in this section do not constitute a comprehensive list of all the possibilities, but include most of the conditions that are seen from time-to-time in a busy craniofacial unit, and which are usually amenable to some form of surgical correction, albeit with variable degrees of success. The disorders are variable in extent, the spectrum extending from discrete areas to massive involvement of a large portion of the craniofacial region.

Dysplasias of bone

The most interesting and extensive of these conditions are *fibrous dysplasia* and *cherubism*.

Fibrous dysplasia

Fibrous dysplasia of bone may affect the bones of the cranium and face in three ways:

(1) as a monostotic lesion
(2) as one or more of the lesions of polyostotic disease
(3) as one or more of the lesions of *Albright's syndrome*, in which the polyostotic lesions are accompanied by such manifestations as cutaneous pigmentation, endocrine disorders with precocious puberty and premature skull maturation.

The nature and aetiology of fibrous dysplasia are unknown, but the consensus of opinion at present regards it as a developmental defect. There is no evidence to suggest that the lesions are neoplastic, and they tend to become inactive or stabilized after the normal period of skeletal growth has come to an end. Fibrous dysplasia is not inherited, but there is a definite sex predilection, two to three times as many females being affected.

Distribution of lesions

In monostotic cases, practically any bone may be involved, but limb bones, ribs, jaws and cranial bones are those most frequently affected. In polyostotic fibrous dysplasia the skull is involved in about half the cases in which there is a moderate degree of skeletal involvement, while in severe cases the skull is constantly involved. While almost any combination of lesions may occur, there is a well marked tendency for the lesions to occur segmentally, with localization in one limb or on one side of the body. When the jaws are involved, the lesion is usually solitary, occurring more often in the maxilla than the mandible. Multiple jaw lesions are less frequent, but when they occur may be accompanied by lesions in the facial and cranial bones (*Figure 16.51*).

Clinical features

Patients with polyostotic disease that is at all extensive practically always present as children, usually with deformity or pathological fracture (*Figure 16.52*). When solitary or relatively few lesions exist, presentation is usually in childhood or adolescence, but occasionally this is delayed until adult life. Jaw lesions occur as bony hard, non-tender swellings that expand the jaw, producing a gradually increasing facial asymmetry that may be first noticed by the parents. Often the deformity is slight, even when the lesion has ceased to be active. However, in some cases growth is more rapid and extensive, and in a comparatively short time there may develop a large mandibular swelling or a maxillary lesion that causes marked swelling of the cheek, exophthalmos or nasal obstruction. Such a case is shown in *Figure 16.55*. It is probable that many of the cases previously termed *leontiasis ossea* were examples of fibrous dysplasia.

Radiology

Radiographic appearances in the jaws (*Figure 16.53*) are generally similar to those seen in other bones. Both radiolucent and ground glass appearances are seen. On intraoral films a characteristic orange peel picture is seen in those areas that appear as a ground glass appearance in extraoral films. Diffuse lesions in the maxilla and facial bones may extend up to, and distort, the suture lines, but do not cross them. Skull radiographs in jaw cases frequently show that there is an increased density at the base of the skull (*Figure 16.54*).

260

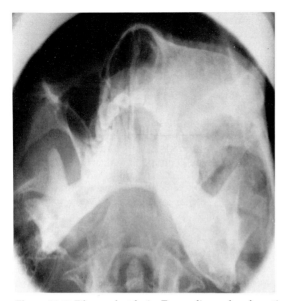
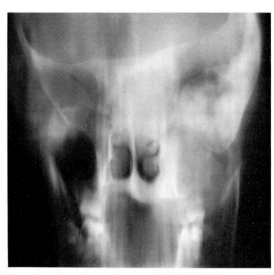

Figure 16.51 Fibrous dysplasia. Two radiographs of a patient showing extensive involvement of both facial bones and skull

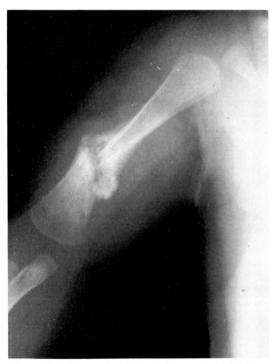

Figure 16.52 Fibrous dysplasia. Radiograph of a child with polyostotic disease demonstrating a pathological fracture of the humerus

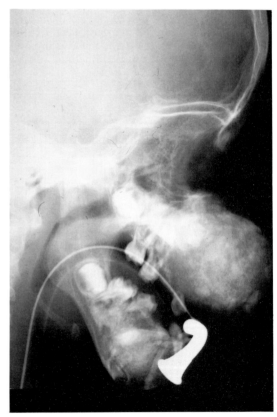

Figure 16.53 Fibrous dysplasia. Extraoral radiograph revealing a gross lesion in the maxilla and a smaller lesion in the mandible; both radiolucent and radiodense areas are seen

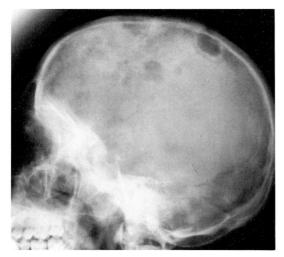

Figure 16.54 Fibrous dysplasia. Lateral skull radiograph of a young adult patient showing radiolucent lesions in the skull vault and increased density of the base of the skull

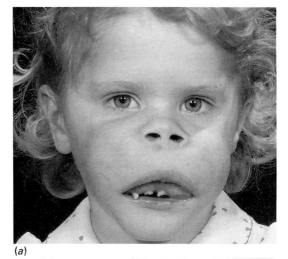

(a)

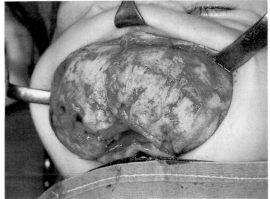

(b)

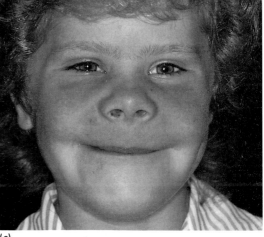

(c)

Figure 16.55 Fibrous dysplasia. (*a*) A 3-year-old girl with polyostotic disease, including gross involvement of the maxilla; (*b*) intraoperative photograph revealing the gross appearance of the affected bone; (*c*) early postoperative appearance. Further enlargement of the maxilla may be anticipated as facial growth proceeds

Pathology

The lesions are yellowish or greyish-white, and impart a gritty sensation to the knife when cut. Microscopically they consist of fibrous tissue that replaces normal bone and gives rise to osseous trabeculae. The proportion of fibrous to bony tissue varies from case to case and in different areas of the same lesion. It has been suggested that the proportion of fibrous tissue diminishes with the increasing age of a lesion, while calcification increases; this is no more than a trend, and is not necessarily a regular occurrence.

Differential diagnosis

This condition is sometimes confused with cherubism, but a careful family history and clinical examination of the jaws augmented by radiographic examination should clarify the situation. Fibrous dysplasia occurs in a totally different age group from Paget's disease, and the serum chemistry is within normal limits. Examination of biopsy material by an experienced oral pathologist should clinch the diagnosis.

Treatment

In the craniofacial region treatment is usually instituted for cosmetic reasons rather than for functional disability. Whenever possible, treatment should be deferred until after puberty when the progressive enlargement of the affected areas usually ceases. In some cases, due to the rapid progress of disease, it is necessary to intervene before maturation of the lesions (*Figure 16.55*); in this situation it may be necessary to repeat the surgery, sometimes several times, and at varying intervals.

Contouring of the affected areas is the treatment of choice. The consistency of lesions varies widely, some being amenable to paring with a scalpel, while others are hard enough to require shaping with osteotomes or mechanical instruments. Resection is both mutilating and unnecessary. On rare occasions, orbital and frontal bone involvement may necessitate a transcranial surgical approach (*Figure 16.56*).

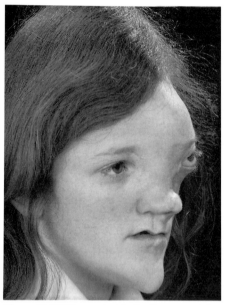

Figure 16.56 Fibrous dysplasia. Gross craniofacial involvement in an 11-year-old girl which will require a transcranial surgical approach for correction

Cherubism

This condition was first described by Jones in 1933 as familial multilocular cystic disease of the jaws, but the term *cherubism*, coined by the same author, has gained wider acceptance. Lucas (1984) provided a good review of the condition. The familial incidence of cherubism is one of its characteristic features, probably being inherited as a dominant trait with variable expressivity. Males are affected twice as frequently as females. Children with cherubism appear normal at birth, but swellings appear in the jaws between 1 and 4 years of age; the mandible is always affected, and very often the maxilla. The lesions rapidly increase in size up to the age of about 7 years, then enter a static phase or progress slowly up to puberty. The facial

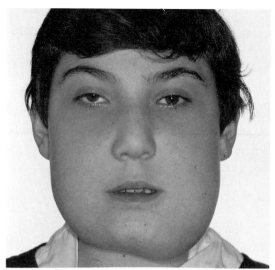

Figure 16.57 Cherubism. A 13-year-old child with asymmetrical cherubism

appearance is then said to improve, despite abnormal radiological appearances.

Clinical features

Facial deformity is the chief complaint (*Figure 16.57*). There is a characteristic fullness of the cheeks and jaws, and there is often a slightly upturned appearance to the eyes, with a rim of sclera visible beneath the iris. This latter sign is due to involvement of the orbital floor causing upward displacement of the eyeball and loss of support for the lower eyelid. The upturned eyes and full cheeks produce a cherubic appearance. The submandibular lymph nodes are generally enlarged, and the cervical nodes are also sometimes involved. There is fibrous enlargement of large areas of the jaws, resulting in gross expansion and irregularity. The resulting irregular bulges are painless and non-tender. Expansion of the mandible may elevate the tongue and cause a degree of speech impairment. The maxillary involvement is variable, sometimes being sufficiently extensive to produce nasal obstruction or ocular proptosis (*Figure 16.58*). The dentition is almost always abnormal.

Radiology

Radiographic appearances in the jaws are characteristic (*Figure 16.59*). Multiloculated radiolucencies produce considerable expansion of the bone; the loculi are sharply defined, and crossed by bony septa. The thinned and expanded cortex may be deficient in some areas without periosteal new bone formation.

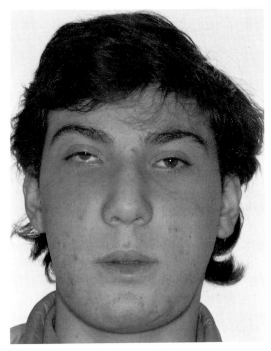

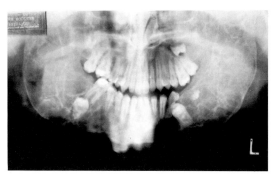

Figure 16.59 Cherubism. Orthopantomogram showing the typical radiographic appearance of cherubism

Pathology

The tissue that replaces normal bone is soft, fibrous or friable, and mottled reddish-brown or greyish-brown. The main constituent of the lesion is fibrous tissue arranged in a whorled pattern. Giant cells are concentrated around the numerous thin-walled blood vessels that permeate this vascular lesion. The enlarged lymph nodes show reactive changes only.

Differential diagnosis

The main distinction is from fibrous dysplasia. Cherubism is almost always familial, and the lesions are bilateral. As in fibrous dysplasia, it is important that any biopsy material is examined by an experienced oral pathologist.

Treatment

Management is essentially the same as that described for fibrous dysplasia. Surgery should be conservative, and only performed before puberty when absolutely necessary.

Angiomatous malformations

Haemangioma

The appellation *haemangioma*, although generally accepted, is taxonomically erroneous, as the anomaly is a hamartoma rather than a true neoplasm. Haemangiomata are usually classified as capillary and cavernous, although mixed types are common. It is beyond the scope of this chapter to deal with them in a systematic way; rather, the discussion will be limited to those large, cavernous or mixed haemangiomata that occupy a substantial area in the craniofacial region and produce a significant deformity.

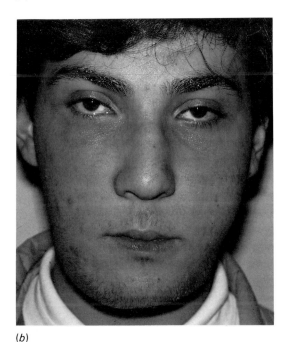

Figure 16.58 Cherubism. (*a*) The patient shown in *Figure 16.57* underwent surgical correction of the facial deformity, but subsequently developed proptosis and elevation of the right globe due to involvement of the orbital floor; (*b*) same patient following surgical reduction of the enlarged orbital floor

Clinical features

Facial cavernous and mixed haemangiomata may present as a very superficial, comparatively flat tumour at birth. They may enlarge slowly, but 60–70% of lesions regress completely by the age of 8 years if the parents will permit this approach. The occasional overwhelming lesion that has microarteriovenous fistulae demonstrates no regression, but continues to grow and expand. It rapidly develops (a deeper cavernous element) until the whole or large part of the face becomes involved (*Figure 16.60a*). The distended tissues may bulge out in the eyelids and around the mouth, so that the eye is completely hidden and the mouth may be partially obstructed. The skin and musculature of the face are greatly stretched, and feeding may become very difficult.

Differential diagnosis

This condition may be confused with lymphangioma, neurofibroma and congenital hemihypertrophy of the face. In young children it is important to exclude rhabdomyosarcoma (50% occur before the age of 5 years, and 25% are in the head and neck region). If any doubt exists, a biopsy is justified.

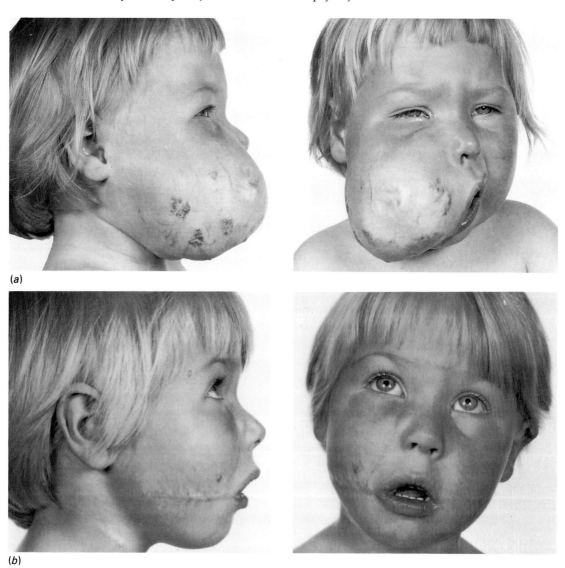

(a)

(b)

Figure 16.60 Haemangioma. (*a*) Expanding lesion of the right side of the face in a 16-month-old child; (*b*) appearance 9 months after surgical excision

Treatment

Treatment of large facial haemangiomata should be embarked upon with considerable circumspection. The help of a neuroradiologist can be invaluable, both in terms of defining the extent and nature of the lesion, and also carrying out microembolization with muscle or microspheres. This latter procedure is seldom anything other than transitory in its effect, but it permits surgery under much more favourable conditions, thus reducing the operative risk. The results of surgery in such large lesions are usually disappointing. Occasionally, however, favourable results are obtained (*Figures 16.60b–16.60d*). For cavernous lesions that are not excessively large, Matthews (1968) advocated the use of saturated saline as a sclerosing fluid. The use of radiotherapy in children is to be condemned.

Klippel–Trenaunay–Weber syndrome

The aetiology of this syndrome, also called vascular gigantism, is unknown, and almost all cases are sporadic. The original description defined the Klippel–Trenaunay–Weber syndrome as consisting of unilateral extremity enlargement with cutaneous and subcutaneous haemangiomata, varicosities, phlebectasia and occasionally arteriovenous fistulae. The syndrome has since been expanded to include almost every body area; many additional abnormalities have been recognized, including lymphangiomatous anomalies, macrodactyly, syndactyly, polydactyly, oligodactyly and abdominal haemangiomata (Gorlin, Pindborg and Cohen, 1976).

Craniofacial involvement (*Figure 16.61*) is rare, but when present is similar to that seen in Sturge-Weber syndrome, both in distribution and

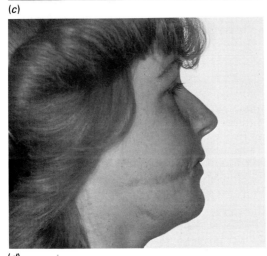

(c)

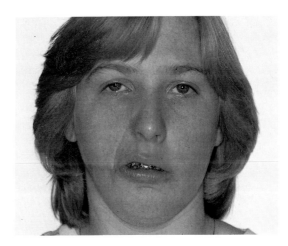

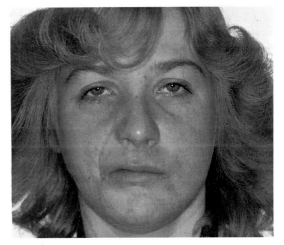

(d)

Figure 16.60 (*c*) Same patient at the age of 20 years; (*d*) following orthognathic surgical correction of the facial disproportion

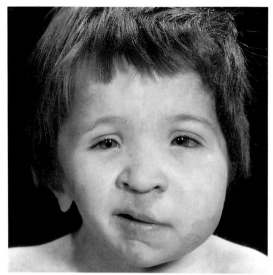

Figure 16.61 Klippel–Trenaunay–Weber syndrome. A 6-year-old boy with the rare craniofacial involvement

the degree of variability. Patients may exhibit mental retardation when cutaneous involvement is present. Occasionally the jaws may exhibit bony enlargement.

Differential diagnosis

Neurofibroma must be excluded, since limb hypertrophy and cutaneous haemangiomata may be associated with it; café-au-lait spots do not occur in Klippel–Trenaunay–Weber syndrome. Hemihypertrophy and cutaneous haemangiomata occur in both Beckwith–Weidemann syndrome and Maffucci syndrome. Vascular anomalies of the skin have also been reported in true congenital hypertrophy.

Treatment

Most patients do reasonably well. Some form of soft-tissue reduction such as filletting may be necessary; care should be exercised, as wound healing is usually delayed and skin infarction is common. For this reason, considerable circumspection is necessary when dealing with facial lesions. In cases with severe disproportionate growth in a limb, epiphyseal fusion or removal of a gigantic digit may be necessary. When gigantic extremities are gross enough to produce disseminated intravascular coagulation or evidence of high-output cardiac failure, amputation may be essential (Thomson, 1979).

Sturge–Weber syndrome

This syndrome is a non-hereditary condition that has neither sex nor ethnic predilection. It is characterized by:

(1) unilateral venous angiomatosis of the leptomeninges
(2) ipsilateral facial angiomatosis
(3) ipsilateral gyriform calcifications of the cerebral cortex
(4) seizures, hemiplegia and mental retardation
(5) ocular defects.

A port-wine stain on the ipsilateral side of the face (*Figure 16.62*) occurs in 90% of individuals, and this may extend onto the neck, chest and back. The colour varies from pink to purplish-red, and rarely decreases in intensity with age.

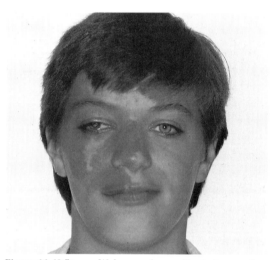

Figure 16.62 Sturge-Weber syndrome. Typical port-wine stain of the ipsilateral side of the face which affects 90% of affected individuals

Seizures, usually focal and rarely generalized, have been observed in 90% of patients. The symptoms appear during infancy on the side contralateral to the angiomatosis. Hemiparesis is less frequent. Mental impairment affects at least 30% of patients, being more severe with widespread cerebral involvement. Ophthalmic complications include choroidal angioma and glaucoma, both of which are fairly common.

Differential diagnosis

The relationship between Sturge–Weber and Klippel–Trenaunay–Weber syndromes is not usually a problem, but the two may coexist, and could represent the same basic disorder in a different site (Goodman and Gorlin, 1983). Transitory port-wine stains are very common in the neonatal period, but dark supraorbital involvement should arouse suspicion. The association of macrocephaly and angiomatosis may occur in disseminated haemangiomatosis, neurofibromatosis, Beckwith–Wiedemann syndrome, Klippel–Trenaunay–Weber syndrome and cutis marmorata telengiectatica congenita.

Treatment

Satisfactory treatment of the patient with a port-wine stain has escaped all investigators (Thomson, 1979). Various modalities of treatment have been tried, but all have failed the patients' needs. These treatments include radiotherapy, cryotherapy, argon laser therapy and surgical tattooing. Cosmetic camouflage remains the mainstay of treatment. However, surgical tattooing may enable the patient to use a lighter cosmetic coverage, but fading or leaking out of the pigment is the major drawback; such fading appears less in adult patients. Seizures are managed using standard anticonvulsant therapy.

Lymphangioma

About 75% of cases of lymphangioma are found in the head and neck region. Like haemangiomata,

these hamartomata are almost always evident by the age of 3 years. They may be present as unilocular or multilocular (more common) masses, with thin, often transparent walls enclosing a straw-coloured fluid. Such lesions are known as *cystic hygromata* (*Figure 16.63*).

Cystic hygromata are usually slow-growing, unless there is an associated internal venous haemorrhage or infective lymphangitis. Most lesions appear in the posterior triangle of the neck, often occupying the supraclavicular fossa. When they occur in the submandibular region or in the cervical prevertebral region, there may be severe respiratory distress in the neonatal period, especially if the disease is bilateral.

On rare occasions there is a rapid increase in growth. This can result in a grotesque enlargement of the affected side of the face, with the eye becoming obscured and gross distortion of the mouth. Hypertrophy of the maxilla and mandible may develop, but not to any marked extent.

There appears to be considerable disagreement about whether or not these lesions undergo spontaneous regression.

Treatment

This condition responds poorly to both radiotherapy and cryotherapy. Apart from the long-term danger of irradiating the neck in a child, radiotherapy produces extensive fibrosis, and this renders

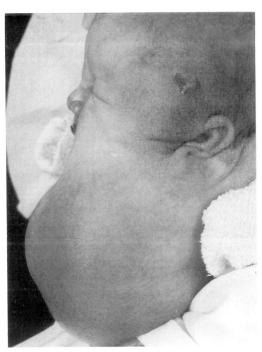

Figure 16.63 Cystic Hygroma. Bilateral involvement in a neonate: any signs of respiratory distress will necessitate emergency surgical treatment (Courtesy of Mr Ivor Broomhead, FRCS)

subsequent surgical dissection extremely difficult. Similar difficulty is experienced following the injection of sclerosing fluids. Thus radiotherapy, cryotherapy and sclerosing fluids should be avoided in the management of lymphangiomata.

Surgery remains the mainstay of treatment. Lymphangiomata of the neck and upper mediastinum which produce neonatal respiratory distress require to be treated as acute surgical emergencies. A preoperative chest radiograph is mandatory in order to exclude mediastinal extension. A tracheostomy and wide surgical excision is the treatment of choice. Cystic hygroma has an apparent disregard for anatomical planes, making total excision very difficult, and sometimes impossible. For this reason, some surgeons prefer less radical means of surgical decompression, employing vacuum drains or marsupialization of the cysts (Thomson, 1979).

In gross cases, a radical approach should be made without regard for the facial nerve (Mustardé, 1979). Not only is it extremely difficult to dissect out the functioning branches of the nerve, but more importantly, gross involvement and stretching of the facial muscles renders their preservation pointless and usually impossible. A series of planned resections is necessary, and subsequent reconstruction involves the standard techniques for dealing with facial palsy. Readers are directed to Mustardé's account for information regarding management of grossly involved eyelids.

Benign neoplasms

Neurofibroma

This benign tumour of the nerve sheath is an important, if rare, cause of gross facial deformity. It occurs only rarely as a solitary tumour. Much more often there are multiple tumours (neurofibromatosis) occurring in connection with the nerves of the skin and subcutaneous tissues and also those of internal organs. Neurofibromatosis (von Recklinghausen's disease) is an hereditary disorder transmitted as an autosomal dominant trait. It has the highest mutation rate known to man, 50% of cases representing a fresh mutation. The commonest presentation of this disease to the surgeon is that of facial deformity, and on rare occasions this may result in a gigantic overgrowth of one side of the face (*Figure 16.64*). While café-au-lait skin pigmentation may have been present since birth or early childhood, tumour formation becomes evident during childhood, and is usually most aggressive at the time of puberty. The condition is progressive, not subject to

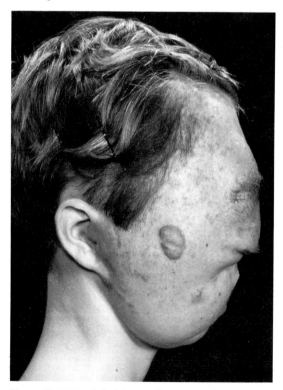
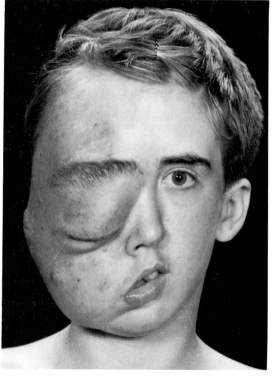

Figure 16.64 Craniofacial neurofibroma resulting in gross facial deformity with displacement of the right eye; the skin pigmentation is evident on the affected side of the face

spontaneous regression, and the pathology is that of plexiform neurofibroma. Both the fifth and seventh cranial nerves are involved, and it is impossible to dissect them out from the mass of tumour tissue. In gross facial lesions the facial bones are involved, and may show considerable enlargement and deformity. The skin is grossly expanded, and may hang down in tumour-filled folds over the eye or cheek; the eyelids may be considerably elongated.

Differential diagnosis

A gigantic plexiform neurofibroma of the face bears a resemblance to gross haemangiomata and lymphangiomata, but is usually distinguished by the simultaneous presence of café-au-lait spots. Polyostotic fibrous dysplasia with grossly enlarged facial bones may also have café-au-lait patches, but the enlargement is bony rather than soft tissue. Hemifacial hypertrophy is an enlargement of all the elements of the face, and this should make it easy to distinguish from neurofibroma.

Treatment

Treatment is directed at serial resection, access being gained via an extended parotidectomy incision, with secondary incisions in the nasolabial folds and eyelid margins. No attempt is made to preserve neurological function, and excess skin should be excised. The neurofibromatous tissue is extremely vascular, but preliminary carotid ligation does not usually result in a significant reduction in peroperative bleeding. Complete removal of all the involved tissue is virtually impossible. Resection of grossly involved parts of the maxilla and mandible may be necessary. There is considerable skeletal deformity in the orbital region; surgery is, of necessity, crude, and enucleation of the globe may be required.

Prodigious efforts are usually expended over a number of years to effect an improvement in appearance, but this is seldom acceptable to the patient or his relatives. The prognosis is poor, as growth of the incompletely excised tumour tissue is unavoidable. In addition, there is the risk of malignant transformation.

Miscellaneous malformations

Congenital hemihypertrophy of the face (facial gigantism)

Asymmetrical growth or development of the body or any of its parts is not too unusual; this may be trivial or very obvious. It may result from localized overgrowth of a single tissue or of all the tissues within a part.

Marked asymmetry caused by localized overgrowth of all the tissues within a part is rare. It is probably due to faulty cell division of the zygote which results in two daughter cells of unequal size, and has been considered a form of incomplete twinning (Norman, 1983).

Congenital hemihypertrophy may be of several types, and these have been classified by Rowe (1962):

(1) complex hemihypertrophy involving an entire half of the body, or at least an arm and a leg; enlarged parts may be all on the same side of the body (complex ipsilateral hemihypertrophy) or crossed, in which case enlarged parts may be found on both sides (complex contralateral hemihypertrophy)
(2) simple hemihypertrophy, involving part or the whole of a limb
(3) hemifacial hypertrophy, involving one side of the face (*Figure 16.65*).

The criteria for the hemifacial type of congenital hypertrophy are as follows:

(1) unilateral enlargement of the viscerocranium bounded superiorly by the frontal bone (not including the eye), inferiorly by the inferior border of the mandible, medially by the facial midline and laterally by the ear, the pinna being involved
(2) enlargement of *all* tissues – bone, teeth and soft tissue – within this area.

Almost all instances of this condition are sporadic, but a few familial cases have been reported. The incidence is about one per 15 000 births. Rowe (1962) recorded that the enlargement results from an increased number of cells rather than increase in cell size.

Asymmetry is usually evident at birth, but may become accentuated with age, especially at puberty. Occasionally there is unilateral enlargement of a cerebral hemisphere, and mental retardation is reported in 15–20% of cases. When the hemihypertrophy is restricted to the face, there is usually macroglossia. The lips, palate, maxilla and dentition (especially the permanent teeth) are all enlarged. Unlike both hard and soft tissues, the teeth are unique in that their form and size are determined early and thereafter are not modified. A consideration of the size of the teeth on the affected side, therefore, is significant in this condition, as it establishes it as being congenital. Of special interest is the association with various neoplasms such as adrenocortical carcinoma, nephroblastoma, hepatoblastoma, adrenal adenoma, adrenal neuroblastoma and undifferentiated sarcoma of the lung. Neoplasia and renal dysplasia may be the cause of a reduced life span.

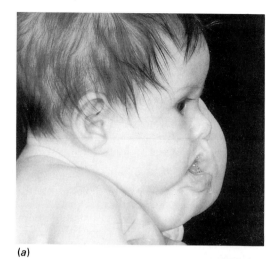

(a)

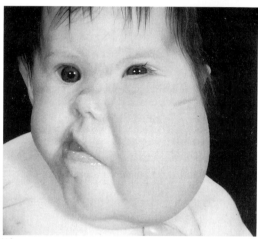

(b)

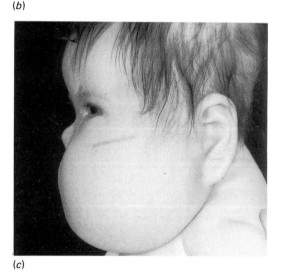

(c)

Figure 16.65 Congenital hemihypertrophy of the face in a 3-month-old girl

Differential diagnosis

Congenital facial hemihypertrophy may be confused with lymphangioma, haemangioma, neurofibroma and lipoma. It is usually distinctive due to involvement of *all* the tissues in the region, and it is the only condition where the teeth are enlarged.

Treatment

Due to the involvement of all facial tissues, surgical correction can be difficult, and as a result of the extreme paucity of cases, few surgeons gain much experience in treating such patients.

Progressive hemifacial atrophy

This disorder is also called Romberg's disease, Parry–Romberg syndrome and progressive facial hemiatrophy. Although it was mentioned by Parry in 1825 (Gorlin, Pindborg and Cohen, 1976), credit for its description is usually given to Romberg (1846). The condition consists of:

(1) slowly progressive atrophy of the soft tissues of essentially half the face, accompanied most often by
(2) contralateral Jacksonian epilepsy
(3) trigeminal neuralgia
(4) changes in the eyes and hair
(5) associated atrophy of half the body.

Nearly all cases are sporadic, but a few familial cases have been noted. There is no proven cause for progressive hemifacial atrophy. After a review of the various hypotheses, Rogers (1977) has concluded that a sympathetic nervous system cause is the most likely. It is postulated that sympathetic tracts are affected centrally, perhaps directly in their centres in the diencephalon. There is a long-standing debate about the relationship between progressive and hemifacial atrophy and scleroderma, some authors asserting that the *coup-de-sabre* form of scleroderma is a special type of progressive hemifacial atrophy.

Clinical features

Progressive hemifacial atrophy classically starts during the first decade with atrophy of the subcutaneous fat in the paramedian area of the face (*Figure 16.66a*). The process slowly spreads, so that atrophy of the underlying muscle, bone and cartilage becomes apparent. From the initial site, frequently in the area covered by temporalis and buccinator muscles, involvement extends to include the brow, angle of the mouth, neck or even half the body (*Figures 16.66a* and *16.66b*). There is a marked predilection for left-sided involvement,

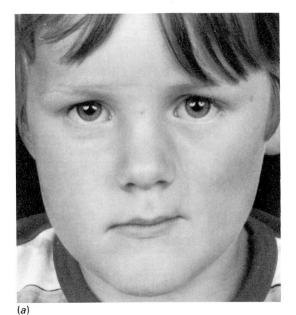

(a)

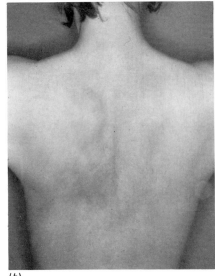

(b)

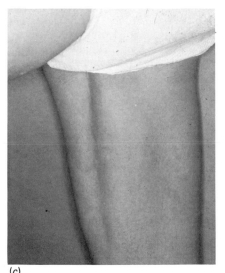

(c)

Figure 16.66 Progressive hemifacial atrophy. (*a*) Early onset of the condition in a 4-year-old child with left-sided facial involvement; (*b*) dorsal view to show atrophy on the left trunk in a mature female; (*c*) same patient as (*b*) exhibiting atrophy in the left thigh

and the overlying skin often becomes darkly pigmented. Changes in the hair may precede those in the skin; the scalp on the affected side may exhibit complete alopecia limited to the paramedian area, eyelashes and medial part of the eyebrow. Poliosis (blanching of the hair) has been observed.

Loss of periorbital fat produces enophthalmos and the outer canthus may be displayed due to loss of the underlying bone. Muscular paresis, lagophthalmos and ptosis have all been reported, as well as a variety of inflammatory, intraocular conditions.

The bone and cartilage of the face are underdeveloped to a degree directly related to the age of onset of progressive hemifacial atrophy. The bony involvement is thus most severe when the disorder commences in early childhood. When the mandible is involved, both ramus and body are shorter than the contralateral side, and teeth on the involved side may be retarded in eruption or may have atrophic roots. Atrophy of half the tongue and upper lip are common, sometimes resulting in exposure of the teeth.

The commonest neurological abnormality is epilepsy, usually of the Jacksonian variety, which often appears late. Conversely, trigeminal neuralgia and/or facial paraesthesia appear early, and may precede the rest of the changes. Migraine is a common finding.

Progressive hemifacial atrophy usually commences in late childhood or adolescence, and 75% of cases appear before the twentieth year. The atrophy is slowly progressive, and is usually limited to one side of the face, although bilateral disease has been reported. The 'active' period of the disease progression lasts for 2 to 10 years, but may stop at any time, leaving minimal deformity. Some cases of progressive hemifacial atrophy continue beyond a period of 10 years.

Differential diagnosis

The main conditions with which progressive hemifacial atrophy may be confused are scleroderma and craniofacial microsomia.

Treatment

Little information is published about the treatment of this condition, and the results are frequently disappointing. The main problem is that the same unknown factors which cause the initial atrophy frequently act against the success of the various forms of graft that have been used in reconstructive surgery; this is clearly a major problem when surgical procedures are undertaken during the 'active' phase of the disease. If at all possible, treatment is better delayed until the atrophy is no longer progressive.

Dimethylpolysiloxane fluid injections

This liquid form of silicone has been widely used in the USA, and is advocated by Grabb (1979) as the best treatment for progressive hemifacial atrophy. Plastic surgeons in the UK, however, have found this method of treatment less satisfactory. Inflammatory reactions, excessive fibrosis and migration of the fluid have all caused problems, and the technique has largely been abandoned.

Grafts

Dermo-fat grafts are still widely used. When they are inserted in areas not affected by progressive hemifacial atrophy, the resorption rate is unpredictable, and 50% or more of the original bulk is often lost. The resorption rate of dermo-fat grafts in tissues affected by the atrophy is even greater, and patients with severe forms of the disease have to be regrafted many times.

Flaps

Pedicled flaps of omentum have been used, but if this tissue is chosen, it is now more frequently used as a 'free' microvascular transfer. Temporalis muscle has been transferred on its pedicle in cases where the upper face has been largely spared, but this technique is clearly unsatisfactory in patients with extensive and severe involvement of the face.

The recent development of microvascular techniques has offered the best chance for reconstruction in progressive hemifacial atrophy. Each microvascular surgeon has his own preference in selecting the donor site. The main problems are the maintenance of an even distribution of soft tissue so transferred (it frequently 'sags') and variation in the bulk of the flap with changes in the weight of the patient due to its content of adipose tissue.

Moebius syndrome

This condition, while rare, is one of the commoner disorders of oromandibular limb hypogenesis. Moebius (1888), in attempting to classify multiple congenital cranial nerve palsies, created a division in which palsies of the sixth and seventh cranial nerves were combined. Subsequently the concept of Moebius syndrome has been expanded to include:

sixth and seventh cranial nerve palsies, usually bilateral
occasionally other cranial nerve involvement (third, fifth, ninth and twelfth)
reductive limb anomalies (30%)

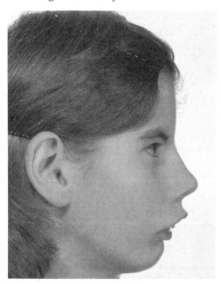 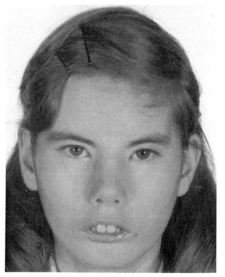

Figure 16.67 Moebius syndrome. Typical facies of patient with bilateral facial nerve involvement; the mask-like appearance is accompanied by mandibular retrusion, accentuated by the midfacial prominence

Poland anomaly (15%) i.e. abnormality of pectoralis major muscle and ipsilateral syndactyly mild mental retardation (10–15%).

The aetiology of Moebius syndrome is unknown, and all cases are sporadic. Post-mortem studies have demonstrated nuclear agenesis.

Clinical features

The mask-like facies is characteristic (*Figure 16.67*). Bilateral facial palsies usually impart a symmetrical appearance, but variation in the degree of involvement of each side of the face can cause significant

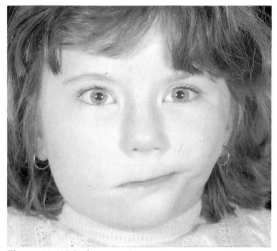

Figure 16.68 Moebius syndrome. Appearance of child with asymmetrical facial nerve involvement

asymmetry (*Figure 16.68*). Occasionally the facial palsy is unilateral.

Most patients cannot abduct either eye beyond the midline, but unilateral sixth nerve palsy does occur. Ptosis, nystagmus or strabismus may accompany the above features, and epicanthal folds are common (*Figure 16.69*). Some patients are unable to close their eyelids, resulting in conjunctivitis or corneal ulceration.

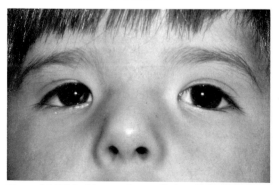

Figure 16.69 Moebius syndrome. Epicanthal folds

The nasal bridge is often high and broad, especially during infancy and childhood. The broadness of the bridge extends downwards in a parallel fashion to include the nasal tip, thus providing midfacial prominence which is accentuated by the retruded mandible (*Figure 16.67*).

The angles of the mouth droop, allowing saliva to escape. The mouth aperture is small, and mandibular opening may be restricted; this tends to improve spontaneously as the child develops. Unilateral or bilateral tongue hypoplasia is seen, and when combined with poor palatal mobility, can result in impaired feeding or speech. The mandible is frequently hypoplastic, adding to these problems. The pinnas may be hypoplastic, normal or large, and frequently protrude laterally.

Unilateral, bilateral or asymmetrical hypoplasia or aplasia of pectoralis major muscle or complete Poland anomaly occurs in 15% of cases. Limb defects occur in 50% of affected individuals, 30% constituting talipes deformities and the other 20% include hypoplasia of digits, syndactyly or more severe reductive deformities (*Figure 16.70*). Mental retardation, usually of a mild nature, occurs in 10–15% of patients with Moebius syndrome.

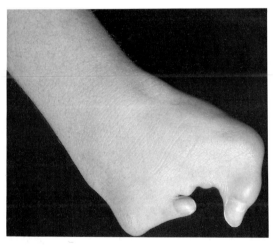

Figure 16.70 Moebius syndrome. Left hand of patient with severe reductive deformity

Differential diagnosis

There are variable degrees of overlap between the oromandibular limb hypogenesis syndromes. Thus Moebius syndrome must be distinguished from Charlie M. syndrome, glossopalatine ankylosis syndrome, Hanhart syndrome and hypoglossia-hypodactylia syndrome; all these are much rarer than Moebius syndrome. Similar limb defects are seen in the Poland anomaly, amniotic band syndrome and other reductive limb anomalies.

Superficially, Moebius syndrome may be confused with craniofacial microsomia, Treacher Collins syndrome and Pierre Robin syndrome. Isolated facial palsy may occur as an inherited disorder, or may result from birth trauma.

Treatment

The treatment of Moebius syndrome has received scant attention. Much has, however, been written about the management of facial palsy. It is outside the scope of this chapter to cover this challenging field of reconstructive surgery. Static sling procedures and reanimation techniques each have their advocates. It is the author's experience that results of reanimation are inconsistent and often disappointing, although satisfactory results are occasionally presented. If advances in this field are to continue, it is essential that patients with facial palsy are referred to those surgeons with an interest in and experience of these problems.

If static slings are employed, it is preferable that they are delayed until after any orthognathic surgery has been performed, as they usually severely restrict access to the oral cavity. The same principle applies to orthodontic treatment which is usually necessary.

The upper lip is short and immobile. The only satisfactory way of managing this problem is by means of a Le Fort I osteotomy to intrude the maxilla. This will have to be accompanied by an osteotomy of the mandible which usually needs advancement. Surgical details of the various orthognathic techniques are well described by Henderson (1985). Repositioning of the jaws may have a beneficial effect on feeding and speech, although the results are frequently disappointing in this respect.

The facial appearance can be further improved by correcting the wide nasal bridge and epicanthal folds when present.

References

APERT, E. (1906) De l' acrocéphalosyndactylie. Le Bulletin de la Société Medicine du Hôpital de Paris, **23**, 1310–1330

ARLT, F. von (1881) *Klinische Darstellung der Krankheiten des Auges.* Vienna: W. Braunmüller

BOO-CHAI, K. (1970) The oblique facial cleft: a report of 2 cases and a review of 41 cases. *British Journal of Plastic Surgery,* **23**, 352–359

CARONNI, E. P. (1985) Editor. *Craniofacial Surgery.* Boston: Little, Brown and Company

COHEN, M. M. (1979) Craniosynostosis and syndromes with craniosynostosis: incidence, genetics, penetrance, variability and new syndrome updating. *Birth Defects,* **XV**, 13–63

COLLINS, E. T. (1900) Cases with symmetrical congenital notches in the outer part of each lid and defective development of the malar bones. *Transactions of the Ophthalmological Society of the United Kingdom,* **20**, 190–192

CONVERSE, J. M., McCARTHY, J. G., WOOD-SMITH, D. and COCCARO, P. J. (1977) Craniofacial microsomia. In *Reconstructive Plastic Surgery,* 2nd edn, edited by J. M. Converse, pp. 2359–2400. Philadelphia: W. B. Saunders

CROUZON, O. (1912) Dyostose craniofociale héréditaire. Le Bulletin de la Société Medicine du Hôpital de Paris, **33**, 545–555

DAL PONT, G. (1961) Retromolar osteotomy for the correction of prognathism. *Journal of Oral Surgery, Anaesthesia and Hospital Dental Services,* **19**, 42–47

DAVID, D. J., POSWILLO, D. and SIMPSON, D. (1982) *The Craniosynostoses – Causes, Natural History and Management.* Berlin: Springer-Verlag

DELAIRE, J., GAILLARD, A., BILLET, J., LANDAIS, H. and RENAUD, Y. (1963) Considérations sur les synostoses prématurées et leur conséquences au crâne et à la face. Revue de Stomatologie, **64**, 97–106

DROMMER, R. B. (1986) The history of the Le Fort I osteotomy. *Journal of Maxillofacial Surgery,* **14**, 119–122

FRANCESCHETTI, A. and KLEIN, D. (1949) The Mandibulofacial dysostosis: new hereditary syndrome. *Acta Ophthalmologica,* **27**, 143–224

FRIEDENWALD, H. (1893) Cranial deformity and optic nerve atrophy. *American Journal of Medical Science,* **105**, 529–535

GILLIES, H. D. and HARRISON, S. H. (1950) Operative correction by osteotomy of recessed malar maxillary compound in a case of oxycephaly. *British Journal of Plastic Surgery,* **2**, 123–127

GOODMAN, R. M. and GORLIN, R. J. (1983) *The Malformed Infant and Child.* New York: Oxford University Press

GORLIN, R. J., JUE, K. L., JACOBSEN, U. and GOLDSCHMIDT, E. (1963) Oculoauriculovertebral dysplasia. *Journal of Paediatrics,* **63**, 991–999

GORLIN, R. J., PINDBORG, J. J. and COHEN, M. M. (1976) *Syndromes of the Head and Neck,* 2nd edn. New York: McGraw-Hill

GRABB, W. C. (1979) Some anomalies of the head and neck. In *Plastic Surgery,* 3rd edn, edited by W. C. Grabb and J. W. Smith, pp. 115–130. Boston: Little, Brown and Company

GREIG, D. M. (1924) A hitherto undifferentiated congenital cranio-facial deformity. *Edinburgh Medical Journal,* **31**, 560–593

HENDERSON, D. (1985) *A Colour Atlas and Textbook of Orthognathic Surgery – The Surgery of Facial Skeletal Deformity.* London: Wolfe Medical Publications

HUNSUCK, E. E. (1968) A modified intraoral sagittal splitting technique for correction of mandibular prognathism. *Journal of Oral Surgery,* **26**, 249–252

JONES, W. A. (1933) Familial multilocular cystic disease of the jaws. *American Journal of Cancer,* **17**, 946–950

KREIBORG, S. and BJORK, A. (1982) Description of a dry skull with Crouzon syndrome. *Scandinavian Journal of Plastic and Reconstructive Surgery,* **16**, 245–253

LUCAS, R. B. (1984) *Pathology of Tumours of the Oral Tissues,* 4th edn, pp. 408–412. Edinburgh: Churchill Livingstone

MARCHAC, D. and RENIER, D. (1981) Cranio-facial surgery for craniosynostosis. *Scandinavian Journal of Plastic and Reconstructive Surgery,* **15**, 235–243

MARSH, J. L. and VANNIER, M. W. (1985) Editors. *Comprehensive Care of Craniofacial Deformities.* St Louis: C. V. Mosby Co

MATTHEWS, D. N. (1968) Haemangiomata. *Plastic and Reconstructive Surgery,* **41,** 528–535

MOEBIUS, P. J. (1888) Über angeborene doppelseitige abducens-focialis lahmung. *Münchene Medizinische Wochenschrift,* **35,** 91–94 and 108–111

MOSS, J. P. and JAMES, D. R. (1984) An investigation of a group of 35 consecutive patients with a first arch syndrome. *British Journal of Oral and Maxillofacial Surgery,* **22,** 157–169

MUSTARDÉ, J. C. (1979) Editor. Acquired hemifacial hypertrophy (hemifacial gigantism). In *Plastic Surgery in Infancy and Childhood,* 2nd edn, pp. 372–379. Edinburgh: Churchill Livingstone

MYRIANTHOPOULOS, N. C. (1982) Epidemiology of craniofacial malformations. In *Clinical Dysmorphology of Oral-Facial Structures,* edited by M. Melnick, E. D. Shields and N. J. Burzynski, pp. 1–27. Bristol: John Wright

NORMAN, M. E. (1983) The bones and joints. In *Nelson Textbook of Pediatrics,* edited by R. E. Behrman and V. C. Vaughan, pp. 1614–1662. Philadelphia: W. B. Saunders

OBWEGESER, H. L. (1969) Surgical correction of small or retrodisplaced maxillae. *Plastic and Reconstructive Surgery,* **43,** 351–365

PETERSON, M. Q., COHEN, M. M., SEDANO, H. O. and FRERICHS, C. T. (1971) Comments on frontonasal dysplasia, ocular hypertelorism and dystopia canthorum. *Birth Defects,* **VII,** 120–124

PFEIFFER, R. A. (1964) Dominant erbliche akrocephalosyndaktylie. *Zeitschrift für Kinderheilkunde,* **90,** 301–320

POSWILLO, D. (1973) The pathogenesis of the first and second branchial arch syndrome. *Oral Surgery, Oral Medicine, Oral Pathology,* **35,** 302–328

POSWILLO, D. (1974) Otomandibular deformity: pathogenesis as a guide to reconstruction. *Journal of Maxillofacial Surgery,* **2,** 64–72

ROMBERG, M. H. (1846) Trophoneurosen. In *Klinische Ergebnisse,* pp. 75–81. Berlin: A. Forstner

ROGERS, B. O. (1977) Embryology of the face and introduction to craniofacial anomalies. In *Reconstructive Plastic Surgery,* 2nd edn, edited by J. M. Converse, pp. 2296–2358. Philadelphia: W. B. Saunders

ROWE, N. H. (1962) Hemifacial hypertrophy: a review of the literature and addition of four cases. *Oral Surgery, Oral Medicine, Oral Pathology,* **15,** 572–587

ROWE, N. L. (1960) The aetiology, clinical features and treatment of mandibular deformities. *British Dental Journal,* **108,** 45–64 and 97–115

SEDANO, H. O., COHEN, M. M., JIRASEK, J. and GORLIN, R. J. (1970) Frontonasal dysplasia. *Journal of Paediatrics,* **76,** 906–913

TESSIER, P. (1967) Ostéotomies totales de la face; syndrome de Crouzon; syndrome d'Apert; oxycéphalies, scaphocéphalies, turricéphalies. *Annales de Chirurgie Plastique,* **12,** 273–286

TESSIER, P. (1976) Anatomical classification of facial, cranio-facial and lateral-facial clefts. *Journal of Maxillofacial Surgery,* **4,** 69–92

TESSIER, P., GUIOT, G., ROUGERIE, J., DELBERT, J. P. and PASTORIZA, J. (1967) Ostéotomies cranio-naso-orbito-faciales – hypertélorisme. *Annales de Chirurgie Plastique,* **12,** 103–118

THOMSON, H. G. (1979) Hemangioma, lymphangioma, and arteriovenous fistula. In *Plastic Surgery,* 3rd edn, edited by W. C. Grabb and J. W. Smith, pp. 518–529. Boston: Little, Brown and Company

TOWERS, J. F. (1976) The management of congenital and acquired deformity of the mandibular condyle in children. *Cartwright Prize Essay,* London: Royal College of Surgeons of England

TRAUNER, R. and OBWEGESER, H. L. (1957) Surgical correction of mandibular prognathism and retrogenia with consideration of genioplasty. *Oral Surgery, Oral Medicine, Oral Pathology,* **10,** 677–689

ZINS, J. E. and WHITAKER, L. A. (1983) Membranous versus endochondral bone; implications for craniofacial reconstruction. *Plastic and Reconstructive Surgery,* **72,** 778–784

17

Foreign bodies in the nose

Joselen Ransome

Foreign bodies in the nose do not feature largely in otolaryngological literature, yet on occasions they may pose a considerable challenge to both the diagnosis and surgical skills of the otolaryngologist.

Aetiology

Mode of entry

Foreign bodies may enter the nose by several different means including:

(1) the anterior naris (accounting for the vast majority)
(2) the posterior naris, during vomiting, coughing, and regurgitation, or in patients with palatal incompetence – when the foreign body will consist of stomach, oesophageal or mouth contents, and occasionally a roundworm (ascaris)
(3) penetrating wounds and nasal surgery
(4) a palatal perforation as in cleft palate or following a gumma of the hard palate or surgery of the palate for malignant disease
(5) sequestration of bone *in situ* after trauma (which may be operative), and syphilis
(6) calcification *in situ* of inspissated mucopus or of exogenous foreign material, leading to the formation of a rhinolith.

Incidence

Children constitute the large majority of patients with foreign bodies in the nose. The foreign body will be any small object encountered by the child, and it will usually be introduced through the

anterior naris. Children with cleft palate will also have food from the mouth entering the nose, and occasionally other foreign material which the child is exploring with the mouth. Children of low socio-economic groups living in tropical climates may also be the victims of myiasis (disease due to maggots, larvae and flies), particularly if they already suffer from debilitating disease.

Adults and older children with foreign bodies in the nose are usually mentally disturbed; but they may also be the victims of penetrating injuries caused by bullets or shrapnel, or of operations on the nose, in which swabs, particles of tissue or instruments may be left behind.

Site of the foreign body

If it has been inserted by the patient it is more commonly in the right nasal cavity, since right-handedness predominates in the general population. The foreign body may be in any part of the nasal fossa.

Types of foreign body

Foreign bodies in the nose may be animate or inanimate (vegetable, mineral, arising from surgery, sequestra, or rhinoliths).

Animate

Maggots, screw worms and their larvae, and black carpet beetles may all infest the nose (myiasis) in tropical climates, and occasionally a roundworm (ascaris) may be coughed or regurgitated through the posterior naris.

Inanimate

Vegetable foreign bodies are commonly peas, beans, dried pulses, nuts, paper and pieces of pencils. *Mineral* matter may be parts from metal and plastic toys, washers, nuts, nails, screws, buttons, sponge, studs, plasticine, pebbles, beads and cotton wool, to name but a few. *Arising from surgery,* pieces of polyps, bone, cartilage, swabs, instruments, or packs may be left behind. *Sequestra* occur in syphilis and neoplasm, and after trauma. *Rhinoliths* occur *in situ* (*see above* and *below*).

Pathology

Some foreign bodies are inert and may remain in the nose for years without mucosal changes. Many however lead to inflammation and infection of the mucous membrane, which in turn leads to fetid mucopurulent discharge and epistaxis, these symptoms being unilateral, except with animate infestations. Ultimately granulation tissue is formed, and there may be ulceration of the mucosa, and occasionally necrosis of bone or cartilage.

These changes impact the foreign body, which may not be visible on either anterior or posterior rhinoscopy because of surrounding oedema, granulations and discharge. This is particularly so with vegetable foreign bodies which not only absorb water from the tissues and swell, but also evoke a very brisk inflammatory reaction. Occasionally the inflammatory reaction is sufficient to produce toxaemia.

Maggots and screw worms attack both nasal cavities and may give rise to a severe inflammatory reaction. During maturation, larvae burrow into the tissues. The mature larva of the screw worm has rings around its body, giving the appearance of a screw. If untreated they may attack nasal bone and cartilage and also involve the sinuses, orbits, adjoining skin, meninges, and brain (Gupta and Nema, 1970). Ascaris produces less inflammation but gives the patient a feeling of irritation and movement in the nose.

Sharp foreign bodies may occasionally penetrate the sinuses and give rise to sinusitis.

If a foreign body is buried in granulations or firmly impacted, it may act as a nucleus for concretion, that is it receives a coating of calcium, magnesium phosphate and carbonate and becomes a rhinolith. Occasionally this process may occur round an area of inspissated mucopus, or even a blood clot. Rhinoliths usually form near the floor of the nose and are radiopaque.

Symptoms and signs

Mineral and vegetable foreign bodies

These generally give rise to a unilateral fetid discharge, usually mucopurulent and sometimes blood-stained. There is frequently unilateral nasal obstruction, and there may be pain, epistaxis, and sneezing. A few foreign bodies are inert and cause either no symptoms, or unilateral nasal obstruction if sufficiently large.

Examination of the nose shows reddened congested mucosa, mucopus and sometimes granulations, ulceration and necrosis. The foreign body may or may not be visible, depending on its size and nature, and on the degree of surrounding oedema.

Animate foreign bodies

The symptoms are often bilateral, and nasal obstruction, headaches and serosanguineous fetid discharge may occur within a few days of infestation. In the larval stage pyrexia may occur. The patient has a constant feeling of formication in the nose. In poor communities the patients adapt surprisingly well to the condition, and instead of being driven to despair, have to be persuaded to seek treatment, on the grounds that complications may occur.

Examination shows marked swelling of the mucosa, which is fragile and bleeds easily. In heavy infestations there is an appearance of constant motion, which on closer inspection is seen to be due to masses of worms, which are firmly attached and difficult to remove. In long-standing infestation there may be destruction of bone and cartilage.

Due to secondary infection and bone destruction complications are not rare, and patients may present with orbital infection or meningitis. In the rare case of ascaris in the nose, the worm is large (15–25 cm) and easy to remove. There is minimal mucosal reaction.

Rhinoliths

As they increase in size slowly and are relatively inert, rhinoliths are initially symptomless, and later cause nasal obstruction if they become large enough. They may be discovered when a cause is sought for an unresolved sinus infection.

Examination of the nasal cavity shows a brown or greyish irregular mass, usually near the floor of the nose, which feels stony hard and gritty on probing (*Figure 17.1*). X-rays will reveal the extent of the rhinolith, which may attain a very large size, and may occasionally extend into the antrum.

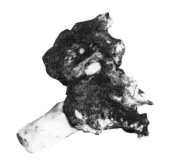

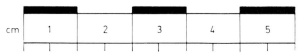

Figure 17.1 Rhinolith from a case described by Mr R. McNab Jones

Diagnosis

The diagnosis of animate foreign bodies is usually all too apparent on inspection.

With inanimate foreign bodies, the suspicion usually arises because of a unilateral purulent nasal discharge, and in children this must be regarded as due to a foreign body until proved otherwise. Frequently the foreign body will be seen on anterior rhinoscopy (and sometimes on posterior rhinoscopy), but on occasions the mucosal oedema or granulations will hide it. If such unilateral changes are seen but no foreign body, in cooperative older children and adults, the nose should be sprayed with a vasoconstrictor to shrink the mucosa and the fossa re-examined. Sometimes a foreign body will then be seen. If not, the nose should be X-rayed as many foreign bodies are radiopaque. In younger or very apprehensive children it may be necessary for the search to be carried out under a general anaesthetic, and this procedure is described below.

Other conditions to be excluded are neoplasm (by biopsy of granulations), unilateral sinusitis (by X-ray), syphilis (by serology), diphtheria (by nasal swab), and unilateral choanal atresia (by passing a catheter through the nasal fossa or by X-ray after instilling a contrast medium).

Management

Animate foreign bodies

Infestations with maggots and screw worms are treated by instilling a 25% chloroform solution into the nasal cavities. This is repeated two or three times a week for about 6 weeks until all larvae are killed. After each treatment the patient blows his nose to clear the dead worms and larvae. Sometimes treatment is given under general anaesthesia (with a cuffed endotracheal tube and throat pack), when repeated irrigation followed by suction can be carried out.

Ascaris is managed by removal of the worm with forceps, followed by treatment of the general condition with piperazine and magnesium sulphate purges to clear dead worms from the bowel.

Inanimate foreign bodies (except rhinoliths)

If the foreign body is easily seen, and the patient is a cooperative child or an adult, it is usually possible to remove the object through the anterior naris, either with no anaesthetic, or after spraying with a local anaesthetic solution such as lignocaine.

However, it cannot be too strongly emphasized that unskilled attempts to remove the foreign body in the accident and emergency department, by personnel without appropriate training, may result in disaster: the foreign body may be displaced backwards and may even reach the nasopharynx with risk of inhalation; marked epistaxis may occur; and a docile child may become terrified and require a general anaesthetic and admission to hospital which might have been avoided.

The patient is placed in the usual upright position for routine otolaryngological examination, and the nasal fossa illuminated with a head mirror or fibrelight headlight. It is important that the light source should be very bright. The following instruments should be available: nasal speculum, curved hook, Jobson Horne probe, selection of angled crocodile forceps, angled nasal dressing forceps of various sizes, nasal sucker and source of suction. A jar to receive specimens to send to the pathology department should also be prepared.

The nasal speculum is inserted with the left hand, and with the right hand the curved hook is passed beyond the object and the tip rotated to rest just posterior to the object. The object is then gently drawn forwards and removed completely, or brought almost to the nasal vestibule and then removed with forceps. The above technique should be used whenever there is a risk of displacing the object backwards into the nasopharynx, as with spherical objects such as beads. Rough semi-impacted objects such as bits of paper and sponge, and objects placed very near the vestibule, can be removed directly with forceps.

A general anaesthetic will be required in the following circumstances:

(1) if the patient is uncooperative or very apprehensive
(2) if there is likely to be troublesome bleeding, for instance if the foreign body is firmly embedded in granulation tissue
(3) if the foreign body is posteriorly placed with a risk of pushing it back into the nasopharynx
(4) if a foreign body is strongly suspected but cannot be found, and more extensive examination of the nose is required, with the opportunity to deal with whatever is found. It must be emphasized that there is *no need for haste* on these occasions. The foreign body may have been in the nose for a considerable period and it is important to wait for ideal facilities, especially an experienced anaesthetist. Unskilled manipulation in adverse conditions can lead to inhalation of the foreign body or of blood.

The patient is anaesthetized and a cuffed oral endotracheal tube and a pharyngeal pack are inserted . With the patient in the usual position for nasal surgery, the nose is examined using a nasal speculum, headlight, and suction to remove secretions. To minimize bleeding, the affected nasal fossa is then sprayed with 1 ml of a mixture of 5% cocaine and 1/1000 adrenaline (50% of each), in consultation with the anaesthetist. After waiting for this to take effect, the nose is then re-examined, and the foreign body is gently withdrawn.

If the object is wedged posteriorly and cannot be brought out through the anterior naris, it is occasionally necessary to push the foreign body backwards into the nasopharynx. Before doing so the patient is placed in the tonsil position, a Boyle Davis gag is inserted, and the palate gently retracted with a soft catheter passed through the unaffected side of the nose and out through the mouth. An assistant holds the catheter while the surgeon pushes back the foreign body, at the same time watching the nasopharynx with a small laryngeal mirror. The foreign body cannot fall into the larynx because of the patient's position and the cuffed tube, and can readily be picked out of the nasopharynx with curved forceps.

Rhinoliths

These present a different problem as they are impacted and often large. It may be necessary to break up the rhinolith within the nasal fossa with forceps, and then to remove it piecemeal. This procedure should be carried out under a general anaesthetic. Rarely a rhinolith is so large that it can only be removed through a lateral rhinotomy approach. Occasionally one may even extend into the antrum, in which case a Caldwell-Luc approach is required.

References

GUPTA, S. K. and NEMA, H. V. (1970) Rhino-orbital-myiasis. *Journal of Laryngology and Otology*, **84,** 453–455
McNAB JONES, R. (1971) In *Scott-Brown's Diseases of the Ear, Nose and Throat*, 3rd edn, vol. 3, p. 41. London: Butterworths

18

The catarrhal child

A. B. Drake-Lee

The period of a child's development between the ages of 4 and 8 years, is often described as the catarrhal stage. This is because of the increased incidence of upper respiratory tract infections which is associated with the start of schooling. The otolaryngologist will spend much of his time advising the parents of normal children with these infections and it is his job to provide reassurance and to prevent unnecessary surgery, at the same time treating those whose life is handicapped by their nasal problems.

While excessive or apparently excessive mucus normally occurs between these years, it may be present from birth and continue throughout adolescence. Mucus hypersecretion is rarely found alone but is frequently associated with other nasal symptoms, particularly blockage, which may be real or apparent. It is important to evaluate all the nasal symptoms, signs and investigations, in order to give a working diagnosis and to tailor the treatment effectively. It is pointless to perform multiple nasal operations for a problem such as the immotile cilia syndrome. Children should be grouped into those who are handicapped but essentially normal and those who have a persistent underlying pathology such as allergy, cystic fibrosis and immotile cilia syndrome.

Social conditions have an effect on a child's response to illness. If they are poor and the diet inadequate, a child's resistance will be lower. Parents may also not be concerned that a child cannot clear his nose. Passive smoking may irritate the nasal mucosa in children whose parents smoke.

A rational approach will produce effective treatment and this chapter will be orientated along these lines rather than describing all the syndromes which may cause mucus hypersecretion (*Table 18.1*).

Table 18.1 The main causes of a catarrhal child

Infective rhinitis
  acute viral (recurrent)
  acute bacterial
Sinusitis
  secondary to infective rhinitis
  secondary to allergic rhinitis
  cystic fibrosis
Allergic rhinosinusitis
  inhaled
    pollinosis
    moulds
    animal danders
    house dust mite, etc.
  ingested
    animal proteins (milk)
    eggs
    additives (colourings and preservatives)
Structural
  trauma
  small nasal size (Down's syndrome)
  septal deviation
  posterior choanal stenosis and atresia
  adenoids
  tonsils
  high arched palate
Mucosal abnormalities
  abnormal mucus (Young's syndrome)
  immotile cilia (Kartagener's syndrome)
  exocrine glands (cystic fibrosis)
Immune deficiencies
  IgA and IgG subclasses

Protective function of nasal mucus

The word catarrh is derived from the Greek and means to 'flow down'. In essence it is the increased production of mucus in the upper respiratory tract and it most frequently follows infection and allergic reactions.

Mucus is the product of secretions from the nasal glands, the goblet cells and transudation from the nasal vasculature. The anterior serous glands provide little to the main secretions of the nose. Mucus contributes to all the nasal functions. It covers the nasal mucosa and provides a very effective protection from the environment. It helps physiologically to humidify the air during respiration and it aids in the transport of olfactory molecules to the special sense organs which monitor smell. Its protective function will be considered further.

Mucus is a complex substance which coats the surface of the nose and is propelled backwards by ciliary action to the nasopharynx. Mucus has two definable layers: the outer more viscous layer is above the cilia and underneath is a watery layer in which the cilia move. Abnormality or deficiency may be found in mucus or in the cilia and result in the breakdown of protection which may be temporary or, in more severe cases, permanent.

Constituents of mucus (Table 18.2)

As nasal mucus has been little studied, much of the work on it is conjectural resulting from studies of the lower airway (Widdicombe and Wells, 1982).

Table 18.2 Constituents of mucus

Water and ions from transudation
Glycoproteins: sialomucins, fucomucins, sulfomucins
Enzymes: lysozymes, lactoferrin
Circulatory proteins, complement: macroglobulin, C reactive protein
Immunoglobulins: IgA, IgE, IgG, IgM, IgD
Cells: surface epithelium, basophils, eosinophils, leucocytes

Glycoproteins

There are three main groups of glycoproteins produced by the goblet cells – the sialomucins, fucomucins and the sulfomucins. The sialomucins have some antibacterial activity over and above their contribution to the physical characteristics of mucus which provide a mechanical barrier.

Enzymes

Mucus contains a variety of enzymes and the lysozymes are particularly important. Lysozymes are produced locally from the glandular tissue and from tears which pass down the nasolacrimal duct

into the nose. The cells which are present in the mucus may contribute to the production of lysozymes, particularly macrophages and polymorphs. Lysozymes may be both bactericidal and bacteriostatic and act also with more specific systems such as complement activation and IgA-mediated immune reactions. The other main enzyme is lactoferrin which is produced by serous cells in the glands. Its mode of action is to remove iron ions from mucus and it is bacteriostatic particularly for staphylococci and pseudomonas. It is not present in serum. There are a number of other antiproteases and macromolecules which may affect bacterial colonization of the nose.

Complement

All members of the complement cascade system are found in mucus. Reactions may be triggered specifically by immunological reactions and non-specifically by non-immunological reactions. The immunological reactions require time, whereas non-immunological reactions are immediate. Both pathways act on C3 which is produced mainly in the liver, but is also found in macrophages, and the reactions cause a variety of cellular and mucosal changes. Bacterial lysis can be produced by both pathways through the action of C9. Fragments C3a and C5a act on mast cells and the resulting inflammation causes transudation of plasma protein, chemotaxis of leucocytes, activation of mast cell degranulation and phagocytosis.

Specific immunological substances

The immunoglobulins and interferon are found in nasal secretions. All the immunoglobulins may be produced locally but IgA and IgE are the main types in the surface epithelia.

IgA

This is the specific immunoglobulin for mucosal surfaces and is produced throughout the respiratory and gastrointestinal tracts. IgA is divided into two subtypes IgA_1 and IgA_2 but both will be considered together here. Nasal IgA is produced by plasma cells in the lamina propria and it is also derived from the circulation. Levels in nasal secretions are well above those of sera and show that most is produced locally. In the mucus the immunoglobulin is a dimer of two IgA molecules which are connected by a junctional chain. When it passes through the surface epithelium and glands a secretory piece is attached. The molecule is stable in mucus and forms an insoluble complex with antigen. The complexes are transported backward, swallowed and then destroyed in the stomach.

IgE

Levels of this immunoglobulin are much lower than the other classes. IgE is produced locally and is usually considered in the light of its allergic reactions which are pathological. IgE is firmly attached to the tissue mast cell and circulating basophils and two molecules of allergen-specific IgE must be located on adjacent receptor sites in the mast cell for degranulation to occur. Degranulation has two phases – the immediate, when preformed elements in the granules such as histamine are released, and the delayed, when arachidonic acid is mobilized from the cell membrane into the prostaglandins and leukotrienes. Although mast cells and circulatory basophils are found in mucus, mast cells and occasional basophils are mainly subepithelial and thus require allergen to penetrate the epithelium in normal individuals to mount a response.

IgG

This group of four subclasses is produced mainly in the lymph nodes and levels in mucus are below those found in sera. Plasma cells which produce IgG are found in nasal tissue and numbers increase during infection.

IgM

This is a large less specific macromolecule which can be produced locally but is mainly present as a result of diffusion. It is produced first, before the IgG specific to the allergen, is fabricated.

Cells in mucus

A variety of cells are present in mucus. Epithelium is continually being sloughed off and debris is particularly frequent. Infection increases the rate of turnover and other cells are found more frequently at that time. Macrophages, polymorphs, mast cells, basophils and eosinophils may be seen when mucus is stained. Numbers of each cell type vary and no cell type is diagnostic when encountered in a nasal smear. The value of nasal smears is considered later.

Conclusions

Mucus and its constituents give the respiratory tract its first line of defence. When it is penetrated the subsequent inflammation results in mucus hypersecretion which is an attempt to achieve homeostasis. The viscosity of this mucus will vary from normal depending on the different proportion of mucins present (which account for 80% of the viscosity and elasticity) and the cellular components of their products.

Microorganisms in the nose

The normal nose is not sterile and great care must be exercised when bacterial cultures are taken both from the nose and the paranasal sinuses. The main problem is to decide when an organism is truly pathological. Most information has been obtained from the anterior nares and the postnasal space; there is little information on the nasal passages. Unless technique is meticulous the postnasal swab may reflect organisms encountered in transit.

The normal nasal vestibule in a child is more frequently colonized with staphylococci, diphtheroids and Gram-negative bacteria. The nasopharynx has streptococci, *Haemophilus influenzae*, staphylococci, Gram-negative bacteria and occasionally the meningococcus. These organisms are found to a lesser extent in the normal adult. A balance exists between the organisms cultured and nasal defences. If this is lost, infection will occur as is frequently seen following a cold or in otitis media in children (Gwaltney and Hayden, 1982).

Clinical symptoms

Anterior and posterior nasal discharge

The most prominent feature of the catarrhal child is an anterior nasal discharge. It is usually bilateral and the age of onset will give some indication of the underlying pathology. It is unusual to start in the first year of life and early onset suggests a structural problem or major deficit in nasal protection. It most commonly starts around 3 years of age or later and is frequently worse in the winter when upper respiratory tract infections are more common. Normally, a child will be able to breathe through the nose to some extent even when it is severely blocked by adenoids. The presence of bubbles in the mucus on respiration indicates a patent airway. A unilateral discharge with no evidence of an airway suggests unilateral choanal atresia. Bilateral choanal atresia presents soon after birth and does not present problems with later diagnosis. A degree of stenosis will produce stasis of secretions and anterior discharge. Unilateral discharge with airflow should indicate the need for a full examination to exclude a foreign body, because, sometimes unknown to their parents, younger children put objects in their ears and noses.

Mucus is usually white or off white in colour and a change in colour can indicate infection. It is an error to assume that all yellow or green mucus is infective. Large numbers of eosinophils will colour the mucus yellow or light green. If infection is to be diagnosed and mucus evaluated correctly then a culture should be taken and a smear made of the material. It is a very easy and a frequently made mistake to dismiss children with greenish secretion and abnormal sinus radiographs as suffering from sinusitis and then to submit them for surgery. Results are unimpressive because allergic reactions may well be at the root of the problem particularly since a large number of children suffer from allergic diathesis.

Frequent colds with a greenish discharge do suggest infection which is usually a secondary bacterial infection and probably colonized from the organisms normally resident in the anterior and postnasal space (*Table 18.3*). It is unfortunate

Table 18.3 Bacterial contamination of the nasal cavities by potential pathogens

Staphylococcus aureus	30%
Streptococcus pneumoniae	50%
Streptococcus pyogenes	50%
Haemophilus influenzae	20%
Neisseria meningitidis	5%
Gram-negative bacilli	6%

Some noses contain more than one pathogen.
These figures are approximate.

that many children make no effort to clear their noses and so the infection persists for longer than is necessary. Usually such children are not distressed by their nasal condition and cope perfectly satisfactorily at school. They have no demonstrable airway obstruction and surgery is inappropriate. The upper respiratory tract infections which start around the onset of schooling may be very frequent and distress the parents. They may be improved surgically if the child is handicapped for more than 2 years and has airway obstruction.

If the discharge is associated with nasal irritation, eye problems, eczema or asthma, it is probably caused by an allergic diathesis. Children either rub their noses upwards or sideways depending on habit. Similarly they can cause traumatic epistaxis by putting their fingers up their noses to relieve the irritation and to improve the nasal congestion. Cautery does not solve this problem except temporarily.

The natural ciliary action should clear the mucus backwards. An anterior discharge when the airway is patent either indicates excessive mucus with which the normal mechanisms cannot cope or impaired ciliary mobility.

Postnasal drip is much more common in adults: this may be because children do not complain of the problem. Parents will complain that the child is often full of catarrh, snorts, sniffs or clears his throat. The mucus hypersecretion may be present in the pharynx and trachea and produce a chronic cough. There is no evidence that nasal mucus

flows down into the larynx and the trachea. Adenoidectomy has not been shown to improve a chronic cough.

Nasal blockage

Nasal blockage is frequently encountered in children and it is up to the surgeon to determine whether the blockage is real or apparent. Young children do not complain of nasal blockage and usually it is only significant if the child has problems eating and persistent snoring. Snoring may be present even when the airway is apparently satisfactory. The problem is caused by the tonsils prolapsing backwards at rest. This may only become apparent during induction of anaesthesia, and is easily overcome by the insertion of an oral airway. Blockage may fluctuate or be seasonal and even young children may develop hay fever. A considerable number of children have apparent blockage and this can be demonstrated easily with a metal spatula which shows a normal misting pattern and thus prevents the unnecessary removal of a child's adenoids. Some children will have an exaggerated nasal cycle and the blockage will fluctuate. If in doubt a lateral radiograph of the postnasal space will indicate the size of the adenoids.

The nasal cycle

The nasal cycle is easy to demonstrate in adults and occurs every 4–12 hours (Kayser, 1895). Roughly, the overall airflow is constant for both sides when added together but varies from side to side. It is easily suppressed by exercise, emotion, infection and medication. The effect of infection is temporary. The cycle is more difficult to demonstrate in children but there is evidence to suggest it does occur in the majority of children (Cawenberg and Deleye, 1984). It is important to bear this in mind when examining a child's nose because the cross-sectional area is small. Any structural abnormality such as a slight septal deviation will cause complete blockage at times. Treatment to cure the nasal cycle will end in failure.

Epistaxis

Nose bleeds are common in children and it is assumed generally that these are the result of congested or abnormal vessels in Little's area. Children with chronic rhinitis have nose bleeds simply because they traumatize the nasal mucosa with their fingers while trying to stop the irritation. Crusting and picking also cause trauma and bleeding. It is pointless to cauterize such noses and control of the rhinitis solves the problem. Sprays may also dry the mucosa excessively and cause bleeding; in particular freon propellants have been implicated.

Pain

Children do not tend to complain of maxillary or facial pain. Its absence is similar to lack of symptoms in otitis media where children may have an acute episode with apparently little pain. Anatomically, the sinuses are smaller or absent and so may not produce as much in the way of symptoms as in adulthood.

Sneezing

The most frequent cause of repeated sneezing is allergy. Children suffer both irritation and sneezing and tend to rub their noses. Sneezing is associated with foreign bodies, viral rhinitis, chemical and other irritants. Older children may have fake sneezing and apparently sneeze for weeks. It is an hysterical symptom comparable to aphonia.

Anosmia

Children do not complain of anosmia and parents are unable to gauge how well a child can smell because they rarely notice any problem.

Halitosis

Bad breath results from excessive mucus, infection in the nose and paranasal sinuses, from nasal blockage and secondary obstruction by the tonsils and adenoids, and is usually worse in the morning. Parents frequently complain about this condition. Treatment depends on the underlying problem.

General health and development

When any child who is catarrhal is assessed it is most important to evaluate the general health, social skills and development of the child. If a child is healthy, socially adjusted and performing well at school there is little that probably needs to be done apart from reassuring the parents. Nasal and upper aerodigestive problems may cause severe educational and social problems and debilitate a child so that he or she does not grow

well. These children need prompt action which is frequently surgical if they are to develop their full potential. The ill child needs to be assessed carefully to ensure that there is no more serious pathology underlying the cause of his upper respiratory problems.

Examination

An overall assessment of the child will show if there is any developmental syndrome which may be associated with nasal problems, such as Down's syndrome. The general size, development and facial features should be evaluated.

It is most useful clinically to divide children into those who have nasal symptoms, particularly anterior discharge with nasal obstruction, and those who have a patent airway. It is pointless giving inhalational sprays to completely obstructed noses. When children suffer from nasal obstruction, the doctor should have the site of obstruction clearly in his mind by the end of the consultation. Obstruction may be a consequence of the size of the nose, the anterior nasal valve, the turbinates, septum, foreign body, the posterior choana, the postnasal space, and finally the oropharynx and palate. Once the level of obstruction is known then the decision has to be made whether the obstruction is the major symptom or if it is secondary to an underlying problem which, when cured, will relieve the obstruction.

The nasal airflow can be assessed very simply and objectively by asking the child to breathe through the nose and by watching the misting pattern on a nasal spatum (*Figure 18.1*). Many children who mouth breathe will have no nasal obstruction and the habit has been picked up following previous episodes of obstruction. Children will continue to mouth breathe after ade-

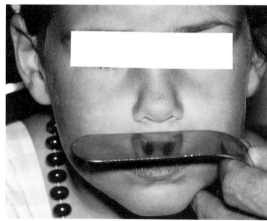

Figure 18.1 Normal misting pattern

noidectomy but the symptom eventually will resolve.

The thumb can be used to turn the tip of the nose upwards and because the structures are so elastic a metal speculum is rarely needed. The secretions, septum and turbinates and colour of the mucosa may be assessed.

Secretions

Secretions may be obvious at the time of examination and are either unilateral or bilateral. They may be profuse or scanty, mucoid or clear. If they are infected or if an eosinophilia is present they may be yellow or green. Often the secretions are not present at the time of interview. They may be confined to the nasal passages or may be seen to originate from the middle meatus. If the secretions come from the middle meatus then the maxillary sinuses are involved. When the oral cavity is examined, mucus may be seen in the postnasal space.

Intranasal examination

Besides the airflow and secretions, it is important to examine the mucosa and the nasal structure. The mucosa may be normal, congested or hypertrophied and its colour may vary from bright red to deep blue. The septum, lateral cartilages, turbinates and postnasal space should be examined. The postnasal space is frequently difficult to examine in younger children and the child should not be upset by any medical procedure if at all possible.

It is possible to obtain some idea of structural obstruction and it may be caused by previous nasal trauma resulting in nasal or septal deformity. The anterior nasal valve may be small and the nose generally smaller. Polyps are unusual and if present in the infant may be caused by herniation or ectopic tissue from the anterior cranial fossa. Polyps in older children should be investigated to exclude cystic fibrosis. An antrochoanal polyp may be seen and is associated with an opaque maxillary sinus radiograph. It may be possible to determine the presence of choanal stenosis, but usually this requires general anaesthesia. Unilateral choanal atresia may be diagnosed radiologically when radiopaque dye is placed in the nose. A computerized tomographic scan will show whether the obstruction is membranous or bony. The remaining examination will show if the adenoids and tonsils are contributing to nasal obstruction and adenoid enlargement may restrict palatal movement. The soft palate may also be poorly developed and the hard palate highly arched restricting the nasal size. Syndromes such as Down's, are associated with small noses, large tongues and such children are catarrhal.

The examination will give four different parameters which may be assessed in making the diagnosis and initiating the subsequent treatment: the airflow, the nature and extent of secretions, the state of the mucosa, and the structure of the nose itself.

Investigations (*Table 18.4*)

Many children require no investigation to evaluate their nasal problems. The following investigations may be of benefit in selected cases.

Table 18.4 Investigations for the catarrhal child

Full blood count and differential white cell count
Serum immunoglobulins, IgA and IgG subclasses
Complement levels
Radioallergosorbent test (RAST), allergen specific IgE
Radiographs of the sinus, postnasal space and chest
Ultrasound of the maxillary sinuses
Nasal clearance
Nasal smears
Skin tests

Blood investigations

A full blood count will demonstrate acute infection, anaemia or eosinophilia which may be present occasionally in gross allergic disease. Recurrent infections may be a consequence of leukaemia or more rarely immune deficiency. If the latter is suspected then the serum immunoglobulins may prove useful. A temporary deficiency may occur during some infections so any abnormal result requires confirmation. Any obvious medical problem should be corrected before surgery is contemplated. Total and allergen specific levels of serum IgE may be helpful occasionally in difficult allergic problems or if the diagnosis is unclear. Unfortunately there is considerable overlap in the levels of total IgE between the normal and allergic patients. The radioallergosorbent test which is allergen specific is of more value in cases where multiple skin tests are positive or food allergy is suspected.

Radiology

Routine sinus radiographs including the postnasal space may be of value, particularly when there is some degree of nasal obstruction. The relative size of the adenoids may be determined and this helps when the nasal mucosa is congested as a result of secondary stasis of secretions. Unfortunately, one-third of all children have some degree of mucosal thickening of the maxillary antrum which makes interpretation difficult. Assessment should be made of the development of all the sinuses, the bony walls, the presence and degree of mucosal thickening and fluid levels. A completely opaque sinus suggests a significant problem. In the older male an angiofibroma may cause anterior bowing of the posterior wall of the maxillary sinus. If bony erosion is suspected then computerized tomography is needed. Any suspected neoplasm or anterior cranial fossa defects also require computerized tomography to be undertaken.

A normal sinus radiograph does not exclude maxillary sinusitis if mucopus or pus is seen to originate from the middle meatus. The necessary steps should be taken to exclude infection by proof puncture.

A chest X-ray may show changes of bronchiectasis, and dextrocardia which is associated with cilial abnormalities.

Transillumination and ultrasound

The vogue for transillumination of the maxillary sinuses with an oral light source has now passed. The subject was studied in a darkened room, the side with less light suggesting more antral disease. Unfortunately, there are too many variables such as different tissue thickness, bony development, teeth development and inter- and intrasubject variability for any reliability to be placed on the results.

Ultrasound now occupies the place of transillumination. There is little published work confined to children, but studies of adults show it to be no better than radiology for patients with chronic sinus disease (Pfleiderer, Drake-Lee and Lowe, 1984). It gives far less structural information and its only theoretical advantage is the lack of a minute dosage of radiation.

Nasal clearance

If ciliary abnormality is suspected, the simplest test of nasal ciliary clearance is the saccharine transit time. It has been thought to be unreliable but when performed by someone familiar with nasal anatomy and able to use both hands to examine a patient, it is reproducible. The saccharine should be placed behind the first 1 cm of the inferior turbinate. Only a small particle is used and the time taken for the patient to notice a sweet taste is noted. The usual interval is under 20 minutes. Older children will be able to undertake

the test, and it is possible to perform it on 5 year olds and sometimes on 4 year olds (Andersen *et al.*, 1974).

Nasal smears

The value of nasal smears is underrated in the UK. Mucus may be collected by blowing out or mopping the inside of the nose and smearing the swab on a slide. When fixed and stained the slide may be evaluated to see the number of eosinophils, polymorphs, leucocytes, basophils and epithelial cells. The presence of polymorphs and leucocytes indicates infection whereas eosinophils indicate either allergy or rhinitis. Its value lies in helping to categorize nasal disease and preventing unnecessary surgery. It also requires someone who is experienced at examining the films.

Skin tests

Many parents are worried that allergy may be responsible for the symptoms in their child. Skin tests by the prick method are simple to perform, cause no significant morbidity and, if negative, help reassure parents. The tests provide a simple working classification by categorizing patients into two groups: those who are atopic and liable to have allergic reactions and those who are non-atopic where allergy is much less likely. While they give limited information on the nature of the allergen they demonstrate the type of reaction occurring in the nose and are useful when counselling parents.

Differential diagnosis

The causes of nasal symptoms are many, only the common and more frequently found of the rarer causes will be discussed. Although the causes may be divided into congenital or acquired ones, the approach used here will consider the different areas from which disease may arise, such as infection, allergy, structural variability and abnormality, and finally mucosal abnormalities (*see Table 18.1*).

Two causes may coexist in the same child, for example an allergic child may suffer from recurrent viral rhinitis.

Infective rhinitis

There are a large number of viruses which can cause infective rhinitis and rhinoviruses have many different antigenic serotypes. The main groups are rhinoviruses, coronaviruses, respiratory syncytial virus, influenza and parainfluenza viruses, enteroviruses, and adenoviruses. All except the last are RNA viruses. Adenoviruses may chronically infect the lymphoid tissue of children and may explain some chronic symptoms in the absence of any response to antibiotics. The most common cause of chronicity is recurrent infection. Viral infections lower the normal nasal resistance to bacterial invasion, thus a secondary bacterial infection may develop. It can become persistent in the nose and sinuses. Infection causes mucus hypersecretion, and as a result of prolonged infections a child becomes catarrhal, particularly if adenoidal hypertrophy is marked and prevents the free drainage of mucus posteriorly. Unfortunately, recurrent viral infections do not respond to treatment and there is a great degree of variability between individuals and their susceptibility.

If the adenoids are causing problems because of obstruction then removal will help to resolve the prolonged catarrhal stage.

Sinusitis

Perhaps the most overworked diagnosis in current otolaryngological practice is chronic bacterial sinusitis. Undoubtedly in the preantibiotic era it was a common entity and was associated with poor nutrition and social conditions. It is similar in this respect to recurrent acute otitis media and mastoiditis. Mucosal congestion, oedema and mucus hypersecretion may affect the sinuses as well as the nose, but unless the ostia of the sinuses are blocked for a prolonged period, infection will not persist. The contents of the sinuses are rarely purulent on wash out and no studies have shown conclusively that surgical enthusiasm in the sinuses is effective in hastening resolution of the mucosal changes.

Allergic rhinitis

Although rhinitis can be caused by a large number of allergens a simple classification can be devised if the allergens can be identified from the history and investigations. Three main groups of inhaled allergens are:

(1) grass and tree pollens and moulds
(2) animal allergens
(3) the perennial allergens, house dust mite, its faeces and moulds.

Ingested allergens such as food additives and dyes, and milk products may also cause nasal symptoms and diagnosis is by exclusion and re-introduction into the diet. Treatment is by avoidance and, in selected cases, topical nasal medication, systemic therapy and, in a very few cases, surgical procedures.

Non-allergic or vasomotor rhinitis

This condition is less common in children, but in some there is an eosinophilia in the nasal secretion in the absence of any allergen. The condition is sometimes labelled non-allergic rhinitis with eosinophilic secretions (NARES!). All that can be said is that non-allergic rhinitis probably comprises a miscellaneous collection of entities. If turbinate obstruction is the major problem then these patients may be best treated surgically.

Structural variation and abnormality

Considerable variation of nasal size is encountered both within and between racial groups. The smaller the nose the more likely obstruction becomes. Change in diameter will cause symptoms and in a certain number of children it will be the main contributing factor. The smallest cross-sectional area is the external nasal valve, trauma will cause trouble if the septum is dislocated or a haematoma develops and organizes. The child's nose is smaller and more malleable than the adults and is also more resistant to trauma.

Although the anterior diameter is smallest, posterior stenosis or atresia will cause stasis of secretions. If atresia is bilateral it presents at or soon after birth. Unilateral atresia may not be diagnosed until the early teens. Adenoids, if grossly enlarged, will block the posterior choana as will hypertrophy of the posterior ends of the turbinates. An antrochoanal polyp will block both sides of the nose if very large.

Palate size and mobility may cause symptoms, and this may be a problem in Down's syndrome. Children with Down's syndrome have nasal symptoms for a variety of reasons including small nasal size, increase in connective tissue bulk and a large tongue which restricts palate movement. The problem is refractory.

Mucosal abnormalities

Nasal disease may result from abnormalities of the protective mechanisms. The commonest faults are immotile cilia, exocrine gland abnormality and immunodeficiency. They are not found frequently and may be overlooked.

Temporary ciliary paralysis occurs with acute infection but quickly reverts to normal. In chronic infection it may be difficult to determine whether paralysis is primary or secondary. The abnormality involves both the nose and the paranasal sinuses. The value of the intranasal antrostomy has been questioned as a result of ciliary motility studies in the normal sinuses: it must be remembered that ciliary paralysis is one of the first mucosal abnormalities in infection, and this invalidates these studies. Stasis of secretions with ciliary paralysis causes the maxillary sinus to act as a sump. Treatment by either indwelling cannulae or antrostomy may well aid resolution.

Immotile cilia syndrome

This was first described by Kartagener (1933) and it is now seen to be related to a primary ciliary abnormality. The internal ultrastructure of the cilia is responsible for activity. A central pair of microtubules is surrounded by nine similar pairs which are connected by dynein arms. The central microtubules are connected to the peripheral pairs by radial spokes and the dynein arms are arranged in inner and outer pairs. An inherited lack of intracellular ATPase is the cause of immotile cilia in those where there is no obvious ultrastructural deficit. In severe cases marked abnormalities of the microtubular system are seen.

The syndrome may present as infertility, with immotile sperms, sinusitis and bronchitis, and situs inversus in one-half of the cases. A chest X-ray is useful in diagnosis.

Patients can present from infancy onwards and any child who has had mucopurulent nasal discharge for a long time, particularly if there is no obvious nasal obstruction, should have chest and sinus radiographs taken. If the radiograph is normal and the child is old enough ciliary clearance and biopsy of the inferior turbinates may be carried out. Material is best fixed for electron microscopy in gluteraldehyde 2.5% with magnesium phosphate buffer (Fox, Bull and Arden, 1980). Ciliary abnormality is frequently observed in normal nasal mucosa and so over one-half of the cilia should be abnormal.

Treatment of the condition is difficult. The maxillary antrum acts as a sump and drainage may be required. Removal of the mucosa will rarely produce any more than the most temporary benefit. A long-term patent antrostomy is difficult to achieve in children.

The rhinosinusitis and bronchitis occur together and treatment of the sinus appears to have little effect on the chest. Vigorous antibiotic therapy will improve both conditions and long-term therapy may be required.

Young's syndrome

Sinusitis, bronchitis and infertility result from abnormally viscous mucus. The condition is similar to Kartagener's syndrome but spermatazoa are mobile and ciliary activity is normal unless destroyed by recurrent infection.

Cystic fibrosis

One-third of children with cystic fibrosis have nasal symptoms and under 10% develop nasal polyps (Shwackhman *et al.*, 1962). In mild cases, nasal polyps may be the first sign of the disease. They are rare in children under 10 years of age and when seen, children should have cystic fibrosis excluded by a sweat test. Mucopurulent rhinorrhoea is the commonest symptom and is associated with blockage. The endocrine glands produce an abnormal mucus which does not give the usual protection and leads to recurrent infection.

Radiographs of the sinuses are abnormal in virtually all children with cystic fibrosis. Culture of wash out material is sterile or similar to those organisms usually encountered in the sinuses. There is no correlation between bacterial culture from the sputum and those from the sinus which indicates that the sinuses do not constitute a reservoir for chest infection.

Glue ear is no more frequent than to be expected for the general population and argues against the belief that sinus disease predisposes to glue ears (Taylor, Evans and Hope, 1974).

Treatment of cases is symptomatic and conservative, extensive sinus surgery has not been shown to be of any benefit in children with severe recurrent nasal polyps. If mucosal disease is

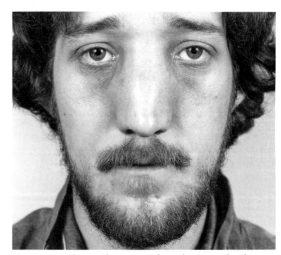

Figure 18.2 Hypertelorism resulting from nasal polyps which developed before the symphyses of the bones of the facial skeleton had fused

severe and occurs before the symphyses are fused, the pressure in the ethmoids results in expansion in the base of the skull and so hypertelorism will be produced (*Figure 18.2*).

Glue ear (otitis media with effusion)

Glue ear is frequently called catarrhal otitis media. Changes in the respiratory mucosa of the middle ear cleft result in goblet cell hyperplasia and the prolonged presence of mucus in the middle ear cleft. Its pathogenesis and management is considered elsewhere (Chapter 12).

Treatment

The treatment of the catarrhal child depends on the underlying cause. Many children will not be easily classified and so a general approach to treatment is required.

Although many medical practitioners feel that chronic rhinitis is trivial, it causes morbidity and distress to children and parents. Children will put up with symptoms which are treatable and the general ill health may affect schooling and subsequent achievements. The first goal is to determine which children require treatment and which parents have difficulty in coping with normal children.

Chronic rhinitis may be divided conveniently into three types – allergic, non-allergic and infective – which may be found singly or in combination.

Allergic rhinitis

Avoidance

The inhaled allergens can be avoided to some degree. Domestic animals should be excluded from the sleeping area if symptoms are trivial or removed from the home altogether if severe asthma coexists. It may be possible to minimize seasonal allergic symptoms by keeping the child indoors and the windows closed. Children who are sensitive to house dust mite can have their lives made a misery by excessive allergen avoidance. Changing the bedding, vacuuming the mattress weekly and covering it with polythene reduces the contamination of allergen.

Food allergy can cause problems, but although it is a fashionable diagnosis, it is difficult to prove and can only be satisfactorily diagnosed by removing the suspected allergen from the diet and reintroducing it after a period of 2–4 weeks. Diets may be worth trying if the parents are willing, the rhinitis does not have an inhaled allergic element

and is non-infective. Books on diets are available but the allergens can be simply grouped into areas – milk and its products, eggs, animal meat proteins and finally dyes and added preservatives. Certain products advertise the lack of colouring and preservatives and if in doubt books can be bought listing all the E numbers used for identifying additives; for example E102 is tartrazine. Very occasionally spectacular results are achieved if one of these major groups is excluded from the diet.

Desensitizing

The only allergen which has been shown to be effectively controlled by desensitization is mixed grass pollen. There is a definite risk of anaphylaxis and so adrenaline, corticosteroids, and antihistamines should be available when desensitizing injections are administered. Desensitization should only be given to older children and to adolescents. Dust mite desensitization has no proven place in management and is not used by the author.

Non-allergic rhinitis

Topical medical treatment

Both allergic and non-allergic rhinitis respond to topical medical medication. Children under the age of 5 years do not comply well with sprays or nose drops.

Vasoactive compounds

These are of use occasionally in recurrent acute infection, unfortunately they are freely available and, although not subject to the same misuse as in adults, may cause rhinitis medicamentosa.

Corticosteroids

Corticosteroids may be used after the age of 5 years and have not been shown to have any side-effects even if used for up to 3 months. A 3-month trial may cause a break in the cycle of congestion and secretion and resolve the rhinitis completely. The same sprays may be used as in adults, for example flunisolide and beclomethasone. The dose should be halved for younger children.

Sodium cromoglycate

This may be tried for the treatment of non-allergic and allergic rhinitis but its main disadvantage is the need for application four times a day. It has the theoretical advantage of being free from the side-effects that corticosteroids may induce.

All sprays should be given one week before the presumed start of the hay fever season since this gives better control. If patients have nose and eye symptoms it is preferable to use two topical medications than an oral antihistamine.

Systemic medication

Systemic medication may be divided into decongestants, antihistamines, mucolytics and antibiotics. Apart from antibiotics which have a distinct role in infection, there is little evidence that other medications have a proven place in the management of the catarrhal child. Pressure from parents ensures that they are widely prescribed. If the child has an allergic history the antihistamines may be useful in some cases. There are no guidelines on when and how to prescribe decongestants, mucolytics and antihistamines and personal choice plays a large part in therapy. Except in the severest cases the author does not prescribe any medication, and usually starts with a decongestant followed by a combined preparation which includes an antihistamine. There are virtually no indications for systemic corticosteroids in younger children although they may improve nasal symptoms dramatically.

Antibiotics

Antibiotics are widely and indiscriminately prescribed to children with nasal symptoms. Unless there is a diagnosed disease such as cystic fibrosis, mucociliary abnormality or immunodeficiency, antibiotics should be withheld in the first instance.

Since the anterior nares harbour bacteria in health, nasal swabs are of limited value. A nasal cytology smear gives more reliable evidence of infection. Despite parental pressure to prescribe, most mucoid discharge is not infective and there is no evidence that antibiotics help in this condition. A persistent profuse bilateral green discharge in the absence of allergy should be treated with broad spectrum antibiotics for 10 days. Other factors such as poor housing, and nutritional and social factors may be more important in the perseverance of symptoms.

Systemic antibiotics may be required in chronic disease states and may help prevent chronic sinusitis and irreversible lung disease in patients with mucociliary abnormality.

Surgery

Unfortunately much unnecessary surgery is performed on children, and often on an *ad hoc* basis before the surgeon is clear in his own mind exactly why the child is having symptoms. The indica-

tions for adenoidectomy and tonsillectomy are discussed elsewhere in this volume as is surgery for other problems such as choanal atresia.

Chronically hypertrophied inferior turbinates respond to submucus diathermy if the child is not allergic. Some surgeons prefer to trim or remove turbinates.

Unless there is major nasal deformity following trauma, the septum should not be corrected or resected since deformity will be increased during the pubertal growth spurt.

Infection of the maxillary sinus may be improved by irrigation and the insertion of indwelling cannulae. The intranasal antrostomy is of limited value since it will be closed within 12 months.

Conclusion

The catarrhal stage is common and many children outgrow it without any treatment. The place of the otolaryngologist is in recognizing those patients who are abnormally handicapped or who have an underlying abnormality. A logical approach will prevent unnecessary surgery and will give the correct diagnosis.

References

ANDERSEN, I., CAMNER, P., JENSEN, P., PHILIPSON, K. and PROCTOR, D. (1974) A comparison of nasal and tracheobronchial clearance. *Archives of Environmental Health*, **29**, 290–293

CAWENBERG, P. B. and DELEYE, L. (1984) Nasal cycle in children. *Archives of Otolaryngology*, **110**, 108–110

FOX, B., BULL, T. and ARDEN, G. (1980) Variations in the ultrastructure of human nasal cilia including abnormalities found in retinitis pigmentosa. *Journal of Clinical Pathology*, **30**, 277–335

GWALTNEY, J. and HAYDEN, F. (1982) The nose and infection. In *The Nose: Upper Airway Physiology and the Atmospheric Environment*, edited by D. Proctor and I. Andersen, pp. 399–422. Amsterdam: Elsevier

KARTAGENER, M. (1933) Zur pathogenese der bronchiektasien, I Bronchiektagein bei situ inversus. *Beitrage zur Klinik Tuberkulose und Spezifishem Tuberkulose-forschung*, **83**, 489–501

KAYSER, R. (1895) Die exacte messung der luftdurchgangikeit der nase. *Archives of Laryngology*, **3**, 101–210

PFLEIDERER, A., DRAKE-LEE, A. and LOWE, D. (1984) Ultrasound of the sinuses: a worthwhile procedure. *Clinical Otolaryngology*, **9**, 335–339

SHWACKHMAN, H., KUKZYCHI, I., MUELLER, H. and FLAKE, C. (1962) Nasal polyps in patients with cystic fibrosis. *Paediatrics*, **30**, 389–401

TAYLOR, B., EVANS, J. and HOPE, G. (1974) Upper respiratory tract in cystic fibrosis. *Archives of Diseases in Childhood*, **49**, 133–136

WIDDICOMBE, E. and WELLS, H. (1982) Airway secretions in the nose. In *The Nose, Upper Airway Physiology and the Atmospheric Environment*, edited by D. Proctor and I. Andersen, pp. 215–244. Amsterdam: Elsevier

19

Angiofibroma

O. H. Shaheen

Definition

The term *angiofibroma* denotes a vascular swelling presenting in the nasopharynx of prepubertal and adolescent males and exhibiting a tendency to bleed. Alternative titles such as juvenile angiofibroma, nasopharyngeal fibroma, bleeding fibroma of adolescence and fibroangioma have largely been superseded by the simpler label of angiofibroma. They are, nevertheless, acceptable since they refer to the basic features of the condition and are not likely to be misinterpreted.

Much of the previous literature concerning aetiology and treatment was speculative and controversial, but a clearer picture of the nature of these swellings, their site of origin, behaviour, and safer management has emerged in recent years.

Background

At one time, the impression existed that the prevalence of angiofibromata was higher in certain parts of the world, for example the Middle East and the Americas, than in northwestern Europe where it was considered to be quite low. It is probable that such an assumption was arrived at by equating large reported series from specific centres with a high geographical prevalence. The series reported by Shaheen (1930), Figi (1940) and Handousa, Farid and Elwi (1954) are classical examples of major centres drawing cases from far and wide and suggesting a disproportionately high incidence of angiofibromata for the areas in question.

The ratio of angiofibromata to other ear, nose and throat conditions, as culled from diagnostic registers, is likely to show wide variations, even

between hospitals within a single large conurbation, and is therefore valueless as a guide to the prevalence of the condition. Martin, Ehrlich and Abels (1948) reported an annual admission rate of one or two cases for the 2000 or so cases seen in the head and neck service of the Memorial Hospital, New York, but with a formidable reputation such as that of the Memorial Hospital, it would not be surprising if it received a far larger number of referrals than a lesser institution of comparable size within the same city.

In London, Harrison (1976) recorded the figure of one per 15 000 patients at the Royal National Throat, Nose and Ear Hospital which might prompt one to conclude that there are fewer angiofibromata in London than in New York. However, the two situations are not comparable and, in any case, the large number of London teaching hospitals, existing as a counterweight to the Royal National Hospital, are likely to share in a fairer distribution of cases, so that even if the influx of tumours per hospital is small, the collective total might match that of any large metropolis.

Some doubt has been cast about the authenticity of certain of the series reported in the past, the main objections being questionable histology, and the inclusion of females and patients of extreme age among genuine cases.

There is now general agreement that this is exclusively a disease of males and that the mean age at presentation is around 14 years (Harrison, 1976). The range, however, is wide and varies between 7 and 19 years (Martin, Ehrlich and Abels, 1948) with isolated cases presenting earlier or later.

Many of the older reports implied that patients suffering from the condition displayed signs of delayed maturity as judged by secondary sexual characteristics, and that tumour pathogenesis was somehow linked to this. The regression which was observed with age or supposedly under the influence of hormones, was cited as evidence of an hormonal aetiology, but was never supported by objective biochemical signs of hormonal insufficiency.

The suggestion that total regression occurs in the late teens or early twenties has never been convincingly demonstrated, although most authorities concede that some shrinkage, hardening and loss of vascularity of the swellings occur with age.

The lack of complete regression could well explain the inclusion of older patients in some of the earlier reports, and would exonerate their authors of the charge of having misdiagnosed such cases.

Pathology

Grossly, angiofibromata appear as firm, slightly spongy lobulated swellings, the nodularity of which increases with age. The colour varies *in vivo* from pink to white. That part which can be seen in the nasopharynx and is therefore covered by mucous membrane is invariably pink, whereas those parts which have escaped to adjacent extrapharyngeal areas are often white or grey. On section, the tumour has a reticulated, whorled or spongy appearance, and lacks a true capsule. The edge, however, is sharply demarcated and easily distinguishable from the surrounding tissues.

Microscopically, the picture is of vascular spaces of varying shape and size abounding in a stroma of fibrous tissue, the relative proportions of which alter with the age of the swelling. In the younger lesion, the vascular component stands out as an all-pervasive feature, whereas in the older swellings collagen predominates. It would seem that, as one strays from the heart of the tumour, the fibrous tissue element overshadows the vascular.

The vascular pattern consists of large thin-walled sinusoidal vessels lined by flattened epithelium, unsupported by a muscular coat, and the closer these are to the surface of the swelling, the smaller they become.

In older swellings, there is a tendency towards gradual compression of the sinusoids so that the lining endothelial cells are pushed against each other like cords, while in others intravascular thrombosis occurs (Hubbard, 1958).

The stroma is composed of coarse parallel wavy or interlacing bundles of collagen in which stromal cells are seen to radiate outwards from the vessels (Steinberg, 1954) and in which localized areas of myxomatous degeneration may be observed.

Pathogenesis

A number of theories have been propounded over the years to explain the origin of angiofibromata and, although one or two are seemingly plausible, none is entirely convincing.

Ringertz (1938) suggested that the tumour arose from the periosteum of the nasopharyngeal vault, while Som and Neffson (1940) believed that inequalities in the growth of the bones forming the skull base resulted in hypertrophy of the underlying periosteum in response to hormonal influences. Bensch and Ewing (1941) thought that the tumour probably arose from embryonic fibrocartilage between the basiocciput and basisphenoid, whereas Brunner (1942) suggested an origin from the conjoined pharyngobasilar and buccopharyngeal fascia.

More plausibly, Osborn (1959) considered two alternatives, namely the possibility that the swellings were either hamartomata, or residues of fetal erectile tissue which were subject to hormonal influences.

Girgis and Fahmy (1973) noted cell nests of undifferentiated epithelioid cells or 'zellballen' at the growing edge of angiofibromata, an appearance which they likened to paragangliomata. They also commented on the existence of paragangliomatous tissue around the terminal part of the maxillary artery in the pterygopalatine fossa of stillborn infants and put forward the view that these might be the forerunners of angiofibromata.

With the possibility of vascular malformations still in mind, it would not be too far fetched to suggest that angiofibromata might arise from vestiges of the atrophied stapedial artery, although clearly it is not possible to validate such an assertion.

Site of origin and behaviour of angiofibromata

It was previously assumed that the vault of the nasopharynx was the most likely site of origin because of the broad-based attachment to the skull base which is so typical of the majority of swellings. Others considered the choana to be a more probable site in view of the frequency with which both nasopharynx and nasal fossa are involved, but failed to specify the precise point of origin.

Modern methods of investigation and ambitious surgical procedures have focused attention on the region of the sphenopalatine foramen as the site of origin which would most reasonably explain the subsequent behaviour of angiofibromata. This is based on the observation that larger tumours present as bilobed dumb-bell swellings straddling the sphenopalatine foramen, with one component filling the nasopharynx and the other extending out into the pterygopalatine and infratemporal fossae. The central stalk joining the two portions occupies the sphenopalatine foramen at the upper end of the vertical plate of the palatine bone, without appearing to enlarge it very much. In the absence of any significant degree of erosion of the sphenopalatine foramen, the only logical way that such a dumb-bell arrangement can come about is if the rudiment of the swelling were to be either in or very close to the foramen.

The seedling swelling arising from such a site would migrate medially beneath the mucous membrane of the nasopharynx, displacing it downwards in the process, and eventually growing to fill the postnasal space. As the process of growth continues, the anterior face of the sphenoidal sinus is encroached upon and eroded, and the sinus is invaded. The swelling then follows the line of least resistance and grows forwards into the nasal fossa where it may acquire secondary attachments. Having filled the nasal fossa it will displace the nasal septum over to the opposite side, so that the healthy side of the nose also becomes blocked.

Growth in a lateral direction may take place in some cases, and the starting point is once again the sphenopalatine foramen. The pterygopalatine fossa is thus invaded and, once filled, causes forward bowing of the posterior wall of the antrum. Eventually, the swelling comes to occupy the infratemporal fossa and when insufficient room remains for further expansion, it will encroach on the orbital fissures.

However, this is not to say that every angiofibroma behaves in this way; indeed, some remain confined to the nasopharynx but usually with a bias towards one side.

That portion of a bilobed angiofibroma which lies outside the nasopharynx eventually becomes very hard and nodular, and in the course of its spread into the pterygopalatine and infratemporal fossae may well erode the anterior face of the greater wing of the sphenoid so as to make contact with the dura of the middle fossa. It may displace the maxillary nerve upwards, and less commonly the optic nerve, and if it invades the orbit through the posteriorly placed fissures of that cavity, will eventually cause proptosis. The main blood supply to angiofibromata comes by way of an enlarged maxillary artery, but other arteries, such as the ascending pharyngeal, vidian, unnamed branches of the internal carotid and rarely the vertebral, may contribute to its vascularization.

Symptoms and signs

The two cardinal symptoms of angiofibroma are nasal obstruction and intermittent epistaxis. The latter may vary in severity from the occasional show to an alarming and sometimes life-threatening torrent. Chronic anaemia is thus a common feature of the established condition.

It should be stressed that the bleeding which is so characteristic of much of the surgery of angiofibroma is caused by breaking into the parenchyma of the swelling or by disrupting the feeding vessels, whereas the bleeding which occurs prior to operation is entirely spontaneous and usually unconnected with trauma.

The completeness of nasal obstruction is such that stasis of secretions and sepsis are virtually inevitable, followed by hyposmia or anosmia.

The voice acquires a nasal intonation and, if the swelling is large enough to force the soft palate down, there may be an added plummy quality to it. Blockage of the eustachian tube is not uncommon in such a situation and leads to deafness and otalgia.

Anterior rhinoscopy is likely to confirm the presence of abundant purulent secretions together with bowing of the nasal septum to the uninvolved side. Posterior rhinoscopy in the cooperative relaxed patient should display a pink or red mass filling the nasopharynx, but the bulk of the lesion is generally such that it is not often possible to ascertain the site of attachment.

Gross physical signs are evident when extensive disease has involved the nose and infratemporal fossa, the nasal bones being splayed out and there is obvious swelling in the temple and cheek. Intraoral palpation in the interval between the ascending ramus of the mandible and the side of the maxilla may also reveal the tell-tale thickening of disease which has crept round the back of the antrum.

Impaction of bulky disease in the infratemporal fossa results in extreme signs such as trismus and bulging of the parotid gland, while proptosis is a definite sign that the orbital fissures have been penetrated. The classical frog face as displayed in older publications is the ultimate picture of massive escape of disease.

Headache is not uncommon in long-standing cases and is attributable to chronic sinusitis in some patients. In other instances the cause is not so obvious and explanations, such as dural compression at sites of bone erosion or invasion of the sphenoidal sinus, can only be speculative.

Failing vision has been seen by the author on two occasions and indicates tenting of the optic nerve over a substantial extrapharyngeal extension of the tumour.

Investigations

Standard X-rays of the paranasal sinuses taken in the occipitofrontal or lateral projections may sometimes be misleading in that opacity of the maxillary sinus, in association with a soft tissue shadow of the postnasal space, may be mistaken for an antrochoanal polyp.

On the other hand, tomography in the fronto-occipital plane may be helpful in localizing the position of the mass, and showing areas of bone destruction or invasion of the sphenoidal sinus–findings which are inconsistent with an antrochoanal polyp. Lateral tomograms are desirable as they may reveal forward bowing of the posterior antral wall which is typical of angiofibroma filling the pterygopalatine fossa.

The introduction of computerized tomographic scanning with enhancement, and more recently, the technique of magnetic resonance imaging, has to some extent pre-empted the routine use of arteriography (Levine *et al.*, 1979).

Invasion of the sphenoidal sinus, erosion of the greater wing of the sphenoid, and extension into the pterygopalatine and infratemporal fossae is detectable with remarkable clarity on the latest generation of scanners. When doubt exists about the accuracy of the imaging, or in cases of recurrent angiofibroma, selective arteriography should be performed and the results displayed to the best advantage using subtraction techniques.

The vascular blush, which shows up in the postnasal space and adjacent areas, is diagnostic of the condition and obviates the need for biopsy (*Figure 19.1*). Useful information is obtained from the arteriograms on the size and site of the lesion and the size and location of feeding vessels, some of which arise from unusual sources such as the internal carotid or vertebral arteries (Thomas and Mowat, 1970; Ward *et al.*, 1974).

Biopsy is no longer justifiable in view of the risk of severe and protracted haemorrhage and since

modern radiological techniques will establish the diagnosis with a high degree of accuracy.

Differential diagnosis

The list of possible diagnoses with which angiofibroma may be confused includes antrochoanal polyp, large adenoids, tumours of the postnasal space and chordoma. In practice there is rarely any doubt about the issue once the patient has been fully investigated.

Treatment

The treatment of angiofibroma has been subject to considerable change over the years, but appears to be coming round full circle.

In the earlier part of the century treatment comprised surgery, but one suspects only because safer alternatives were not available. These surgical efforts were thwarted by the inadequacies of preoperative investigations and the torrential haemorrhage which accompanied the surgical endeavours. The anaesthetics of the era were unsophisticated or poorly administered, often adding to the problem of bleeding, and septic complications were all too common.

It was not universally appreciated that the severe bleeding which accompanied operations for angiofibroma was, in large measure, due to the surgeons' failure to avoid breaching the surface of the swelling during the course of the dissection. This is hardly surprising in the light of present knowledge about its tendency to fill nooks and crannies and to invade adjacent areas. Even as late as the 1960s, the practice of grasping angiofibromata with giant bone-holding forceps and wrenching them out was still in evidence in some centres.

The disillusionment created by the uncertainties and dangers of surgery led to a search for alternative and safer methods of treatment.

Attention was directed at hormone therapy and external beam irradiation, often as a preliminary to surgery, on the basis that such treatment promoted collagen formation and thereby reduced vascularity.

Testosterone was used on its own (Martin, Ehrlich and Abels, 1948) for the treatment of some swellings, as were oestrogens (Patterson, 1973; Jafek *et al.*, 1973), and a combination of the two was advocated by Schiff (1959). There is some evidence, in fact, to support the view that either type of hormone may encourage maturation of collagen while, at the same time, reducing vascularity (Arolde and Schatzle, 1971), but whether this contributes significantly to the safety

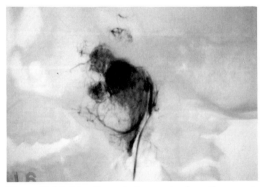

Figure 19.1 Subtraction arteriogram to show the vascular blush of a typical angiofibroma

of surgery is impossible to determine. It makes no sense, however, to use hormones prior to radiotherapy since the latter is known to be an effective method of reducing the vascularity of tissues when used on its own.

Therefore, the case for using radiotherapy exclusively as a definitive treatment for angiofibroma is not without merit. Briant, Fitzpatrick and Book (1970) advocated it on the grounds that surgery carries a high recurrence rate, but others have felt that radiotherapy should be reserved for selected patients, such as those with inoperable intracranial extensions and recurrent tumours (Ward *et al.*, 1974). The effect of ionizing radiation on angiofibromata has been studied in those patients who subsequently undergo surgery, and is judged to bring about a shrinkage and hardening of the tumours with a resultant reduction of their vascularity. Many clinicians, however, view the prospect of irradiating young adolescents with considerable diffidence and feel that it cannot be justified in the face of possible future carcinogenicity.

The resurgence of interest in surgery as definitive treatment has gathered momentum in recent years, largely because of improvements in preoperative assessment and a better understanding of the condition. There is some reason to suppose that preoperative embolization may reduce bleeding provided that the timing is right, although its hazards should not be minimized (Lasjaunias, 1980; Lang, McKellar and Lang, 1983).

The argument as to which surgical approach is best for the removal of angiofibromata implies that all swellings are identical – a notion which is nonsensical. Empiricism has no part in surgical judgements, and each case should be approached on the results of the preoperative findings. The transpalatal operation, favoured exclusively by many, would be rational if all angiofibromata were confined to the nasopharynx, a state of affairs which borders on the exceptional (English, Hemenway and Cundy, 1972).

An alternative and possibly more adaptable approach combines a transpalatal route with a gingivobuccal incision for access to the pterygomaxillary region (Jafek *et al.*, 1973), but even this entails a degree of empiricism which is incompatible with the philosophy of tailoring the operation to the disease.

Clearly, every case is judged on its merits and the surgical approach planned on the basis of the preoperative findings. A tumour which is confined exclusively to the postnasal space should be removed transpalatally, but one which has escaped into the pterygopalatine fossa, or beyond, requires a more ambitious approach. This must entail adequate access to the extensions in question and allow dissection between swelling

and surrounding structures in such a way as to ensure that the tumour parenchyma is not breached in the process (Shaheen, 1984). It should also provide the surgeon with sufficient room to ligate the principal feeding vessel to the tumour, and not compromise his ability to deal with major haemorrhage.

For tumours which encroach on the nasal fossa and just spill over into the pterygopalatine fossa, a lateral rhinotomy combined with resection of the medial antral wall may suffice to deliver the tumour and its extensions. For larger angiofibromata which invade the infratemporal fossa, a Weber-Ferguson incision combined with a transmaxillary-nasal approach is favoured (Shaheen, 1982).

Once the cheek flap has been reflected, the anterior, lateral, posterior, and medial walls of the maxilla are removed, leaving the orbital floor and upper alveolar arch as two intact shelves separated by a void (*Figure 19.2*). By ensuring that all of the

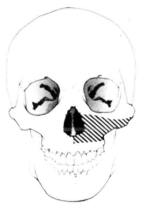

Figure 19.2 The area of bony removal of the maxilla to provide access to the lateral extension of the angiofibroma outside the nasopharynx

medial antral wall is removed – including the vertical plate of the palatine bone – the nasal cavity, antrum, infratemporal fossa, pterygopalatine fossa and nasopharynx are thrown into one large continuous space, a state of affairs which affords access to both the components of the swelling and its central stalk.

Starting laterally, the infratemporal part of the swelling is first identified and the maxillary artery found and ligated. The tumour is then mobilized in a medial and forward direction towards the antrum and nasopharynx. Removal of the perpendicular plate of the palatine bone serves to uncap the central stalk of the dumb-bell, which previously occupied the sphenopalatine foramen, and facilitates the subsequent mobilization of the nasopharyngeal component of the swelling.

The latter is dissected free from the base of the skull and from within the sphenoidal sinus, and the mucous membrane covering its undersurface is then divided at its periphery in order to complete the detachment of the tumour. No attempt is made to strip the mucous membrane off the inferior aspect of the swelling because of the intimacy of attachment between the two.

Complications

A palatal fistula may result when the transpalatal route is used, especially if the incision is sited directly over the junction of hard and soft palates. With the Weber-Ferguson approach, anaesthesia of the cheek is inevitable, although it rarely assumes troublesome proportions in this age group. Slight ectropion of the lower lid occasionally results and crusting of the nose may occur in some cases for some time afterwards.

The frequency of recurrence is very much dependent on the adequacy of the approach, the conditions at operation, and the experience of the surgeon.

References

AROLDE, R. and SCHATZLE, W. (1971) Histologisch histochemische untersuchungen juveniler nasenbachenfibrome vor und nach hormon behandlung. *H.N.O.*, **19**, 69–74

BENSCH, H. and EWING, J. (1941) *Neoplastic Disease*, 4th edn. Philadelphia: Saunders & Co.

BRIANT, T. D. R., FITZPATRICK, P. J. and BOOK, H. (1970) The radiological treatment of juvenile nasopharyngeal angiofibromas. *Annals of Otology, Rhinology and Laryngology*, **79**, 108–113

BRUNNER, H. (1942) Nasopharyngeal fibroma. *Annals of Otology, Rhinology and Laryngology*, **51**, 29–65

ENGLISH, G. M., HEMENWAY, W. G. and CUNDY, R. L. (1972) Surgical treatment of invasive angiofibroma. *Archives of Otolaryngology*, **96**, 312–318

FIGI, F. (1940) Fibromas of the nasopharynx. *Journal of the American Medical Association*, **1115**, 665–671

GIRGIS, I. H. and FAHMY, S. A. (1973) Nasopharyngeal fibroma: its histopathology. *Journal of Laryngology and Otology*, **87**, 1107–1123

HANDOUSA, A. S., FARID, H. and ELWI, A. M. (1954) Nasopharyngeal angiofibroma and its treatment. *Journal of Laryngology and Otology*, **68**, 647–666

HARRISON, D. F. N. (1976) Juvenile postnasal angiofibroma – an evaluation. *Clinical Otolaryngology*, **1**, 187–197

HUBBARD, E. M. (1958) Nasopharyngeal angiofibromas. *Archives of Pathology*, **65**, 192–204

JAFEK, B. W., NAHUM, A. M., BUTLER, R. M. and WARD, P. H. (1973) Surgical treatment of juvenile nasopharyngeal angiofibroma. *The Laryngoscope*, **83**, 707–720

LANG, D. A., McKELLAR, N. J. and LANG, W. (1983) Juvenile nasopharyngeal angiofibroma. The preferred treatment. *Scottish Medical Journal*, **28**, 64–66

LASJAUNIAS, P. (1980) Nasopharyngeal angiofibromas. Hazards of embolization. *Radiology*, **136**, 119–123

LEVINE, H. L., WEINSTEIN, M. A., TUCKER, H. M., WOOD, V. G. and DUCHESNEAU, T. M. (1979) Diagnosis of juvenile nasopharyngeal angiofibroma by computed tomography. *Otolaryngology: Head and Neck Surgery*, **87**, 304–310

MARTIN, H., EHRLICH, H. E. and ABELS, J. G. (1948) Juvenile nasopharyngeal angiofibroma. *Annals of Surgery*, **127**, 513–536

OSBORN, D. A. (1959) The so-called juvenile angiofibroma of the nasopharynx. *Journal of Laryngology and Otology*, **69**, 295–316

PATTERSON, C. N. (1973) Juvenile nasopharyngeal angiofibroma. *Otolaryngologic Clinics of North America*, **6**, 839–861

RINGERTZ, N. (1938) Pathology of malignant tumours arising in the nasal and paranasal cavities and maxilla. *Acta Oto-Laryngologica Supplementum*, **27**, 1–405

SCHIFF, M. (1959) Juvenile nasopharyngeal angiofibroma. *The Laryngoscope*, **69**, 981–1016

SHAHEEN, H. (1930) Nasopharyngeal fibroma. *Journal of Laryngology and Otology*, **45**, 259–264

SHAHEEN, O. H. (1982) Swellings of the infratemporal fossa. *Journal of Laryngology and Otology*, **96**, 817–836

SHAHEEN, O. H. (1984) *Problems in Head and Neck Surgery*, p. 100. London: Bailliere Tindall

SOM, M. L. and NEFFSON, A. H. (1940) Fibromas of the nasopharynx: juvenile and cellular types. *Annals of Otology, Rhinology and Laryngology*, **49**, 211–218

STEINBERG, S. S. (1954) Pathology of juvenile nasopharyngeal angiofibroma – a lesion of adolescent males. *Cancer*, **7**, 15–28

THOMAS, M. I. and MOWAT, P. D. (1970) Angiography in juvenile nasopharyngeal haemangiofibroma. *Clinical Radiology*, **21**, 403–406

WARD, P. H., THOMPSON, R., CALCATERRA, T. and KADIM, M. R. (1974) Juvenile angiofibroma, a more rational therapeutic approach based upon clinical and experimental evidence. *The Laryngoscope*, **84**, 2181–2194

20

Branchial cleft anomalies, thyroglossal cysts and fistulae

P. D. M. Ellis

Branchial cleft anomalies and thyroglossal cysts and fistulae are the end result of defects in development in the neck area of the embryo. In this chapter an attempt is made to show how such defects occur and the mechanisms by which various well recognized clinical conditions are created. It should be remembered that the development of the neck is complex and that our knowledge of the rapidly changing anatomical relationships between the various structures is incomplete. Nonetheless, when embryological knowledge is combined with a study of established clinical conditions, some degree of certainty and logic can emerge.

Branchial cleft anomalies

Embryology

In the early embryo, the foregut develops between the brain above and the primitive heart below (Hamilton, Boyd and Mossman, 1972). The mouth is separated from the pharynx by the buccopharyngeal membrane which disappears around the end of the third week when a series of bars appears in the walls of the pharynx. These bars are formed by mesodermal condensations and are known as the branchial arches. The arches fuse ventrally, thus forming U-shaped structures which support the pharynx. Initially there are six of these arches, but the fifth is vestigial and rapidly disappears.

Figure 20.1 shows how four branchial pouches internally, and four branchial grooves (clefts) externally, separate the remaining five branchial arches. Each branchial pouch is lined by endoderm and each branchial groove by ectoderm, and these pouches and grooves are separated by a

thin layer of mesoderm. In fish this endoderm–mesoderm–ectoderm layer breaks down so that a branchial cleft or gill-slit is formed. This does not normally occur in man but, should it do so, a branchial fistula may result.

A central core of cartilage develops in each arch and muscles differentiate from the surrounding mesoderm. Each arch is supplied by a cranial nerve and by an artery (aortic arch artery) which connects the ventral aortic sac to the dorsal aorta. Our knowledge of the exact derivatives of the arches is detailed in the more cranial arches, but becomes progressively less so in the caudal arches.

The first branchial arch gives rise to the maxilla, incus, malleus, anterior ligament of malleus, sphenomandibular ligament and mandible. The muscles are the muscles of mastication and the nerve is the mandibular branch of the trigeminal nerve. The artery is the first aortic arch artery from which is formed the maxillary artery.

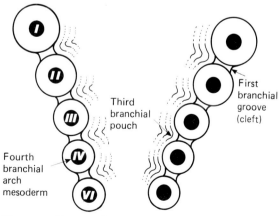

Figure 20.1 Diagram showing coronal section of 4-week-old embryo

The second arch forms the stapes, styloid process, stylohyoid ligament and the lesser cornu and upper part of the body of the hyoid bone. Its muscles are the muscles of facial expression which are supplied by the facial nerve. The artery is the second aortic arch artery which, rarely, may persist as the stapedial artery.

The third arch gives rise to the greater cornu and lower part of the body of the hyoid bone. Its nerve is the glossopharyngeal nerve and its artery is the third aortic arch artery which persists as part of the internal carotid artery.

The fourth and sixth arches form the laryngeal cartilages and the muscles of the pharynx and larynx which are supplied by the superior laryngeal (fourth arch) and recurrent laryngeal (sixth arch) branches of the vagus nerve. The fourth aortic arch artery forms the adult aorta on the left and the subclavian artery on the right while the sixth arch artery becomes the pulmonary trunk.

Between the branchial arches are the branchial pouches internally and the branchial grooves externally.

First branchial pouch and groove

The first pouch grows laterally to form the eustachian tube and middle ear while the groove is deepened to form the external auditory meatus. The pouch and groove meet at the tympanic membrane where they are separated by a thin layer of mesoderm. This mesoderm persists as the middle fibrous layer of the tympanic membrane. Note that only the dorsal part of the first groove takes part in forming the external auditory meatus. The remainder of the groove normally disappears but may persist as a preauricular sinus or a collaural fistula. The pinna is formed from a number of tubercles which appear at the dorsal ends of the first and second branchial arches. These tubercles surround the dorsal end of the first groove which is to form the external auditory meatus (*Figure 20.2*).

Second, third and fourth branchial pouches and grooves

The dorsal part of the second pouch contributes to the middle ear while the ventral part forms the supratonsillar fossa. The dorsal part of the third pouch forms the inferior parathyroid gland while the ventral part forms the thymic duct. The dorsal part of the fourth pouch forms the superior parathyroid gland while the ventral part probably contributes to the thyroid gland. Externally, the second branchial arch grows caudally and covers over the third, fourth and sixth arches, thus creating a deep pit or sinus lined by ectoderm

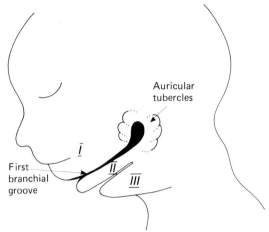

Figure 20.2 Diagram showing first, second and third branchial arches at about 7 weeks. (Modified from Frazer, J. E., 1926, *Journal of Anatomy*, **61**, by courtesy of Cambridge University Press)

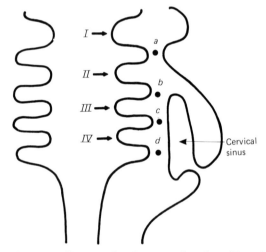

Figure 20.3 Diagram showing coronal section of 5-week-old embryo. a, b, c, d = sites of possible breakdown leading to a first, second, third or fourth branchial cleft fistula

(*Figure 20.3*). The opening to this cervical sinus is normally closed by fusion of its lips so that an ectoderm-lined cystic space is produced; later the cyst is resorbed and disappears.

Pathogenesis and pathology

Abnormal development of the branchial pouches and grooves may result in cysts, sinuses or fistulae.

A cyst is defined as a collection of fluid in an epithelium-lined sac. It may occur when part of a branchial groove or pouch becomes separated from the surface and fails to resorb. A cyst derived from a branchial groove will be lined by squamous epithelium; one derived from a branchial pouch will be lined by respiratory epithelium which may undergo squamous metaplasia after recurrent infections.

A sinus is a blind-ended track leading from an epithelial surface into deeper tissues. Such a sinus will occur when a branchial groove or pouch fails to resorb and remains open onto its epithelial surface.

A fistula is an abnormal communication between two epithelial surfaces. A branchial fistula is the human equivalent of the gill-slit in fishes and passes from the skin externally to the pharynx or larynx internally.

It is important to note that inclusion dermoids can closely mimic cysts derived from branchial grooves. In both cases the cyst will be lined by squamous epithelium and may contain skin adnexae. Only if cartilage is present can the cyst be certainly ascribed to a branchial groove origin. Inclusion dermoids occur especially in relation to the tubercles which appear at the cranial ends of the first and second arches and form the pinna. Here it is often impossible to be certain whether a cyst or sinus is an inclusion dermoid or a true branchial groove abnormality.

Anomalies of the first branchial cleft

Abnormal development may result in periauricular sinuses, cysts and collaural fistulae. Accessory tragi are also conveniently considered here although they develop from branchial arch tissue rather than the branchial cleft itself.

Accessory tragi

Accessory tragi are the result of anomalous growth of the tubercles of the first or second branchial arches and are therefore not true *cleft* anomalies. They are usually found in the preauricular region but may also occur anywhere along a line passing down to the sternoclavicular joint. They often contain cartilage and may be associated with other first and second arch abnormalities such as cleft palate and mandibular hypoplasia. If they do not contain cartilage they may be indistinguishable from a simple skin tag. Unsightly accessory tragi should be removed.

Periauricular sinuses and cysts

It may be difficult to decide whether these sinuses and cysts are inclusion dermoids resulting from

epithelium trapped between the developing auricular tubercles or whether they are remnants of first branchial groove epithelium which has failed to resorb. Attempts have been made by Work (1972) and Batsakis (1980) to support one or other pathogenesis but the present author remains unconvinced, especially as there may be no pathological differences between the two. Perhaps one should simply state that superficial lesions may be a consequence of either, while the deeper lesions and especially those passing to the nasopharynx are more certainly branchial cleft in origin.

The sinus or cyst is usually preauricular in site, although inferior and posterior lesions do occur. The commonest lesion is the preauricular sinus with its opening just in front of the ascending limb of the helix (*Figure 20.4*). Preauricular cysts are less

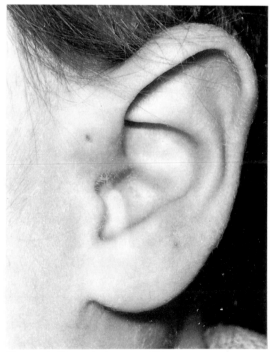

Figure 20.4 Preauricular sinus. This sinus was asymptomatic and required no treatment

common and, unless large, may only present when they become infected. An infected cyst may rupture or be drained onto the surface and thus be converted into a sinus. Both sinuses and cysts are lined by squamous epithelium and may contain skin adnexae in their walls. Many preauricular sinuses cause no trouble or may be kept quiescent by regular expression of any sebaceous material that collects. Others, however, become infected and cause recurrent pain, swelling and offensive discharge. Similarly, preauricular cysts often cause no symptoms and simply appear as an incidental finding in a routine otolaryngological examination. If symptoms are sufficiently troublesome, excision of the cyst or sinus with its track must be considered. The difficulty, of course, is that an apparently simple cyst or sinus may have extensive and deep branching ramifications which pass close to the facial nerve. The patient or parent, must fully understand the risk of facial nerve damage before agreeing to operation. He or she must be sure that the severity of symptoms justifies the risk of facial paralysis.

At operation, in the case of a cyst, a vertical incision is made over the cyst just anterior to the pinna. In the case of a sinus a similar incision is made but it should be split to include the opening of the sinus (*Figure 20.5*). Injection of the sinus with methylene blue may be of help, but care should be taken as any extravasation of dye outside the track will make dissection more difficult. The vertical incision can be extended into a standard parotidectomy incision if necessary.

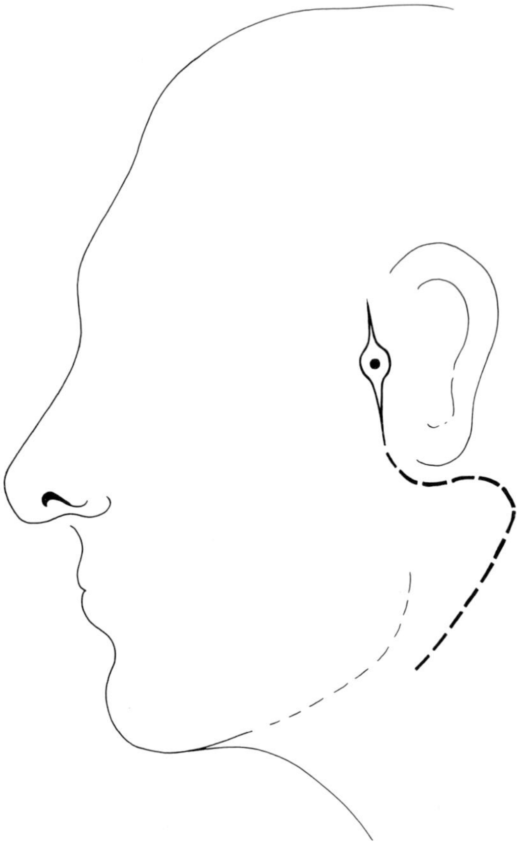

Dissection should now proceed medially until the whole cyst or sinus has been excised. Usually the track peters out above the level of the bony tympanic plate but, if it passes deeply into the parotid gland, it is best to carry out a superficial parotidectomy, displaying the facial nerve and its branches. It will now be possible to excise the track completely while preserving the facial nerve.

Collaural fistula

A collaural fistula is the least common of the first branchial cleft anomalies. It runs from the external auditory meatus or tragal notch down into the

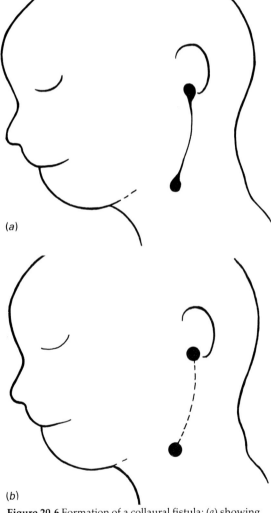

Figure 20.5 Incision for preauricular cyst and sinus. Note that it can be extended into a standard parotid incision if necessary

Figure 20.6 Formation of a collaural fistula; (*a*) showing the first branchial groove; (*b*) showing how the lips of the groove have fused causing a fistula which opens dorsally into the external auditory meatus and ventrally into the neck

neck where it opens at a point between the angle of the mandible and the sternomastoid muscle. The fistula is caused by a failure of resorption of the ventral part of the first branchial groove (*Figure 20.6*). The fistulous track runs through the parotid gland and may pass medial to, lateral to, or through the facial nerve.

If the fistula is causing sufficient symptoms it should be excised. A modified parotidectomy incision is made which should include the ear opening at its upper end and the neck opening at its lower end. After the facial nerve has been displayed by a superficial parotidectomy, the track can be dissected and excised. It must be remembered, however, that recurrent infections and previous attempts at removal often cause extensive scarring and cystic masses. The facial nerve may be embedded in such tissue rendering it likely to damage. Patients *must* be warned of a possible facial paralysis.

Lastly, it should be noted that it is possible for the endoderm–mesoderm–ectoderm layer between the first branchial groove and first branchial pouch to disappear so that the two become continuous as a branchial fistula (*see Figure 20.3*). Should such a fistula persist there will be an internal opening in the region of the eustachian tube orifice and the fistula will pass to the surface between the internal and external carotid arteries. The author has no personal experience of such a case, but suggests that the medial extent of the fistula could be explored in the same way as other lesions in the parapharyngeal space.

Anomalies of the second branchial cleft

Anomalous development of the second branchial cleft can result in fistulae, sinuses or cysts. A fistula occurs when the cervical sinus persists and the layer of endoderm–mesoderm–ectoderm between the second branchial pouch and groove breaks down (*see Figure 20.3*). If the fistulous track is incomplete an internal or external sinus is formed. Rarely, a true branchial cyst is caused by incomplete resorption of the cervical sinus after closure of its lips. Most so-called 'branchial cysts', however, are probably due to epithelial inclusions in lymph nodes; this controversy, and 'branchial cysts' in general, are further discussed in Volume 5, Chapter 15.

A second branchial cleft fistula opens externally into the lower third of the neck just anterior to the sternomastoid muscle (*Figure 20.7*). This external opening will have been present since birth unless it has been produced by incision and drainage of an abscess. Other members of the patient's family may be affected and the lesion is occasionally bilateral. Recurrent infection with abscess forma-

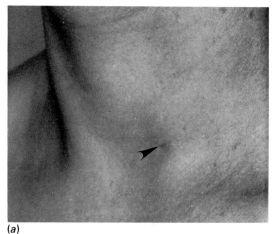

(*a*)

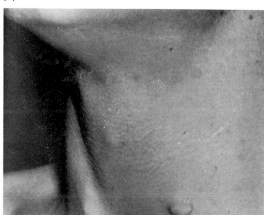

(*b*)

Figure 20.7 External appearances of second branchial cleft anomaly. (*a*) Fistulous opening; (*b*) skin tag

tion may occur in the fistulous track or there may be an intermittent clear mucoid discharge through the external opening onto the skin of the neck. Pathologically, the fistula consists of a muscular tube lined by respiratory or squamous epithelium, the latter being more common after recurrent infection. There are often cystic dilatations along the course of the fistula and the submucosa may contain glandular elements as well as nerves and lymphoid tissue.

Fistulae which are the site of recurrent infection or discharge should be excised, but other fistulae can be left unless the external opening is cosmetically unacceptable. The extent of the track can be assessed preoperatively by injection of a radiopaque dye. A complete fistula is uncommon and most sinuses end well before the pharynx is reached. At operation (*Figure 20.8*), a horizontal skin crease incision is made to include the external opening. Dissection follows the track as it pierces

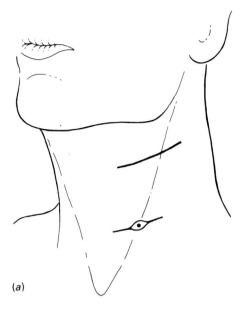

(a)

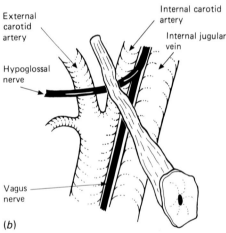

External
carotid
artery

Internal carotid
artery

Internal jugular
vein

Hypoglossal
nerve

Vagus
nerve

(b)

Figure 20.8 Operation for second branchial cleft fistula (a) showing two horizontal incisions, the lower one to include the fistulous opening; (b) the fistula is seen crossing the hypoglossal nerve to pass between the internal and external carotid arteries

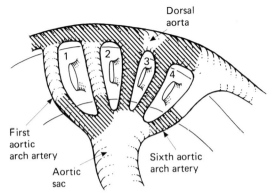

Dorsal
aorta

First
aortic
arch artery

Aortic
sac

Sixth aortic
arch artery

Figure 20.9 Diagram showing the relationship of branchial clefts to the developing aortic arch arteries. The branchial clefts are numbered 1, 2, 3, 4. The common carotid artery is formed from the aortic sac; the external carotid artery is formed from the roots of the first and second aortic arch arteries; the internal carotid artery is formed from the third aortic arch artery, then the dorsal aorta, then the cranial prolongation of the dorsal aorta. The fourth aortic arch artery forms the arch of the aorta on the left and the subclavian artery on the right. Note that derivatives of the first and second clefts will pass between the internal and external carotid arteries; derivatives of the third cleft will pass caudal, that is posterior to the internal carotid artery; derivatives of the fourth cleft will pass caudal, that is inferior to the arch of the aorta on the left and the subclavian artery on the right

the investing layer of deeper cervical fascia and ascends along the carotid sheath. After recurrent infection the track may be firmly adherent to the internal jugular vein or carotid artery so it is best to define these structures carefully as dissection proceeds. In long necks, and especially in complete fistulae, a further horizontal incision will be needed higher in the neck. The track is delivered into the upper incision and can be followed as it passes to the pharyngeal wall. *Figure 20.9* shows how the track must pass between the internal and external carotid arteries and how it will be cranial or anterior to the glossopharyngeal and vagus nerves which are the nerves of the third and fourth arches. To ensure that symptoms will not recur, the whole track should be excised up to and including its opening into the pharynx.

Anomalies of the third and fourth branchial clefts

Third and fourth branchial cleft fistulae are rare and only a handful have been reported in the literature.

The author has treated one patient with a third cleft fistula and the case history will serve as a description.

The patient was a 12-year-old girl who had had 13 operations for drainage of recurrent neck abscesses. She presented to the author with a discharging opening in the neck just anterior to the sternomastoid muscle. At operation a fistulous track was found which passed between the common carotid artery and the vagus nerve and ended in the pyriform fossa. The track was completely excised and histological examination

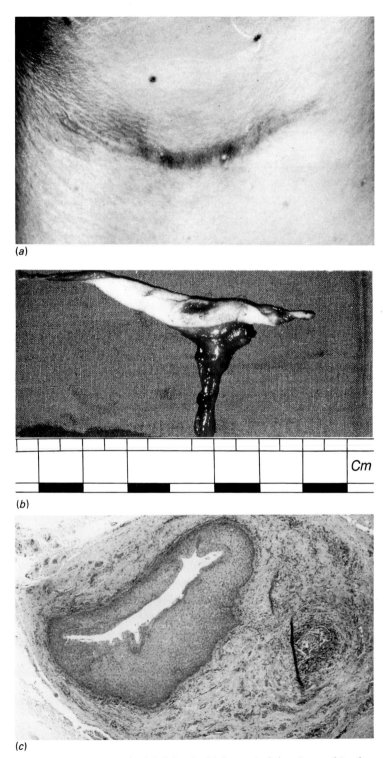

(a)

(b)

(c)

Figure 20.10 Third branchial cleft fistula. (*a*) Cosmetic deformity resulting from previous attempts at removal; (*b*) surgical specimen including ellipse of skin and fistulous track; (*c*) transverse section of fistula showing stratified squamous epithelium and surrounding scar tissue

showed it to be lined by stratified squamous epithelium (*Figure 20.10*).

A fistula of the fourth cleft would have to pass caudal to the arch of the aorta or right subclavian artery and end in the upper oesophagus or pyriform fossa. Isolated branchial cleft remnants have been described along this anatomical pathway (Downey and Ward, 1969; Tucker and Skolnick, 1973) but no complete fistula has yet been described.

Thyroglossal cysts and fistulae
Embryology

Towards the end of the third week of embryonic life a thickening of endoderm appears at the site of the tuberculum impar in the floor of the primitive pharynx. This endodermal thickening soon be-

comes evaginated to form the thyroglossal duct which descends into the neck between the first and second branchial arches so that it comes to lie in close relationship to the primitive aorta. Later the duct solidifies and is then known as the thyroglossal tract (*Figure 20.11*). When the thyroglossal tract reaches the front of the trachea it becomes bilobed to form the two thyroid lobes which are connected by the isthmus; each thyroid lobe may also receive a contribution from the ventral part of the fourth pharyngeal pouch. Normally, the rest of the tract disappears leaving the foramen caecum at the base of the tongue as the only adult indication of its place of origin.

Any part of the thyroglossal tract may persist into adult life. Much the commonest finding is a persistence of the lowest part of the tract as the pyramidal lobe of the thyroid gland. Less frequently, the tract may fail to descend into the neck from the base of the tongue so that it persists as a lingual thyroid. Because of the early relationship of the tract to the aortic arch, islands of thyroid tissue have also been found in the superior mediastinum. The most common clinical condition resulting from persisting tract remnants is the thyroglossal cyst. The precise embryology of the

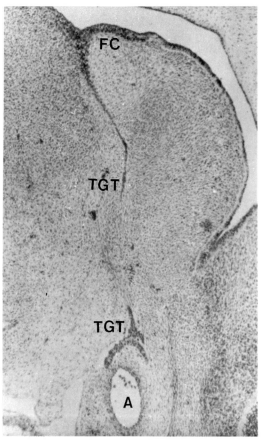

Figure 20.11 Three-week-old embryo showing the thyroglossal tract passing down through the tongue to the aorta. (TGT) thyroglossal tract, (FC) foramen caecum, (A) arch of aorta. (From Ellis, P. D. M. and van Nostrand, A. W. P., 1977, *The Laryngoscope*, **87**, by courtesy of the authors and publisher)

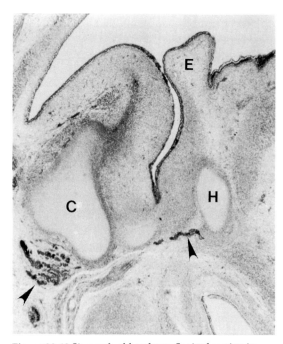

Figure 20.12 Six-week-old embryo. Sagittal section in which the thyroglossal tract (arrowed) is shown to remain anterior to the developing hyoid bone. (E) epiglottis, (H) hyoid bone precursor and (C) cricoid cartilage. (From Ellis, P. D. M. and van Nostrand, A. W. P., 1977, *The Laryngoscope*, **87**, by courtesy of the authors and publisher)

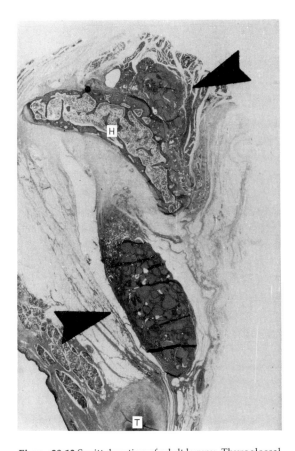

Figure 20.13 Sagittal section of adult larynx. Thyroglossal tract remnants are arrowed. (H) hyoid bone and (T) thyroid cartilage. Note: (1) crescentic shape of the hyoid bone; (2) intimate relationship of tract remnants to the hyoid bone; (3) the tract hooks around the inferior border of the hyoid bone to lie posterior to it before descending to the isthmus. (From Ellis, P. D. M. and van Nostrand, A. W. P., 1977, *The Laryngoscope*, **87**, by courtesy of the authors and publisher)

thyroglossal tract is fundamental to an understanding of surgical treatment and so will be described in detail.

As mentioned previously the tract descends into the neck between the first and second branchial arches. This means that it must descend between the developing mandible (first arch) cranially and the hyoid bone (second and third arches) caudally. *Figure 20.12* confirms that the track passes into the neck, cranial or anterior to the hyoid bone and laryngeal cartilage.

Frazer in 1940 discussed the intimate relationship between the tract and the hyoid bone. He noted that the hyoid bone changes from an ovoid shape in the embryo (*Figure 20.12*) to a crescentic shape in the adult (*Figure 20.13*). He suggested that this change of shape was a result of the downward pull of the strap muscles producing a downward projection of the body of the hyoid bone which thus indented the tract. In the adult, therefore, a persisting thyroglossal tract will pass down in front of the hyoid bone and then hook up around its inferior border to lie posterior to the bone before finally descending to the isthmus. Several authors (Ward, Hendrick and Chambers, 1949; Lawson and Fallin, 1969) have stated that the tract may descend posterior to or even through the hyoid bone. They do not, however, supply pathological evidence nor do they refute the embryological studies of Frazer (1940) and Hamilton, Boyd and Mossman (1972) which show conclusively that the tract descends cranial or anterior to the second and third branchial arches in which the bone develops. Ellis and van Nostrand (1977) studied 30 embryos at varying stages of development, 200 adult larynges and 20 thyroglossal cyst specimens; in no instance did the tract pass down posterior to or through the hyoid bone. They suggested that reports of the tract passing through the hyoid bone could be due to misinterpretation of pathological specimens (*Figure 20.14*). All are agreed, however, that the tract

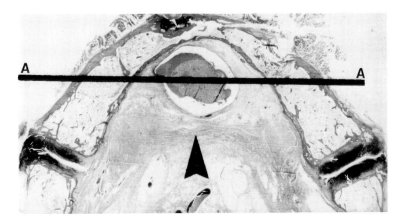

Figure 20.14 Horizontal section of an adult larynx at the level of the hyoid bone. The thyroglossal tract remnant is arrowed. As a result of the concavity of the posterior surface of the bone a section taken at (AA) may show thyroid tissue in a ring of bone. Note also the unusual finding of a jointed hyoid bone. (From Ellis, P. D. M. and van Nostrand, A. W. P., 1977, *The Laryngoscope*, **87**, by courtesy of the authors and publisher)

is intimately related to the bone and that attempts to dissect the tract from its surface are likely to fail. The best way to remove all tract remnants and thus avoid recurrence is to excise the central part of the hyoid bone as recommended by Sistrunk in 1920 (*see below*).

Clinical features and management of thyroglossal tract remnants

Lingual thyroid

The thyroglossal tract may fail to descend into the neck so that the adult thyroid gland comes to lie at any point from the foramen caecum to the front of the trachea. The most common clinical condition is the so-called lingual thyroid. These patients usually present in childhood when a symptomless lump is noticed on the base of the tongue (*Figure 20.15*). Obstructive symptoms such as dysphagia or dysarthria are rare and usually occur only when the lump enlarges as a result of pregnancy, thyrotoxicosis or neoplasia. A thyroid scan must

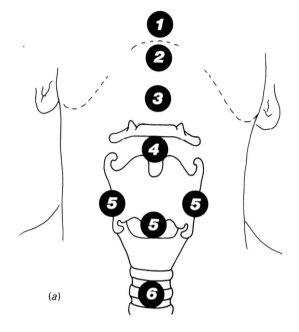

(a)

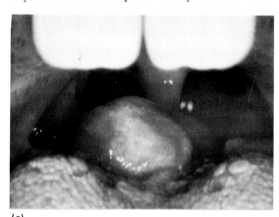

(a)

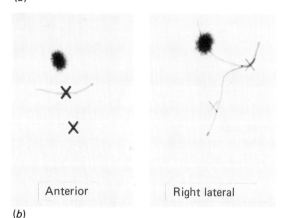

(b)

Figure 20.15 (*a*) A 10-year-old girl with a lingual thyroid. (*b*) The thyroid scan shows this to be her only functioning thyroid tissue

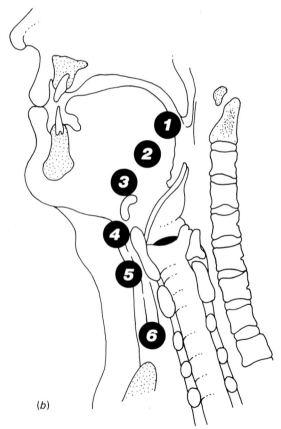

(b)

Figure 20.16 Possible sites of thyroglossal cysts. 1, base of tongue; 2, intralingual; 3, suprahyoid; 4, infrahyoid; 5, prethyroid; 6, pretracheal

be performed if surgical excision is contemplated as the lingual thyroid may be the only functioning thyroid tissue present. Usually, however, no treatment is required and patients can be confidently reassured.

Thyroglossal cysts

Thyroglossal cysts occur equally in men and women and are usually noted in childhood,

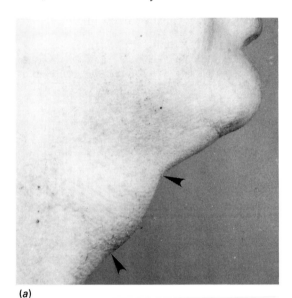

(a)

(b)

Figure 20.17 Large thyroglossal cyst (arrowed). Note that the cyst has risen on tongue protrusion (*b*). This physical sign is best demonstrated by palpating the cyst while the patient protrudes his tongue

although they may present at any age. The cyst can occur at any point along the path of the tract from the base of the tongue to the thyroid isthmus, the commonest site being just above, or just below the hyoid bone (*Figure 20.16*). Most cysts are midline, but those at the level of the thyroid cartilage may be pushed to one or other side, usually the left.

Most patients present complaining of a symptomless lump in the midline of the neck. Examination will show that it is freely mobile from side to side and that it may transilluminate. The lump will rise on swallowing (on account of its attachment to the hyoid bone via the thyroglossal tract) and will also rise on protrusion of the tongue (because of its attachment to the base of the tongue via the thyroglossal tract) (*Figure 20.17*). No other midline neck lump rises on tongue protrusion, so this physical sign is virtually pathognomonic. Some patients present with acute infection and abscess formation (*Figure 20.18*) which may result in a sinus or fistula with intermittent discharge of a clear glairy mucus. Such a sinus or fistula is always acquired and may also be caused by inadequate surgical excision.

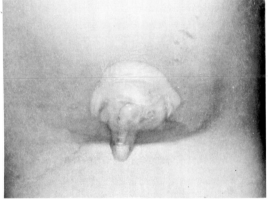

Figure 20.18 Infected thyroglossal cyst with spontaneous rupture and discharge

If the cyst is cosmetically unacceptable or is the site of recurrent infection and fistula formation it should be excised. Gross and Connerley (1940) have argued that small symptomless cysts may be left *in situ*. However, many cysts do eventually become the site of recurrent inflammation and, very occasionally, a carcinoma may develop within the cyst. In most cases, therefore, surgical excision is the treatment of choice. A preoperative thyroid scan should be performed and this will usually show a normal thyroid gland in the normal position. Perhaps surprisingly, it is uncommon to find functioning thyroid tissue in relation to the cyst.

Sistrunk's operation for the removal of thyroglossal cysts

In 1920, Sistrunk described his technique for the removal of thyroglossal cysts. He had found that simple excision of the cyst was often followed by further cyst formation or a chronically discharging sinus at the operative site; he argued that these recurrences could be avoided only by removing the whole of the thyroglossal tract. To do this he advised excision of the central part of the body of the hyoid bone and a core of tongue muscle up to the foramen caecum. Using this technique on 270 patients at the Mayo Clinic, Brown and Judd (1961) were able to reduce the previously high recurrence rate to only 4%.

A horizontal skin crease incision is made at the level of the cyst including, if necessary, the external opening of any sinus or fistula. The cyst is easily defined lying anterior to the larynx and it will usually be possible to find a well-defined fibrous cord passing to the body of the hyoid bone (*Figure 20.19*). Using bone-cutting forceps, the body of the hyoid bone is transected on either side of the midline, thus freeing a central portion of about 1–2 cm in length. Patients seem to suffer no disadvantage through losing most of the body of the hyoid bone and there is no need to attempt to suture the cut ends of bone together. It may be possible to follow the fibrous cord superiorly through the tongue musculature to the base of the

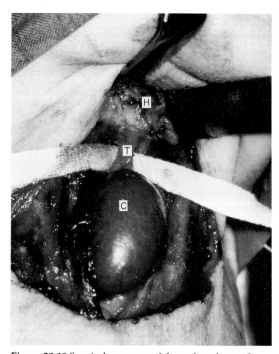

Figure 20.19 Surgical exposure of thyroglossal cyst (C), tract (T) and hyoid bone (H)

tongue but, more usually, the cord peters out above the hyoid bone. In all cases, however, a core of tongue tissue comprising parts of geniohyoid and genioglossus should be excised, thus ensuring that all tract remnants are removed. A useful manoeuvre at this stage is to place the index finger of the left hand in the mouth on the foramen caecum. This removes any uncertainty concerning which part of the tongue should be excised and allows dissection right up to the foramen caecum. Ideally dissection should stop just short of the mucosa at the foramen caecum. If the mucosa should be breached, a catgut purse string suture will produce satisfactory closure. During closure, great care should be taken to halt any bleeding and to drain the wound. A postoperative haematoma may cause respiratory obstruction and be life threatening. Close supervision is essential in the early postoperative period and stitch scissors and sinus forceps should be kept at the bedside so that any necessary drainage can be carried out.

Pathological examination of the cyst will show it to be lined by columnar epithelium, squamous epithelium or, occasionally, no epithelium at all. When the epithelium is columnar it is usually pseudostratified, ciliated and associated with mucous glands in the submucosa; the cyst itself contains mucus. When the epithelium is squamous it keratinizes so that the cyst contains keratin. After recurrent infections, epithelium is often absent and the cyst contains inflammatory exudate. Lymphoid tissue is not normally found in the cyst wall (contrast 'branchial cysts'), so that infection of the cyst is probably either blood-borne or spreads down a patent thyroglossal tract from the foramen caecum. The cyst may be in continuity with a tubular or solid thyroglossal tract and the tract may be duplicated or branching, emphasizing again the importance of excising a wide core of tongue tissue with the specimen.

Thyroid carcinomata are occasionally found in thyroglossal cysts. Page *et al.* (1974) reviewed the literature and found 656 such cases, all of which were papillary carcinomata. Most had presented as simple cysts and were diagnosed only on pathological examination. Treatment is adequate surgical excision followed by suppressive doses of thyroid.

References

BATSAKIS, J. G. (1980) *Tumours of the Head and Neck*, 2nd edn, pp. 514–520. Baltimore: Williams and Wilkins

BROWN, P. M. and JUDD, E. S. (1961) Thyroglossal duct cysts and sinuses. *American Journal of Surgery*, **102**, 494–501

DOWNEY, W. L. and WARD, P. H. (1969) Branchial cleft cysts in the mediastinum. *Archives of Otolaryngology*, **89**, 762–765

ELLIS, P. D. M. and van NOSTRAND, A. W. P. (1977) The applied anatomy of thyroglossal tract remnants. *The Laryngoscope*, **87**, 765–770

FRAZER, S. E. (1926) The disappearance of the precervical sinus. *Journal of Anatomy*, **61**, 139

FRAZER, S. E. (1940) *A Manual of Embryology*, 2nd edn, pp. 236–238. London: Balliere, Tindall and Cox

GROSS, R. E. and CONNERLEY, M. L. (1940) Thyroglossal cysts and sinuses: a study and report of 198 cases. *New England Journal of Medicine*, **223**, 616–624

HAMILTON, W. J., BOYD, J. D. and MOSSMAN, H. W. (1972) *Human Embryology*, 4th edn, pp. 151–192. Cambridge: W. Heffer

LAWSON, V. G. and FALLIS, J. C. (1969) Surgical treatment of thyroglossal tract remnants. *Canadian Medical Association Journal*, **100**, 855–858

PAGE, C. P., KEMMERER, W. T., HAFF, R. C. and MAZZAFEVRI, E. L. (1974) Thyroid carcinomas arising in thyroglossal ducts. *Annals of Surgery*, **180**, 799–803

SISTRUNK, W. E. (1920) The surgical treatment of cysts of the thyroglossal tract. *Annals of Surgery*, **71**, 121–122

TUCKER, H. M. and SKOLNICK, M. L. (1973) Fourth branchial cleft (pharyngeal pouch) remnant. *Transactions of the American Academy of Ophthalmology and Otolaryngology*, **77**, 368–371

WARD, G. E., HENDRICK, J. W. and CHAMBERS, R. G. (1949) Thyroglossal tract abnormalities. *Surgery, Gynecology and Obstetrics*, **89**, 727–734

WORK, W. P. (1972) Newer concepts of first branchial cleft defects. *The Laryngoscope*, **82**, 1581–1593

21

The management of cleft palate

R. W. Pigott and D. S. McManamny

Successful treatment of congenital and acquired conditions affecting the palate depends on an understanding of its functions. As the floor of the nose, it provides part of the airway, isolating the nasal cavity from obstruction by food during mastication, and as the roof of the mouth, it provides a surface against which food may be broken up by the tongue and neatly passed back as manageable boluses for swallowing. In man its smooth surface is also concerned with the production of distinguishably different sounds which can be combined together to produce intelligible speech. The soft palate has the additional ability to contribute to closure of the velopharyngeal isthmus to prevent food entering the nose in swallowing and also to conserve and direct respired air through the mouth under pressure for speech.

Speech analysis

One of the main aims of the management of patients with cleft palate is the provision of an anatomical and physiological environment in which comprehensible speech can be produced. The speech of a patient with an unrepaired cleft palate is characterized by features which are instantly recognizable by most people, lay public and medical professionals alike. However, it is misleading to assume that the speech defects of patients with this problem are identical. The speech of any individual patient will alter, depending on such factors as the inability to bring the lips together, necessary to pronounce /p/ and /b/; the configuration of the hard palate and alveolar arch and the integrity of the dental arcade which may affect sounds such as /s/ and /z/; the

presence of fistulae at different points in the palate which can alter air escape affecting consonants such as /d/ /g/ and /k/ made against the hard or soft palate and, most importantly, the competence of the velopharyngeal isthmus which conserves the air stream and directs it past the articulators or allows it to escape through the nose to produce nasal consonants. In this light, speech analysis may seem a difficult and complicated task, but it becomes straightforward when an ordered approach is taken.

As well as analysing the various components of speech, the degree to which the patient becomes breathless on talking is one of the first aspects to be noted. This can be assessed by asking the patient to count up to twenty rapidly. With velopharyngeal competence it should be unnecessary for the patient to take more than one breath to complete the task; with severe incompetence a breath may be taken for every few digits.

For the purposes of defining various speech defects with greater precision, and comparing different methods of treatment, articulation, velopharyngeal function and intelligibility are considered separately (*see* Chapter 11 on Disorders of speech).

Closure patterns of the velopharyngeal isthmus

From a few well documented direct observations following maxillectomy, but mainly from radiological and endoscopic studies, normal and abnormal patterns of closure of the velopharyngeal isthmus have been defined both for swallowing and for speech (Calnan, 1952; Astley, 1958; Massengill *et al.*, 1966; Pigott, 1969; Skolnick,

McCall and Barnes, 1973). Further information has come from electromyography (Fritzell, 1969, Bell-Bertie, 1976; Mulder, 1976).

These patterns may be summarized as follows.

Swallowing

Swallowing is a relatively slowly developed, powerful sphincteric movement involving approximation of the posterior third of the palate to the pharyngeal wall. The action of swallowing is innervated by the ninth, tenth and eleventh cranial nerves via the pharyngeal plexus and invariably functions normally in the group of patients whose behaviour is considered in this chapter. One principal muscle is the superior constrictor with assistance from palatopharyngeus and to a lesser extent levator palati. Closure is below the level of the area of the atlas.

Speaking

Closure for speech, by contrast, occurs rapidly, (for example the palate must rise and fall eight times to produce the 13 syllables in counting from 15–20 at a normal speed (in 3 seconds). If the movements were equally distributed this would give a cycle open-closed-open of 0.36 seconds, but very much higher speeds have been recorded. The role of the palate depressors is very important under these circumstances. The sacrifice of all the fibres of the palatopharyngeus muscle in certain pharyngoplasties may lead to the palate remaining up for open nasal sounds with resultant hyponasality; at least part of this muscle should be conserved during surgery. The closure takes place above the level of the arch of the atlas in adults, at the level of the basiocciput in children, and at the level of the basisphenoid in infants (Calnan, 1959). These changes are due to descent of the maxilla, and with it the hard palate and attached soft palate, with age and also to atrophy of the adenoids against which they actually make contact in infants and younger children. In these younger groups the palate rotates up as a fixed length structure to touch the adenoid mass, but with increasing age, it also lengthens (velar stretch).

Muscular control

The principal muscle is the levator palati and when this contracts alone the palate rises as a simple valve (*Figure 21.1*). More often there is a contribution to closure from the superior constrictor and/or the horizontal fibres of the palatopharyngeus which originate in the soft palate and sweep around the pharynx as the palatopharyngeal sphincter (Whillis, 1930; Calnan, 1952). It is likely that velar stretch is due to these horizontal fibres. Whatever muscle is responsible, the effect is advancement of the lateral and posterior walls, each to a greater or lesser degree, resulting in a final pattern of closure which may be coronal, sagittal or sphincteric (Skolnick, McCall and Barnes, 1973; Shprintzen *et al.*, 1979) and is as idiosyncratic to that person as the movements of their mouth (*Figure 21.2*).

The less the movement of the palate, the greater the movement of the lateral and posterior walls, which may be compensatory, since in cases of unrepaired or inadequately repaired palate clefts, a well-defined semicircular shelf develops on the posterior wall, known as Passavant's ridge (after Gustav Passavant, a Frankfurt surgeon, who first described it in 1869).

Evidence from neurological syndromes (Sedlakova, Lastovka and Scram, 1973), observations on patients with facial palsy (Podvinec, 1952), from human observation studies (Nickl, 1950), and from animal experiments (Nishio *et al.*, 1976a,b) supports the view that the seventh cranial nerve innervates the levator for speech, possibly via the chorda tympani, or the greater superficial petrosal nerves, sphenopalatine ganglion and lesser palatine nerves, in addition to fibres from the pharyngeal plexus.

The vertical fibres of the palatopharyngeus actively depress the palate, assisted by elastic fibres in the palatoglossus, the muscle fibres, like those of salpingopharyngeus, being small and inconstant (Kuehn and Azzam, 1978).

The upper surface of the soft palate is convex at the level of the levator eminence over its median

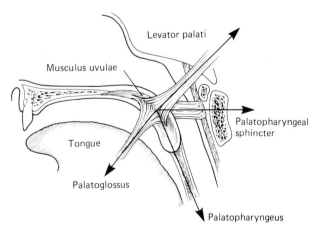

Figure 21.1 Muscle vectors. Palatoglossus and palatopharyngeus are seen to be antagonists to levator palati. The palatopharyngeal sphincter aids closure by advancing the lateral and posterior walls and causing velar stretch

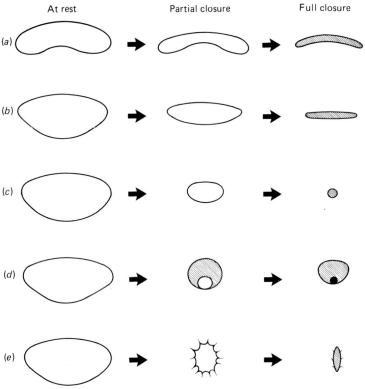

At rest   Partial closure   Full closure

(a)

(b)

(c)

(d)

(e)

Figure 21.2 Patterns of velopharyngeal closure (Skolnick, 1973). Basal view.
(*a*) Normal subject. Note musculus uvulae bulge; (*b*) coronal pattern.
Repaired cleft palate subject; (*c*) circular closure pattern, repaired cleft palate;
(*d*) circular closure pattern with Passavant's ridge (shaded area); (*e*) sagittal
closure pattern, repaired cleft palate

third, due to the bulk of the paired musculus uvulae and the associated mass of mucosal glands (Pigott, 1969; Azzam and Kuehn, 1977). This allows it to fit snugly into the concavity of the posterior pharyngeal wall. Laterally, the inconstant ridges of salpingopharyngeus advance medially to fit against the sides of the musculus uvulae ridge.

Diagnostic techniques

Oral examination

Direct observation of the oral cavity provides essential but limited information about the cleft palate patient. Unfortunately, the competence or otherwise of the velopharyngeal sphincter cannot be determined by looking into the mouth, since the point of closure lies above the soft palate, not directly behind it. Examination of the oral cavity must include a good view right back to the uvula and pharyngeal walls. If there is an unrepaired

cleft, note is made of the extent and the width of the defect.

The examiner should look particularly for signs of a submucous cleft. Not all the signs are found in each patient. There is often a translucent stripe running down the centre of the soft palate. This represents an area devoid of muscle. The posterior border of the palate should be palpated for a notch in place of the nasal spine. This is pathognomonic of submucous cleft and probably represents the anterior insertion of the palate muscles exactly as seen in overt clefts. The levator lift dimples should be examined as the patient says 'ah'. Lateral placement also indicates muscle separation. The uvula is bifid in four out of five cases of submucous cleft, but this is not a reliable sign of a submucous cleft, as it occurs in more than 1% of the population. Irregularities of the dental arcade and collapse of the arch should be noted as they will make articulation more difficult.

In the case of a repaired palate, examination will reveal the quality of the resultant scar and apparent mobility, and the presence or absence of a fistula. Although nasopharyngeal closure cannot be confirmed by oral examination, a fair assessment of palate mobility can be achieved. The time-honoured sound the patient is asked to utter, /ah/, is not as effective in achieving maximum velar elevation as the vowel /ee/. Formation of this sound normally lifts the soft palate to a level well above the hard palate, and should be used instead. Both Calnan (1952) and more recently Sommerlad (1981) have pointed out that in the normal palate, elevation is accompanied by the presence of dimples on the oral surface at points of attachment of the levator palati muscles to the soft palate. In the cleft palate, these dimples may be displaced laterally, or grooves running forward to the posterior edge of the hard palate may be seen instead. Large tonsils may be responsible for obstruction of either nasal or oral air flow which can lead to hyper- or hyponasality or to a 'hot potato' quality of the patient's speech.

Some idea can be gained of the relative sizes of the oral cavity, palate and pharynx. In a small group of patients with velopharyngeal incompetence no abnormality will be found other than a disproportionately large pharynx. Passavant's ridge is sometimes visible on saying /ah/, but even if the ridge itself cannot be seen, bunching of the mucosa may be visible below the palate. Mirror examination will confirm this. Although further investigations are required, a provisional diagnosis of pharyngeal disproportion can be made on oral examination.

Nasopharyngoscopy

Historical

The anatomical position of the velopharyngeal isthmus has rendered it inaccessible to direct observation until relatively recently. Borel-Maisonny (1937) was able to view the isthmus during the production of isolated sounds using a laryngopharyngoscope and nasopharyngoscope, introduced over the dorsum of the tongue. In 1966, Taub introduced the use of an oral panendoscope with which cine and video recording was possible. It is a right-angled viewing instrument and has a 50° cone of acceptance. However, conversational levels of speech muscle activity cannot be assessed, and in particular, /s/ and /s/ blends, the sounds most likely to be mispronounced by cleft patients cannot be tested.

An instrument which enables observation of the velopharyngeal isthmus from the nasal site is required in order to do this. Using this approach, observation of soft palate function does not interrupt the normal flow of air during random connected speech. The ideal endoscope for nasal pharyngoscopy does not exist at present, but the introduction of light conduction by solid cable has at least made this technique feasible. There are several instruments available, of both rigid and flexible type.

Rigid endoscopes

One of the most important features of a rigid nasoendoscope is its angle of view. In the sitting patient with the head positioned so that the hard palate is horizontal, the plane of the nasopharyngeal isthmus can be related to the plane of the hard palate. The plane of the isthmus is defined when the point of contact, or attempted contact, between the genu of the soft palate and the posterior pharyngeal wall is known (Pigott and Makepeace, 1982). A tangent drawn to that point on the posterior wall lies at right angles to the plane of the isthmus. This tangent is termed the presumptive closure plane. The angle between the presumptive closure plane and hard palate is termed the 'presumptive closure plane angle' (*Figure 21.3*). If an accurate assessment of closure

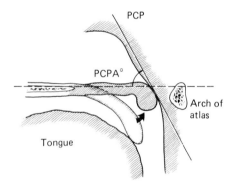

Figure 21.3 Presumptive closure plane (PCP). Presumptive closure plane angle (PCPA)

is to be made the endoscopic view must be at an angle normal to the presumptive closure plane angle. During growth the hard palate descends relative to the base of the skull, and therefore the presumptive closure plane angle will increase with age. This must be considered when selecting a suitable instrument for a given patient (*Figure 21.4*). A direction of view that is not parallel to the presumptive closure plane will lead to foreshortening of the endoscope image and the isthmus may even be out of sight. The presumptive closure plane of 60 randomly selected patients with an age range of 7 to 23 years varied from 32° in the youngest to 112° in the eldest. The mean angle was in the region of 70°. A rigid endoscope can be tipped up, to decrease the angle of view,

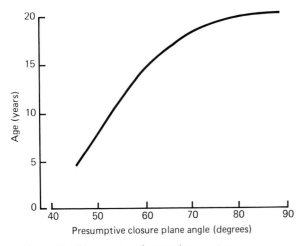

Figure 21.4 Presumptive closure plane angle increasing with age

but it cannot be tipped down without causing significant discomfort to the patient.

The Storz Hopkins 70° nasopharyngoscope is the most commonly used rigid nasopharyngoscope. The optics are excellent. The angle of view is similar to the presumptive closure plane of the isthmus in an average examination. It has a cone of acceptance of 110°, which makes orientation and siting of the instrument quite straightforward (*Figure 21.5*). The tip can be lifted, and the field of view increased. The wide angle enables the circumference of the isthmus to be viewed in one field from quite close. The shaft of the endoscope is oval in cross-section, and measures 4.2 × 3.5 mm. This means that rotation beyond 30° may be uncomfortable, especially in children. Consequently, visualization of the eustachian tube orifices may not be possible.

For smaller children, the Storz 30° endoscope is useful. The cone of acceptance is smaller, but its 3.0 mm diameter requires less room for it to be

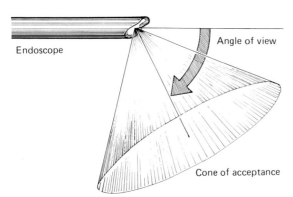

Figure 21.5 Mean angle of view and cone of acceptance of the endoscope

passed, and its circular cross-section allows rotation to view the eustachian tubes.

Flexible endoscopes

The new Machida (3 mm o.d.) fibreoptic endoscope (Wolff 7200) has an outside diameter of 3.0 mm and a small radius of flexion, which make it a very versatile instrument. A range of closure planes can be examined, and its small size makes it more acceptable to younger patients than the larger endoscopes. It is therefore a suitable instrument for a large number of patients. Shprintzen (personal communication, 1984) has achieved considerable success using the Machida endoscope in children from 3 years of age and, in practice, a child who will tolerate topical nasal anaesthesia will almost always tolerate endoscopy.

The technique of endoscopy

Patient selection

Patients must be conscious and cooperative to obtain speech samples. A child who cries produces mucus in the nose which obstructs the view. Using the Storz 70° nasopharyngoscope Pigott and Makepeace (1982) found that the success was proportional to age, with 30% success in 3 year olds rising to nearly 100% in 10 year olds, providing gross nasal obstruction was not present.

Equipment

The examination is performed in a dental chair with facilities for raising and lowering, and head rest adjustment. It is very important that the head is well supported as movement when the endoscope is in place can disturb the image or the recording, and can be quite uncomfortable.

The endoscope is attached to a rigid multiarticulated teaching attachment (Storz) or to a fibreoptic teaching attachment which connects to a high resolution black and white camera, if video recording is to be undertaken. Radiographic equipment, television monitor, video recorder and image integration unit should be available under ideal circumstances, to allow simultaneous fluoroscopic and endoscopic recording which permits a later review of findings (Pigott and Makepeace, 1982).

Anaesthesia

Patients are asked to rub a small quantity of cocaine paste (25%) on their little finger into both nasal vestibules 5 minutes before examination (Henderson, personal cummunication, 1983). Ciliary action carries this back to the inferior turbinate. For more posterior anaesthesia the two commonly used agents are 4% lignocaine hydrochloride solution, and 5% cocaine solution. Cocaine is the more effective of the two, however, a dangerous drug register must be used, and resuscitation facilities must be available.

Prior to anaesthesia the patient is asked to clear the nasal passages as much as possible by sniffing and blowing the nose, until it sounds quite dry, since mucous interferes with the effectiveness of the local anaesthetic.

One millilitre of cocaine solution is drawn up in a syringe, to which is attached a no. 10 Portex catheter. At the other end of a catheter a twist of cotton wool is held in place with Micropore tape. The cotton wool bud should be of a diameter similar to that of the endoscope. The nostrils are inspected, and the airway with the greater aperture is chosen. The tip of the catheter is inserted along the nostril floor and a few drops of anaesthetic are released. The catheter is advanced, slowly, and the entire nasal cavity floor is covered with solution, until the posterior pharyngeal wall is contacted. For flexible endoscopy it is useful to anaesthetize above the inferior turbinate. When examining children it may help to offer them a sweet to suck while this part of the procedure is being carried out, as the anaesthetic solution tastes bitter.

Examination

Previous experience of inserting an endoscope with adult volunteers is essential before undertaking clinical work. After allowing adequate time for the anaesthetic to take effect, the tip of the endoscope is placed on the nostril sill, and gently advanced with the free hand. Insertion is achieved by gently feeling for resistance and watching the angle of the endoscope and the head. In the case of a unilateral cleft, the non-cleft nostril should usually be used. However, the endoscope often requires angulation around the posterior border of the vomer because of the convexity of the septal midzone into the cleft nostril. If fluoroscopic screening is available, the position of the tip of the endoscope can be accurately sited to obtain the correct view of the nasopharyngeal isthmus. Care should be taken not to contact the posterior pharyngeal wall. This can cause severe bilateral earache despite otherwise adequate local anaesthesia, and if even a spot of blood contacts the light emission pupil or objective lens of the endoscope, the examination is impossible.

The patient is asked to swallow. Velopharyngeal closure in this instance will be lower in the nasopharynx than that achieved in speech. The endoscope tip is manoeuvred until the best position for observation is obtained.

The following speech sequence is then used to test closure effort with the tongue in different positions. Each sequence is demonstrated and the patient then attempts to reproduce the sound.

Pah, pah, pah	(bilabial plosive)
Tah, tah, tah	(alveolar plosive)
Sah, sah, sah	(alveolar fricative)
Cha, cha, cha	(palatal affricative)
Kah, kah, kah	(velar plosive, unvoiced)

The patient is then asked to count up to 20 slowly, and finally, as fast as possible.

The eustachian tube orifices may be examined, and the other nostril may be used for further viewing if indicated. During the examination, the size and shape of the resting isthmus are observed, as well as the degree and type of velopharyngeal movement. The presence of bubbles in the nasopharynx on attempted closure suggests failure of a complete seal. Movement of the lateral pharyngeal walls, or the development of a Passavant's ridge are noted.

Simultaneous recording of endoscopy with lateral fluoroscopy permits absolute measurements to be calculated (Pigott and Makepeace, 1982).

Fallacies of endoscopic assessment

The apparent size of an object in the field of view is misleading, since it is inversely proportional to the square of the distance between the object and the endoscope tip.

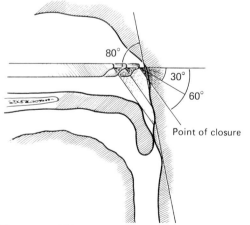

Figure 21.6 Oblique view fallacy. Point of velopharyngeal closure cannot be seen if angle of view of endoscope is inappropriate. For example, a 30° viewing foreoblique telescope with a cone of acceptance of 60° will not view the point of closure where the presumptive closure plane angle is 80°

Misinterpretation may occur because of the angle of view of the endoscope to the closure plane. A tangential view will give the impression of a smaller isthmus and to prevent this, the endoscope should be gently manipulated until the best tip position is achieved. If there is a gross discrepancy between the angle of the presumptive closure plane, the point of closure may be missed completely (*Figure 21.6*). Movement may be underestimated if the instrument is maintained in one position. As objects move closer to the lens, they become more brightly illuminated, but the distance traversed is difficult to estimate unless the instrument is 'panned' across the isthmus.

The wide angle effect of the lens of the 70° Storz endoscope must be taken into account (*Figure 21.7*). Objects in the outer annulus of the field of view will have an image that is compressed be a factor of two to three. Thus, one is especially likely to underestimate the area of failure of a port to close on the far side of a pharyngeal flap, because it is viewed obliquely, and its image is compressed by the peripheral image distortion effect of the wide angle lens.

X-ray examination

Historical

Velopharyngeal function has been investigated by means of radiology for many years. Scheier used single-exposure lateral radiographs in 1897, and since that time basal and frontal views have been found to provide valuable information. The disadvantage of single films, including tomograms, is the uncertainty over timing of the exposure.

Cineradiography became available in the 1950s (Carrell, 1952; Ardran and Wyatt, 1954), and to a large extent, this overcame the problem of coordinating exposure and palate movement. However, it involved relatively high doses of radiation. With the use of an image intensifier and videotape recording, the radiation factor can be reduced by a factor of ten, and exposure during an average one minute assessment is reduced to less than that of one chest film. Care must be taken to screen the eyes and thyroid.

Lateral pharyngeal view

Ideally a radiological examination will be performed during the same session as nasopharyngoscopy, but if this is not possible, a plain lateral view obtained prior to endoscopy allows the presumed isthmus closure plane to be seen and an appropriate endoscopy selected. In any case both uncoated and barium-coated lateral views should be obtained. Lateral fluoroscopy can be used during introduction of the endoscope to ensure correct positioning of the tip of the instrument for

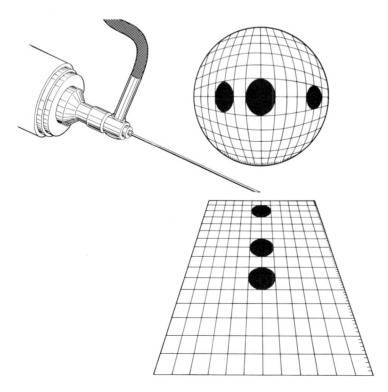

Figure 21.7 Wide angle fallacy. Apparent size of objects in periphery of endoscope view are reduced by a one-half to one-third of normal

observation of the isthmus. The radiological shadow of the endoscope is measured and related to the known width of the endoscope. The dimensions of the hard and soft palate, the range and timing of gross velar movement, and the presence of Passavant's ridge can then be assessed.

After the endoscopic examination is completed, barium sulphate (mixed as for a barium swallow) is instilled into each nostril in turn using a no. 8 FG catheter passed 2.5 cm back along the nasal floor. About 2 ml of the mixture are injected from a 10 ml syringe. The patient is asked to sniff and swallow. This helps to coat the entire nasopharynx. The patient repeats the phoneme sequence used during nasopharyngoscopic assessment, and palatal mobility is observed with a true lateral fluoroscopic view. Posterior wall activity and especially the presence of Passavant's ridge is noted.

Because X-rays are two dimensional, velopharyngeal closure may appear adequate on lateral projection with air contrast. This impression can be false and significant gaps may exist centrally or laterally. Two layers of barium (on the shoulder and in the valley) are frequently seen in submucous cleft and failed repaired cleft palate patients. Obviously, this diagnosis can only be made having checked that the image is a true lateral.

Basal view

X-rays of the isthmus at right angles to the lateral view overcome this problem. Skolnick (1970) showed that the velopharyngeal isthmus could be viewed *en face* by positioning the patient with head and neck extended, and the X-ray beam at right angles to a line passing from the corner of the mouth to the external auditory meatus.

Difficulties may arise in attempting to execute this view. Even with the use of a Philips 'C' arm BV image intensifier, some adults with short necks are incapable of extending sufficiently, and some children have an isthmus orientated in a plane that is too horizontal to obtain an *en face* view. Also, patients in whom closure is barely adequate with head and neck in the normal position may become incompetent when the neck is hyperextended. The basal view is least reliable when incompetence is being investigated following pharyngeal flap surgery. The lateral ports may become blocked by barium and give the impression of closure when in fact they are open. The axis of the port may be at an angle to the vertical plane, and several barium rings may be seen. In the absence of previous endoscopic information, accurate interpretation is impossible.

Fronto-occipital view

The plane of the isthmus in young children is disposed more horizontally, and closure occurs against the basisphenoid rather than the posterior pharyngeal wall. The basal view will not show the isthmus adequately, but a fronto-occipital view, despite the superimposition of the occipital bone, will do this.

Frontal view

This view is used to demonstrate the level at which maximal movement of the lateral pharyngeal walls occurs in order to place a pharyngeal mucomuscular obturator between the pharyngeal wall and palate at that level, against which the lateral wall can adduct, although the level at which the flap finally lies is largely beyond the surgeon's control.

Split screen recording

There are obvious advantages associated with simultaneous recording of nasopharyngoscopy and fluoroscopy, some of which have already been mentioned. Nasopharyngoscopy provides the best method of qualitatively assessing velopharyngeal closure, and radiology the best quantitative method.

Simultaneous recording provides a three-dimensional concept of what takes place and has contributed much to our understanding of the strengths and weaknesses of both systems. Neither form of investigation can be performed for more than one minute because of the invasive nature of endoscopy and the radiation hazard of X-rays. Repeated viewing of even brief records, particularly with stop and slow motion facilitates accurate diagnosis and research. A split screen unit provides a very convenient method of doing this.

Ideally, three personnel – an endoscopist, a radiographer, and an audiovisual supervisor – are required to run the examination, and must perform tasks simultaneously. A number of pieces of audiovisual equipment are used during investigation. These include a video camera, teaching attachment, video recorder and monitor. The image intensifier has its own video camera and a split screen unit allows the images to be combined.

The simplest method (David *et al.*, 1982) uses one half of a commercial split screen unit for the endoscope image, recorded on a colour video camera. The X-ray image is recorded by the other half by placing a second camera in front of the X-ray image intensifier monitor since commercial units (at a reasonable price) cannot displace the images from the centre of the screen. The two video cameras must be synchronized. The alternative system used by the authors involves a custom-built unit (Leendertz, Makepeace and Pigott, 1982) in which the images can be displaced. This obviates the degradation of the X-ray image involved in recording from the monitor. The brightness of both images is controlled independently and an electronically generated display provides a unique examination identification number and timing information to permit identification of a specific video frame.

The routine examination has the following parts:

(1) endoscopy with uncoated lateral pharyngeal X-ray
(2) portrait view of the patient with barium-coated lateral X-ray (using another video camera mounted 3 m in front of the patient with a 300 mm zoom lens)
(3) basal and/or fronto-occipital and/or frontal views.

Anemometry

A number of devices have been developed to measure nasal air flow during attempted velopharyngeal closure. Although the presence or absence of nasal escape can be determined subjectively by ear, quantitative data are helpful to allow objective comparison before and after treatment and between series treated at different centres.

Blowing devices, U-tube manometers and mirrors that record nasal fogging are among the clinical tools that have been used to record the presence or absence of nasal escape, but the results are lacking in standardization and cannot be used in random connected speech. During manoeuvres such as blowing and sucking, apparently satisfactory nasopharyngeal closure can often be achieved by utilizing contact between the tongue and palate.

Using an analogue study of nasal escape and by taking oral and nasal air pressure and flow measurements, Warren and Devereaux (1966) and Warren *et al.* (1985) were able to measure orifice size. They showed that for areas of incompetence more than 20 mm², there is poor correlation between area of incompetence and perceived levels of nasal escape, but good correlation below this. However, over 20 mm² nasal escape is likely to be perceived as moderate and therefore surgery will be indicated. Between 10 and 20 mm² escape will be perceived as slight to moderate and surgery may be indicated. Below 10 mm² escape will be perceived to be slight or nil and surgery is unlikely to be needed.

The equipment required for these measurements is expensive and more complex than that required in clinical context, and Warren (1979) has

developed a simpler instrument – PERCI (palatal efficiency rating computed instantaneously) – to confirm the presence of and quantify velopharyngeal incompetence. The technique also involves recording simultaneous pressures in the mouth and nose. Using this instrument reproducible pressure differences can be measured between the mouth and nose, and values for inadequate closure can be derived. However, the instrument cannot be used to measure incompetence in the not infrequent situation where the isthmus functions perfectly on plosives, but totally fails to attempt closure on fricatives particularly /s/ and /s/ blends.

Electromyography

This technique is not used extensively because of technical difficulties associated with the procedure, and the complex arrangement of the muscles of the region.

Fritzell (1969) and Lubker (1975) have undertaken some of the more extensive electromyographic studies of palatal function. Their investigations have required the insertion of electrodes via the nasal and oral cavities. They concluded that velopharyngeal musculature functions in a predictable fashion. However, the pattern of function depends on the order of the phonemes in the speech sequence and the action of individual muscles in the palate and pharynx are influenced by others about them.

Primary management of cleft palate
Classification

Kernahan and Stark (1958) termed the premaxillary complex the primary palate, because it

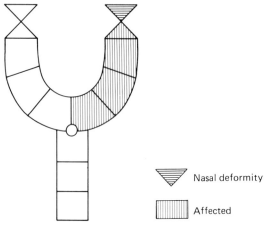

Figure 21.8 Striped Y classification (Kernahan, 1971) incorporating Millard's modification to represent nasal deformity. A complete cleft of the left side of the primary palate is represented

Table 21.1 Kernahan and Starke's classification of clefts

Cleft of primary palate only
Unilateral (right or left)
  complete
  incomplete
Median
  complete (premaxilla absent)
  incomplete (premaxilla rudimentary)
Bilateral
  complete
  incomplete

Clefts of secondary palate only
  complete
  incomplete
  submucous

Clefts of primary and secondary palates
Unilateral (right or left)
  complete
  incomplete
Median
  complete
  incomplete
Bilateral
  complete

develops in the embryo at 4–7 weeks, and the maxillary part the secondary palate, because it develops at 7–12 weeks. These structures combine at the incisive foramen to form the definitive palate. In this classification (*Table 21.1*), there is no facility for differentiation between clefts of the hard palate and the soft palate and, in an attempt to avoid sometimes confusing descriptions, Kernahan (1971) suggested a graphic method of representing clefts of the prepalate and palate, called the 'striped Y' classification (*Figure 21.8*).

Cleft palate repair

Timing

During the normal development of speech patterns, the first phonemes that require velopharyngeal closure are used between 6 and 9 months of age, suggesting that repair should precede this period. In 1927 Veau demonstrated that patients who underwent repair of the palate after 2 years of age had notably worse 'speech' than those whose palates were repaired before that age. Personal experience has indicated that there is a statistically significant higher rate of velopharyngeal sufficiency in children operated on under the age of one year compared with those operated on between one and 2 years (unpublished data). As infant nutrition and management of cardiac anomalies or diabetes, for example, improves, and as the experience of surgical, anaesthetic and nursing

teams increases, the dangers of early operation become less.

However, there are arguments against operating on the palate before the age of 12 months. As the infant grows older, the blood volume increases, leaving a greater margin of error in resuscitation. A larger airway reduces the risk of airway obstruction postoperatively and at one year of age the bulk of muscle in the palate is much larger than at 3 months, making tension-free repair easier.

Extent of repair

Controversy still exists regarding how much of the palate should be repaired at the primary procedure. The most common approach is to repair the soft palate, and all of the hard palate in need of closure. This avoids the postoperative requirement of an obturator. Surgeons who advocate this approach believe that simple elevation of mucoperiosteum to close the hard palate is only one factor causing maxillary retrusion. Inherent lack of growth potential in some cases and simple repair of the lip cleft may be of far greater significance. However, a number of authors are still of the opinion that a two-stage plan is better. Gillies noted that the maxillae of skulls which had not been operated upon grew virtually normally. This led Gillies and Fry (1921) to favour closure of only the soft palate before 2 years of age, and to leave a defect in the hard palate which was filled with an obturator. The remaining defect was sometimes repaired at 4 or 5 years of age, but many patients lived with their obturators until dental decay made this impossible. Others found that an obturator was a nuisance to manage, and preferred to be without one. Frequent remodelling of the plate is required as the palate grows and teeth erupt and are lost. Advocates who favour early repair of the soft palate and delayed repair of the hard palate, varying between 4 and 12 years, point out that considerable narrowing of the cleft takes place so that extensive mucoperiosteal undermining and displacement are not required (Hotz *et al.*, 1978; Schweckendiek, 1978). Since maxillary retrusion does not become fully evident until after the pubertal growth spurt, carefully planned long-term studies of speech and growth require completion before this issue can be resolved.

Technique

Surgery is performed at 6 months of age unless there are any contraindications.

A modified von Langenbeck (1861) technique will be described. The use of this method depends

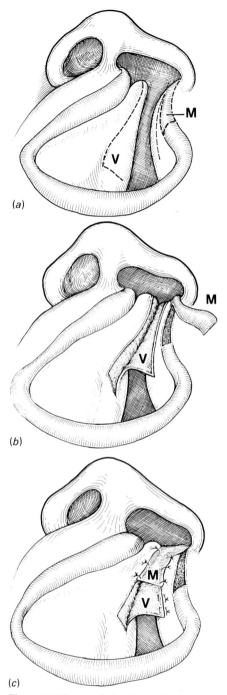

Figure 21.9 Repair of alveolus and anterior hard palate. (*a*) Lines of incision in palatal mucoperiosteum, of vomer and lesser segment for nasal layer closure and lines of incision in lateral labial mucosa for oral flap; (*b*) cleft is closed by approximating mucoperiosteal layers of alveolus and vomerine flap (V) of major segment beneath the mucoperiosteum of lesser flap; (*c*) a two-layer closure is achieved anteriorly by using the labial mucosa flap (M)

on closure of the anterior palate at the same time as the lip is repaired in those cases of complete cleft lip and palate. This is usually performed 3 months before palatal repair (*Figure 21.9*).

Longitudinal studies of facial growth (Ross, 1970) have shown a significantly greater proportion of midface retrusion in the patients who underwent the Veau procedure (*Figure 21.10*) compared with the von Langenbeck procedure (*Figure 21.11*). This has been attributed to the reduced amount of dissection of the hard palate in the von Langenbeck procedure, anteriorly. Veau's technique has, in the past, been considered to give superior speech results because it lengthened the palate. However, in 1959 and 1960 Calnan reported that the palatal lengthening achieved by the Veau V to Y pushback operation, modified by Wardill and Kilner, is not sustained. Reports of better speech results with the Veau operation over Langenbeck's and vice versa abound but some authors find no real difference (Jolleys, 1954; Witzel *et al.*, 1979).

Preoperative preparation

Bacteriological swabs are taken from the nose and throat 3 days preoperatively. The operation is postponed if group A β-haemolytic streptococci are cultured, and treatment with penicillin is commenced. Staphylococci are treated with nasal chlorhexidene and flucloxacillin.

Operation

Under endotracheal anaesthesia using a non-cuffed tube, gauze swabs soaked in 3% cocaine are placed along the margins of the cleft, and are inserted into the nostrils. Care is taken not to exceed a dose of 3 mg/kg body weight. An intravenous drip is inserted. The patient is positioned with a sandbag placed beneath the shoulders, and the head extended on the neck.

Both headlight and magnification with 2.5 loupes are used by the surgeon. Suction apparatus is available with a paediatric measuring facility. A Dott mouth gag and a throat pack are inserted. The palate is infiltrated with a solution of 1% lignocaine hydrochloride with 1:250000 adrenaline. Seven minutes are allowed for the vasoconstrictor to take effect.

The initial incision is made in the oral mucosa down to bone just medial to the sulcus between alveolar and palatal mucosa, from a point a little anterior to the forward limit of the cleft, back to the maxillary buttress, then laterally to the outer margin of the alveolus and then back again to the tip of the hamulus.

A second incision is made on the oral side of the margin of the cleft, along a line between oral and

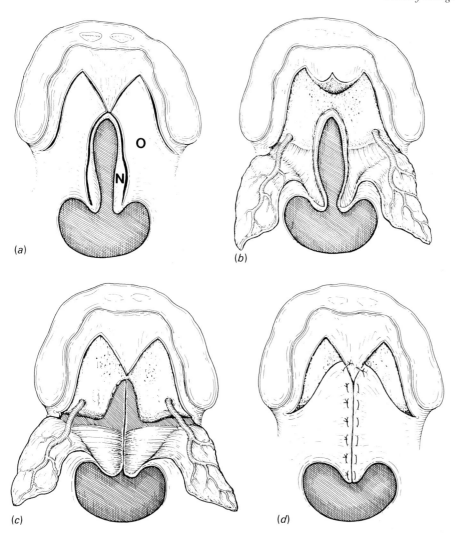

Figure 21.10 Veau technique of cleft palate repair, with veloplasty. (*a*) Lines of incision in palatal mucosa; (*b*) flaps are elevated based on the greater palatine arteries; (*c*) musculature of the soft palate is approximated; (*d*) mucosal closure, with V-Y pushback. O: oral mucosa; N: nasal mucosa

nasal mucosa where a distinct colour change from the redder nasal to the whiter oral mucosa exists. A small periosteal elevator such as a Mitchell's trimmer is used to separate the mucoperiosteum from the underlying bony palate starting from the lateral incision and working across to the cleft margin. Care must be taken to avoid damage to the greater palatine vessels. After exposure of the bony cleft margin, the nasal mucosa is mobilized blindly for a short distance laterally from the cleft margin.

With the posterior border of the hard palate in view, the soft palate musculature is gently mobilized at the line of attachment to the posterior margin of the hard palate using a combination of sharp and blunt dissection. Laterally, fibres of tensor palati can be seen passing around the hook of the hamulus. The tensor is preserved and the hamulus is not fractured. The lesser palatine nerve which supplies musculus uvulae is also preserved, if possible. The nasopharyngeal mucosa is mobilized from the medial surface of the pterygoid plate up to the base of skull. Both oral mucosa and mucous glands are separated from the muscular layer of the soft palate for about 1 cm to permit displacement of the musculus uvulae onto the palatal dorsum while uniting the levator and depressors beneath it. Oral and nasal flaps must

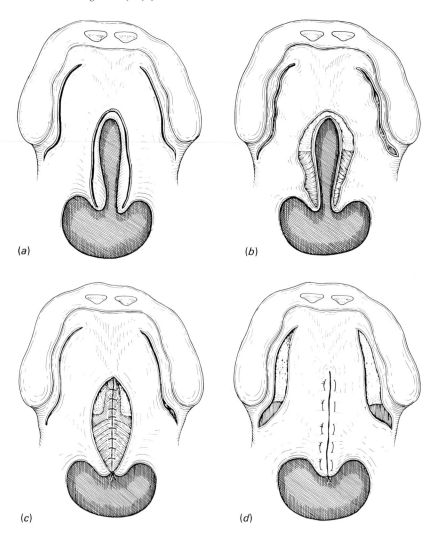

(a)

(b)

(c)

(d)

Figure 21.11 Von Langenbeck repair incorporating author's modifications. (*a*) Lines of incision in palatal mucosa; (*b*) flaps are elevated. Muscle layer of soft palate is defined but not dissected completely. Nasopharyngeal mucosa adherent to medial pterygoid plate is mobilized; (*c*) muscle layers are sutured in the midline, and the nasal mucosa everted with a horizontal mattress suture; (*d*) oral mucosa closure. No pushback, and minimal exposure of palatal bone occurs.

reach easily to the midline. A similar procedure is performed on the remaining side.

The nasal layer is closed first using interrupted absorbable sutures, beginning anteriorly and working back. Then a heavy (3.0 chromic) horizontal mattress suture is placed at the junction of the middle and posterior thirds of the soft palate. It passes through both muscle and nasal mucosa layers lateral to the musculus uvulae fibres, with the aim of bunching up the tissue on the dorsum midline of the palate to recreate the uvula muscle ridge (*Figure 21.12*).

The oral layer is then closed with interrupted mattress sutures, one suture being placed between oral and nasal layers at the junction of the hard and soft palate to obliterate a potential dead space. Small wedges of absorbable haemostatic agent (Oxycel) are placed in the lateral defects, which heal rapidly by secondary intention.

Postoperatively thumb sucking is prevented by armsplints for 2 weeks. The patient remains in hospital for 10 days after surgery.

A routine postoperative follow-up is arranged for 6 months, and the first formal speech

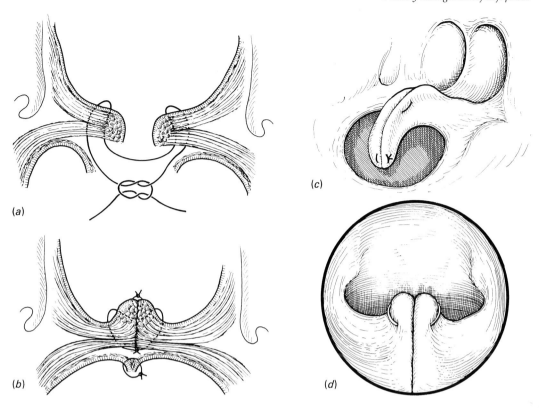

Figure 21.12 Musculus uvulae eversion suture. (*a*) Placement of suture; (*b*) and (*c*) eversion achieved; (*d*) endoscopic view of eversion achieved

assessment is carried out at 18 months. By this time it is already possible to assess velopharyngeal competence in some children, but most children can be reliably assessed at 30 months (van Demark and van Demark, 1970).

Early complications

The majority of children recover quickly from cleft palate repair, and the incidence of complications is low in experienced hands. Of the problems that can occur postoperatively, airway obstruction and bleeding are the two most dangerous.

Difficult intubation due to micrognathia, subglottic stenosis, cervical spine anomalies or incorrect tube selection may cause oedema of the glottis and tracheostomy may be required. More often, a tongue-stitch may be used to hold the tongue forward for a few hours in some micrognathic infants. It also facilitates pharyngeal suction. Humidification has been found useful in about 10% of infants and betamethasone has produced dramatic improvement on rare occasions.

Usually, bleeding can be controlled in the ward with direct pressure, using a swab placed over the bleeding point and digital compression. Haemorrhage sufficient to require return to theatre has occurred in approximately 5% of cases. Secondary haemorrhage is very uncommon, but if it occurs it can be life-threatening. Return to theatre and surgical control of the bleeding is necessary, as are antibiotics. The most common pathogen under these circumstances is the group A β-haemolytic streptococcus and penicillin is the drug of choice for treatment, but mixed infections are not uncommon and flucloxacillin should be added pending swab results. Group A streptococcal infection may also result in wound breakdown and fistula formation. Fistula repair should be deferred for a minimum of 6 months to allow scars to mature and the tissues to soften.

Late complications

Maxillary retrusion

The significant long-term problem following early total cleft palate repair is the effect that this surgery has on the growth of the midface. Some 80% of children with total clefts will require orthodontic correction for dental arch collapse and

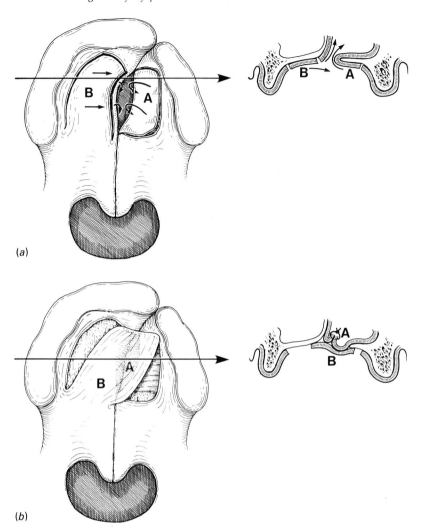

(a)

(b)

Figure 21.13 Local flap repair of hard palate fistula. The turnover flap is based on a scar at the edge of the fistula and must be elevated with great caution

10% will require surgery in the late teens for severe maxillary hypoplasia. Against this must be set evidence suggesting that early repair of the palate may reduce the incidence of ear infections and deafness and also reduce the incidence of severe articulatory disturbances leading to markedly impaired intelligibility.

Fistulae

Symptoms

While many fistulae remaining after cleft palate repair are small and asymptomatic, the following symptoms may be sufficient to merit surgery. Nasal dribbling, especially of ice cream or choco-late rubbed against the palate for taste, is a significant social disability and may occur with pinhole fistulae. Alteration of nasal resonance and loss of oral air pressure may occur. The tongue may naturally occlude the fistula for some sounds but trick movements to occlude it for other sounds distort articulation. Symptoms of rhinitis are not uncommon and ironically an enlarged turbinate may obturate a large fistula. Fistulae are described as being pre-, per- or postalveolar, hard palate, soft palate or a combination.

Treatment

Treatment may be by dental obturation or surgical closure. Dental obturation is particularly suitable if the patient must wear a partial denture due to loss of teeth. However, retention with cribs causes eventual tooth decay. While some patients wish to avoid surgery if at all possible, others may find the need to wear a plate unacceptable.

Surgical management to close the fistula requires tissue which may be available locally or may need to be imported. A surprisingly large flap of oral mucosa may be 'hinged' on the scar and turned up to line the nose. This is then reinforced, often as a double-breasting manoeuvre, with a flap transposed from the opposite side (*Figure 21.13*). Another local flap may be developed by advancing a segment of palatal mucoperiosteum on the greater palatine artery. After teasing out the vessel from the foramen, up to 2 cm of anterior displacement may be obtained. This operation described by Widmaier in 1973 has been christened, most aptly, the tadpole flap by Henderson (1982).

Where local tissue is considered to be too scarred or insufficient in area, distant flaps may be obtained from the buccal sulcus or tongue. Buccal sulcus mucosa may be transposed on a posterior base round behind the maxillary tuberosity, or anteriorly through the alveolar cleft.

The tongue provides a major reservoir of tissue where previous surgery has rendered repair with local tissue impracticable. A flap of mucosa with a shaving of muscle is raised, usually on an anterior base which should be sited beneath the posterior margin of the fistula and rotated through 180° to be sutured to the freshened edges of the fistula. Detachment of the pedicle is usually possible at 10–14 days. The mucosa retains its papillae and if a very large flap is taken sensation of the tongue may be impaired (Pigott, Reiger and Frazer Moodie, 1984).

Velopharyngeal incompetence

The concept of velopharyngeal incompetence or insufficiency has been covered, together with methods of investigation (*see also* Chapter 23). The incidence after cleft palate repair varies from less than 10% (Morley, 1970) up to more than 50% in other series, but many authors accept a figure in the region of 20% for patients operated upon in the first 2 years of life.

Improved velopharyngeal function in speech can be achieved by modifying one or more of the walls of the velopharyngeal isthmus.

Anterior wall

The failed repaired cleft palate shares several stigmata with submucous cleft (*see below*). In particular, the points of lift seen on the oral side of the palate are more widely separated than normal causing the palate to assume a square, rather than a Gothic pointed arch or the lift may be diffuse, producing a Norman or rounded arch. At the same time, ridges of muscle may be seen to build up towards the posterior nasal spine from the region of the eustachian tubes (Boorman and Sommerlad, 1985). The dorsal surface seen endoscopically has a V-shaped midline valley and this may be the site of failure to close as the palate shoulders reach the posterior wall. Alternatively, there may be a total failure of the palate to reach the posterior wall, a pharyngeal disproportion, indicating a degree of hypoplasia of the palate. Restoration of normal function may require some or all of the following (*Figure 21.14*):

(1) realignment of muscles by intravelar veloplasty (Kriens, 1975)
(2) reconstruction of the musculus uvulae ridge (Pigott, unpublished data)
(3) correction of the disproportion by lengthening the palate (Honig, 1967)
(4) augmentation of the palatal dorsum (Moore, 1960).

Posterior wall

The posterior wall may be advanced by insertion of materials such as cartilage, muscle, bone or synthetics such as Teflon and silastic. Alternatively the wall may be advanced by construction of a mucomuscular ridge on the posterior wall above the level of the arch of the atlas vertebra (Hynes, 1953; Orticochea, 1967). In order to perform this part of the operation the soft palate is retracted out of the way, and a transverse incision is made across the posterior wall as far above the level of the arch of the atlas as possible.

Bilateral flaps of posterior tonsillar pillar are raised, with bases orientated superiorly, at the same level as the transverse pharyngeal incision. The posterior margins of the flaps are continuous with this transverse incision. The flaps must contain some palatopharyngeus fibres if they are to be dynamic, but some muscle must be left behind, otherwise active palatal depression is reduced, with subsequent hyponasality. The flaps are transposed through 90° and sutured end to end. The inferior border of this newly created horizontal bar is then attached to the inferior border of the transverse incision in the posterior pharyngeal wall.

The pharyngoplasty is given time to heal and, although it may initially be immobile, on reassessment some months later, it will be seen to contract during speech. There are two possible explanations for the delay in function of this muscle bar. One is that cortical representation of the muscle activity, which was originally concerned with palatal depression, must have time to reorganize to coordinate with palatal elevation, and velopharyngeal closure. Another explanation is that during elevation and transposition of the

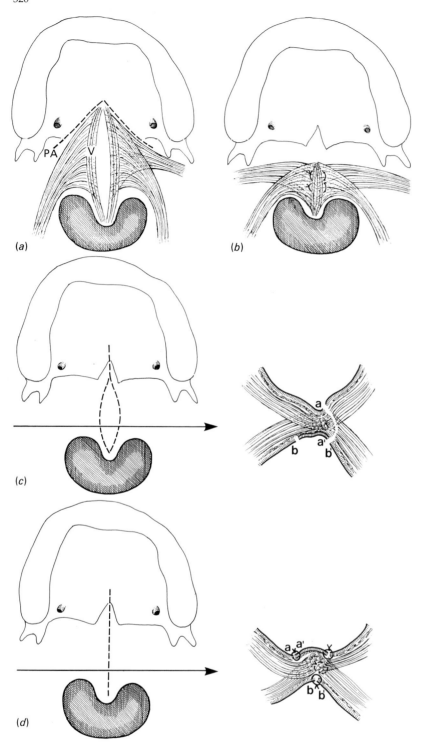

Figure 21.14 Techniques for restoring velopharyngeal competence. (*a*) Re-repair of the palate by intravelar veloplasty. Dotted line indicates incision through the palatine aponeurosis (PA) and Veau's muscle (V); (*b*) muscles retroposed and sutured in the midline; (*c*) oral mucosal island based on the muscles of one side; (*d*) after transposition to the nasal layer carrying the fibres of the musculus uvulae onto the dorsum

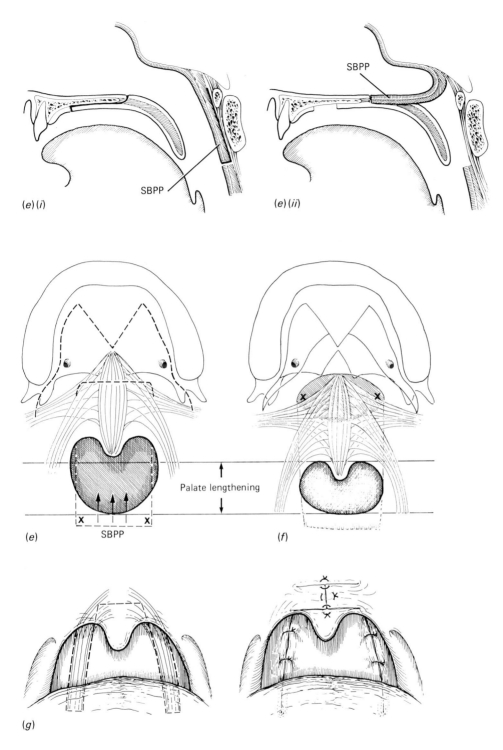

(e)(i)

SBPP

(e)(ii)

SBPP

(e)

SBPP

Palate lengthening

x   x

(f)

x

x

(g)

Figure 21.14 (e) palate lengthening by V-Y push back (Veau) of oral layer combined with inset of tip of pharyngeal flap, with superior base (SBPP) into the nasal layer (Honig); (f) flap inset into nasal layer; (g) lateral wall flaps containing palatopharyngeus and salpingopharyngeus transposed into a horizontal incision above the level of the arch of the atlas (Hynes). Incisions outlined and flaps transposed

muscle flaps, they become denervated, and they do not become active again until they have reinnervated with nerve fibres from the posterior pharynx. This muscle ridge will usually produce a static advancement of 5 mm, but in some cases it is dynamic, thus permitting sphincteric closure of the isthmus (Lendrum and Dhar, 1984).

Surgical obturation by pharyngeal flap

A superiorly or inferiorly based trapdoor of mucosa and muscle from the posterior wall (Schoenborn, 1876) is attached to the soft palate to obstruct the central part of the isthmus. These operations rely on adduction of the lateral pharyngeal walls to the flap to complete closure. The defect on each side of the bar is known as a port or gutter. The bridge of the mucosa is usually passive, although a few studies have suggested residual activity of the accompanying superior constrictor muscle. The width of the flap may be adjusted to take advantage of observed mobility of the lateral pharyngeal walls which provide the opening/closing element as they adduct against the bridge.

A method of employing several of these techniques dependent on the endoscopic and radiological findings is given in *Table 21.2*. Although good success has been reported with any one of the above operations, better results follow selection of the operation to fit the individual patient.

Complications particular to these operations include hyponasality, due to overclosure of the isthmus or inability of the palate to descend rapidly between phonemes; pooling of mucus occurs and may be due to impaired nasal drainage or to importing oral mucosal glands onto the nasal

surface of the palate; difficulty in eating may be experienced due to inability to inspire air with the mouth full due to overclosure of the isthmus. While snoring may occur due to altered air flow and turbulence, some patients who snore before operation are cured by pharyngoplasty.

Prosthetic obturation

An alternative approach is the non-surgical obturation of the defect with an acrylic mould. A piece of softened gutta-percha or other suitable dental impression material is introduced into the velopharyngeal isthmus on a bent wire attached to the back of the denture and the patient is asked to make a prolonged closure sound such as S-S-S, thus 'muscle trimming' the obturator. When the muscles relax there should be adequate space for nasal respiration and mucus drainage. Accurate addition and subtraction from the obturator is facilitated by nasal endoscopic control. Once a satisfactory shape has been achieved, the obturator is cast in acrylic.

Submucous cleft palate

Submucous cleft palate is an infrequently diagnosed condition, and anatomically is the least obvious form of cleft palate. However, it can be the cause of infant feeding difficulty, otitis media, deafness, and velopharyngeal incompetence, and treatment may be necessary. The term submucous cleft palate was first used by Kelly in 1910, although the condition had been described by Roux in the nineteenth century.

The incidence of this condition was thought to be quite rare. However, in 1972 Weatherley-White

Table 21.2 Method of pharyngoplasty selection

Observation	Deduction	Operation
(1) V-shaped upper surface of palate Anteroposterior gap less than 2 mm	Inadequate muscle union No disproportion Lateral wall movement irrelevant	Re-repair palate
(2) V-shaped upper surface of palate Anteroposterior gap of 2–5 mm	Inadeqaute muscle union Moderate disproportion Lateral wall movement irrelevant	Re-repair palate plus Hynes pharyngoplasty
(3) Anteroposterior gap greater than 5 mm	Severe disproportion Lateral wall movement irrelevant	Palate re-repair with lengthening by pharyngeal flap (Honig)
(4) Lateral walls adduct to close lateral ⅙ isthmus each	Disproportion irrelevant	Wide pharyngeal flap
(5) Lateral walls adduct to close lateral ⅓ isthmus each	Disproportion irrelevant	Narrow pharyngeal flap
(6) Asymmetrical movement	Modification of one of above to close residual defect	

et al. studied all 10836 children enrolled in the Denver school system. As a result, nine submucous cleft palates were identified, providing an incidence of 1:1200. This is roughly equivalent to the incidence of complete clefts of the secondary palate. Seven of those nine pupils were entirely asymptomatic, and only one required surgery for correction of a speech problem.

Aetiology

The cause of submucous cleft palate is unknown, but cleft palate is hereditary, with variable penetrance, and submucous cleft should probably be considered the mildest form, with recessive autosomal inheritance.

Classification

Submucous clefts may be considered overt or occult. They may also be associated with pharyngeal disproportion (*see also* Chapter 23).

In 1954, Calnan described the classic triad of examination findings associated with this condition:

(1) bifid uvula
(2) palatal muscle diastasis giving a translucent zone
(3) bony notch in the hard palate.

Essentially the same abnormal muscle configuration as seen in overt clefts leads to inadequate soft palate movement. This produces, initially, difficulty in feeding in a small number of cases, and subsequently, nasal escape on speaking. In addition, the same abnormality results in poor eustachian tube function.

As Kaplan (1975) has pointed out a spectrum of severity exists with regard to clefts of the secondary palate. This ranges from the complete overt cleft of both hard and soft palates, through to the classical submucous cleft and eventually to an entity termed the 'occult' submucous cleft in which velar function is abnormal, but there are no oral signs. The diagnosis is indicated by the symptomatology and must be confirmed by endoscopy, basal view X-rays and eventually by surgery. It is important to appreciate that submucous cleft may also be associated with pharyngeal disproportion, hypoplasia, etc.

Hypoplasia occurs in submucous cleft as it does in overt clefts and probably becomes worse with age (Skoog, 1965). Well developed adenoids may mask the disproportion. It is most important, therefore, to be aware of submucous cleft prior to adenoidectomy, in order to warn the patient or family of the possibility of speech impairment. Furthermore, if adenoidectomy had been recommended for recurrent otitis media there is a real possibility that the deranged musculature is responsible and not the adenoidal cushion.

Diagnosis

The diagnosis should be considered in all children with evidence of palatal incompetence, especially if there is a history of feeding difficulty in infancy, and it becomes almost certain if there is also a history of otitis media. The corollary is that it should always be excluded before treating cases of otitis media. An oral examination allows the diagnosis to be made on Calnan's criteria. In addition, on induction of a gag reflex, or if the patient is capable of saying 'ee-ee', the vault of the soft palate may be seen to rise and assume a box shape rather than the usual Gothic arch configuration, due to separation of the levator lift points (*Figure 21.15*). The soft palate itself may be seen to be short in comparison to the pharynx.

Kaplan has pointed out the association of the following facial features as characteristic of

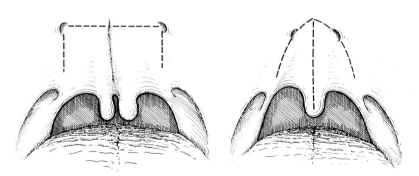

Figure 21.15 (*a*) Submucous cleft palate. Bifid uvulae and 'box-like' soft palate elevation with laterally placed dimples are demonstrated; (*b*) normal palate. 'Gothic arch' elevation is demonstrated

patients with classic submucous cleft, occult submucous cleft, and some overt clefts of the secondary palate; they are present to varying degrees:

(1) maxillary hypoplasia – 'dish face'
(2) lip contour deformity at vermilion border – 'gull wing'
(3) drooping of oral commissure
(4) hypodynamic facial muscles
(5) external ear abnormality – flat arc of superior helix
(6) alveolar arch abnormality.

Submucous clefting has been associated with a number of conditions. These include cleft lip, Treacher Collins, Klippel-Feil and Fanconi syndromes, congenital rubella, albinism, choanal atresia, Moebius syndrome, ring 18 chromosome and mental retardation. If any of these conditions is diagnosed early in life and a submucous cleft is recognized as well, speech development can be monitored carefully, and at the first signs of ear symptoms or speech problems associated with velopharyngeal incompetence appropriate measures can be taken.

Investigation

A speech assessment is undertaken, and if surgery is considered appropriate radiological and endoscopic assessments are made. The shape, size, and level of the incompetent velopharyngeal isthmus are recorded as for patients with an overt cleft.

Repair

Timing

Inevitably most submucous clefts are diagnosed late compared with overt clefts. The speech or ear problems with which they present will dictate correction as early as possible. Aberrant speech patterns may have become fixed, with grossly impaired intelligibility, and treatment can be quite difficult. Surgery should be combined with intensive speech therapy, in a residential course if progress is slow. However, a child with a submucous cleft may have normal articulation and intelligibility where nasal escape has been masked by large adenoids. If adenoidectomy is performed with subsequent intractable nasal escape and hypernasal resonance, an excellent result can be achieved by repair of the submucous cleft with or without pharyngoplasty.

Technique

A number of options are available in the surgical management of these patients. The choice of procedure depends on the findings at investigation.

If a palate with good length and mobility has been demonstrated radiographically (reaching to within 3 mm of the posterior pharyngeal wall), a standard cleft palate repair is undertaken. The soft palate is split in the midline and the velar musculature mobilized. The muscles of the two halves of the palate are brought together in the midline. The nasal midline bulge is carefully reconstructed with judicious placement of a horizontal everting mattress suture and the palate closed. For a gap of 3–5 mm a Hynes-type pharyngoplasty is added to the procedures above. Palates so short that they fail to achieve closure by more than 5 mm are comparatively rare and may require a Honig pharyngoplasty.

Results

The results of surgery for submucous cleft palate are variable and in general are not as good as for cleft palate repair. The most important aetiological factor in this regard is that surgery is not undertaken until significantly later compared with surgery for the overt cleft, and it has already been mentioned that the earlier a cleft is repaired, the more likely a satisfactory outcome will be achieved.

Only one-third of patients over 2 years of age achieve palatal competence if no additional manoeuvre is undertaken. However, with intensive speech therapy, good hearing and intelligence and, perhaps most important, the incentive to relearn articulation patterns, dramatic improvements often follow quickly (within 6 months) of the provision of a competent velopharyngeal mechanism.

The cleft palate clinic

Because children with a cleft palate in particular, but also the condition of velopharyngeal incompetence in general, frequently suffer with problems of deafness and otitis, of speech difficulty, of dental arch malformation and maxillary growth impairment, the families will be faced with many separate clinics and locations to visit. These visits can be very disruptive of schooling and family life. Associated congenital deformities, such as cardiac and ophthalmic conditions, will require yet more visits, and secondary problems such as school placement for the partially hearing, partially sighted or mentally retarded can add yet more.

Cleft palate clinics can go a considerable way to reducing this burden for the child and family. They can also provide an invaluable forum for the interchange of ideas and aims between the specialists involved and reduce the amount of contradictory information received by the families. The group of specialists may also find it desirable to run update courses for other professionals who come across the problem infrequently. Pamphlets for parents and books for use of those who occasionally have to treat these children can be developed and are more likely to provide a coherent concept. The secretary with a specialist member of the clinic in whose department the clinic is held, will become an invaluable liaison point for enquiries from patients and coordination between professionals.

It is worth considering who should be a member of the team, where and how often clinics should be held. In principle each member should feel that they have an input to most of the patients who attend on a particular occasion. Children without a cleft of the primary palate (approximately 25% of clefts) are unlikely to have a dental problem. The cleft palate team at Frenchay Hospital, Bristol (serving a population of about 800 000) therefore finds it useful to hold a monthly 'alveolar' cleft clinic. Here the orthodontist, plastic surgeon, speech therapist and clinical medical officer in audiology with an audiometrician, will find a high percentage of patients who require their advice. A second clinic called the 'speech' clinic will not require the orthodontist. The viability of this second monthly clinic depends partly on the special interest of one of the author's (RWP) in velopharyngeal incompetence.

These limited groups of specialists can sit together with the patient and family and, although each professional only contributes for about 25% of the time, on average, decisions are taken in concert and the family leaves with reasonably complete information. About three or at most four patients can be seen per hour, so about 12–15 patients would be the maximum per session. Routine records can often be obtained at the same visit. Audiometry is performed in a separate room and speech recordings, photographs, models and X-rays may be taken, ideally, before the consultation. If larger groups of professionals attend, it becomes impossible to sit in together, staffing meetings are required after the clinic and the patient does not receive the complete information for some time.

Clearly such clinics are for review only and are not working clinics. The actual visits for treatment tend to be relatively short bursts of time in the 20 year span of the child's association with the clinic. The exception may be the problems of otitis. Certainly it poses the greatest problem in providing adequate screening.

To keep the review clinic workload manageable, careful thought is required to avoid unnecessary visits. After primary repair of the lip and palate certain landmarks can be considered. Two and a half years is about the earliest reliable age to assess adequacy of palate function for speech. At 4 years, a general assessment of acceptability of all treatment is useful to allow time for desirable therapy or surgical revision prior to school. At 9 years, orthodontic assessment and treatment may be required over some 18–24 months as the permanent dentition erupts. Often this will be combined with bone grafting to the alveolus to allow optimal final tooth positioning. In the late teens, final orthodontic treatment will be combined with assessment of maxillary growth and possibly osteotomy of the mandible or maxilla. Soft tissue surgery for appearance, breathing and speech can often be combined with the two periods of bony surgery. In addition, children will be asked to attend for general record taking at the nationally agreed timing of 5, 10, 15 and 20 years to permit interunit comparisons.

Against these isolated occasions it is necessary to provide a relentless review system to maintain hearing levels during the critical years up to puberty. Such a high density review will not usually be practicable at a general cleft clinic. However, a parallel clinic would be ideal for cross-referral at the same session.

The venue of the clinic will be dictated by local factors of available space, special interest, etc. The authors have found that childrens' centres, and orthodontic and speech therapy departments have all provided excellent locations. The location secretary and professional must be enthusiastic about the work and prepared to give time unstintingly to ensure efficiency of the service. The question of a clinic leader or chair person will often resolve itself quite effortlessley as some specialists would not wish to take the chair. Where several members are keen to chair the clinic, rotation would seem to be eminently sensible. No member of the team has a monopoly of responsibility for a successful outcome.

Cleft lip and palate and related anomalies are rare in the total of each professional's work spectrum. To make efficient use of time a certain minimum case load is desirable and the senior author has been privileged to treat a major share of the cases from the sub region served by the Department of Plastic Surgery at Frenchay Hospital, Bristol. In turn, this has made it possible to confine referral of the patients to only one otolaryngologist in each of four areas visited so that they should be enabled to develop a special interest, leading to adoption of a specific otolaryngological cleft palate review clinic. These are vital concepts since it has been seen that where individual specialists treat these complicated cases but rarely, rather poor results frequently follow.

References

ARDRAN, G. M. and WYATT, D. G. (1954) 35 mm cine camera incorporating a Philips X-ray image intensifier. *Journal of Physiology*, **126**, 1–2

ASTLEY, R. (1958) The movements of the lateral walls of the nasopharynx: a cineradiographic study. *Journal of Laryngoscopy*, **72**, 325–328

AZZAM, N. A. and KUEHN, D. P. (1977) The morphology of musculus uvulae. *Cleft Palate Journal*, **14**, 78–87

BELL-BERTIE, F. (1976) An electromyographic study of velopharyngeal function in speech. *Cleft Palate Journal*, **19**, 225–240

BOORMAN, J. G. and SOMMERLAD, B. C. (1985) Levator palati and palatal dimples: their anatomy, relationship and clinical significance. *British Journal of Plastic Surgery*, **38**, 326–332

BOREL-MAISONNY, S. (1937) Resultats phonetiques obtenus dans les fissures palatines. *Revue de Stomatologies*, **39**, 733–754

CALNAN, J. S. (1952) Movements of the soft palate. *British Journal of Plastic Surgery*, **5**, 286–296

CALNAN, J. S. (1954) Submucous cleft palate. *British Journal of Plastic Surgery*, **6**, 264–282

CALNAN, J. S. (1959) The surgical treatment of nasal speech disorders. *Annals of the Royal College of Surgeons England*, **25**, 119–141

CALNAN, J. S. (1960) Cleft palate: lengthening of the soft palate following the V-Y repair. *British Journal of Plastic Surgery*, **13**, 243–248

CARRELL, J. (1952) A cinefluorographic technique for the study of velopharyngeal closure. *Journal of Speech and Hearing Disorders*, **17**, 224–228

DAVID, D. J., WHITE, J., SPROD, R. and BAGNAL, A. (1982) Nasendoscopy: significant refinements of a direct-viewing technique of the velopharyngeal sphincter. *Plastic and Reconstructive Surgery*, **70**, 423–428

FRITZELL, B. (1969) The velopharyngeal muscles in speech. *Acta Oto-Laryngologica Supplementum*, **250**, 48

GILLIES, H. D. and FRY, W. K. (1921) A new principle in the surgical treatment of congenital cleft palate and its mechanical counterparts. *British Medical Journal*, **1**, 335–338

HENDERSON, H. P. (1982) An advancement island flap for the closure of anterior palatal fistulae. *British Journal of Plastic Surgery*, **35**, 163–166

HONIG, C. A. (1967) The treatment of velopharyngeal insufficiency after palatal repair. *Archivum Chirurgicum Neerlandicum*, **19**, 71–81

HOTZ, M. M., GNOINSKI, W. M., NUSSBAUMER, H. and KISTLER, E. (1978) Early maxillary orthopaedics in cleft lip and palate cases: guidelines for surgery. *Cleft Palate Journal*, **15**, 405–411

HYNES, W. (1953) The results of muscle transplantation in 'failed cleft palate' cases, with special reference to the influence of the pharynx on voice production. *Annals of the Royal College of Surgeons*, **13**, 17–35

JOLLEYS, A. (1954) A review of the results of operations on cleft palates with reference to maxillary growth and speech function. *British Journal of Plastic Surgery*, **7**, 229–241

KAPLAN, E. N. (1975) The occult submucous cleft palate. *Cleft Palate Journal*, **12**, 356–368

KELLY, A. B. (1910) Congenital insufficiency of the palate. *Journal of Laryngology, Rhinology and Otology*, **25**, 281–342

KERNAHAN, D. A. (1971) The striped Y-A symbolic classification for cleft lip and palate. *Plastic and Reconstructive Surgery*, **47**, 469–470

KERNAHAN, D. A. and STARK, R. B. (1958) A new classification for cleft lip and palate. *Plastic and Reconstructive Surgery*, **22**, 435–441

KRIENS, O. (1975) Anatomy of the velopharyngeal area in cleft palate. *Clinics in Plastic Surgery*, **2**, 261–283

KUEHN, D. P. and AZZAM, N. A. (1978) Anatomical characteristics of palatoglossus and the anterior faucial pillar. *Cleft Palate Journal*, **15**, 349–359

LEENDERTZ, J., MAKEPEACE, A. P. W. and PIGOTT, R. W. (1982) A television split screen unit for recording combined endoscopic and X-ray image intensifier views of the human nasopharynx for the investigation of palato-glossal malfunction. *Proceedings of the Physiological Society*, **327**, 23

LENDRUM, J. and DHAR, B. K. (1984) The Orticochea dynamic pharyngoplasty. *British Journal of Plastic Surgery*, **37**, 160–168

LUBKER, J. F. (1975) Normal velopharyngeal function in speech. *Clinics in Plastic Surgery*, **2**, 249–259

MASSENGILL, R., QUINN, G., BARRY, W. F. and PICKRELL, K. (1966) The development of rotational cinefluorography and its application to speech research. *Journal of Speech and Hearing Research*, **9**, 259–265

MOORE, F. T. (1960) A new operation to cure nasopharyngeal incompetence. *British Journal of Surgery*, **47**, 424–428

MORLEY, M. E. (1970) *Cleft Palate and Speech*, 7th edn, ch. 3, pp. 124–127. Edinburgh: Livingstone

MULDER, J. W. (1976) Velopharyngeal function and speech. *Doctoral thesis*. Amsterdam: Van Gorcum & Co. B.V. Assen

NICKL, A. (1950) Uber die Innervation des musculus levator veli palatini durch den N. facialis. *Archiv für Psychiatrie und Zeitschrift Neurologie*, **184**, 117–132

NISHIO, J., MATSUYA, T., MACHIDA, J. and MIYAZAKI, T. (1976a) The motor nerve supply of the velopharyngeal muscles. *Cleft Palate Journal*, **13**, 20–30

NISHIO, J., MATSUYA, T., IBUKI, K. and MIYAZAKI, T. (1976b) Roles of the facial, glossopharyngeal and vagus nerves in velopharyngeal movements. *Cleft Palate Journal*, **13**, 201–214

ORTICOCHEA, M. (1967) Construction of a dynamic muscle sphincter in cleft palates. *Plastic and Reconstructive Surgery*, **41**, 323–327

PIGOTT, R. W. (1969) The nasendoscopic appearance of the normal palato-pharyngeal valve. *Plastic and Reconstructive Surgery*, **43**, 19–24

PIGOTT, R. W. and MAKEPEACE, A. P. (1982) Some characteristics of endoscopic and radiological systems used in elaboration of the diagnosis of velopharyngeal incompetence. *British Journal of Plastic Surgery*, **35**, 19–32

PIGOTT, R. W., REIGER, F. W. and FRAZER MOODIE, A. (1984) Tongue flap repair of cleft palate fistulae. *British Journal of Plastic Surgery*, **37**, 285–293

PODVINEC, S. (1952) The physiology and pathology of the soft palate. *Journal of Laryngology and Otology*, **66**, 452–461

ROSS, R. B. (1970) The clinical implications of facial growth in cleft lip and palate. *Cleft Palate Journal*, **7**, 37–47

SCHEIER, M. (1897) Uber die Verwerthung der Rontgen-strahlen in der Rhino-und Laryngologie. *Archiv für Laryngologie*, **6**, 57–66

SCHOENBORN, D. (1876) Uber eine neue methode der staphylorrhaphie. *Archiv für Klinistre Chirurgie,* **19,** 527

SCHWECKENDIECK, W. (1978) Primary veloplasty: long term results without maxillary deformity. *Cleft Palate Journal,* **15,** 268–274

SEDLAKOVA, E., LASTOVKA, M. and SCRAM, F. (1973) Contribution to knowledge of soft palate innervation. *Folia phoniatrica,* **25,** 434–441

SHPRINTZEN, R. J., LEWIN, M. L., CROFT, C. B., DANILLER, A. I., ARGAMASO, R. V., SHIP, A. G. et al. (1979) A comprehensive study of pharyngeal flap surgery. Tailor made flaps. *Cleft Palate Journal,* **16,** 46–55

SKOLNICK, M. L. (1970) Videofluoroscopic examination of the velopharyngeal portal during phonation in lateral and base projections – a new technique for studying the mechanics of closure. *Cleft Palate Journal,* **7,** 803–816

SKOLNICK, M. L., McCALL, G. N. and BARNES, R. T. (1973) The sphincteric mechanism of velopharyngeal closure. *Cleft Palate Journal,* **10,** 286–305

SKOOG, T. (1965) The management of the bilateral cleft of the primary palate (lip and alveolus). *Plastic and Reconstructive Surgery,* **35,** 35–44

SOMMERLAD, B. (1981) Nasendoscopy. In *Recent Advances in Plastic Surgery,* edited by I. T. Jackson, vol. 2, pp. 11–27. Edinburgh: Churchill Livingstone

TAUB, S. (1966) The Taub oral panendoscope: a new technique. *Cleft Palate Journal,* **3,** 328–346

VAN DEMARK D. and VAN DEMARK, A. (1970) Speech and sociovocational aspects of individuals with cleft palate. *Cleft Palate Journal,* **7,** 284–299

VEAU, V. (1926-1927) The treatment of cleft palate by operation. *Proceedings of the Royal Society of Medicine,* **20,** 1916–1926

VON LANGENBECK, B. (1861) Operation der Angeborenen totalen Spaltung des harten Gaumens nach einer neuer Methode. *Dtsch. Klin.,* **8,** 231

WARREN, D. W. (1979) Perci: a method for rating palatal efficiency. *Cleft Palate Journal,* **16,** 279–285

WARREN, D. W., DALSTON, R. M., TRIER, W. C. and HOLDER, M. B. (1985) A pressure-flow technique for quantifying temporal patterns of palatopharyngeal closure. *Cleft Palate Journal,* **22,** 11–19

WARREN, D. W. and DEVEREAUX, J. L. (1966) An analogue study of cleft palate speech. *Cleft Palate Journal,* **3,** 103–114

WEATHERLEY-WHITE, R. C. A., SAKURA, C. Y., BRENNER, L. D., STEWART, J. M. and OTT, J. E. (1972) Submucous cleft palate. *Plastic and Reconstructive Surgery,* **49,** 297–304

WHILLIS, J. (1930) A note on the muscles of the palate and the superior constrictor. *Journal of Anatomy,* **65,** 92–95

WIDMAIER, W. (1973) Beitrag zum Verschluss schwieriger Restperforationen am Gaumen mit Insellappen und Lyodura. In *Fortschritte der Kiefer- und Gesichts-Chirurgie,* edited by K. Schuchardt, G. Steinhardt and N. Schwenzer, pp. 299–320. Stuttgart: Thieme

WITZEL, M. A., CLARKE, J. A., LINDSAY, W. K. and THOMSON, H. G. (1979) Companion of results of pushback or Von Langenbeck repair of isolated cleft of the hard and soft palate. *Plastic and Reconstructive Surgery,* **64,** 347–352

22

Orthodontics

D. A. Plint

The relationship between dentistry and the speciality of otolaryngology is a close one. They share common ground, and pathology affecting one area encroaches on, or may arise from, conditions more immediately associated with the other speciality.

Orthodontics is a branch of dentistry that can be defined as a dental science concerned with genetic variations, development and growth of facial forms, and the manner in which these factors affect the occlusion of the teeth, and function of associated organs.

Growth and development

Growth of the face takes place at the circum-maxillary sutures, and also by surface deposition. Growth is mainly in a forward and downward direction from the anterior cranial base. Interference with the growth of the cranial base will, therefore, have an influence on the development of the maxilla and mandible – the former because of its direct relationship to the cranial base, the latter due to aberrant position of the glenoid fossae.

The mandible moves downwards from the cranial base with bone formation at the condylar and coronoid processes. There is also surface deposition to the posterior borders of the ascending rami, with corresponding resorption of the anterior surface. Direction of growth of the mandible is important, and here environmental factors may play a part (posture of the head and mouth breathing).

In both jaws, alveolar bone keeps pace with the downward and forward growth of the maxilla and mandible, and also to provide support for the teeth.

Abnormalities of the cranium, for example Apert's syndrome, and facial complex, for example first arch anomalies, affect the relationship of the jaws and, in turn, the occlusion of the teeth.

Orthodontic treatment mainly takes place during the growing period of the individual and, therefore, an understanding of normal growth is important. However, growth is not fully predictable. Where pathology exists it is even more important to be able to assess the underlying cause, and carry out corrective measures at the appropriate time.

Aetiology of malocclusion of the teeth

Both inherited and environmental factors play a part in the establishment of malocclusion of the teeth. For many years genetic factors were considered to be more important. Recently, environmental factors have been gaining ground – but not to the exclusion of inherited ones. Whatever the underlying cause, the position of the teeth is mainly dependent on three factors:

(1) skeletal pattern
(2) soft tissue morphology
(3) ratio of tooth to jaw size.

Skeletal pattern

Differences in size, shape and position or adverse growth of the bones of the face and skull, whether due to inherited, environmental or pathological reasons, can result in an unfavourable relationship of the maxilla to the mandible. This may lead to malocclusion of the teeth. A controversy exists as

334

to whether the inherent growth pattern has a greater influence on growth and development of the facial skeleton than the environmental factors put forward in the functional matrix theory (Moss and Salentijn, 1969). This theory postulates that bony growth of the face is greatly influenced by soft tissues and changes in size of the spaces in the head, for example mouth, sinuses, pharynx. A comparison is made with the cranium which is influenced by normal and pathological changes within it, for example hydrocephalus.

In discussing the relationship of the maxilla to the mandible, three planes must be considered:

(1) anteroposterior (sagittal) plane
(2) vertical plane
(3) transverse plane.

Adverse position of, or growth, in any one plane, or a combination of planes, will contribute towards the establishment of a malocclusion of the teeth.

(1) The most commonly observed and measured plane is the anteroposterior one. This and the vertical plane can be judged clinically and by special radiographic techniques (*Figure 22.1*). It is important to be able to assess whether the underlying skeletal problem is due to the position of the maxilla or mandible – or a combination of the two. These cephalometric radiographs can be taken at regular intervals to monitor growth. They also record changes to the position of the teeth, brought about by orthodontic treatment, and to the jaws by surgical procedures.
(2) Vertical anomalies will be discussed in more detail under Mouth breathing, but two main types of facial form are described – the broad short brachycephalic face (*Figure 22.2*), and the long thin dolichocephalic one (*Figure 22.3*).

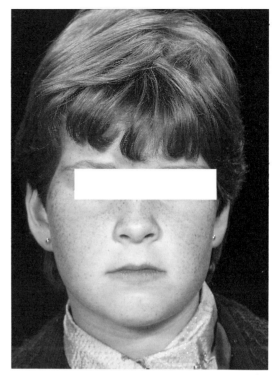

Figure 22.2 Broad or brachycephalic face

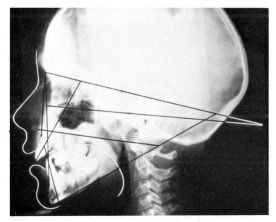

Figure 22.1 Cephalometric radiograph showing planes used for angular measurements

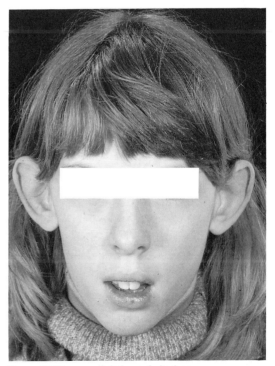

Figure 22.3 Long or dolichocephalic face

There may also be differences in proportion between the upper and lower facial heights. This must be taken into account when planning treatment for the correction of facial anomalies.

(3) Transverse relations are best assessed clinically. Basically, the upper jaw can be too wide or too narrow to match the too wide or too narrow lower jaw (*Figure 22.4*). Transverse

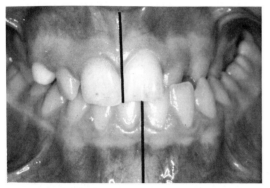

Figure 22.4 Crossbite of buccal teeth with displacement of mandible to the left

basal bone discrepancies are compensated for in some cases by buccal and/or lingual tilting of the maxillary and mandibular teeth, and supporting alveolar bone. If this does not result in normal intercuspation of the buccal teeth, the result is what is termed 'a crossbite'. A severe example of this is where maxillary teeth occlude completely buccal to the lower teeth in a scissor-bite relationship, for example some thalassaemia patients suffer this due to expanded maxillary bone (*Figure 22.5*).

There is no clear evidence that orthodontic treatment can alter the skeletal pattern – the changes that take place are mainly in respect of the supporting alveolar bone.

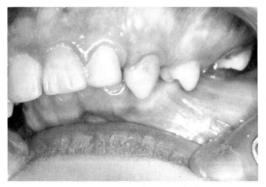

Figure 22.5 Scissor-type crossbite in a thalassaemia patient

Soft tissue morphology

Lips

The position of the teeth is also dependent on the soft tissue environment of the lips, cheeks, and tongue. There is debate as to whether the activity of the surrounding musculature is the main factor influencing this, or whether position and size of lips, tongue, etc. are of equal importance in guiding and maintaining the teeth in occlusion. Objective measurements are difficult – so most observations are subjective.

The position of the incisor teeth is governed by the lips anteriorly, and by the tongue posteriorly. Both activity and posture probably play a part in incisor position. The lower lip is probably the more important. Lip line is defined as the position on the upper incisors where the upper and lower lips meet. In a patient where the upper incisors are proclined, the lip line is low on the upper incisors, or the lower lip may even be behind the incisors at rest and during activity (*Figure 22.6*). Where the upper incisors are retroclined, the lower lip usually covers most of the crowns of the incisors during rest and activity.

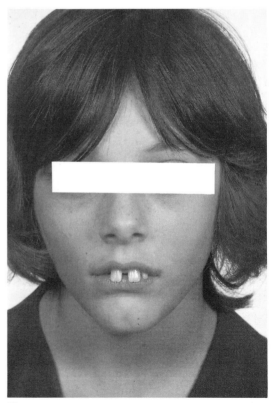

Figure 22.6 Incompetent lips with lower lip trapped behind upper incisors

The terms 'competent' and 'incompetent' have been used to describe the morphology of the lips. By definition, lips that can be opposed with minimal muscular contraction, with the mandible in the rest position, are said to be competent (*Figure 22.7*). These are poor terms – no other valve or orifice in the body is termed 'incompetent' if it can achieve adequate opening and closing. A better method of describing the lip morphology would be to note how a lip seal is achieved, for example visible contraction of the orbicularis oris and mentalis muscles, with or without forward posturing of the mandible. The use of the tongue to help achieve a seal should also be noted as this may influence the orthodontic prognosis.

Where there is a habitual lack of a lip seal, it must *not* be assumed that the patient is a mouth breather (*Figure 22.8*). It is possible to achieve an anterior oral seal between tongue and lower lip and/or a posterior seal between dorsum of the tongue and soft palate (*Figure 22.9*).

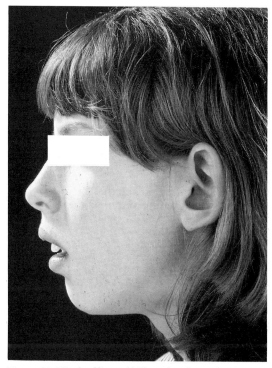

Figure 22.8 Lack of lip seal in long faced case

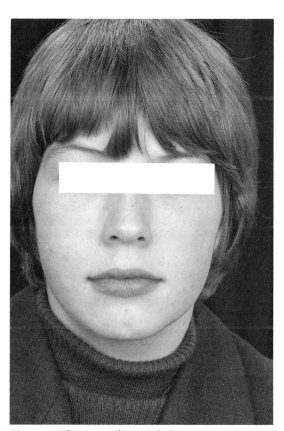

Figure 22.7 Competent lip morphology

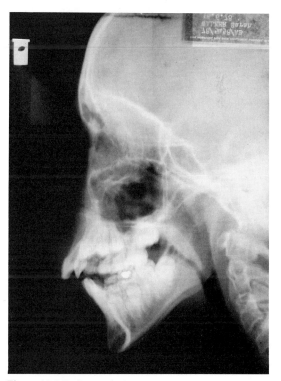

Figure 22.9 Radiograph showing posterior seal between dorsum of the tongue and palate – same case as *Figure 22.8*

Tongue

Size, position and activity are even more difficult to assess for the tongue than for the lips.

The tongue normally adapts to the size and form of the oral cavity but, in certain circumstances, appears not to be able to be accommodated. Examples are in Down's (*Figure 22.10*) and Beckwith's syndromes, tumours of the tongue (*Figure 22.11*) and hemifacial hypertrophy. In the case of Down's syndrome, the fault may be due to the small oral cavity, or to the tongue posture. The other three examples are true tongue enlargements.

Where the tongue is held habitually forward, there will be an interference with the developing occlusion – proclination of upper incisors and a tendency towards an anterior open bite.

Tongue *posture* may be influenced by anomalies such as a narrow upper arch, as seen in some repaired cleft palate patients – here the tongue position will be low. In mouth breathing, the mandible is lowered, and the tongue again adopts a low position to facilitate breathing. Some believe that enlarged tonsils contribute to a forward tongue position. Regression in respect of size of

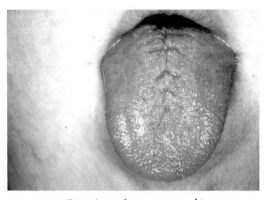

Figure 22.10 Down's syndrome – grooved tongue

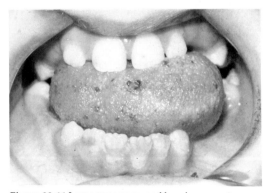

Figure 22.11 Large tongue caused by a haemangioma

the tonsils may allow the tongue to adopt a more normal position in the mouth. Enlargements of the tongue will interfere with the position of the teeth – unilateral examples demonstrate this clearly as seen in haemangiomata (*Figure 22.11*).

Tongue activity

In the new-born baby the tongue lies between the gum pads, and in contact with the lips anteriorly. Swallowing takes place with the tongue in this position. The eruption of teeth leads to a change from this infant type of swallowing to the adult form. Here the teeth are brought lightly together and the tongue is contained by the teeth and the alveolar processes. The infant type of swallow sometimes persists. Where it does, there may be an interference with the position of the teeth. The majority of children eventually adopt a normal swallowing behaviour; this allows for spontaneous correction of the occlusion unless other factors, such as digit sucking, gross anomalies of jaw relationship, or adverse soft tissue lip factors, prevent it. An atypical swallowing behaviour described as an endogenous tongue thrust, probably due to abnormal neuromuscular activity, is sometimes seen. Fortunately, this is not common. It is difficult to diagnose and sometimes only appreciated when treatment fails to produce a stable result. Some pointers are the force of the tongue thrust, and the extent of the resulting malocclusion. Also, an associated speech defect, such as a lisp, may help in diagnosis.

To summarize, the teeth are held in a balanced position between the soft tissues of lip and tongue. If the position of the teeth is altered, a new position of balance must be achieved, if a stable result is to be the outcome of treatment.

Tooth tissue ratio

The third important factor as a cause of malocclusion is the relation in size between the teeth and available bone to accommodate them. Unfavourable relationships will lead to crowding or spacing of the teeth. Crowding is a more common problem than spacing especially in the UK – possibly the result of a mixed population group (*Figure 22.12*). However, crowding is an aetiological factor that can be dealt with effectively by the extraction of teeth.

Evolutionary changes are slow in bringing about the reduction of teeth to match the jaw size. The full complement of teeth in man is 32. Missing permanent teeth are fairly common, third molars and upper lateral incisors being the most frequent to be absent. Where a number of teeth are absent the terms 'hypodontia' or 'oligodontia' are used

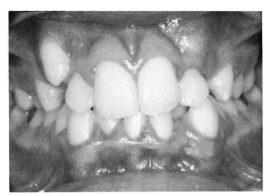

Figure 22.12 Crowding of teeth, the result of disproportion between tooth and arch size

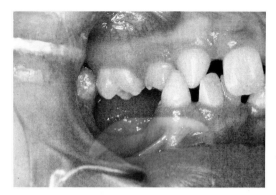

Figure 22.13 Spacing of teeth, caused by the absence of a number of teeth, known as hypodontia

(*Figure 22.13*). This is seen in syndromes, such as ectodermal dysplasia and orofacial digital syndrome.

Extra teeth, called supernumeraries, are less of a problem. If interfering with the occlusion, they can be removed. The upper incisor region is the most common site (*Figure 22.14*).

There are a few other local anomalies that can lead to malocclusions: habits, such as dummy and finger sucking, can cause or aggravate the malposition of teeth (*Figure 22.15*). Early loss of deciduous teeth where crowding is present will lead to a loss of space at the site of the extraction, and may interfere or prevent eruption of the permanent successor. Occasionally pathological conditions such as cysts or odontomes may interfere with the normal eruption of teeth. These can be dealt with by surgery.

Malocclusion is the result of many complex factors, and careful diagnosis and treatment planning are required in order to bring about a satisfactory and stable result. This will be discussed in the next section.

Classification of malocclusion and treatment objectives in orthodontics

Malocclusion will be discussed under the following headings:

(1) dental base relationship
(2) dental arch relationship
(3) individual tooth positions.

Dental base relationship

The dental base relationship is termed 'skeletal pattern'. It is most commonly used to describe the anteroposterior relationship, but vertical and transverse dimensions should also be taken into

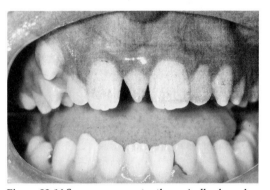

Figure 22.14 Supernumerary tooth, conically shaped extra tooth in the midline

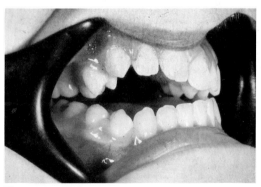

Figure 22.15 Malposition of teeth, resulting from a thumb sucking habit

account. Anteroposterior relationships are divided into three groups – skeletal I, II and III.

Skeletal I is where there is a normal relationship between the maxilla and mandible, that is in fact where the maxilla is slightly anterior to the mandible (*Figure 22.16*).

Skeletal II is where the maxilla is placed anteriorly to the mandible. This may be due to a

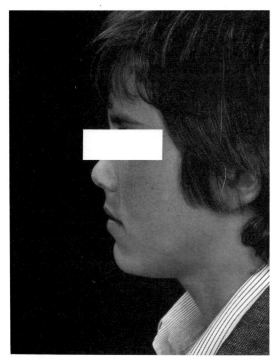

Figure 22.16 Skeletal I facial profile. Normal maxillary/mandibular relationship

prominent maxilla or, more commonly, to a small and/or retrusive mandible (*Figure 22.17*).

Skeletal III is where the maxilla is placed posteriorly to the mandible and this can be due to a retrusive maxilla or prognathic mandible (*Figure 22.18*).

Cases which have a skeletal I dental base are usually easier to treat and have a better prognosis than those on skeletal II or III bases.

Dental arch relationship

Here we are dealing with the relationship of the teeth in one jaw to those in the opposing jaw, that is how they occlude.

The most widely used classification is one where the relationship of the upper and lower first permanent molars is used to classify the occlusion. This is called the Angle classification after Edward Angle. However, a more useful one which is simple and unambiguous is the British Standard Incisor Classification. This is a record of the relationship of the upper and lower incisor teeth.

As with skeletal pattern there are three divisions:

Class I is where the lower incisors occlude (or would meet, if not in contact) with the middle

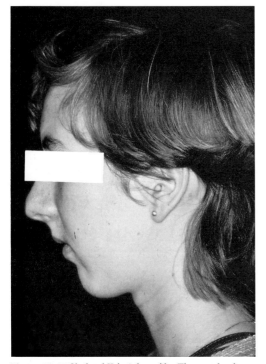

Figure 22.17 Skeletal II facial profile. The result of maxillary prognathism or mandibular retrusion or a combination of the two

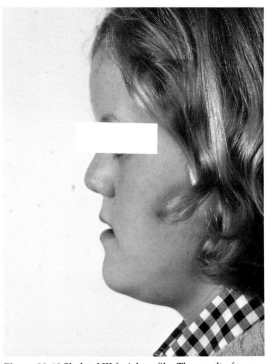

Figure 22.18 Skeletal III facial profile. The result of maxillary retrusion or mandibular prognathism, or a combination of the two

part of the palatal surface of the upper central incisors (*Figure 22.19*).

Class II is where the lower incisors lie posterior to the middle part of the palatal surfaces of the upper central incisors (*Figure 22.20*).

Class III is where the lower incisors lie anterior to the middle part of the palatal surfaces of the upper central incisors (*Figure 22.21*).

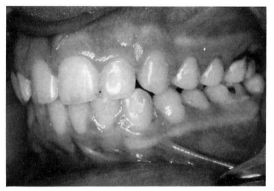

Figure 22.19 Class I occlusion. Normal incisor relationship

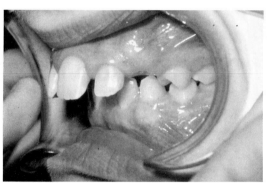

Figure 22.20 Class II malocclusion. Usually associated with prominent upper incisors, but may only involve an increase in the overbite

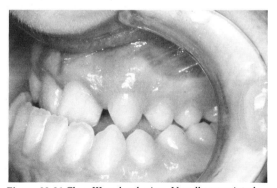

Figure 22.21 Class III malocclusion. Usually associated with lingual occlusion of the upper incisors

Individual tooth positions

Tooth positions can be further described in groups or individually. Inclinations of incisor teeth in the sagittal plane are described as being proclined or retroclined to average figures. Crowding or spacing of teeth is usually noted with specific reference to the site.

Rotations, malpositions and malformations of teeth are recorded, as this often gives an idea of the complexity of the problem when it comes to treatment planning.

It can, therefore, be seen that a malocclusion may involve malalignment of teeth within an arch and/or malrelationship between the arches.

Treatment objectives

The main objective of orthodontic treatment is to improve facial and dental aesthetics. In doing this, other objectives are achieved – better alignment of teeth allows for easier cleaning, overcomes traumatic irregularities and improves function. It is doubtful whether orthodontic treatment can greatly influence growth of the facial skeleton.

Claims and counterclaims are put forward as to the advantages of one type of appliance or technique over others, or whether treatment in the mixed dentition is better than in the early permanent dentition. Some operators advocate extractions, others non-extraction treatment. The fact that so much controversy exists points to considerable doubt in the understanding of the individual response to treatment. However, certain factors limit the scope of orthodontic treatment. Chief among these is the skeletal pattern. Where there is a severe discrepancy between maxillary and mandibular dental bases, a combined orthodontic/surgical approach is often indicated. Unfavourable soft tissue behaviour, such as an endogenous tongue thrust, points to a poor prognosis, and may limit treatment to the relief of crowding.

Appliances

Various types of appliance can be used. *Removable appliances* (*Figure 22.22*) consist of a plastic base with wire auxiliaries to retain the appliance and to bring about the tooth movements. *Functional appliances* (*Figure 22.23*) are a form of removable appliance where the orofacial musculature is used to bring about the tooth movements. *Fixed appliances* (*Figure 22.24*) consist of bands and brackets cemented or bonded to the teeth; wires attached to the brackets adjust the position of the teeth.

Fixed appliances with direct attachments to individual teeth allow for more precise control of tooth movements. However, greater skill and training is required in their use.

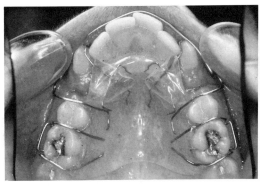

Figure 22.22 A removable appliance. This consists of a plastic base plate with stainless steel wires for retention and springs to bring about the movement of teeth

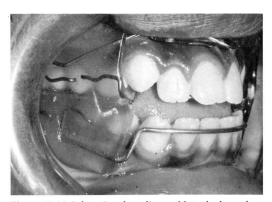

Figure 22.23 A functional appliance. Note the buccal shield, this holds the cheek away from the teeth, thus altering the muscle balance between the tongue and cheek

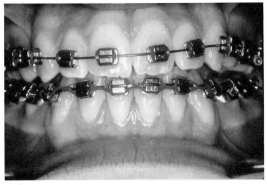

Figure 22.24 A fixed appliance with brackets bonded to the teeth. These allow precise movements of individual teeth

Special groups of mutual interest

In this section areas of special interest to the otolaryngologist and the orthodontist will be discussed. It is by no means intended that this should cover all aspects of mutual interest.

Facial growth and mouth breathing

The relationship between the growth of the face and the mode of respiration has been debated for many years. At the centre of the controversy is the issue of chronic nasal obstruction and mouth breathing. There is disagreement as to what degree of adenoidal enlargement should be defined as obstruction, and also the methods of assessing mouth breathing and the effect that obstruction and mouth breathing may have on the development of facial form.

A brief outline follows of the theories that have been put forward in respect of the effect that an impaired nasal airway has on dental development and facial form. This is a preliminary to the discussion of the problem.

(1) An impaired nasal airway is a factor in producing the so-called 'adenoidal facies'. This is brought about by an alteration in the normal air currents and pressures in the nasal and oral cavities. The result is interference with downward growth of the palate, and associated facial form.
(2) An impaired nasal airway results in mouth breathing. Mouth breathing is made easier by lowering the mandible with the tongue kept low in the oral cavity. The result is that the maxilla, lacking the support of the tongue, is narrow and the teeth crowded. The lower and total face heights are increased.
(3) An impaired nasal airway and mouth breathing do not produce deformities of the jaws and malocclusions. They do not result in the development of the adenoidal facies, that is facial form which is genetically determined.

When discussing mouth breathing, the problem is to assess whether the patient is a mouth breather. It has already been pointed out that a lack of lip seal does not necessarily mean that the patient is a mouth breather.

Vig and coworkers (1981) in North Carolina using sophisticated equipment established that there were few true mouth breathers in their adult study. They concluded that most people fell between two extremes of nasal and mouth breathing.

Linder-Aronson (1979), although agreeing that there are difficulties in diagnosing mouth breathing (except in cases of bilateral choanal atresia or insufficiency of nostrils), used subjective methods to assess mouth breathing in his studies.

Most observations are subjective. Some clinicians use a mirror to detect misting – or a wisp of cotton wool. These tests are perhaps best done with the patient asleep, but cannot be considered as objective.

Adenoid size

Adenoid size is usually assessed by orthodontists by the use of lateral skull radiographs. This has disadvantages as it only reflects the size of the nasopharynx and adenoid mass in two dimensions (*Figure 22.25*). However, Holmberg and Linder-Aronson (1979) have found a significant relationship between the size of the adenoids as measured on lateral skull radiographs and assessed clinically by nasopharyngoscopy.

Tonsil size

It is also difficult to be certain whether the size of tonsils interferes with respiration – unless grossly enlarged. Enlarged tonsils could result in forward posture of the tongue and lowering of the mandible. This would provide a more adequate oropharyngeal space for mouth breathing.

The question is, when does impairment with the normal pattern of breathing interfere with the development of the dentofacial complex?

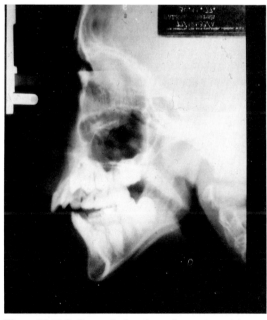

Figure 22.25 Radiograph showing enlargement of the adenoids

The evidence is far from conclusive, particularly concerning at what level the ratio of oral to nasal respiration becomes an important aetiological factor.

The animal experiments of Harvold *et al.* (1981) showed that, in primates with artificially obstructed nares, mouth breathing developed which in some cases led to alteration in skeletal pattern, dental occlusion and muscular activity. The skeletal changes seen consistently included an increased facial height and a steep gonial angle. Occlusal and muscular changes were less uniform.

Linder-Aronson (1979) has compared a group of children with obstructed nasal airways with a control group. He stated that the obstructed nasal airway group has certain characteristics: a narrow upper jaw with upright incisors and a tendency to crossbites and open bites. Following adenoidectomy and change from mouth to nose breathing, Linder-Aronson showed that normalization of arch width, inclination of incisors to the sella-nasion plane, and the depth of the nasopharynx took place. The steeper angle of the mandible to the rest of the face also improved. The other changes mentioned took place mainly in the first year following adenoidectomy, whereas the changes in the direction of mandibular growth took longer. There has been some criticism about Linder-Aronson's subjective method of assessing mouth breathing, and also the make-up of his control groups (Ryan *et al.*, 1982). Linder-Aronson, however, says his results clearly support the view that disturbed nasal respiration can affect both facial morphology and the dentition. He is careful to point out that the changes that take place following the elimination of nasal obstruction must not be overrated. These may be small in relation to the genetic influences, and only indicate that the mode of breathing is one factor in a multifactorial complex which can alter facial growth. Linder-Aronson's diagram depicting the possible changes in mandibular posture resulting from nasal obstruction is of interest (*Figure 22.26*).

More recently, attention has been drawn to the possible effect of the mode of respiration and the vertical development of the face. In order to facilitate breathing, individuals with nasal obstruction may extend the head. This leads to stretching of the muscles and soft tissues of the neck, which in turn is said to result in a more vertical pattern of growth of the mandible and face (Solow, 1980).

The evidence relating the method of breathing to dentofacial form is inconclusive. It cannot reliably be predicted at what point mouth breathing, in excess of nasal breathing, is a significant aetiological factor. It would, therefore, seem unwise at this stage for orthodontists to recommend surgery with the hope of bringing about favourable occlusal and growth changes. In turn

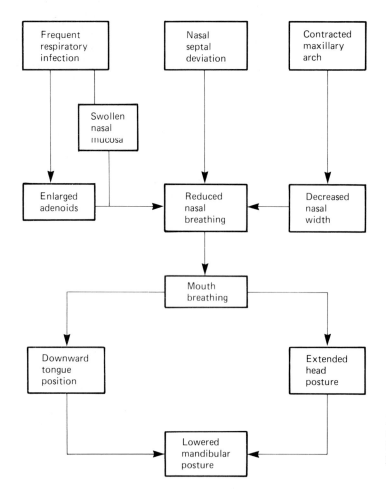

Figure 22.26 Linder-Aronson's diagram depicting the possible changes resulting in nasal obstruction. (Reproduced with permission from Linder-Aronson, 1979)

the otolaryngologist should not completely exclude the possible effects that severe nasal obstruction may have on growth when assessing the indications for surgery in the growing individual.

Rapid maxillary expansion: can orthodontists influence the pattern of respiration?

Some years ago, mouth shields (*Figure 22.27*) were recommended to encourage patients to achieve a lip seal, with the hope that this might lead to nasal respiration. A patent nasal airway was confirmed prior to the fitting. The result depended on the reason for the patient's inability to achieve a seal. However, in many cases the lack of seal was due to a disproportion between the size of the bony skeleton and the available soft tissue covering, that is a long-faced individual. Here the screen will not be successful in achieving a lip seal without

considerable muscular effort, but might encourage a change from predominantly mouth breathing to nasal respiration.

A more generally employed orthodontic procedure used to improve the nasal airway is the method of rapid maxillary expansion.

This method of expansion is carried out by fitting metal cap splints or orthodontic bands to

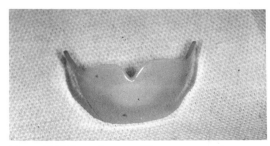

Figure 22.27 An oral screen. These were popular some years ago to encourage patients to change from mouth to nasal breathing

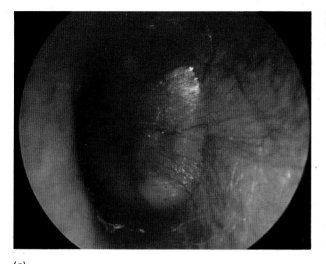

(a)

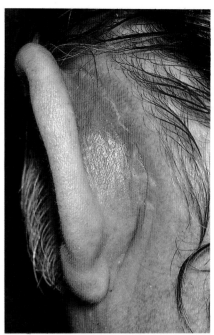

(b)

Plate 1 (*a*) Acute suppurative otitis media. Note acute inflammation of parts of the tympanic membrane, and bulging posteriorly; (*b*) acute mastoiditis with postauricular swelling and redness, and protuberance of the pinna. Note that there is a previous mastoidectomy incision, as in this patient there was a recurrence of acute mastoiditis following a previous cortical mastoidectomy. (Reproduced from T. R. Bull, 1986, *A Colour Atlas of ENT Diagnosis*, 2nd edn, with permission of the Publishers, Wolfe, London)

Plate 2 (*a*) Bifid nose; (*b*) nasal dermoid

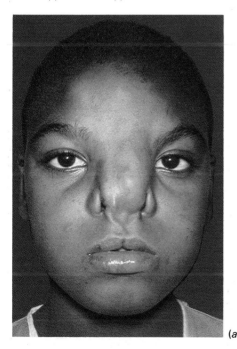

(a)

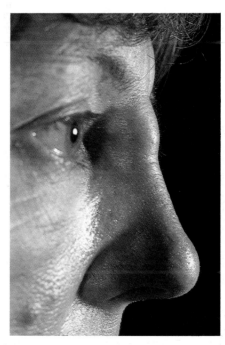

(b)

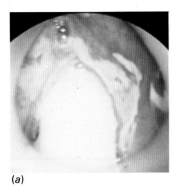

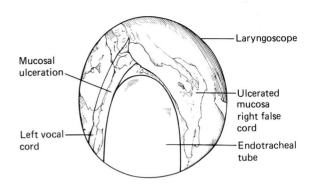

(a)

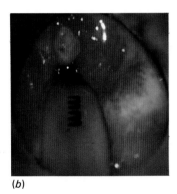

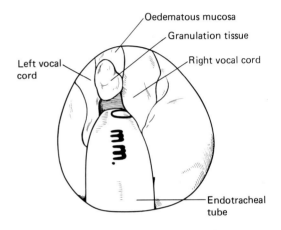

(b)

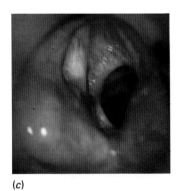

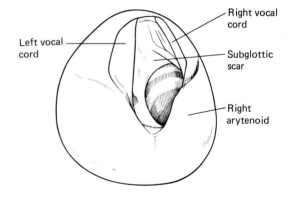

(c)

Plate 3 Microlaryngoscopy showing (a) mucosal ulceration of the vocal cords and right false cord 24 hours after intubation for ventilatory support for respiratory distress; (b) granulation tissue filling the glottis in front of the endotracheal tube; (c) a fibrous subglottic stenosis

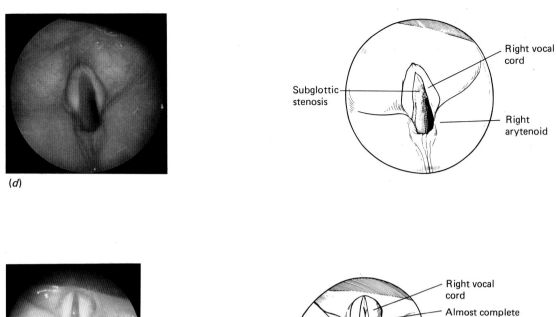

(d)

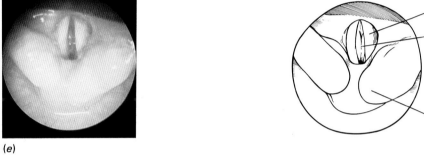

(e)

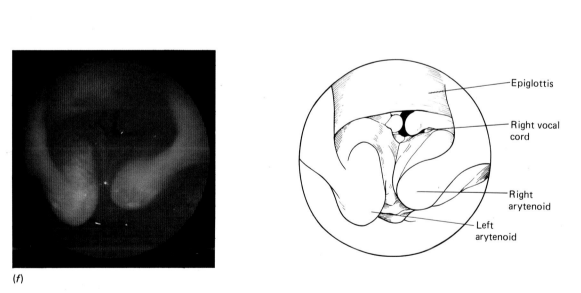

(f)

Plate 3 (*continued*) Microlaryngoscopy showing (*d*) mild congenital subglottic stenosis; (*e*) severe congenital subglottic stenosis; (*f*) mucus retention cysts after intubation

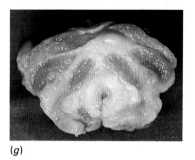

(g)

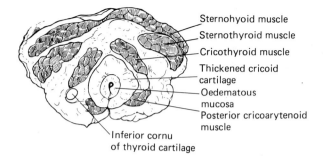

Sternohyoid muscle
Sternothyroid muscle
Cricothyroid muscle
Thickened cricoid cartilage
Oedematous mucosa
Posterior cricoarytenoid muscle
Inferior cornu of thyroid cartilage

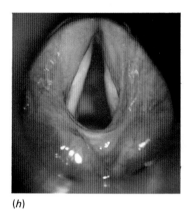

(h)

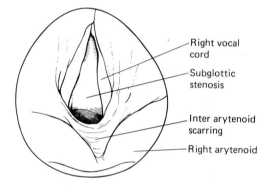

Right vocal cord
Subglottic stenosis
Inter arytenoid scarring
Right arytenoid

Plate 3 (*continued*) (*g*) post-mortem specimen showing an abnormally thick cricoid and hyperplasia of the submucosa (courtesy of Mr R. Pracy); (*h*) microlaryngoscopy showing interarytenoid fixation

the maxillary teeth. The appliance incorporates a special screw between the two lateral segments (*Figure 22.28*). Conventionally when expanding an arch during orthodontic treatment using a screw-plate, the screw is turned a quarter or half turn *per week*. In rapid maxillary expansion, it is turned a half to three-quarters turn *per day*. Thus, in a 2–3 week period the maxillary arch can be expanded by 7 mm. In the non-cleft palate case, expansion leads not only to dentoalveolar movement, but also to separation of the midpalatal suture.

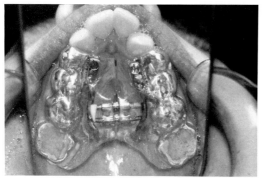

Figure 22.28 Rapid expansion splint used to widen a maxillary arch

It is claimed that rapid maxillary expansion, by increasing the width of a narrow maxillary arch, reduces nasal resistance, and thus encourages nasal respiration. Rapid maxillary expansion is also said to correct septal deformities, by the lowering of the palatal vault which is attached to the septum.

Timms (1980) claimed that rapid maxillary expansion can have an effect on areas as remote as the pterygoid processes of the sphenoid.

The changes in the nasal airway resistance brought about by rapid maxillary expansion are said to improve respiratory physiology (Hershey, Steward and Warren, 1976). Claims are also made that, in selected cases, rapid maxillary expansion may be responsible for hearing improvement in those patients who have conductive hearing loss, due to middle ear and eustachian tube problems, the expansion leading to changes in the muscle tension of tensor and levator palati muscles (Laptook, 1981).

The difficulty in recommending this procedure is twofold:

(1) the problem of stability of the expansion following the removal of the appliance
(2) the method of assessing and recording the improvement in respiratory function.

In respect of the stability it is generally agreed that most cases relapse to a certain extent. The degree is a debatable issue.

Many of the claims regarding the improvement in nasal breathing are judged by subjective methods, and some by patient questionnaires.

Therefore the long-term effectiveness of rapid maxillary expansion must be treated with caution, but if carried out to treat an occlusal anomaly, it is probably vindicated, but only in very carefully selected cases.

Cleft lip and palate patients

This group of patients comes under the care of many specialists including the otolaryngologist and the orthodontist. Both therefore have a part to play from birth to maturity. The orthodontist is chiefly interested in how the timing and type of surgery will influence growth of the face. The otolaryngologist is concerned about how the timing and type of surgery will influence hearing, speech and growth.

Interference with postnasal drainage related to the cleft is known to result in ear problems. This has encouraged some plastic surgeons to carry out an early repair of the palate. Desai (1983) repairs the palate at 16 weeks and claims that this reduces middle ear problems dramatically without interfering with growth. The usual age for palatal closure is at about one year.

Otitis media with effusion in children aged 2–20 months with cleft palate diagnosed by myringotomy has been confirmed in a high percentage of cases in a multicentre prospective study (Grant *et al.* personal communication).

In the orthodontic field there is little that can be done in the early years of the child's life that can be of help to otolaryngologists.

There are claims that presurgical orthopaedic appliances (*Figure 22.29*) promote better growth (Hotz and Gnoinski, 1979), improve feeding and, by encouraging more normal tongue behaviour from an early date, will in turn lead to improved

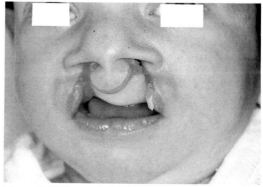

Figure 22.29 Presurgical orthopaedic appliance in a patient with bilateral cleft lip and palate

speech (Huddart and Stuffins, personal communication, 1984). This latter claim must also depend on the skill of the surgeon in obtaining an adequate hard and soft palate repair. Presurgical orthopaedic appliances are acrylic plates fitted prior to lip repair, to encourage improved alignment of the divided palatal segments.

A frequent result of palatal repair is contraction of the maxillary arch. In the early teenage patient rapid maxillary expansion and bone grafting was a form of treatment advocated by plastic surgeons (Matthews, 1975) (*Figure 22.30*). The claim was that, in the cleft palate case, expansion of the maxilla led to an improved nasal airway and that the bone graft stabilized the expanded segments. There are doubts about the efficacy of this in several respects.

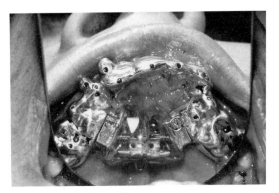

Figure 22.30 Rapid maxillary expansion splint used in patients with cleft palate to widen the maxilla, prior to bone grafting

First there is no valid evidence in the cleft patient that expansion leads to enlargement of the nasal cavities. It would appear that the nasal floor may rotate upwards as the alveolar bone and teeth move buccally (Rune *et al.*, 1980). Second, the bone graft does not lead to stability of the expanded buccal maxillary segments (Plint and Nicholson, 1985, personal communication). So even if patients reported an initial improvement in breathing, this would not persist as a result of the expansion. Bone grafted maxillae, when not permanently retained by an appliance, relapse almost entirely to their pre-expansion positions (Plint and Nicholson, 1985, personal communication).

Finally, in cleft patients an additional problem exists in respect of the nasal airway – this is the commonly found deviated nasal septum. This, and deformed nares, are as likely to result in an impaired nasal airway as a narrow maxillary arch (*Figure 22.31*).

Two other bone grafting procedures have been carried out on cleft lip and palate patients with an

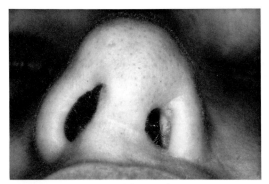

Figure 22.31 Narrow and distorted nares in a patient with cleft lip and palate

alveolar defect. These are primary and alveolar bone grafting. The primary bone grafting was usually done at the time of the lip repair, or soon after. A small section of rib was removed and wedged into the alveolar gap. It was hoped that this would stabilize the maxillary segments and also provide bone for teeth to migrate into. Unfortunately, this has not proved to be successful in many cases. The research work of Robertson and Jolleys (1968) in Manchester and Friede and Johanson (1974) in Gothenburg has shown that grafting interfered with growth of the maxilla. However, there are still some units that advocate this procedure, reporting success in terms of migration of teeth into the grafted area, without interference with growth (Rosenstein *et al.*, 1982; Nordin *et al.*, 1983).

The alveolar bone grafting technique was first suggested by Boyne and Sands (1972) and has been developed by the Oslo unit (Abyholm, Bergland and Semb, 1981). The optimal age for the graft is before the eruption of the permanent canine teeth ($\pm$ 10 years of age). It involves the use of cancellous bone obtained from the iliac crest. The bone is placed in a pocket in the alveolar defect (it is important to have an intact nasal layer). The oral flap design is different from flaps previously used to repair alveolar fistulae in that it is of keratinized mucosa brought forward from the buccal gingivae (*Figure 22.32*). The dental advantages are:

(1) an intact bony ridge is established
(2) depending on the timing of the procedure, unerupted teeth may migrate into the grafted area or, if erupted, can be moved into the grafted area, by orthodontic appliances; this in many cases avoids the need for a denture or bridge work (*Figure 22.33*)
(3) the repair of the alveolar fistula excludes the need for an obturator-type denture, and facilitates bridgework construction, should it not be possible to bring anterior teeth into

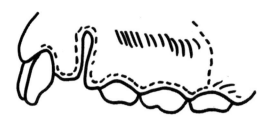

Figure 22.32 Diagram of incision used to raise keratinized buccal flap to repair alveolar cleft following bone grafting

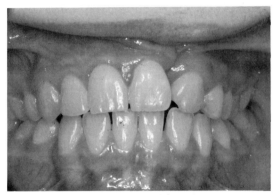

Figure 22.33 The occlusion, showing approximation of teeth following alveolar bone grafting in a case of cleft lip and palate

contact by orthodontic methods, that is the cleft segments are stabilized by the graft

(4) no reported interference with maxillary growth.

As in many handicapped patients, cleft lip and palate cases require the continued effort of a number of specialities in order to obtain a satisfactory result.

Other orofacial anomalies

First arch or facial microsomia

First arch anomalies affect the structures derived from the first branchial arch. They are now known as hemifacial microsomia – however, a number of cases are bilateral. There is a disturbance of the maxilla and mandible on the affected side(s). The severity varies from case to case. In the most severe, the ramus of the mandible may be absent. In the less severe, the mandible is reasonably formed, but diminished in size. The soft tissues are also affected, and some of the muscles of mastication may be absent, or only vestigial in form. Alveolar growth is also deficient, and molar

teeth may be unerupted or only partly erupted. The mandible deviates to the affected side and there is quite a marked cant of the occlusal plane in the transverse direction (*Figure 22.34*).

Various procedures have been carried out in order to correct the asymmetry. In the growing child, bone grafting has been tried both by inserts to the ramus or body to increase the length and by costochondral rib grafts to the condylar region to encourage growth. The latter procedure is usually followed by orthodontic treatment to encourage the eruption of teeth on the affected side, following the rotation of the mandible into its more symmetrical position. The success of the graft and the improvement of the occlusion appear to depend on the severity of the deformity. Where there is adequate soft tissue and muscle the response is favourable. Where there is lack of soft tissue the results are less good.

It is difficult to measure growth changes accurately in these cases due to the degree of asymmetry. Rune, Sarnas and Selvik (1975) have developed a technique which allows three-dimensional movements of sections of the skeleton to be studied using X-ray stereometry.

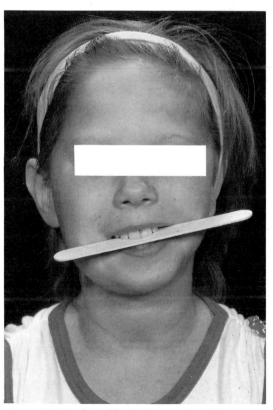

Figure 22.34 Unilateral facial microsomia: note the cant of the occlusal plane

The technique involves the placement of small tantalum implants in the forehead, maxillae and mandible. (This is done at the time of a minor surgical procedure such as removal of accessory ear tags.) Lateral and posteroanterior facial radiographs are then taken simultaneously, with the patient's head in a calibration cage. This allows the three-dimensional measurements to be made. The technique is most valuable as it is now possible to monitor growth for a period to assess the need for grafting and subsequently to measure the changes in growth following the costochondral grafts.

Bilateral cases may have respiratory problems which could need tracheostomies. Early intervention by way of bone grafting may be helpful in advancing the mandible and tongue, thus providing a larger pharyngeal space. Postoperatively, orthodontic methods are used to help maintain the mandible in its new position.

The more severe cases usually require further surgery at about the time of the completion of growth. The surgery involves maxillary and mandibular osteotomies to correct the asymmetry. Pre- and postsurgical orthodontic treatment is often necessary in order to obtain a satisfactory occlusion.

Treacher Collins syndrome

These patients are difficult to treat. The deformity of eyes, ears, zygomae, maxillae and mandible lead to a rather bird-like face (*Figure 22.35*). There is usually a small mandible with quite a steep gonial angle. This, together with the abnormal maxillary growth, results in an open bite which sometimes extends to the molar region.

Orthodontic treatment is limited to treating the crowding of the teeth which usually exists. The skeletal deformity cannot be helped by orthodontic methods. The child usually undergoes a number of surgical procedures. The most beneficial, from an aesthetic point of view, are those involving the bony framework by operations which follow the completion of growth.

The occlusion is the least important of the many problems found in this condition – hearing loss and facial deformity being the main problems.

Infection and trauma to the mandibular condyles

In the past, interference in growth to the mandibular condyles, resulting from infection in the middle ear, was not uncommon. This is now seldom seen in the UK, but is still occasionally seen in children born abroad (*Figure 22.36*). There is speculation as to whether the condyle is a true growth site – some believe that growth in this area merely represents a 'filling in' as the mandible is propelled downwards and forwards by the in-

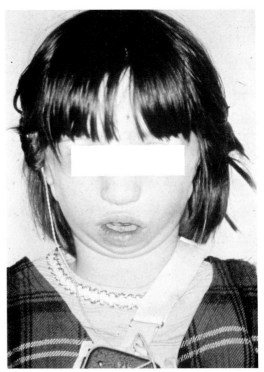

Figure 22.35 A case of Treacher Collins syndrome with recessive mandible

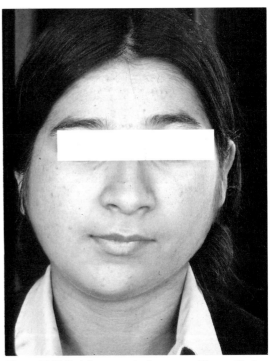

Figure 22.36 Facial asymmetry in a case with mandibular ankylosis

crease in size of the oral cavity (theory of functional matrices). However, infection in the condylar region may lead to ankylosis of the temporomandibular joint and, whether the resulting deformity is due to scarring or interference with a growth site, is only of academic interest.

In children where infection or trauma leads to ankylosis, surgery should take place as early as possible to release the ankylosis. Costochondral grafts are usually inserted, and early movement of the mandible encouraged to restore function. The occlusion in the late diagnosed case may be quite markedly disturbed, and will need adjustment following the treatment of the ankylosis.

The prognosis in respect of restoring function and aesthetics is more favourable in these cases than in the first arch syndrome. Here the soft tissues, although scarred, are otherwise normal.

Conclusion

Liaison between the specialists of otolaryngology and orthodontics has many advantages. Both groups see a large number of young patients. Recognition of problems of mutual interest, and early referral for advice, should provide a better service. If this is allied to well-planned research, this may in time lead to an improvement in the treatment of patients.

References

ABYHOLM, F. E., BERGLAND, O. and SEMB, G. (1981) Secondary bone grafting of alveolar clefts. *Scandinavian Journal of Plastic Reconstruction Surgery*, **15**, 127–140

BOYNE, P. J. and SANDS, N. R. (1972) Secondary bone grafting of residual and alveolar and palatal clefts. *Journal of Oral Surgery*, **30**, 87

DESAI, J. H. (1983) Early cleft palate repair completed before the age of 16 weeks: observations on a personal series of 100 children. *British Journal of Plastic Surgery*, **36**, 300–304

FRIEDE, H. and JOHANSON, B. (1974) A follow-up study of cleft children treated with primary bone grafting. *Scandinavian Journal of Plastic Reconstructive Surgery*, **8**, 88

HARVOLD, E. P., VARGERVIK, K., CHIERICI, G. and TOMER, B. S. (1981) Primate experiments in oral respiration. *American Journal of Orthodontics*, **79**, 359–372

HERSHEY, H. G., STEWARD, B. L. and WARREN, D. W. (1976) Changes in nasal airway resistance associated with rapid maxillary expansion. *American Journal of Orthodontics*, **69**, 274–284

HOLMBERG, H. and LINDER-ARONSON, S. (1979) Cephalometric radiographs as a means of evaluating the capacity of the nasal and nasopharyngeal airway. *American Journal of Orthodontics*, **76**, 363–375

HOTZ, M. M. and GNOINSKI, W. (1979) Effects of early maxillary orthopaedics in coordination with delayed surgery for cleft lip and palate. *Journal of Maxillofacial Surgery*, **7**, 201–210

LAPTOOK, T. (1981) Conductive hearing loss and rapid maxillary expansion. Report of a case. *American Journal of Orthodontics*, **80**, 325–331

LINDER-ARONSON, S. (1979) Respiratory function in relation to facial morphology and the dentition. *British Journal of Orthodontics*, **6**, 59–71

MATTHEWS, D. (1975) Rapid expansion in clefts. *Plastic Reconstructive Surgery*, **56**, 396–401

MOSS, M. L. and SALENTIJN, L. (1969) Functional matrices in facial growth. *American Journal of Orthodontics*, **55**, 566–577

NORDIN, K. E., LARSON, O., NYLEN, B. and EKLUND, G. (1983) Early bone grafting in complete cleft lip and palate cases following maxillofacial orthopaedics. *Scandinavian Journal of Plastic Reconstructive Surgery*, **17**, 51–62

RYAN, F. S., GALLAGHER, D. M., La BLANC, J. P. and EPKER, B. H. (1982) The relation between nasorespiratory function and dentofacial morphology. A review. *American Journal of Orthodontics*, **82**, 403–410

ROBERTSON, N. R. E. and JOLLEYS, A. (1968) Effects of early bone grafting in complete clefts of lip and palate. *Plastic Reconstructive Surgery*, **42**, 414–421

ROSENSTEIN, S. W., MONROE, C. W., KERNATAW, D. A., JACOBSON, B. H., GRIFFITH, B. H. and BAUER, B. S. (1982) The case for early bone grafting in cleft lip and palate. *Plastic Reconstructive Surgery*, **70**, 297–306

RUNE, B., SARNAS, K. V. and SELVIK, G. (1975) Analysis of motion of skeletal segments following surgical–orthodontic correction of maxillary retrusion application of a new roentgen stereophotogrammatic method. *Dentomaxillofacial Radiology*, **4**, 90–94

RUNE, B., SARNAS, K. V., SELVIK, G. and JACOBSSON, S. (1980) Movements of the maxillary segments after expansion and/or secondary bone grafting in cleft lip and palate: a roentgen stereophotogrammatic study with aid of metallic implants. *American Journal of Orthodontics*, **77**, 643–653

SOLOW, B. (1980) The dentoalveolar compensatory mechanism: background and clinical implications. *British Journal of Orthodontics*, **7**, 145–161

TIMMS, D. J. (1980) A study of basal movement with rapid maxillary expansion. *American Journal of Orthodontics*, **77**, 500–507

VIG, P. S., SARVER, D. M., HALL, D. J. and WARREN, D. W. (1981) Quantitive evaluation of nasal airflow in relation to facial morphology. *American Journal of Orthodontics*, **79**, 263–272

23

Stertor, sleep apnoea and velopharyngeal insufficiency

C. M. Bailey and C. B. Croft

Stertor

Definition

Stertor may be defined as noisy respiration caused by partial airway obstruction above the level of the larynx. It is a low-pitched, snoring or snuffly sound, in contrast to the higher pitched musical sound of stridor which characterizes partial airway obstruction at or below the level of the larynx. The noise is produced by turbulent airflow through the narrowed airway, setting up vibrations in the surrounding tissues.

Pathophysiology

It is helpful to consider the physics of airflow through a tube in order to understand better the way in which the noise of stertor is produced (Cotton and Reilly, 1983).

The pressure exerted by a gas is equal in all directions, except when it is moving. Linear movement of gas through a tube creates additional pressure in the forward direction and, because of the principle of conservation of energy, there is a corresponding fall in pressure laterally against the walls of the tube. The faster the gas flows, the greater the drop in lateral pressure. This phenomenon is termed the Venturi effect.

When air flows rapidly through a passage that is narrowed, the lateral pressure that is holding the lumen open can drop drastically in accordance with the Venturi effect and cause the walls to collapse and the lumen to close momentarily. Closure of the lumen obstructs the flow of air, the intraluminal pressure returns to normal, and the walls spring open again. This cycle rapidly repeats itself, producing a pattern of intermittent flow with associated turbulence and vibration of the lumen wall. This becomes audible as a noise.

Airway narrowing above the level of the larynx produces the low-pitched sound of stertor. The tissues of the tongue and pharynx are relatively loosely supported and can be quite easily drawn into the airway on inspiration. Inspiration is initiated by movement of the thoracic cage and the diaphragm, producing expansion of the lung parenchyma and bronchi, and drawing in air through the upper air passages, larynx and trachea. Narrowing of the airway results in vigorous inspiratory efforts involving the accessory muscles of respiration, in an attempt to draw in a sufficient volume of air. In order to move an adequate volume of air for the child's respiratory needs, high flow rates through the narrowed segment of airway develop with a consequently powerful Venturi effect, thus constricting the airway further.

Thus stertor is an inspiratory noise. Expiration has the opposite effect on the supralaryngeal regions, blowing the airway open, usually with no associated sound.

The high negative pleural pressures which develop during inspiration against an obstructed airway produce marked indrawing of the soft tissues in the subcostal, intercostal, suprasternal and supraclavicular regions. In the suprasternal notch this retraction or recession produces the appearance of the trachea plunging down into the chest with each indrawn breath, the so-called tracheal tug.

The respiratory obstruction which produces stertor can lead to hypoxia, hypercapnia, pulmonary oedema, cor pulmonale, vomiting, aspiration pneumonia and occasionally death. Long-term effects include failure to thrive and permanent brain damage (Heaf et al., 1982).

Aetiology

Any condition which restricts the airway in the nose, nasopharynx or oropharynx is liable to produce stertor.

Congenital conditions

Nasal obstruction

The neonate remains an obligate nose breather for the first 2 or 3 months of life (Stool and Houlihan, 1977), and so nasal obstruction in this age-group is an especially serious problem. Total nasal obstruction, for example caused by complete nasal agenesis or bilateral choanal atresia, is immediately life-threatening. Partial nasal obstruction with stertor produces a less dramatic, but nevertheless serious, clinical picture. Feeding becomes slow and difficult, with frequent interruptions as the infant 'comes up for air', and inspissated nasal secretions may produce near-total nasal obstruction with consequent risk of sudden infant death.

Congenital abnormalities of the external nose are very uncommon, but various degrees of nasal dysgenesis can occur and may produce nasal obstruction: these include nasal hypoplasia (sometimes secondary to one of the mandibulofacial dysostoses), varying degrees of congenital occlusion of the anterior nares, and the group of median facial anomalies classified by De Myer, Zeman and Palmer (1963).

Congenital cysts of the nasal cavity may produce obstruction and stertor, depending upon size and location. They include dermoids, nasoalveolar cysts, dentigerous and mucous cysts of the floor of the nose and Jacobson's organ.

Nasal obstruction in the neonatal period may be caused by a swelling of neural origin extending into the nose. This may be a meningocoele (meninges alone), meningoencephalocoele (meninges plus brain tissue) or encephalocoele (glial tissue with no remaining connection to the brain) (Furstenberg, 1936; Proctor and Proctor, 1979).

Choanal stenosis may produce nasal obstruction with stertorous respiration. In part this is a result of the choanal narrowing itself, and in part caused by secondary stasis of nasal mucus.

Facial skeletal anomalies

Children with craniofacial abnormalities may develop stertor as a result of obstruction in the nose, nasopharynx or oropharynx.

Nasal obstruction occurs, but is seldom severe, in children with unilateral cleft lip and palate. It is caused by a combination of collapse of the ipsilateral alar cartilage and deviation of the nasal septum: the septum is deviated to the contralateral side anteriorly, and to the ipsilateral side posteriorly where it articulates with the malpositioned vomer.

Nasopharyngeal obstruction occurs in Apert's and Crouzon's syndromes as a result of severe posterior displacement of the mid-facial structures and consequent narrowing of the nasopharyngeal airway.

Oropharyngeal obstruction is a feature of glossoptosis, in which there is micrognathia and, as a result, the tongue falls back into the oropharynx. Treacher Collins syndrome is an example of micrognathia in which this may occur. However, the tongue seems to fall back into an obstructing position more readily when there is an associated cleft palate, and the problem is frequently severe in children with the Pierre Robin syndrome where there is both micrognathia and a cleft palate.

Macroglossia

The tongue can produce respiratory obstruction if it is much enlarged, even if the mandible is normal. This can occur in Down's syndrome and as part of the organomegaly of Beckwith's syndrome, or it may be isolated and idiopathic.

Enlargement of the tongue can also occur when it becomes involved in a cystic hygroma or haemangioma of the floor of the mouth, although fortunately it is unusual for the swelling to be so gross that respiratory embarrassment ensues.

Pharyngeal swellings

A large lingual thyroid mass can produce respiratory obstruction and stertor, as may a lingual thyroglossal duct cyst, or any of the rare congenital tumours of the pharynx. The latter include Tornwaldt's bursa, branchial cleft cysts, teratomata, 'hairy polyps', chordomata, craniopharyngiomata, cystic hygromata and haemangiomata (Parkin and Thomas, 1974).

Acquired conditions

Traumatic

A septal haematoma may follow birth trauma, accidental injury or assault, or may develop postoperatively following a septoplasty: the ensuing nasal obstruction may be partial or complete. A septal abscess (often an infected septal haematoma) will be more obvious as a cause of stertor because of the associated pain. Facial fractures often compromise the upper airway.

Inflammatory

The most frequent cause of stertor in childhood is the common cold. Neonates sometimes become 'snuffly' to the point of significant respiratory difficulty and associated feeding problems, but older children generally just mouth-breathe and only snore at night. Sinusitis and nasopharyngitis ('adenoiditis') can produce the same pattern in older children.

Tonsillitis rarely causes respiratory embarrassment, except in children with hugely hypertrophic tonsils. Infectious mononucleosis, however, can produce life-threatening airway obstruction as a result of massive inflammatory swelling of all the pharyngeal lymphoid tissue including the tonsils and adenoids, with grossly stertorous respiration.

It is unusual for a peritonsillar abscess to produce a significant degree of respiratory obstruction, but a parapharyngeal or retropharyngeal abscess may so do. Ludwig's angina is generally accompanied by stertorous, difficult breathing owing to the inflammatory swelling in the floor of the mouth, and there is a danger of laryngeal oedema developing with rapidly fatal consequences.

Various types of rhinitis may produce nasal obstruction with mouth breathing, and snoring during sleep, caused by swelling of the nasal mucosa and over-production of mucus. Chronic infective rhinitis ('chronic catarrhal rhinitis') is characterized by a persistent mucopurulent nasal discharge: commonest in the lower socio-economic groups, it may persist until puberty and usually resists all attempts at treatment. Perennial allergic rhinitis in children usually occurs in atopic individuals who also have asthma, and this can compound their respiratory difficulties. Rhinitis medicamentosa, caused by over-use of topical nasal decongestant drops and sprays, is fortunately rare in childhood. Other specific forms of rhinitis are extremely rare, for example diphtheritic rhinitis, tuberculosis, rhinoscleroma and leprosy.

Neoplastic

The neoplasm that classically produces nasal obstruction and nocturnal stertor in older children and adolescents is the postnasal angiofibroma, which may enlarge to fill the nasopharynx completely. Other tumours may less commonly produce similar symptoms, such as a neuroblastoma, lymphoma or rhabdomyosarcoma.

Other conditions

Hypertrophic adenoids are a common cause of nasal obstruction and stertor, and an important cause of the obstructive sleep apnoea syndrome (*see below*), especially when there are other factors compromising the upper airway such as the cramped nasopharynx of some of the craniofacial anomalies, or the micrognathia of Treacher Collins syndrome.

Nasal polyps in children are usually associated with cystic fibrosis, and there is often a concomitant chronic sinusitis; chronic mucosal swelling and the abnormally thick, tenacious mucus aggravate the obstruction (Baker and Smith, 1970). An antrochoanal polyp may produce stertor during sleep if it is large enough to fill both sides of the nasopharynx.

An important entity in this group of miscellaneous causes of stertor is idiopathic nasal mucosal swelling in the neonate. Many infants have slightly congested nasal mucosa at birth and are 'snuffly', but a very few have severe mucosal swelling with no apparent cause and become stertorous: sometimes the obstruction is so severe that total nasal obstruction ensues and the infant presents the same picture as a case of bilateral choanal atresia (Mugliston and Mitchell, 1984).

Iatrogenic

Nasal obstruction and snoring may result from stenosis of the nasopharyngeal isthmus. This is invariably acquired as a result of surgery: sometimes tonsillectomy and/or adenoidectomy can be responsible, but more usually it is the result of a 'too successful' pharyngoplasty performed for velopharyngeal insufficiency. Nasal and postnasal packing can sometimes cause dramatic stertor and seriously compromise the airway.

Clinical features

Symptoms

The first priority in assessing a child with stertor is to establish whether there is severe respiratory distress requiring urgent action to secure the airway. If there is no immediate threat to the airway, a careful and systematic history should be obtained.

The nature of the noise should be determined first, as parents, nurses (and indeed other physicians) are often extremely vague on this essential point which gives such a useful indication of the site of obstruction. Having established that the noise is stertor rather than stridor, it will invariably become apparent that it is present on inspiration.

Next, the time of onset should be inquired about. Most of the congenital causes of stertor will present with breathing difficulty from birth, and the obstruction will be immediate and dramatic in those neonates with nasal obstruction owing to their obligatory pattern of nasal respiration. A history of preceding trauma or upper respiratory tract infection may be obtained in the older child who rapidly becomes stertorous, indicating respectively the likelihood of faciomaxillary fractures or an inflammatory condition as the cause. Slowly progressive, increasing stertor suggests a neoplastic cause. The older child who mouth breathes during the day and snores at night may have obstructive sleep apnoea, and specific enquiry should be made about sleep patterns.

In the child with long-standing stertor, aggravating and relieving factors should be sought, especially whether the noise is loudest when asleep or awake, and whether it is related to any particular position.

Direct questioning about associated symptoms should include enquiry about the cry or voice. In supralaryngeal obstruction there is no hoarseness, but the cry is characteristically muffled. There is usually no cough. Feeding difficulties are obvious in the infant with nasal obstruction, who will have to come off the nipple frequently to breathe: sometimes this slow, interrupted feeding pattern is so severe that failure to thrive and gain weight becomes apparent. Other children in whom there are no feeding difficulties may fail to thrive simply because of the increased metabolic demand of breathing against resistance (Heaf *et al.*, 1982).

Signs

The primary objective in the physical examination is to assess the severity of respiratory distress. Decreased activity and responsiveness, pallor, sweating, tachypnoea and recession all indicate severe respiratory distress; cyanosis, bradycardia and hypotension are grave signs that herald respiratory arrest and demand immediate action to restore the airway. Such a child should not be disturbed for additional examination lest respiratory arrest is precipitated, but should instead be immediately transferred to the paediatric intensive care unit or operating theatre for intubation, endoscopic examination and possible tracheostomy. The team involved must include a paediatrician, paediatric anaesthetist and otolaryngologist.

The stable, well-oxygenated child can be examined further in a thorough and systematic way. Attention should first be directed towards assessing in more detail the stertorous noise and establishing whether it is present in the inspiratory or expiratory phases of respiration, or both. An attempt should be made to determine whether the noise is arising from the nose or pharynx by listening at the nose and open mouth, and the chest must be auscultated to ensure there is no associated pulmonary pathology. The child should be placed in various positions to establish whether

posture affects the noise: for example, in the Pierre Robin syndrome and other forms of micrognathia or macroglossia the noise is markedly diminished by lying the baby prone with the head extended.

During this general part of the examination, care should be taken to look for any congenital abnormalities.

Next the nose should be examined. Assessment of airway patency can be difficult in the infant, but bubbling of mucus in the nasal cavity indicates that there is airflow, as does misting on a silvered surface held at the nares. Examination of the nasal cavities in the infant is best achieved by using an electric otoscope with a suitably-sized speculum, with the child wrapped in a blanket. Choanal patency is then assessed by ensuring that an 8FG catheter will pass through each side of the nose into the pharynx without difficulty. In the older child, the nose can be examined in the conventional way.

Examination of the throat must include an assessment of the size and position of the tongue and lower jaw. The palate must be checked for a cleft and the size of the tonsils judged. If possible, a view of the oropharynx should be obtained to see if there are any masses or swellings distorting the airway: this can be difficult in the infant, and use of the tongue depressor often induces gagging with simultaneous gastro-oesophageal reflux which instantly obscures the view and induces choking which further threatens the already compromised airway. Great care should therefore be taken, and it is best to avoid use of the tongue-depressor if the child has recently had a feed. If the airway seems precarious, and especially if there is the slightest suspicion of acute epiglottitis, *no attempt* should be made to examine the oropharynx in the clinic or ward: the examination should be delayed until the child is anaesthetized in the operating theatre ready for intubation with anaesthetist, otolaryngologist and paediatrician standing by.

Investigations

Physiological investigations

The usual regular observations of temperature, pulse, respiratory rate and blood pressure must be charted. The resting respiratory rate is a sensitive index of pulmonary function. Neonates have a rate of about 40 breaths/minute; this diminishes with age so that a 2-year-old child has a rate of about 20/minute, and a 6-year-old child 15/minute. With respiratory distress, tachypnoea is an early and important compensatory mechanism. Associated with this is a rise in pulse rate, bearing in mind that the normal heart rate for a neonate is about 140/minute decreasing to around 80/minute in older children. Bradycardia is a late sign that indicates terminal decompensation, and is accompanied by hypotension (although neonates often develop bradycardia as an immediate response to acute hypoxia).

The single most important laboratory test of respiratory efficiency in the critically ill child is measurement of arterial blood gas levels. The P_aO_2 indicates the level of oxygen being delivered to the tissues: this too changes with age, normally being about 9.3 kPa (70 mmHg) in the newborn rising to 11.97 kPa (90 mmHg) in the older child. Serious tissue hypoxia results when the P_aO_2 falls below 6.65 kPa (50 mmHg). The P_aCO_2 is the best indicator of alveolar ventilation, with a normal range of 3.99–4.66 kPa (30–35 mmHg) in the neonate and 4.66–5.99 kPa (35–45 mmHg) in the older child. However, it must be remembered that P_aCO_2 is inversely related to respiratory minute volume, and so if the alveolar minute volume doubles the P_aCO_2 is halved. The pH is a measure of respiratory and metabolic acidosis or alkalosis (range 7.30–7.45).

When serial measurements of arterial blood gases are needed, an indwelling arterial line is necessary. However, a transcutaneous oxygen sensor (ear lobe oximeter) can be invaluable for continuously monitoring tissue oxygenation. Similarly, continuous automatic monitoring of temperature, pulse, blood pressure and ECG can be undertaken if the child's condition is unstable, together with respiratory rate if the patient is intubated. In this situation an intravenous line is mandatory for administration of fluids and drugs.

Radiological investigations

In the child without respiratory distress, radiological evaluation of the upper airway is the next step.

In the assessment of stertor, the soft-tissue lateral X-ray of the neck is the most valuable view, and will demonstrate the size of the nasopharyngeal airway relative to the adenoids, and the size of the oropharyngeal airway relative to the tonsil and tongue position, as well as showing any masses distorting the upper airway. However, the film must be of the highest quality to be meaningful; for example a few degrees of rotation will produce misleading appearances by superimposing normal structures on the air shadow. The X-ray must be taken with the head slightly extended during inspiration; flexed expiratory views, especially if the child is crying, produce dramatic distortions of pharyngeal tissues which can bulge enormously in the infant and mimic the appearance of a retropharyngeal abscess or mass (*Figure 23.1*).

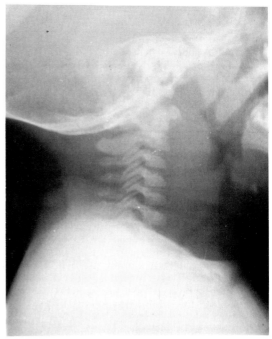

(a)

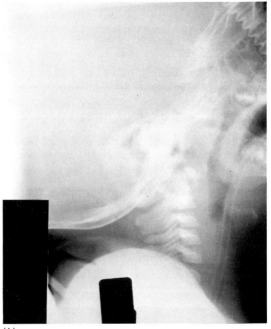

(b)

Figure 23.1 (*a*) Lateral soft-tissue X-ray of a child taken in slight flexion while crying, apparently showing a retropharyngeal mass. (*b*) X-ray of the same child taken shortly afterwards during an examination under anaesthesia. With the head extended and the child relaxed, the retropharyngeal pseudomass has disappeared

The high-kV 'Cincinnati' posteroanterior view of the mediastinum enhances the air column in trachea and bronchi by providing improved contrast between air and soft tissues. This view, together with a plain posteroanterior chest film, should be taken to exclude any unsuspected lower airway pathology.

A barium swallow, essential in the examination of a patient with stridor to look for a vascular ring, is not needed for the patient with stertor alone.

Occasionally, other special X-ray studies can be helpful. Xeroradiography shows the air–soft tissue density interface particularly well, and can sometimes be of value in difficult cases, but has the disadvantage of rather high radiation exposure. Hypocycloidal polytomography shows bone destruction well and is used when a neoplasm is suspected, for example a postnasal angiofibroma. For a vascular tumour such as this, angiography is employed in addition.

Computerized tomography (CT) and more recently magnetic resonance imaging (MR) show soft tissues well and can be complementary to polytomography in demonstrating the extent of tumours or other masses. Computerized tomography is especially valuable in the assessment of choanal atresia and stenosis.

Endoscopy

Sometimes endoscopic examination is needed to confirm the diagnosis. Under general anaesthesia the nose, oral cavity, nasopharynx, oropharynx and hypopharynx are examined.

An orotracheal tube is employed for the anaesthetic. The nasal cavities are inspected directly using a headlight, and with the aid of straight-ahead (0°) and angled (30° or 70°) Hopkins rod telescopes, or a small-bundle flexible fibreoptic nasoendoscope such as the 2.9 mm Olympus ENF 'P'. A Boyle-Davis gag is then inserted to permit viewing of the oral cavity and pharynx. Examination of the postnasal space may be accomplished with a mirror, or a 120° retrograde telescope passed behind the posterior edge of the soft palate.

In some cases it is difficult to decide whether the respiratory noise is stertor alone, or whether there is also an element of stridor indicating pathology in the larynx or tracheobronchial tree. If such doubt exists, then the endoscopic evaluation must be completed by performing a microlaryngoscopy and bronchoscopy.

At the end of the procedure the endotracheal tube should be removed to permit observation of the airway as the child awakens. This may reveal airway obstruction in the dynamic state (such as pharyngeal collapse) that was not apparent when the tube was in place.

Treatment

Medical and conservative measures

Patients with respiratory distress should normally be nursed in a semi-sitting position, as in this posture the abdominal contents fall away from the diaphragm, allowing it to move more efficiently and increasing the functional residual capacity of the lungs. However, in some conditions a different position will greatly improve the airway – for example, the prone position is best for children with the Pierre Robin syndrome.

If necessary, warmed, humidified oxygen should be administered. This is carried out using a blender system that will deliver oxygen in concentrations from 20 to 100%. The concentration is adjusted so that the P_aO_2 is maintained between 7.98 and 11.97 kPa (60 and 90 mmHg) (6.65–10.64 kPa (50–80 mmHg) in neonates to minimize the risk of retrolental fibroplasia). Delivery is best achieved using a head-box for infants and a mist tent or face mask for older children.

Adequate hydration must be maintained with intravenous fluids or tube feeds if oral intake is inadequate. Physiotherapy, to help clear the chest of secretions, should be employed with great caution in the child with a severely compromised upper airway lest complete obstruction be precipitated.

Immediate measures must be taken to improve the airway if it is compromised to the point of respiratory distress. The method employed depends upon the apparent site of obstruction.

Nasal obstruction does not present a great problem in the older child who will simply mouth breathe. However, the neonate, who is an obligate nose breather, will require an oral airway.

Pharyngeal obstruction is often dramatically relieved by employing a nasopharyngeal airway, and this has been well demonstrated in the Pierre Robin syndrome by Heaf *et al.* (1982).

Use of the nasopharyngeal airway ('nasal prong')

A Portex endotracheal tube is employed; for a neonate a 3.0 or 3.5 mm diameter tube is appropriate, and the length required can be estimated from the crown/heel measurement (Heaf *et al.*, 1982). The tube is mounted on a Tunstall connector, passed through the nose and secured with a conventional head band and tapes across the cheeks (*Figure 23.2*). Lateral neck radiography is necessary to check the tube position; ideally the tip should be just above the epiglottis. If the tube is too long, choking and vomiting are induced; if it is too short, relief of airway obstruction is not achieved.

To maintain tube patency, regular suction with a catheter is undertaken, preceded by instillation of

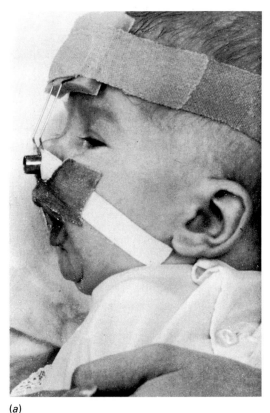

(a)

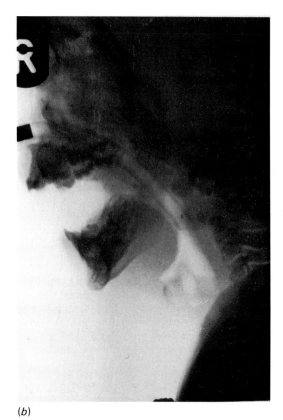

(b)

Figure 23.2 (*a*) A 5-month old infant with Pierre Robin syndrome showing a nasopharyngeal airway in position, secured with a Tunstall connector, head band and cheek tapes. (*b*) Lateral neck X-ray of an infant with a nasopharyngeal airway in place, demonstrating the splinting effect of the tube on the tongue. The position of the anterior tube bevel is seen just above the epiglottis (from Heaf *et al.*, 1982 by kind permission of the Editor and Publisher *Journal of Pediatrics*)

0.5 ml of isotonic saline: this is carried out routinely before feeds and at other times as required. The tube is changed every week and the new tube passed through the opposite nostril.

Occasionally vestibulitis develops around the tube, requiring topical antibiotic therapy. Crusting and blockage may sometimes occur and necessitate a tube change. Parents can be trained to manage the tube at home, with weekly visits to the hospital.

A nasopharyngeal airway may be the only treatment required for some stertorous children. Those with the Pierre Robin syndrome, for example, often grow to develop an adequate airway by the age of about 3 months, and use of the 'prong' can then be discontinued. In other children, the nasopharyngeal airway is an invaluable temporary measure, allowing full assessment of their clinical condition to be made prior to more definitive treatment (for example adenotonsillectomy or tracheostomy).

In some children with severe pharyngeal airway obstruction – for example caused by a craniofacial anomaly with pharyngeal collapse – a nasopharyngeal airway alone is insufficient, but the addition of continuous positive airway pressure overcomes the residual obstruction by distending the pharynx during inspiration. A ventilator is not required: continuous positive airway pressure may be applied via a special valve, or by underwater immersion of the exhalation arm of a T-piece system.

Endotracheal intubation

In some situations airway management with a nasal prong is inappropriate, and endotracheal intubation is necessary. This is the case with patients with faciomaxillary trauma where the tracheobronchial tree must be protected against inhalation of blood, and in children with massive neoplasms compressing the pharyngeal airway.

Surgery

Surgical treatment of the child with stertor depends upon the aetiology. Most of the conditions causing stertor are discussed in depth elsewhere in this volume, and their surgical management described.

In particular, the principles governing adenotonsillectomy in children with stertor are discussed below under the heading of Obstructive sleep apnoea. However, it is important to add that some children with stertor caused by anatomical restriction of the upper airway, for example some of the craniofacial anomalies, may benefit from tonsillectomy and adenoidectomy, even though hypertrophy of the tonsils and adenoids is not the primary cause of the problem. This is because the flow of air through a tube increases as a function of the fourth power of the radius of the tube in accordance with Poiseuille's formula: thus a small increase in radius is accompanied by a large increase in flow. It is therefore often beneficial to remove the tonsils and adenoids in such a situation, and the consequent improvement in respiratory function may avoid the need for tracheostomy.

The neonate with severe idiopathic nasal mucosal swelling can present difficulties in management. If there is associated rhinorrhoea it is important to send nasal swabs for culture and sensitivity to exclude an infective rhinitis. It may be necessary to undertake an examination under anaesthesia in order to exclude absolutely a choanal stenosis. If the cause of the problem is unequivocally established as idiopathic mucosal swelling, topical treatment with nasal drops may be beneficial: 0.5% ephedrine nose drops can be used sparingly, but cause rebound congestion very quickly in infants and so betamethasone drops are more satisfactory, particularly as treatment may have to be continued for several weeks. Occasionally, nasal intubation is the only course. A short nasopharyngeal 'prong' may be used as described above, but if prolonged intubation is contemplated it is better to insert a pair of Portex nasal tubes under general anaesthesia in the same way as for a case of choanal atresia.

Sleep apnoea

Definition

An apnoea has been defined as cessation of airflow at the level of the nostrils and mouth lasting at least 10 seconds. A sleep apnoea syndrome is diagnosed if, during 7 hours of nocturnal sleep, at least 30 apnoeic episodes are observed in both rapid eye movement (REM) and non-rapid eye movement (NREM) sleep, some of which must appear repetitively in NREM sleep (Guilleminault, van den Hoed and Mitler, 1978). It is frequently more convenient to use an 'apnoea index' of the number of apnoeas per sleep-hour: using this notation 5 apnoea/hour or more are needed to diagnose a sleep apnoea syndrome.

Pathological sleep apnoea is classified as central, obstructive or mixed. In central apnoea there are no respiratory movements. In obstructive apnoea there is no airflow despite persistent respiratory effort, with paradoxical movements of chest and abdomen in an attempt to overcome the upper airway obstruction. In mixed apnoea there is initially no airflow or respiratory effort, but after an interval respiratory effort is resumed and eventually re-establishes airflow.

Normal individuals have occasional physiological central apnoeic episodes during REM sleep or at the onset of sleep, but the mean apnoea rate in control subjects is only 0.3 apnoea/hour (women) and 1 apnoea/hour (men) (Guilleminault, van den Hoed and Mitler, 1978).

Normal sleep

Respiration while awake is mainly under voluntary control, but during sleep automatic mechanisms assume greater importance.

At the onset of sleep, respiration is often irregular with short apnoeic episodes. As sleep becomes deeper, breathing becomes more regular. During REM sleep, however, there is decreased muscle tone with diminished responsiveness to hypoxia, hypercapnia and airway obstruction: there is an associated drop in oxygen saturation and a rise in P_aCO_2, with irregular respiration and occasional apnoeic episodes (Apps, 1983).

Pathophysiology and aetiology

Obstructive apnoea

Obstructive apnoea is caused by obstruction of the upper airway, and the possible causes are the same as those already discussed in the section on aetiology of stertor. It is this type of sleep apnoea which is most likely to present to the otolaryngologist.

Fluoroscopy and fibreoptic nasoendoscopy have demonstrated that most episodes of obstructive sleep apnoea are caused by pharyngeal collapse in patients in whom there is already some degree of obstruction of the upper airway (Guilleminault *et al.*, 1978). Diminished pharyngeal muscle tone, especially during REM sleep, precipitates collapse of an already narrowed pharyngeal airway as a result of the Venturi effect already discussed in the section on pathophysiology of stertor. Airway obstruction results in oxygen desaturation and a rise in P_aCO_2, producing increased muscle tone and arousal (often awakening), which terminates the apnoea.

In children, the commonest site of upper airway obstruction is the nasopharynx and oropharynx, caused by large tonsils and adenoids. There is a spectrum of severity in these children, with the fully developed sleep apnoea syndrome at one end of the range; at the other end are children who tend to mouth breathe and snore, but they are often found to have some periods of apnoea when the parents are directly questioned about this possibility.

Central apnoea

Central sleep apnoea is caused by an instability in the automatic control of respiration by the respiratory centre in the medulla. This pattern of respiration can be induced in normal subjects when awake by a voluntary period of hyperventilation, when it is termed periodic breathing. When an individual hyperventilates for 2–3 minutes, and then stops and permits his respiration to continue without exerting any voluntary control over it, there is a period of apnoea. This is followed by a few shallow breaths, and then by another period of apnoea, followed again by a few breaths. The apnoea is the result of hypocapnia induced by the period of hyperventilation. During the apnoea, the alveolar P_{O_2} falls and the P_{CO_2} rises. Breathing resumes because of hypoxic stimulation of the peripheral (carotid and aortic body) chemoreceptors before the CO_2 level has returned to normal. A few breaths eliminate the hypoxic stimulus, and breathing stops until the alveolar P_{O_2} falls again. Gradually, however, the P_{CO_2} returns to normal, the central (medullary) CO_2-driven chemoreceptors come back into play, and normal breathing resumes (Ganong, 1973). Periodic breathing in disease states is called Cheyne-Stokes respiration.

This same imbalance of respiratory control between the central and peripheral chemoreceptors can occur during sleep in some normal individuals at high altitudes, as a result of overbreathing induced by hypoxia. A similar sequence of events is induced by congestive cardiac failure, as a consequence of an imbalance between central and peripheral chemoreceptor responses caused by the prolonged circulation time, and myxoedema can cause central sleep apnoea by the same mechanism.

Neurological lesions in the brainstem or above may produce central apnoea. Some patients with brainstem lesions (for example infarcts) lose automatic control of respiration altogether, and stop breathing when they go to sleep: this is the classical disorder termed Ondine's curse after the mythical water nymph whose human suitor was cursed to stop breathing and die if ever he fell asleep.

Other neurological causes in this category include brainstem encephalitis and supratentorial space-occupying lesions. Some patients with central apnoea have no demonstrable neurological or cardiovascular cause, however, and often are found to have a diminished responsiveness to hypoxia and hypercapnia even when they are awake.

Complications of sleep apnoea

Both central and obstructive sleep apnoea are associated with alveolar hypoventilation, resulting in oxygen desaturation and a rise in P_aCO_2. Very low levels of oxygen saturation can then produce an increase in pulmonary artery pressure and pulmonary vascular resistance. Eventually, irreversible pulmonary hypertension may develop with consequent cor pulmonale. Those patients with some degree of daytime desaturation as well may develop secondary polycythaemia. Systemic hypertension may also ensue (Shephard, 1984). There is some evidence that sleep apnoea may also play a part in the sudden infant death syndrome (Guilleminault *et al.*, 1984).

There are some individuals who present a combination of the complications outlined above associated with obesity. Stool *et al.* (1977) described the 'chubby puffer' syndrome in three children with obesity, airway obstruction caused by enlarged tonsils and/or adenoids, somnolence and cardiopulmonary disturbance. This seems to be closely related to the classical Pickwickian syndrome (so-called after Joe, the fat boy in *The Pickwick Papers*) of obesity, hypoventilation, daytime hypersomnolence, cor pulmonale and polycythaemia. The causation of the Pickwickian syndrome is considered to be multifactorial but some patients have obstructive sleep apnoea due to pharyngeal collapse (Sharp, Barroc and Chokroverty, 1980) as well as hypoventilation secondary to the obesity. Any cause of hypoxia in the waking state, such as obesity, will be associated with worse desaturation during sleep (especially REM sleep), and will be compounded by any element of upper airway obstruction.

Clinical features

Symptoms of obstructive sleep apnoea

The cardinal and universal symptom of obstructive sleep apnoea is snoring. Snoring may be described as the 'stridor of the pharynx' and is produced by vibration of the nearly apposed walls of the pharynx and soft palate. The actual site may vary from the level of the velopharyngeal sphincter down to the tongue base and may involve the soft palate predominantly or the pharyngeal walls primarily.

Snoring is a symptom of airway obstruction and progressive obstruction will lead eventually to shutdown of the airway as increasing velocity of inspiratory airflow through the narrowed pharynx creates an irresistible collapsing force on the pharyngeal walls (Venturi effect) (*see above*: Pathophysiology of stertor). This produces the classical obstructive apnoeic episode which is the second hallmark symptom of obstructive sleep apnoea. The degree of intrinsic airway compromise is of considerable importance in generating these obstructive episodes. Clearly, patients with massive obstructing tonsils and adenoids or narrow pharyngeal dimensions, as in the Treacher Collins syndrome (Shprintzen *et al.*, 1979a), will tend to obstruct with little provocation and the addition of sleep-induced relaxation of the pharyngeal walls completes the embarrassment of the airway.

During periods of apnoea the decrease in oxygen saturation and increasing P_{CO_2} tends to increase muscle tone and produce arousal. The airway is restored as the patient wakes but frequent waking and disturbed sleep are the consequences. This may result in abnormal sleep movements and restlessness with the patient adopting abnormal positions during sleep. The patient may wake, cyanotic and gasping for air. A second, but perhaps major, consequence of disturbed sleep is daytime hypersomnolence. This may become quite extreme in its manifestations, with constant daytime sleepiness in children and adults. The patients tend to fall asleep as soon as their concentration lapses, even when driving a car, with serious effects on concentration and performance at work. There is some evidence that sleep deprivation in children with obstructive sleep apnoea may result in retarded growth and development (Richardson *et al.*, 1980). Feeding is often disrupted both by physical obstruction of the oropharynx and by respiratory difficulties during feeding with a tendency to aspiration.

It is also thought that *nocturnal enuresis* may be exacerbated by obstructive sleep apnoea (Richardson *et al.*, 1980), although hard evidence for these rather soft symptoms is difficult to come by.

Symptoms of central sleep apnoea

There may be few symptoms in patients with central apnoea. Hypersomnolence is unusual. The patient may be aware of stopping breathing at night; awakening in a 'panic or choking attack' or aware of being unable to breathe.

Signs of obstructive sleep apnoea

The great difficulty in diagnosing sleep apnoea is that there may be few, if any, physical signs during the day. However, in the child, a poor nasal airway with constant mouth breathing is usual. The upper lip is often coated with nasal mucus and daytime respiration may be noisy with variable stertor present. The child may be underweight and undersized for his age and there is some evidence that chronic respiratory obstruction is largely responsible for this delay in general development (Richardson *et al.*, 1980), together with real physical problems in swallowing.

Oral examination may show 'midline tonsils' which seem to occupy the oropharynx completely, and nasal airflow may be minimal on objective testing. Physical signs may dramatically increase if the child is asleep, with obvious signs of respiratory embarrassment, sweating, stertor and tracheal 'tug' with intercostal recession.

In the adult, obesity is often present and may be substantial with patients weighing 150 kg plus. The patients may be hypersomnolent and have difficulty concentrating and staying awake during the taking of a medical history. Systemic and pulmonary hypertension may be present. Obstructing pathology in the upper airway in adults is not common, but a diligent search should be made for obstructing nasal pathology – polyps, etc. – and the association of obstructive sleep apnoea with skull base abnormalities and syndromes has already been discussed.

Signs of central sleep apnoea

Central sleep apnoea is very much less common than sleep apnoea of the obstructive type. Patients may present with signs germane to the causal pathology in the central nervous system, that is, patients who have had encephalitis affecting the brainstem, or patients with lesions in the pons, midbrain or above would manifest signs of other neurological disorders. Alternatively, patients may present with signs relating to disruption of their sleep pattern. Hypersomnolence, irritability and, paradoxically, insomnia may be present. However, a proportion of patients with central sleep apnoea have little in the way of signs of neurological or cardiac disease and diagnosis will depend on the history and subsequent positive identification with a sleep study.

Investigations

Sleep studies

Although the history and examination may be highly suggestive of sleep apnoea, observation of the patient during sleep is definitely required if the presence of sleep disordered breathing is to be recognized and quantified. A *polysomnograph* or full sleep study is a detailed examination during sleep, with monitoring of sleep stage (EEG, EMG and eye movement recordings), chest and abdominal movements (for paradoxical movements during efforts to respire), and transcutaneous monitoring of oxygen saturation with measurement of nasal or oral airflow and continuous ECG recording (*Figure 23.3*). Such a study is detailed

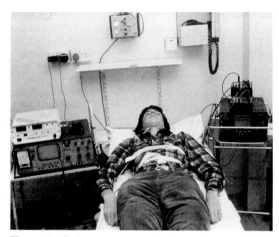

Figure 23.3 Polysomnograph – patient monitoring of PO_2, (airflow/throat microphone), chest movements, with cerebral function monitor

and expensive and the authors believe an initial screening or *'mini-sleep study'*, with observation during sleep and ear lobe oximeter monitoring of oxygen saturation, with an ECG strip and chest X-ray, is useful in identifying those patients who require a full study, and in most children it is sufficient to document the need for adenotonsillectomy without proceeding further. There is no doubt that if major surgery is being contemplated a full sleep study is warranted, and as appropriate treatments are developed for obstructive apnoea, such as uvulopalatopharyngoplasty or tracheostomy, this will increasingly be the case. However, in children a screening study is probably more appropriate unless there are doubts about the site of obstruction.

Radiology

A plain lateral X-ray of the postnasal space and upper airway is extremely useful in identifying and documenting adenoidal obstruction of the nasopharynx and tonsillar obstruction of the oropharynx (*Figure 23.4*). It also shows the position of the lower jaw and tongue base in addition to documenting the airway.

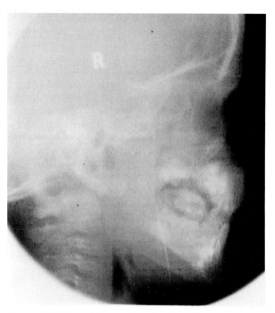

Figure 23.4 Lateral X-ray – head and neck, showing a 3-year old with massive tonsil and adenoid obstruction of the postnasal and oropharyngeal airway

Computerized tomographic scans of the pharyngeal airway in patients with obstructive sleep apnoea (Bohlman *et al.*, 1983) have shown significantly reduced dimensions of the airway at naso- and oropharyngeal level. This is really of research interest only and it is not appropriate to perform CT scanning routinely.

Chest radiography should be performed to exclude cardiopathy and right heart failure.

Nasoendoscopy

The use of the flexible fibreoptic endoscope to examine the physical state and dynamics of the upper airway is extremely valuable in documenting both physical and functional airway obstruction. The Olympus ENF 'P' flexible laryngoscope (*Figure 23.5*) is ideal in having a 2.9 mm bundle which allows examination of the upper airway in the smallest infants. The nasal cavity, postnasal space, velopharyngeal sphincter and hypopharynx and larynx are examined in turn and, if no obvious physical obstruction is seen, a reverse Valsalva or Müller manoeuvre can be performed to try to document areas of functional obstruction. It may even be necessary to perform this examination under light nitrous oxide anaesthesia without intubation to identify pharyngeal airway dysfunction in children (Southall *et al.*, 1986).

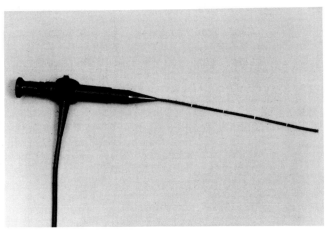

Figure 23.5 Olympus ENF 'P' flexible nasolaryngoscope

Treatment

Medical

Medication has little to offer other than in central apnoea when acetazolamide may be useful in improving respiratory function, by providing central respiratory stimulation.

Continuous positive airway pressure

Continuous positive airway pressure can be helpful in patients with a tendency to pharyngeal airway collapse during sleep. This type of dysfunction can be minimized by increasing the pressure of the inspired air. This requires either a plastic pressure chamber to fit over the head, or alternatively a face mask. There are problems in maintaining treatment in this way, particularly in children, but more major surgical intervention may be avoided (Editorial, 1986).

Surgical

The major complications of obstructive sleep apnoea are potentially reversible, although end-stage cor pulmonale is not; therefore identifiable obstructive lesions in the upper airway should be dealt with surgically as soon as possible. This usually involves simple adenotonsillectomy in the paediatric group, but obstruction may occur at any site from the nasal cavity to the larynx and careful evaluation is required to reveal the site of obstruction (Kravath, Pollak and Borowiecki, 1977).

Tracheostomy

Some children and adults with pharyngeal airway dysfunction experience major nocturnal arterial desaturation (to around 50% P_{O_2}) and may show major cardiac dysrhythmias. These patients represent a high risk group and may well progress to cardiac failure or to life-threatening dysrhythmias (Southall *et al.*, 1986). Tracheostomy is indicated in these unusually severely affected cases and is rapidly effective in reversing the gross cardiorespiratory abnormalities described.

Surgical modification of the major site of pharyngeal airway shutdown is possible and interest has centred on surgical modification of the velopharyngeal sphincter by uvulopalatopharyngoplasty (UPP) as described by Fujita *et al.* (1981). This operation has been performed on quite large numbers of adults and is successful in relieving obstructive sleep apnoea in between 50 and 70% of cases, depending on the criteria involved in selecting the patients (Sher *et al.*, 1985). The operation has not been applied in the paediatric group, where lymphoid obstruction of the upper airway is invariably the rule.

Premedication

Patients with the obstructive sleep apnoea syndrome are extremely sensitive to sedation. Heavy premedication prior to surgery may cause a marked deterioration in the patient's respiratory status and even produce a respiratory arrest. The same strictures apply to postoperative sedation and both should be avoided in patients with obstructive sleep apnoea. Anaesthetists involved in treating these patients should be alerted to the dangers of over-sedation.

Velopharyngeal insufficiency

Definition

Velopharyngeal insufficiency is defined as inadequate closure of the palatopharyngeal sphincter, resulting in nasal escape or rhinolalia aperta and a tendency to nasal regurgitation of fluids and food.

Incidence

Cleft palate and variants

Gross velopharyngeal insufficiency occurs in patients with unrepaired palatal clefts – such cases are increasingly rare in the developed world. Most children with a complete cleft lip and palate undergo lip repair at 3 months or 5 kg and palatal repair at 12–18 months. However, primary repair of a cleft palate fails to secure palatopharyngeal competence in 20–30% of cases (Krause, Tharp and Morris, 1976).

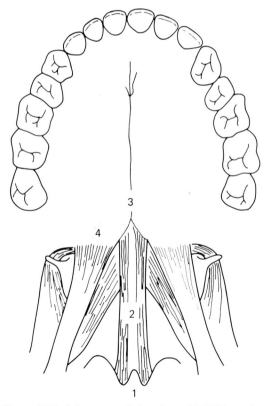

Figure 23.6 Submucous cleft palate. (1) Bifid uvula; (2) diastasis of palatal muscles; (3) notched posterior hard palate; (4) abnormal muscle insertions

Submucous cleft palate

This condition classically consists of a bifid uvula, diastasis of the palatal muscles with separation in the midline and a 'zona pellucida', and a notched posterior border to the hard palate (*Figure 23.6*). The defect may be obvious to the examiner or rather subtle and more difficult to spot. A bifid uvula alone occurs in 1.2% of the population and is a microform of cleft palate. The cleft palate deformity may be regarded as a continuum of defects extending from a complete cleft of the primary and secondary palate down to simple bifidity of the uvula. This latter finding is a visible marker pointing to possible abnormalities of the intrinsic (musculus uvulae) and extrinsic muscles of the palate, which may *not* be obvious on casual inspection. About 20% of these patients will have velopharyngeal insufficiency because of their anatomical deficiency and adenoidectomy will tend to unmask velopharyngeal insufficiency in the remainder and must be avoided (Croft, Shprintzen and Ruben, 1981).

The occult submucous cleft palate

This entity was described by Kaplan (1975) and Croft *et al.* (1978). These are patients with intrinsic muscular abnormalities in the soft palate with absence of the musculus uvulae bulge on the palatal dorsum as seen nasoendoscopically (*Figure 23.7*) (Croft *et al.*, 1978), and abnormal insertion of the levator 'sling' into the posterior border of the hard palate. These patients may only develop velopharyngeal insufficiency after a provocation to the palatopharyngeal sphincter mechanism as in adenoidectomy. There are only occasional reports of velopharyngeal insufficiency developing after adenoidal regression in adolescence in these patients (Mason and Warren, 1980). Kaplan (1975) also noted that some of these patients have abnormal facial characteristics, related to mesodermal deficiencies, and these facial characteristics include:

(1) maxillary hypoplasia   75%
(2) lip deformity at the vermilion border   75%
(3) drooping of the oral commissure   25%
(4) alveolar arch abnormalities (suppressed
     lateral incisors)   5%
(5) external ear abnormalities   10%

Congenital velopharyngeal insufficiency

This condition, present from birth, results in velopharyngeal insufficiency for speech, and is caused by disproportion between the soft palate and nasopharynx. The literature contains many references to ideal functional length of soft palate and depth of nasopharynx (Calnan, 1971), and

pharynx is normal but usually there is gross impairment of velar motion and related pharyngeal wall activity. In a recent series of 120 cases of velopharyngeal insufficiency (Croft, Shprintzen and Ruben, 1981), 17 (14%) had neurological problems including the Arnold-Chiari malformation, myotonic dystrophy, pseudobulbar palsy and isolated pharyngeal paralysis. The degree of velopharyngeal insufficiency may be very severe and it is extremely difficult to help these patients surgically, because of the paucity of function in the palate and related pharynx.

Postoperative velopharyngeal insufficiency: temporary dysfunction

Although emphasis has been already placed on the potential for adenoidectomy to cause postoperative velopharyngeal insufficiency, it, in fact, invariably 'unmasks' an already pre-existing anatomical abnormality in the velopharyngeal sphincter mechanism. The operations which would create velopharyngeal insufficiency are: resection for palatal tumours; palatal damage following 'guillotine' tonsillectomy (which is really of historical interest only); and the new operation for snoring and sleep apnoea, uvulopalatopharyngoplasty. This latter operation involves removal of the tonsils and reduction of the palatoglossus and palatopharyngeus muscles, distal soft palate and uvula. It is a procedure which is only being performed in adults at present. The operation requires careful preoperative assessment as it may lead to velopharyngeal insufficiency. Some series report transient rhinolalia aperta and nasal regurgitation in about 10% of patients following surgery (Sher *et al.*, 1985), and this would match the present authors' experience. Fortunately most of the patients appear to regain velopharyngeal competence with the passage of time.

Pathology

The palatopharyngeal sphincter mechanism consists of palatal muscles – extrinsic and intrinsic – and the pharyngeal wall muscles. The pharyngeal wall muscles which may influence velopharyngeal closure consist of the superior constrictor, the upper fibres of palatopharyngeus and the variably present salpingopharyngeus muscle. There is a difference of opinion about the major muscle component of lateral pharyngeal wall motion; some would feel that levator palatini acts by moving the salpingopharyngeal fold medially on contraction (Isshiki, Harita and Kawano, 1985), whereas others believe that the superior constrictor muscle performs this role. The superior constrictor muscle certainly acts in producing

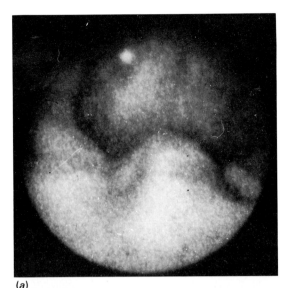
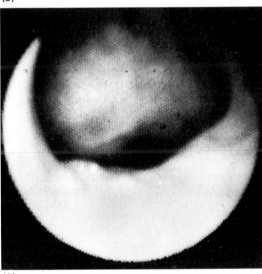

Figure 23.7 Nasoendoscopic view of soft palate. (*a*) Normal musculus uvulae bulge. (*b*) Absence of musculus uvulae bulge = occult submucous cleft palate

there is no doubt that some individuals do have this problem. However, it seems that at least some of the cases diagnosed in the past as velopharyngeal disproportion were probably cases of the occult submucous cleft palate (Croft, Shprintzen and Ruben, 1981) which had gone unrecognized.

Palatal neuromuscular dysfunction

These patients have severe velopharyngeal incompetence which can be extremely difficult to manage. The morphology of soft palate and limited 'sphincteric' contraction of the posterior pharyngeal wall in both normal subjects and patients with cleft palate (Croft, Shprintzen and Rakoff, 1981). However, these fibres may, in fact, be the most rostral fibres of palatopharyngeus which encircle the pharynx within the confines of the superior constrictor muscle (*Figure 23.8*). The prime elevator and mover of the soft palate is the levator palatini which elevates the velum upwards and backwards towards the posterior pharyngeal walls. The musculus uvulae contracts during valving, increasing the dorsal mass of the soft palate and producing the so-called 'levator eminence'. The palate makes contact with the surrounding lateral and posterior pharyngeal walls which are variably dynamic. A recent endoscopic study in 80 normal subjects and 120 patients with velopharyngeal pathology (Croft, Shprintzen and Rakoff, 1981) showed surprising variability of valving patterns with the main closure patterns being coronal (mainly palatal), sagittal (mainly lateral wall), circular, and circular with Passavant's ridge. Interestingly, active posterior wall contraction occurs in 20% of the normal population studied and appears to be more than a 'compensatory' mechanism. Furthermore, much the same spread of attempted closure patterns could be ascertained in the group of individuals with incompetent sphincters.

Clinical features

Symptoms

Velopharyngeal insufficiency is always accompanied by nasal escape or rhinolalia aperta during speech. Reduced intelligibility of speech results from disruption of consonant production. The inability to generate high intraoral pressures creates serious disturbances with fricatives such as /s/ and /z/ and plosives such as /p/ and /b/. These distortions may be accompanied by snorting caused by excessive nasal airway turbulence and 'glottal stops' to try to reduce nasal escape. Extra vocal effort places strain on the larynx and there is an increased incidence of vocal cord pathology in patients with velopharyngeal insufficiency (McWilliams, Lavorato and Bluestone, 1973). Gross velopharyngeal insufficiency may also be accompanied by nasal regurgitation of fluids and food during swallowing.

Signs

Facial

When velopharyngeal insufficiency occurs, a careful search for stigmata of cleft palate or its microforms is required with particular attention to the facies and upper jaw, with palpation of the hard and soft palate. Detection of nasal airflow during connected speech may be straightforward but, in marginal cases, a nasal escape indicator may be helpful. This is a piece of polystyrene foam inside a U-shaped small-bore glass tube. When the tube is connected to the nose, the polystyrene agitates in the presence of abnormal nasal airflow. The use of a small laryngeal mirror or nasal occlusion is less satisfactory.

Otological

Patients with long-standing velopharyngeal insufficiency have been shown to have an increased

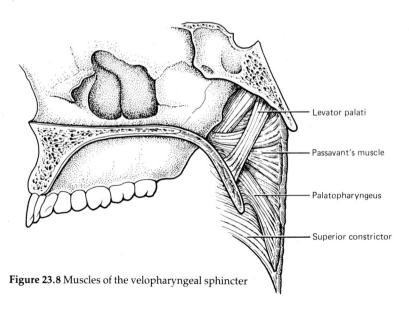

Levator palati

Passavant's muscle

Palatopharyngeus

Superior constrictor

Figure 23.8 Muscles of the velopharyngeal sphincter

incidence of middle ear disease. The incidence (approximately 50%) approaches that seen in the cleft palate population (Heller *et al.*, 1975).

Speech assessment

It is possible to confuse the difference between hyper- and hyponasality. In hyponasality the nasal resonance normally heard in connected speech is missing, there being reduced or absent airflow through the nose. This abnormality or 'rhinolalia clausa' may sound a little like hypernasality with constant and excessive nasal resonance in some cases. Obviously, such a confusion might lead to the wrong treatment being tried and the authors have seen adenoids removed in children with hypernasality in the belief that they really required an increased nasal airway. This confusion may occur in subtle cases and an expert speech therapy opinion should always be sought before resorting to surgery. It is also dangerous to perform adenoidectomy in children who have had major problems requiring speech therapy in the past. A regression may occur and velopharyngeal insufficiency may be precipitated.

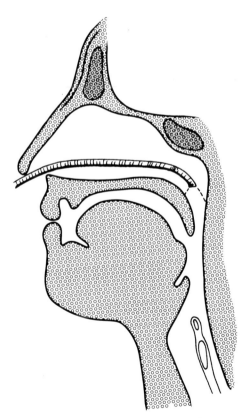

Figure 23.9 Nasoendoscopy – evaluation of the velopharyngeal sphincter

Investigations

Endoscopy

Oral endoscopy

Viewing and assessing function of the velopharyngeal sphincter perorally became popular during the 1960s, but has the major disadvantage of not allowing assessment during connected speech.

Nasoendoscopy

An excellent view of the velopharyngeal isthmus can be obtained pernasally and there is no impediment to connected speech (Pigott, 1969). Rigid or fibreoptic flexible instruments are now routinely used to establish the degree, site and severity of velopharyngeal insufficiency (*Figure 23.9*). This is most important in treatment planning and in subsequent follow-up.

Radiology

Radiographs

Plain lateral X-rays of the soft palate in phonation provide very limited information about the state of the velopharyngeal sphincter, but will give information about velar elevation and posterior wall motion.

Multiview videofluoroscopy

This certainly provides the most comprehensive and functional view of the velopharyngeal sphincter in motion (Skolnick, 1970). The velum and pharyngeal walls are coated with barium via a nasal dropper and the patient examined in lateral, frontal, base and oblique projections. Simultaneous sound recordings are taken and radiation exposure is significantly lower than with cineradiography. An excellent view of the various component movements contributing to velopharyngeal closure is readily obtained.

Audiometry/tympanometry

Approximately 50% of the patients will have middle ear pathology and conductive deafness. Appropriate investigation will include full audiometric assessment.

Treatment

Medical/conservative

Speech therapy

Speech therapy is a vital part of therapy both in its own right and in patients with inconsistent velopharyngeal insufficiency who may well learn to achieve velopharyngeal closure in sustained speech. Even if surgery is required, speech therapy is a vital part of treatment, both pre- and postoperatively.

Biofeedback

Patients with inconsistent velopharyngeal insufficiency who are capable of closure for isolated speech tasks can be helped by nasoendoscopy plus video monitoring to show up the problem and to teach remedial techniques.

Obturators

If there are major contraindications to surgery then prosthetic speech appliances can be constructed and mounted on a dental plate to fit between the palate and pharyngeal walls. These can be difficult to fit and are little used.

Surgical

Cleft palate repair

Repair is usually accomplished between the ages of 12 and 18 months. The major techniques are the Von Langenbeck repair and V-Y retroposition or the Wardill-Kilner technique. These are described in Chapter 21.

Pharyngoplasty

About one in four patients who have primary surgery for the correction of palatal cleft will fail to achieve velopharyngeal competence and most will require further surgery if normal or near normal speech is to be achieved. Although prosthetic management is a possibility, most centres would opt for surgery if there are no contraindications.

Posterior wall augmentation

This technique of narrowing the velopharyngeal port by positioning a non-toxic substance in the posterior pharyngeal wall is long established. Current interest centres on cartilage, Teflon paste or collagen. The authors' experience is that the method can only succeed if the gap in the velopharyngeal sphincter is very small (4 mm), and the vertical positioning of the implant is vital in relation to the variable height of velopharyngeal sphincter closure. Nasoendoscopic control is ideal in securing the correct site and amount of Teflon to be injected (Lewy, Cole and Wepman, 1965).

Pharyngeal flap ± palatal pushback

Although described over 100 years ago, the pharyngeal flap has only come into general use

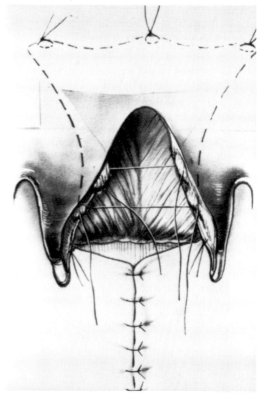

Figure 23.10 Pharyngeal flap surgery. A superiorly based flap being set into the soft palate

during the past 30 years. The method consists of elevating a unipedicle soft tissue flap from the posterior pharyngeal wall and suturing and 'setting' it into the deficient soft palate. The flap may be either superiorly or inferiorly based, but most surgeons now prefer the former (*Figure 23.10*). The flap provides an organic soft tissue obturator for the velopharyngeal sphincter (Shprintzen *et al.*, 1979b). Complete velopharyngeal closure depends on lateral wall movement medially to contact the flap, thus closing off the lateral airways or 'ports'.

Success rates following pharyngeal flap procedures vary from 33 to 100% (Bernstein, 1967; Shprintzen *et al.*, 1979b), but speech is invariably improved.

Sphincter-pharyngoplasty

Sphincter-pharyngoplasty or the Orticochea-Hynes pharyngoplasty is essentially a transfer of the palatopharyngeus muscles into a higher plane in the posterior pharyngeal wall, uniting the two muscles in a sphincteric manner in the plane of velopharyngeal closure. The operation is useful in those patients whose velopharyngeal insufficiency and sphincter gap is modest.

References

APPS, M. C. P. (1983) Sleep disordered breathing. *British Journal of Hospital Medicine*, 339–347

BAKER, D. C. and SMITH, J. T. (1970) Nasal symptoms of mucoviscidosis. *Otolaryngologic Clinics of North America*, **3**, 257–264

BERNSTEIN, L. (1967) Treatment of velopharyngeal incompetence. *Archives of Otolaryngology*, **85**, 67

BOHLMAN, M. E. *et al.* (1983) CT demonstration of pharyngeal narrowing in adult obstructive sleep apnoea. *American Journal of Roentgenology*, **14**, 543–548

CALNAN, J. S. (1971) Congenital large pharynx. *British Journal of Plastic Surgery*, **24**, 263

COTTON, R. and REILLY, J. S. (1983) Stridor and airway obstruction. In *Pediatric Otolaryngology*, edited by C. D. Bluestone and S. E. Stool, pp. 1190–1195. Philadelphia: W. B. Saunders

CROFT, C. B., SHPRINTZEN, R. J., DANILLER, A. and LEWIN, M. L. (1978) The occult submucous cleft palate and the musculus uvulae. *Cleft Palate Journal*, **15**, 150

CROFT, C. B., SHPRINTZEN, R. J. and RAKOFF, S. J. (1981) Patterns of velopharyngeal valving in normal and cleft palate subjects: a multiview videofluoroscopic and nasendoscopic study. *The Laryngoscope*, **2**, 265–271

CROFT, C. B., SHPRINTZEN, R. J. and RUBEN, R. J. (1981) Hypernasal speech following adenotonsillectomy. *Otolaryngology – Head and Neck Surgery*, **89**, 179

DE MYER, W., ZEMAN, W. and PALMER, C. G. (1963) Familial alobar holoprosencephaly (arrhinencephaly) with median cleft lip and palate. *Neurology*, **13**, 913–918

EDITORIAL (1986) PEEP and CPAP. *British Medical Journal*, **292**, 643

FUJITA, S., CONWAY, W., ZORICK, F., *et al.* (1981) Surgical correction of anatomic abnormalities in obstructive sleep apnoea syndrome: uvulo-palato pharyngoplasty. *Otolaryngology – Head and Neck Surgery*, **89**, 923

FURSTENBERG, A. C. (1936) *A Clinical and Pathological Study of Tumours and Cysts of the Nose, Pharynx, Mouth and Neck of Teratological Origin*. Ann Arbor: Edward Brothers

GANONG, W. F. (1973) *Review of Medical Physiology*, 6th edn, p. 507. Los Altos: Lange

GUILLEMINAULT, C., HILL, M. W., SIMMONS, F. B. and DEMENT, W. C. (1978) Obstructive sleep apnea: electromyographic and fiberoptic studies. *Experimental Neurology*, **62**, 48–67

GUILLEMINAULT, C., SOUQUET, M., ARIAGNO, R. L., KOROBKIN, R. and SIMMONS, F. B. (1984) Five cases of near-miss sudden infant death syndrome and development of obstructive sleep apnea syndrome. *Pediatrics*, **73**, 71–78

GUILLEMINAULT, C., VAN DEN HOED, J. and MITLER, M. M. (1978) Clinical overview of the sleep apnea syndromes. In *Sleep Apnea Syndromes*, edited by C. Guilleminault and W. C. Dement, pp. 1–12. New York: Alan R. Liss

HEAF, D. P., HELMS, P. J., DINWIDDIE, R. and MATTHEW, D. J. (1982) Nasopharyngeal airways in Pierre Robin syndrome. *Journal of Pediatrics*, **100**, 698–703

HELLER, J. C., GENS, G. W., MOE, D. and CROFT, C. B. (1978) Conductive hearing loss in patients with velopharyngeal insufficiency. *Cleft Palate Journal*, **151**, 246–251

ISSHIKI, N., HARITA, Y. and KAWANO, M. (1985) What muscle is responsible for lateral pharyngeal wall movement? *Annals of Plastic Surgery*, **14/3**, 224–227

KAPLAN, E. N. (1975) The occult submucous cleft palate. *Cleft Palate Journal*, **12**, 356

KRAUSE, C. J., THARP, R. F. and MORRIS, H. L. (1976) A comparative study of results of the Von Langenbeck and V-Y pushback palatoplasties. *Cleft Palate Journal*, **13**, 11

KRAVATH, R. E., POLLAK, C. P. and BOROWIECKI, B. (1977) Hypoventilation during sleep in children who have lymphoid airway obstruction by nasopharyngeal tube and T and A. *Paediatrics*, **59**, 865–871

LEWY, R., COLE, R. and WEPMAN, J. (1965) Teflon injection in the correction of velopharyngeal insufficiency. *Annals of Otology, Rhinology and Laryngology*, **74**, 874

McWILLIAMS, B. J., LAVORATO, A. S. and BLUESTONE, C. D. (1973) Vocal cord abnormalities in children with velopharyngeal valving problems. *The Laryngoscope*, **83**, 1745

MASON, R. M. and WARREN, D. W. (1980) Adenoid involution and developing hypernasality in cleft palate. *Journal of Speech and Hearing Disorders*, **49**, 469

MUGLISTON, T. A. H. and MITCHELL, D. B. (1984) Nasal obstruction in healthy neonates. *British Medical Journal*, **289**, 1659–1660

PARKIN, J. L. and THOMAS, G. K. (1974) Benign masses of the pharynx. *Rocky Mountain Medical Journal*, **71**, 34

PIGOTT, R. W. (1969) The nasendoscopic appearance of the normal palatopharyngeal valve. *Journal of Plastic and Reconstructive Surgery*, **43**, 19–24

PROCTOR, B. and PROCTOR, C. (1979) Congenital lesions of the head and neck. *Otolaryngologic Clinics of North America*, **3**, 221–248

RICHARDSON, M. A., SEID, A. B., COTTON, R. T., BENTON, C. and KRAMER, M. (1980) Evaluation of tonsils and adenoids in the sleep apnea syndrome. *The Laryngoscope*, **90**, 1106–1110

SHARP, J. T., BARROC, A. S. and CHOKROVERTY, S. (1980) In *Clinics in Chest Medicine*, edited by M. H. Williams, p. 103. Philadelphia: W. B. Saunders

SHEPHARD, J. W. (1984) Pathophysiology and medical therapy of sleep apnea. *Ear, Nose and Throat Journal*, **63**, 24–49

SHER, A. E., THORPY, M. J., SHPRINTZEN, R. J., SPIELMAN, A. J., BURASK, B. and McGREGOR, P. A. (1985) Predictive value of Müller manoeuvre in selection of patients for uvulopalatopharyngoplasty. *The Laryngoscope*, **95**, 1483–1487

SHPRINTZEN, R. J., CROFT, C. B., BERKMAN, M. D. and RAKOFF, S. J. (1979a) Pharyngeal hypoplasia in the Treacher Collins syndrome. *Archives of Otolaryngology*, **105**, 127–131

SHPRINTZEN, R. J., LEWIN, M. L., CROFT, C. B., DANILLER, A., SHIP, A. G. and STRAUCH, B. (1979b) A comprehensive study of pharyngeal flap surgery. Tailor made flaps. *Cleft Palate Journal*, **16**, 46–55

SKOLNICK, M. L. (1970) Videofluoroscopic examination of the velopharyngeal portal during phonation in lateral and base projections – a new technique for studying the mechanics of closure. *Cleft Palate Journal*, **7**, 803

SOUTHALL, O. P., CROFT, C. B., IBRAHIM, H., BUCHDAHL, R. and WARNER, J. (1986) Sleep related upper airway obstruction associated with severe episodes of hypoxaemia in four infants. *Archives of Paediatrics*, (in press)

STOOL, S. E., EAVEY, R. D., STEIN, N. L. and SHARRAR, W. G. (1977) The 'chubby puffer' syndrome. *Clinical Pediatrics*, **16**, 43–50

STOOL, S. E. and HOULIHAN, R. (1977) Otolaryngologic management of craniofacial anomalies. *Otolaryngologic Clinics of North America*, **10**, 41–44

24

Tonsils and adenoids

J. Hibbert

Acute tonsillitis

This is a common disorder in children and it is unusual for a child not to have at least one or two episodes of tonsillitis. These attacks are particularly liable to occur when the child is exposed to large numbers of other children for the first time, that is on entering nursery school or primary school.

The bacteriology of acute tonsillitis and the normal flora of the throat in children is interesting and somewhat puzzling. Several studies (Box, Cleveland and Willard, 1961; Reilly *et al.*, 1981; Toner *et al.*, 1986) have shown that the culture of throat swabs taken from children with a history of acute tonsillitis does not differ, in terms of organisms cultured, from those taken from normal children. Box, Cleveland and Willard (1961), in a study of normal children and those with recurrent tonsillitis showed that a high proportion of normal children grow pathogenic organisms from throat swabs. In this series of normal children, 96% of swabs grew *Streptococcus pneumoniae* (pneumococcus), 50% grew *Staphylococcus aureus*, 30% grew *Haemophilus* and 5% grew a β-haemolytic streptococcus. Similarly, a fair proportion of normal children (10% in a series from Moffett, Siegle and Doyle, 1968) will have viruses present in their throats and also anaerobic organisms (25% in the series of Reilly *et al.*, 1981).

Doubt remains regarding the most common causative organisms in acute tonsillitis in children. It has been stated that a virus infection initiates an attack of tonsillitis and predisposes to a bacterial infection (Everett, 1979). On the other hand, a virus may be the sole agent responsible and adenoviruses, Epstein-Barr virus and herpes simplex virus have been implicated (Sprinkle and Veltri, 1976). Of the bacteria causing acute tonsillitis, β-haemolytic streptococci, *Streptococcus pneumoniae* and *Haemophilus influenzae* are the most frequent. The role of anaerobic organisms in acute tonsillitis remains unknown at the present time.

Clinical features

The classical clinical features of acute tonsillitis are described in Volume 5, Chapter 5. However, in children, particularly young children, the clinical picture may differ. For example, abdominal pain or vomiting may be more significant than sore throat and unless the throat is examined the diagnosis may be missed. Similarly, earache may be a dominant symptom in childhood and this can either be a result of an acute tonsillitis with referred pain to the ears or of coexistent acute tonsillitis and acute otitis media. Examination of the tonsils in classical acute tonsillitis shows erythematous tonsils with pus in the crypts (follicular tonsillitis). Usually there is tender enlargement of the cervical lymph nodes, particularly the jugulodigastric nodes on each side.

Treatment

A child with acute tonsillitis is ill and requires fluids by mouth, paracetamol in a dose of 10 mg/kg 4–6 hourly, and penicillin. The administration of the penicillin may be intravenous, intramuscular or oral. In seriously ill children the best route is intravenous (10–20 mg/kg daily). In hospital, parenteral administration is easy; in the home it is much more difficult and perhaps treatment is best initiated by intramuscular penicillin to be followed by oral dosage. If the patient is allergic to penicillin, erythromycin (25 mg/kg daily) should be used.

Differential diagnosis

Acute tonsillitis may occur in acute diphtheria and infectious mononucleosis and these are the two diseases most likely to be confused with an acute streptococcal tonsillitis. The differentiation is made by Gram staining of a smear made from a throat swab and by examination of a blood film. On occasions, acute leukaemia can present in childhood with a clinical picture like acute tonsillitis, but usually there is more extensive ulceration, particularly in the oral cavity.

Complications of acute tonsillitis

The local complications of acute tonsillitis are discussed in Volume 5 and include respiratory obstruction, peritonsillar and parapharyngeal abscess. In addition, in children, acute otitis media may occur at the same time or be a complication of acute tonsillitis as may an acute retropharyngeal abscess (*see below*).

The systemic or general complications of acute tonsillitis are rare and almost confined to childhood. They are discussed below.

Septicaemia

Untreated acute tonsillitis can result in septicaemia with septic abscesses, septic arthritis and meningitis.

Acute rheumatic fever and glomerulonephritis

These are diseases of unknown aetiology and follow infection with a β-haemolytic streptococcus of Lancefield group A. The current belief as to aetiology is that antibodies produced against the streptococcus may, in some instances, cross-react with the patient's own tissues. Thus the effect on the tissue may be an arthritis, an endocarditis or myocarditis, or a dermatitis, and in rheumatic chorea there is inflammation of the cerebral cortex and basal ganglia. In acute glomerulonephritis there is damage to the glomeruli, possibly caused by immune complexes.

The incidence of acute rheumatic fever following streptococcal tonsillitis is variable but in 1950 was of the order of 2% if the tonsillitis was not treated and 0.3% if the tonsillitis had been treated with penicillin (Denny, Wannamaker and Brink, 1950). The incidence of a second attack of rheumatic fever is approximately 60% and this is reduced to 4% if the patient is on long-term prophylactic penicillin (sulphonamides if the patient is allergic to penicillin). Tonsillectomy does not influence the recurrence rate of rheumatic fever in patients who are given adequate prophylactic penicillin and has no place in the management of this condition.

Tonsillectomy has sometimes been advised for children who are not prepared to take antibiotic prophylaxis (Feinstein and Levitt, 1970), but this certainly does not eliminate streptococcal infections. Acute glomerulonephritis does not recur after a single attack although the effects of the attack may be long-standing. Again, tonsillectomy has no place in the management of this condition.

Peritonsillar abscess in children

As stated above this is a rare condition in childhood. In 1981 Holt and Tinsley reported a series of 41 children seen over a 10-year period in San Antonio, Texas. The interesting facts to emerge from this series are that only 15% of the children had a previous history of recurrent tonsillitis and this is the experience in adults with a quinsy. Of the 41 children, 11 had tonsillectomy and of the remaining children only two had a further quinsy. Here, again, it seems that the chances of having a second quinsy are not very high and certainly do not justify routine tonsillectomy.

Acute retropharyngeal abscess

A collection of pus in the retropharyngeal space occurs in three situations. First, and most commonly in children, it occurs as suppuration in a retropharyngeal lymph node. This is most likely to occur after an upper respiratory tract infection. The other two causes of retropharyngeal abscess are a perforating foreign body (*Figure 24.1*) or following tuberculous disease of the cervical spine (this produces a chronic retropharyngeal abscess and is discussed in Volume 5).

Clinical features

Acute retropharyngeal abscess is most common in infancy and in young children (up to the age of 5 years) (*Figure 24.2*). There may have been a previous upper respiratory tract infection and the child with an abscess is pyrexial and ill. There is dysphagia with marked pain on swallowing and the patient may drool saliva. Respiration is somewhat noisy, in part as a result of accumulated secretions, but also because the abscess obstructs

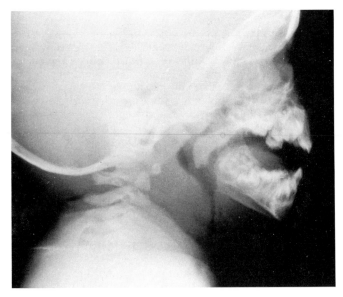

Figure 24.1 Acute retropharyngeal abscess in an infant

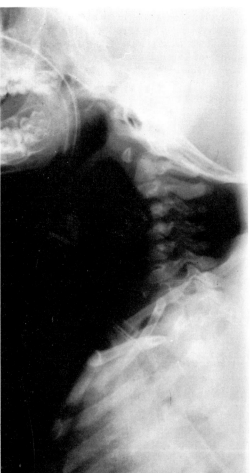

Figure 24.2 Acute retropharyngeal abscess containing gas. The patient has a nasotracheal tube

the airway and causes oedema of the larynx. The patient often holds his neck rigid and resists attempts to move it. There may be cervical lymphadenopathy or a very large abscess may be palpable in the neck. Examination of the child's throat is difficult, but if the posterior pharyngeal wall can be seen this is erythematous and bulging. A lateral radiograph to show the soft tissues of the neck will demonstrate an abscess, initially as an increase in the prevertebral soft tissue shadow, but later, may show an abscess with a fluid level. The dangers of a retropharyngeal abscess are airway obstruction and spread of the infective process to involve the carotid sheath laterally or the mediastinum inferiorly.

Treatment should not be delayed. The child should be started on intravenous penicillin and arrangements made to drain the abscess under general anaesthesia. This is a hazardous general anaesthetic because intubation may be difficult and rupture of the abscess may result in inhalation of infected material into the bronchial tree. Because of these dangers, facilities should be available for emergency laryngotomy or tracheostomy. Tracheostomy may be necessary anyway to safeguard the airway postoperatively if the abscess is large. When the airway has been established the abscess should be drained. This is usually carried out by incising the posterior pharyngeal wall at the point where the abscess seems to be most prominent and breaking down all loculi with artery forceps. In a very large abscess which has extended into the neck, incision of the posterior pharyngeal wall may be insufficient and the abscess may need draining through the neck by a cervical incision and dissection medial to the anterior border of the sternomastoid muscle.

Infectious mononucleosis in children

Infectious mononucleosis is an uncommon but serious illness in childhood. Negative serological tests for infectious mononucleosis are more frequent in childhood than in adults, but the diagnosis is still fairly obvious from the blood film. The major complication of infectious mononucleosis in children is upper airway obstruction resulting from swelling and exudate on the adenoids, tonsil and base of the tongue and the mortality is significant. When the airway is threatened administration of steroids may avoid the need for tracheostomy, although the latter should not be delayed if respiratory obstruction is increasing. It is usual to give hydrocortisone 5 mg/kg intravenously every 6 hours.

Diphtheria in children

Diphtheria is now a rare disease in developed countries with an immunization programme. Two-thirds of patients with diphtheria are children and most of the deaths from the disease occur in this age group. The vast majority of patients who contract diphtheria have either not been or have been inadequately immunized.

Diseases of the adenoids

When considering diseases of the adenoids it is as well to remember that the mass of lymphoid tissue in the nasopharynx generally referred to as the adenoids is a normal structure with a definite function, namely the production of antibodies (IgA locally, and IgG and IgM systemically). Many consider it pedantic to insist on the singular expression, the adenoid, so the more common term, adenoids, will be used here.

The size of the adenoids varies from child to child and also in the same individual as he grows. In general, the normal adenoids attain their maximum size between the ages of 3 and 7 years and then regress. What may be important in considering the harmful effects of the adenoids is not the absolute size, but more size in relation to that of the nasopharynx. The disease processes which affect the adenoids and cause problems are infective.

An acute upper respiratory tract infection affects the adenoids and results in hyperplasia with enlargement and multiplication of the lymphoid follicles. It is certainly possible that recurrent acute infections are the sole cause of abnormally large adenoids, although it has been suggested that allergic disorders also result in adenoidal enlargement. It is likely that most of the harmful effects caused by adenoids are related to size, although it

is often accepted that they may become chronically infected. There is very little evidence that this occurs and histological studies of adenoidal tissue very rarely show septic foci or microabscesses. They simply show hyperplasia of lymphoid follicles. Chronic adenoiditis is therefore not a proven entity and there is even less evidence for its existence as a clinical condition than for chronic tonsillitis. It is safest when considering diseases of the adenoids to limit discussion to acute infection and to chronic enlargement.

Acute infection

It is only relatively recently that the term acute adenotonsillitis has been used with any frequency, but logically it is inconceivable that the adenoids or tonsils can be acutely infected independently of each other. It is easier to see the tonsils during acute infection which is probably why the term acute tonsillitis is most commonly used, but it is almost certain that the adenoids are infected at the same time. Bacteriological culture of tonsils and adenoids removed from the same patient are very similar indeed (Polvogt and Crowe, 1929). Virus cultures of tonsils and adenoids yield similar results, namely adenoviruses, Epstein-Barr virus and herpes simplex virus (Sprinkle and Veltri, 1976).

Enlargement of the adenoids

As stated above it is the size of the adenoids relative to the nasopharynx that may be important, rather than the actual size. The effects of such enlargement produce impairment of nasal respiration and possible obstruction of the eustachian tube openings.

Nasal obstruction

There is no doubt that large adenoids can partially or totally obstruct nasal respiration causing snoring, hyponasal speech and forcing the child to breathe through his mouth. This is well documented and certainly the experience of all otolaryngologists. Unfortunately, there are other causes of nasal obstruction and mouth breathing, and adenoidectomy in these circumstances will be of no benefit. One of the sources of confusion is that a child with an open lip posture, that is with his lips apart at rest, is automatically assumed to be a mouth breather. In fact, a number of studies have shown that this is not the case and that an open lip posture may be totally unrelated to respiration. In 1969, Rasmus and Jacobs showed that children clinically assessed as being mouth breathers by virtue of an open lip posture had identical air flow studies to normal children.

Clinical examination of children with nasal obstruction is notoriously unreliable. Examination of the nasal cavities by anterior rhinoscopy may be normal or may show increased secretion, hypertrophy or congestion (hyperaemia or blueness) of the inferior turbinates. Murray (1972) showed a positive statistical correlation between enlarged adenoids and nasal congestion on anterior rhinoscopy, and while this association may be true in some children, these are precisely the appearances on anterior rhinoscopy of children with allergic rhinitis. In some children examination of the nasopharynx with a postnasal mirror will identify large adenoids. Unfortunately, in many children it is impossible to assess the adenoids in this way.

The most reliable way of assessing the size of the adenoids is to take a lateral radiograph. This will give a measure of the absolute size of the adenoids and also an assessment of the relation to the size of the airway (Hibbert and Whitehouse, 1978; Maw, Jeans and Fernando, 1981; Cohen and Konak, 1985). In an individual child with nasal obstruction, this is the best method of assessing whether adenoidectomy will improve his symptoms (*Figures 24.3, 24.4* and *24.5*).

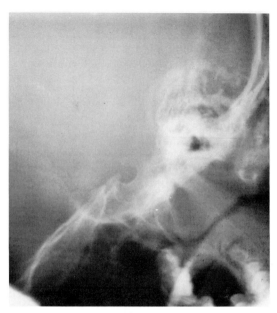

Figure 24.4 Lateral soft tissue radiograph to show partial encroachment of the adenoids on the airway

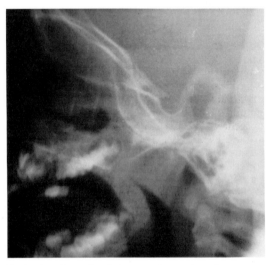

Figure 24.5 Lateral soft tissue radiograph to show apparent total occlusion of the nasopharyngeal airway by the adenoids. There almost certainly is an airway to either side of the main prominence of the adenoids but this, of course, does not show on the radiograph

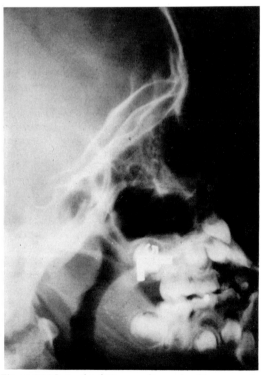

Figure 24.3 Lateral soft tissue radiograph with a normal airway and normal nasopharynx

Adenoid facies

It is generally accepted that a child with enlarged adenoids has a characteristic facial appearance resulting from the effect of nasal obstruction and mouth breathing on the growth of the maxilla. This facial appearance consists of:

(1) an open lip posture with prominent upper incisor teeth and a short upper lip
(2) a thin nose, a hypoplastic narrow maxilla, narrow upper alveolus and a high-arched palate.

These growth abnormalities result in occlusion abnormalities with cross bite and an open bite. In a very detailed and carefully performed radiological study, Linder-Aronson (1970) showed a close relationship between mouth breathing, enlargement of the adenoids and dental and maxillary abnormalities. The alternative argument is that these abnormalities of the upper jaw are, in fact, inherited variations of the normal (Tulley, 1964). It is possible that normal-sized adenoids in an inherited hypoplastic maxilla will give rise to symptoms, whereas this would not occur in a normal maxilla. A causal relationship between enlarged adenoids and maxillary abnormality has never been demonstrated.

Effect of the adenoids on the ear

The classical concept is that enlargement of the adenoids, possibly in association with infection, results in an increased incidence of acute otitis media and of non-suppurative otitis media (glue ear). It has been demonstrated both by radiological techniques (Bluestone, 1971) and by pressure studies (Bluestone, 1975a, b) that the adenoids can mechanically obstruct the eustachian openings and that adenoidectomy relieves the obstruction. The alternative view is that the adenoids may be responsible for recurrent otitis media and otitis media with effusion in only a small proportion of children. If the adenoids are solely responsible, it is difficult to explain the occurrence of ear problems in children with small adenoids, and in those whose adenoids have been removed. Unfortunately, controlled studies of ear disease and adenoidectomy have not resolved this question. In general, the controlled studies have shown that adenoidectomy has little effect on the occurrence of acute otitis media (Rynnel-Dagloo, Ahlbom and Schiratzki, 1978). Two controlled studies have shown some benefit for adenoidectomy in children with otitis media with effusion (Maw, 1983; Bulman, Brook and Berry, 1984) and other studies have shown no benefit (Rynnel-Dagloo, Ahlbom and Schiratzki, 1978; Fiellau-Nicholajsen, Falbe-Hansen and Knudstrup, 1980; Roydhouse, 1980; Widemar *et al.*, 1986). Further discussion of the aetiology of otitis media with effusion is presented in Chapter 12.

Sleep apnoea

The condition known as sleep apnoea was first described by Gastaut, Tassinari and Duron in 1966, and is characterized by apnoeic episodes during sleep associated with hypersomnolence during the day. In normal children brief episodes of apnoea occur during sleep and definition of the abnormal is difficult. This has been arbitrarily chosen as at least 30 episodes of apnoea lasting 10 seconds or more during 6 hours of sleep. Pathological episodes are associated with hypoxaemia and bradycardia which do not occur in normal children (Tilkian *et al.*, 1976).

Apnoeic episodes may be obstructive, central or mixed. Obstructive apnoea is when increasing respiratory effort produces no airflow; central apnoea occurs when respiratory effort ceases and the defect is in the central control mechanism, either in the brainstem or chemoreceptors, or connections of these. The otolaryngologist is concerned with obstructive apnoea and the role that enlargement of the tonsils and adenoids plays in its aetiology. Luke *et al.* (1966) reported a series of children who had developed right ventricular failure and pulmonary oedema. These complications were felt to be related to upper airway obstruction and were completely relieved by tonsillectomy and adenoidectomy in three children and by adenoidectomy in one. Since then a number of reports have confirmed that adenoidectomy alone or combined with tonsillectomy will reverse upper airway obstruction which has caused pulmonary hypertension and right-sided heart failure. In 1977, Mangat, Orr and Smith showed that obstructive apnoea during sleep could be cured by adenoidectomy. Similarly, it has been shown and documented by polysomnography that tonsillectomy and adenoidectomy will improve obstructive apnoea and oxygen desaturation in children (Eliaschar *et al.*, 1980; Mauer, Staats and Olsen, 1983).

The current theory regarding obstructive sleep apnoea is that if untreated, apart from the problems of daytime sleepiness, a proportion of these children will go on to develop pulmonary hypertension and cor pulmonale. The prevalence of pathological sleep apnoea is unknown and the risks of development of cor pulmonale as a result are also unknown and remain to be investigated. These risks must be very small because the number of children who develop cor pulmonale with otherwise normal hearts and respiratory systems is low.

The recognition of sleep apnoea clinically and its treatment are difficult problems. It is surprising how many parents, when questioned about snoring in children, will volunteer the information that as well as snoring their children have apnoeic episodes which, quite naturally, alarm the parents considerably. Clinical examination may confirm noisy respiration even when the child is awake and examination of the throat may show very large tonsils. However, in most children the diagnosis is not nearly so easy to make. Radiology with a soft tissue lateral view may show totally obstructive adenoids and observation in hospital may confirm or refute the diagnosis of sleep apnoea.

Ideally, these children should be monitored during sleep with electrocardiography, strain gauges for chest movement and ear lobe oximetry for oxygen saturation recording. Unfortunately, the facilities for such recordings are rare and in the vast majority of centres observation by nurses and resident medical staff may be all that is available. Such observation, however, is essential to avoid unnecessary and wholesale surgery. Once it has been demonstrated that a child has significant obstructive sleep apnoea and that other conditions such as micrognathia or Treacher Collins syndrome are not responsible, the question still remains as to whether the child should have adenoidectomy alone or whether the tonsils should also be removed. Most authorities in this field favour the combined operation as being the most expedient way of solving the problem. An alternative approach is to assess the size of the adenoids by radiology, and if indeed they are totally obstructing the nasopharynx, then perhaps it is reasonable to perform adenoidectomy alone. This is the author's practice, but it must be admitted that a proportion of children subsequently need tonsillectomy to solve the problem.

Tonsillectomy and adenoidectomy

In the past and sadly, even at the present time, the reasons for subjecting a child to 'Ts and As' (the mere title implies a lack of thought and care) have been and are less than rigid. Large numbers of operations are performed each year and it is the responsibility of every surgeon to be certain that every one of these operations is performed for the correct indications. There is some evidence that the number of operations has been reduced over the last 20 years. In 1963 there were around 200 000 operations per annum in the UK (Tate, 1963). The DHSS statistics on hospital inpatients show that between 70 000 and 90 000 tonsillectomies and/or adenoidectomies have been performed every year in England and Wales between 1978 and 1983. These figures refer to children treated in National Health hospitals. The figures are greater if one includes adults undergoing tonsillectomy and a large number of operations performed in private nursing homes.

The indications for performing this operation, both in general and on every occasion it is done, need to be rigorously examined. The morbidity and mortality associated with such surgery in childhood are not to be taken lightly and thus we are negligent if the operation is performed without very strict indications. Some of the reasons advocated for tonsillectomy and adenoidectomy in the past are plainly ridiculous and it is embarrassing to read them in medical literature. Ideally, an objective way of evaluating the problem is needed before advising any surgical procedure. The more that a surgical procedure relies upon subjectivity either in the patient or the doctor, the less likely is the efficacy of that procedure. In fact, tonsillectomy in particular is the prime example of a surgical procedure the performance of which depends upon the subjective assessment of the parents of the child and, to a lesser extent, of the general practitioner.

Clinical examination is unlikely to be a decisive factor in the assessment of a child for tonsillectomy. Certainly clinical assessment of the size of the tonsils is not particularly reliable and the size is not related to the severity of previous infection (Weir, 1972). Cervical lymphadenopathy is probably related to recurrent tonsillitis and it has been shown that children with a history of tonsillitis are more likely to have large palpable glands in the neck than normal children (Mills and Hibbert, 1983). However, this is a very imprecise method of assessment and 75% of normal children have palpable cervical lymph nodes.

It is most unlikely that bacteriological examination of throat swabs will cast any light on the assessment of children with recurrent tonsillitis. Serological tests have been explored as a possible indicator of recurrent or chronic infection and a report by Veltri *et al.* (1972) seemed to be encouraging. In this study elevated levels of IgG and IgA were found in a small group of children with recurrent tonsillitis or recurrent otitis media. After tonsillectomy and adenoidectomy these levels returned to normal. However, Kerr, Basuttil and Mandell (1977), could not substantiate these findings and found no differences in IgM, IgA or IgG levels in children undergoing tonsillectomy compared with normal individuals. Even if there are changes in immunoglobulins produced by recurrent tonsillitis, these are almost certainly fairly non-specific and unlikely to be a major contribution to the decision of whether or not to remove the tonsils.

We are therefore left with a history of recurrent tonsillitis as the main method of assessing children for tonsillectomy. Based on this history a number of clinical trials have been designed to evaluate tonsillectomy. At the present time five such controlled trials have been published (Kaiser,

1930; McKee, 1963; Mawson, Adlington and Evans, 1968; Roydhouse, 1970; Paradise, 1983), the last one of which is not yet complete. The control patients in these trials are those who, although thought to need operation, have not had surgery and so they are compared with the operated children. Unfortunately, the assessment of the children after surgery is necessarily subjective and therefore the bias introduced by the placebo effect of surgery is not eliminated. This fundamental drawback in such trials is inevitable, the only way round this problem being unethical and not possible, namely the performance of sham operations (that is, the child is anaesthetized but no surgery is performed), and even this would not be blind because it would be obvious which children had had surgery and which had not. Despite this limitation, these trials are of value and, particularly in the case of the Pittsburgh Children's Hospital study, some interesting and relevant facts have been produced.

From the Pittsburgh study it became obvious that a history of recurrent sore throats did not mean that these continued. In fact, of children with a history of recurrent episodes of tonsillitis only 17% continued to have such episodes when supervised and examined at regular intervals by a team of doctors and nurses (Paradise *et al.*, 1978). Since the history of recurrent episodes were quite rigorous (five to seven a year for 2 years), most of these children, if seen by an otolaryngologist, would have been advised to have surgery. If these figures are representative it means that based on history, 80% of tonsillectomies are unnecessary and that we are performing five times as many as are needed. The second fact which has so far emerged from this study is that tonsillectomy does reduce the incidence of sore throats when compared with control children with a similar history of repeated episodes of acute tonsillitis. However, the problems encountered by the control children (that is non-operated children) were not excessive and many of the sore throats which they suffered were classified as mild. This implies that the benefits bestowed by tonsillectomy were not necessarily great, even if it did mean tonsillitis was eliminated.

In many studies, tonsillectomy and adenoidectomy are considered together. This is completely erroneous. Removal of the tonsils and adenoids should be regarded as entirely separate procedures with separate indications. On occasions both tonsils and adenoids will need to be removed but this should not apply to both simply because there are indications that one of these organs needs to be removed. It has been erroneously assumed, with no scientific basis, that if one of these structures is infected or enlarged then the other is inevitably similarly diseased. This is not true; the size of the adenoids in no way relates to the size of the tonsils in a given child (Stearns, 1983). Similarly, it has been felt that if one of these structures is removed then the other will undergo hypertrophy and give rise to problems. In fact, as long ago as 1962, Young showed that in children who had undergone adenoidectomy a further 12% would need tonsillectomy. Looked at another way, if these children had undergone 'Ts and As' instead of adenoidectomy alone, 90% of them would have had an unnecessary tonsillectomy. On occasions indications will exist for both tonsillectomy and adenoidectomy but this should not be a thoughtless ritual.

Indications for tonsillectomy

Recurrent episodes of acute tonsillitis

All children will have one or more episodes of acute tonsillitis and this is not abnormal. A series of many attacks in childhood is unusual and there is no doubt that these can be avoided by tonsillectomy. This has advantages in that if it is possible to prevent these attacks education is not harmed and if a child can be saved these illnesses it is an advantage. It is unlikely that there are any long-term sequelae from recurrent tonsillitis and serious complications of tonsillitis are unusual (*see above*) in the present day because of antibiotics. There is no evidence that recurrent tonsillitis affects growth (Mills and Hibbert, 1983).

When an otolaryngologist sees a child with a history of recurrent acute tonsillitis, a diagnosis possibly supported by examination during acute episodes by the general practitioner and defined as severe illness, pyrexia, dysphagia, lasting at least 5 days, he is asked to predict whether these attacks are going to continue or whether they will cease spontaneously. If it is felt that they are likely to continue then tonsillectomy is reasonable. It is this prediction which is so difficult. However, it is assumed that if a child has had six attacks of genuine tonsillitis per year for at least 2 years then they are likely to continue. This, therefore, is our prime indication for tonsillectomy and doubt is cast even on this by the Pittsburgh Children's Hospital study. It is important to determine that the attacks of sore throat are those of tonsillitis and not an upper respiratory tract virus infection – the latter possibly associated with coryza and usually a shorter-lived infection. If there is doubt the patient can be seen during an acute episode. If the history is questionable then the patient should be reassessed 6 months later. It is surprising how this will reduce parental anxiety and very often avoid the need for surgery.

Tonsillectomy should never be used as a means of placating anxious parents when the indications are not present. On the other hand, parental anxiety is to be respected and can be allayed by careful and sympathetic history taking and examination of the child.

Peritonsillar abscess

As discussed above, quinsies are rare in childhood and the recurrence rate is of the order of 20%. Probably, in the most unlikely event of a child having a recurrent quinsy, tonsillectomy is indicated to prevent further episodes.

Sleep apnoea

Although this is a condition which needs to be evaluated it does seem that a number of children have obstructive sleep apnoea which is cured by tonsillectomy and adenoidectomy.

Contraindications to tonsillectomy

Recent upper respiratory tract infection

A recent upper respiratory tract infection is an absolute contraindication to tonsillectomy and the operation should be postponed for 3 weeks. Primary and secondary haemorrhage are considered to be more likely if an acutely inflamed tonsil is removed. Pulmonary complications of anaesthesia are more likely when the child has an upper respiratory tract infection.

Bleeding

It is essential when considering a child for tonsillectomy that a history of bleeding in the patient or family is excluded. If there is any such history the child must be fully investigated and if a bleeding disorder is discovered the indications for surgery must be reviewed and avoided if at all possible.

If, however, the reasons for surgery are compelling (this must be very rare) then the coagulation deficit must be corrected before surgery.

Cleft palate

A child who has had a cleft palate repair has an abnormal soft palate. Tonsillectomy will result in further scarring of the soft palate and may adversely affect speech. For this reason it should be avoided if at all possible.

The operation of tonsillectomy *(Figures 24.6–24.10)*

The important points about the surgical techniques of tonsillectomy are discussed in the adult in Volume 5 and will not be repeated here. The essential difference in the technique is that, in the

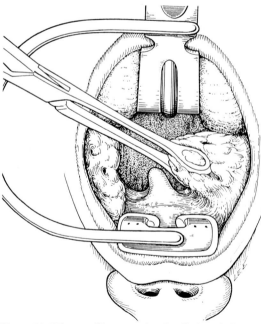

Figure 24.6 The tonsil is grasped and pulled medially. As in all surgery dissection of tissues under tension is the easiest and least traumatic

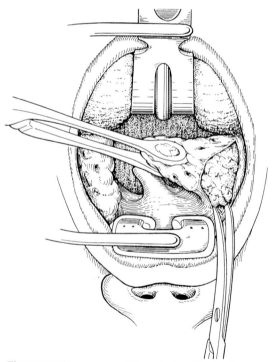

Figure 24.7 The mucosa of the anterior pillar has been incised, the upper pole of the tonsil is being dissected prior to incision of the posterior pillar

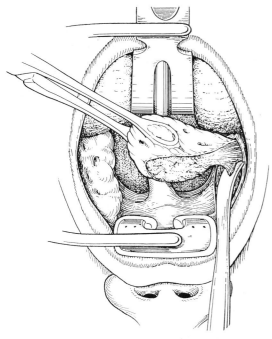

Figure 24.8 The areolar tissue between the tonsillar capsule and the superior constrictor muscle is being dissected. Sufficient tension must be exerted on the tonsil

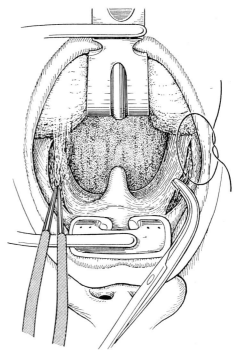

Figure 24.10 Absolute haemostasis must be achieved, either using ligatures or diathermy

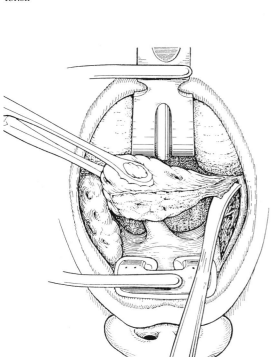

Figure 24.9 The dissection is almost complete but should be continued just onto the base of the tongue

child, an oral endotracheal tube is present. This must be positioned centrally on the dorsum of the tongue and fixed in this position in the slot of the Doughty blade of a Boyle-Davies gag. Unless the tongue is carefully positioned before surgery access to one tonsil will be totally inadequate. It is essential to choose the correct size of Doughty blade. In the average child aged 6 or 7 years a 9 cm (3.5 inch) blade will be found to be appropriate. The cross bar at the tip of a blade which is too small will compress and obstruct the orotracheal anaesthetic tube. A small blade will also allow the base of the tongue to obstruct the view of the lower parts of the tonsillar fossae and make adequate tonsillectomy impossible.

It goes without saying that the blood volume of a child is less than that of an adult and this is an important consideration when performing surgery in children. The average blood loss during a routine tonsillectomy and adenoidectomy is between 100 and 130 ml (Shalom, 1964; Holden and Maher, 1965). If the blood volume of a child is calculated as 75 ml/kg this means that a child weighing 13 kg or less will lose nearly 14% of its blood volume in an uncomplicated procedure; 14% is the point of blood loss in a child at which transfusion is felt to be necessary (Editorial, 1965). Excessive bleeding, postoperative bleeding or preoperative anaemia thus assume great importance in the child, particularly the young child. The blood loss during tonsillectomy should be measured so that excessive loss can be documented and corrected.

The postoperative care of a child undergoing tonsillectomy is of critical importance. The position immediately following extubation should be such that if any bleeding does occur the blood will run out of the mouth and nose and not into an unprotected larynx. Thus the child should lie on his side with his head below the level of the shoulders.

The postoperative observations include regular recording of the pulse rate (every 15 minutes for the first 2 hours, every 30 minutes for the next 2 hours and hourly thereafter) and close observation of the child's breathing pattern. A semiconscious child with blood in the pharynx will always make an audible noise on respiration and this should also be an indication to examine the child's pharynx for haemorrhage. Excessive swallowing or vomiting of blood is a sign that bleeding has occurred and here again the pharynx should be examined. Postoperative sedation should be avoided in children either as a routine or to quieten a restless child because it may well mask haemorrhage. The presence of the parents is the best way of calming an anxious child. Analgesia should be adequate without being excessive and there is little indication for narcotic analgesics. Paracetamol (250–500 mg) as an oral suspension depending on the age of the child is usually sufficient. Aspirin should be avoided as it increases the risk of primary haemorrhage (Carrick, 1984) by reducing the platelet adhesiveness and prolonging the bleeding time. The administration of aspirin has been incriminated in the causation of Reye's syndrome and its use is contraindicated in children under 12 years of age. The vast majority of children can be discharged home 24 hours after tonsillectomy without increasing the risk of haemorrhage (Siodlak, Gleeson and Wengraf, 1985).

Complications of tonsillectomy

These are fully discussed in Volume 5 and will not be restated in detail here. Clearly the most important factor and the cause of most of the deaths associated with tonsillectomy is haemorrhage and the delay in treating it. Tate (1963) investigated the cause of death in 93 children over a 5-year period and stated that this delay was the primary cause of death following tonsillectomy. The death rate was approximately one child per 10 000 operations. The factors which make the operation more serious in a child than an adult are the relative blood volumes, the difficulty in recognition of haemorrhage in children and the problems in coping with it in an uncooperative child. If there is thought to be haemorrhage in a child following tonsillectomy, blood should be prepared for cross-matching and the child should be prepared for anaesthesia. A minor bleed may occur which ceases after a few minutes and, in this situation, a child should be observed very closely with regular inspection of the tonsillar fossae. There is no place for sedation in the treatment of haemorrhage and the idea that this would quieten a restless child and stop the bleeding is not logical. Any child bleeding significantly after tonsillectomy should be re-anaesthetized and the bleeding point dealt with. This second anaesthetic is hazardous (Davies, 1964) and should only be administered by a very experienced anaesthetist.

The psychological effects of operation are likely to be more harmful in children than in adults. In 1945 Levy presented the results of a study of children with behavioural disorders and reached the conclusion that most of these were precipitated by an operation (tonsillectomy and adenoidectomy being the most common). Levy *et al.* (1967) made a number of recommendations to avoid undue psychological trauma:

(1) postponement of surgery if at all possible until the age of 3 years
(2) an explanation of what is going to happen should be given to the child
(3) the child should be with a parent immediately before and after surgery
(4) the child should be adequately sedated before leaving the ward.

Indications for adenoidectomy

Nasal obstruction

Children who have an obstructed nasal airway should be evaluated by clinical examination and by radiography. If the latter shows the airway to be obstructed by the adenoids then adenoidectomy is indicated.

Otitis media with effusion

The evidence that the adenoids are a causative factor in otitis media with effusion is equivocal and was discussed previously. Some surgeons advocate adenoidectomy as primary treatment for otitis media with effusion, either alone or combined with insertion of ventilation tubes. Other surgeons advise the insertion of ventilation tubes possibly reserving adenoidectomy for children whose effusion recurs after extrusion of the tubes. A third approach is to advise insertion of ventilation tubes as primary treatment, only removing the adenoids if they are large.

Recurrent acute otitis media

Although historically adenoidectomy has been advised to prevent recurrent attacks of acute otitis media there is no evidence that it is effective.

Sleep apnoea

As discussed above either adenoidectomy alone or combined with tonsillectomy is valuable in the treatment of obstructive sleep apnoea.

Contraindications to adenoidectomy

Recent upper respiratory tract infection

A recent upper respiratory tract infection is an absolute contraindication to adenoidectomy.

Bleeding

As with tonsillectomy, a suspected bleeding disorder must be investigated before adenoidectomy.

Cleft palate

As discussed in the complications, in certain instances the adenoids assist the soft palate in closure of the nasopharynx from the oropharynx during speech and deglutition, and removal of the adenoids may impair speech. The adenoids should never be removed in a child who has had a cleft palate repair, one who has a congenitally short palate or in one who has a submucous cleft of the palate.

The operation of adenoidectomy

This operation is by no means a minor procedure. Far from being an afterthought following tonsillectomy it should be regarded as a major surgical procedure with significant risks and complications. For example 60–70% of the blood loss during tonsillectomy and adenoidectomy is due to the adenoidectomy and control of excessive bleeding following adenoidectomy is more difficult than after tonsillectomy.

The preoperative considerations and preparation of a child for adenoidectomy are identical to those for tonsillectomy. The anaesthesia is also the same using an orotracheal tube which is stabilized in a Doughty blade using a Boyle-Davies gag.

When performing tonsillectomy and adenoidectomy it is usual to extend the neck of the patient using a sandbag under the shoulders of the child. This accentuates the curvature of the cervical spine and probably makes a complete adenoidectomy more difficult. A more neutral position of the neck, neither flexed nor extended may be preferable.

The adenoids are palpated with an index finger and it is important that the soft palate is relaxed during this manoeuvre or it will be torn. It is usual to dissect, using the finger, the lateral extension of the adenoids towards the midline. A St Clair Thomson curette is then inserted into the nasopharynx, gently positioned against the posterior surface of the nasal septum and swept downwards (*Figures 24.11* and *24.12*). It is important to select the curette of the correct size. Too

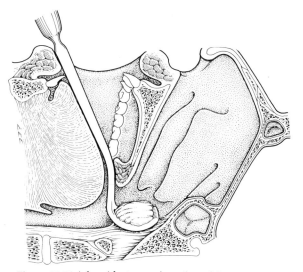

Figure 24.11 Adenoidectomy – insertion of the curette

large a curette will damage the eustachian cushions and one which is too small will mean that the adenoidectomy is incomplete. As the main mass of adenoids has been curetted, the blade of the curette is brought forwards to avoid running it down the posterior pharyngeal wall and stripping the mucosa. On occasions the adenoid mass remains attached by mucosal strands inferiorly. These should be avulsed using Luc's forceps, but the direction of avulsion should be cranial, otherwise the mucosa of the posterior pharyngeal wall will be stripped. The nasopharynx is palpated and any adenoidal remnants are curetted. A pack is then placed in the nasopharynx to help haemostasis. Modifications of this adenoidectomy technique are numerous. Inspection of the nasopharynx with a mirror and removal of remnants of lymphoid tissue have been advocated

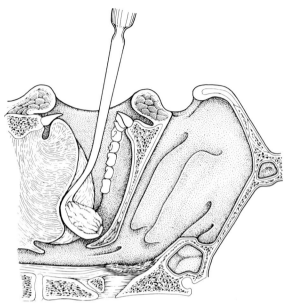

Figure 24.12 Adenoidectomy – curettage of adenoids. The adenoids are shaved away with a firm sweeping movement of the wrist until the curette emerges from behind the soft palate

(Sheridan, 1951). A fundamentally different approach is direct adenoidectomy in which the soft palate is retracted and the adenoids removed under direct vision using punches forceps and scissors (Guggenheim, 1957).

If bleeding continues after removal of the pack a second pack should be inserted and left for a further 5 minutes. If bleeding still continues mirror examination of the nasopharynx may reveal a bleeding point which can be cauterized or an adenoid tag which can be removed. If at this point bleeding continues some surgeons will resort to the use of topical adrenaline (1:1000) on a swab and others will insert a postnasal pack to remain for 24 hours. There must be absolutely no bleeding from the nasopharynx before anaesthesia is terminated.

The complications of adenoidectomy

The possible complications of adenoidectomy are basically the same as for tonsillectomy and will not be considered here in detail. However, there are certain other considerations associated with adenoidectomy.

Excessive haemorrhage

Occasionally there will be excessive haemorrhage at adenoidectomy. Aberrant vessels have been described (Grant, 1944; Duncan, 1963) and occasionally an aberrant internal carotid artery has been damaged at surgery (Harmer, 1914; McKenzie and Woolf, 1959). In general, excessive haemorrhage should be investigated by coagulation studies, blood should be replaced and the haemorrhage corrected by diathermy if possible or with a postnasal pack. Postoperative bleeding from the adenoidal bed is serious and the child should be returned to theatre immediately and a postnasal pack inserted (*Figure 24.13*).

Surgical trauma

The soft palate, particularly if it is not relaxed, can be damaged during adenoidectomy. The eustachian cushions can be injured and stenosis can occur (*see below*). Dislocation of the cervical spine has been described (Gibb, 1969) but usually this is caused by infection affecting the anterior ligaments of the spine and resulting in subluxation of the atlanto-occipital joint about 10 days after surgery.

Effect of adenoidectomy on speech

Children with large obstructive adenoids may have hyponasal speech, that is the speech of nasal obstruction and one would expect this to be improved following adenoidectomy. Hypernasal speech following adenoidectomy has been estimated to occur once every 1450 operations (Gibb, 1958). This is almost certainly a lower figure than the actual incidence because less severe cases may be overlooked or may be only temporary. The reason for hypernasality (nasal escape speech like that with cleft palate) following adenoidectomy is that the adenoids assist the soft palate in closing the nasopharynx during speech. Hypernasality is therefore more likely to occur postoperatively in those children with an abnormal soft palate. This may be congenitally short or its musculature may be defective in a patient with a submucosal cleft. The latter is associated with a bifid uvula and a notch in the hard palate, and adenoidectomy should be avoided in this situation. If the above obvious examples of palatal abnormality are excluded only a small number of children should develop hypernasality following surgery and one would expect these to be only temporary and to respond to speech therapy.

Scarring following surgery

It is not unusual to see fibrous bands or adhesions in the nasopharynx following adenoidectomy and

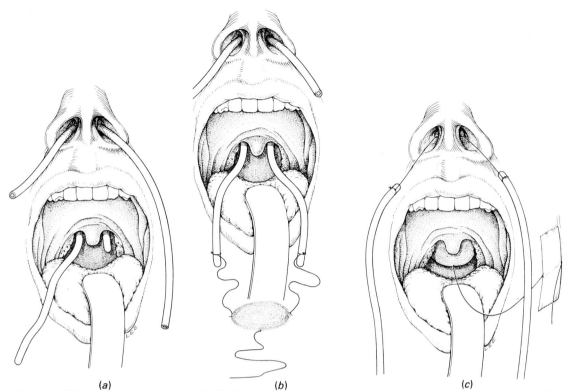

(a)   *(b)*   *(c)*

Figure 24.13 Insertion of a postnasal pack. The illustrations here depict insertion of a pack under local anaesthesia. It is necessary in a child to perform the same manoeuvres under general anaesthesia. (*a*) A small soft rubber or plastic catheter is passed through each nostril via the nasopharynx into the oropharynx. The catheters are drawn out through the mouth; (*b*) a piece of strong thread attached to each side of the pack is tied to the distal end of each catheter; (*c*) the catheters are then withdrawn through the anterior nares and the pack firmly settled into the postnasal space. The threads are tied across the columella and a third piece of thread, previously sutured to the centre of the lower edge of the pack is loosely secured on the cheek with adhesive tape. The pack is removed 24 hours later through the open mouth

normally this will cause no harm. Trauma to the eustachian openings may well produce stenosis and may impair eustachian tube opening and this has been suggested as one of the causes of failure of adenoidectomy to cure ear symptoms. Rarely, adenoidectomy results in total obliteration of the nasopharynx by scar tissue.

Persistence of symptoms following surgery

It is not unusual for symptoms to persist following adenoidectomy. Dawes (1970) has stated that 70% of children in his series with serous otitis had previously had an adenoidectomy. There are three possible explanations for this:

(1) the adenoid was not responsible for the symptoms in the first place
(2) postoperative scarring, particularly of the eustachian openings nullifies any benefit of surgery
(3) lymphoid tissue left in the nasopharynx

following incomplete adenoidectomy results in symptoms. Much has been made of adenoid remnants causing symptoms and the proponents of direct adenoidectomy use it to justify their approach. There is no doubt that some lymphoid tissue must remain in the nasopharynx following adenoidectomy and on occasions this tissue can undergo hypertrophy and cause symptoms. This is probably rare and may be more likely to happen when the child having adenoidectomy is very young.

References

BLUESTONE, C. D. (1971) Eustachian tube in cleft palate. *Annals of Otology, Rhinology and Laryngology,* **80,** (suppl. 2), 1–25
BLUESTONE, C. D. (1975a) Obstructive adenoids in relation to otitis media. *Annals of Otology, Rhinology and Laryngology,* **84,** (suppl. 19), 44–48
BLUESTONE, C. D. (1975b) Certain effects of adenoidectomy on eustachian tube ventilatory function. *The Laryngoscope,* **85,** 113–127

BOX, Q. T., CLEVELAND, R. T. and WILLARD, C. Y. (1961) Bacterial flora of the upper respiratory tract. *American Journal of Diseases of Children*, **102**, 293–301

BULMAN, C. H., BROOK, S. J. and BERRY, M. G. (1984) A prospective randomised trial of adenoidectomy vs. grommet insertion in the treatment of glue ear. *Clinical Otolaryngology*, **9**, 67–75

CARRICK, D. G. (1984) Salicylates and post-tonsillectomy haemorrhage. *Journal of Laryngology and Otology*, **98**, 803–805

COHEN, D. and KONAK, S. (1985) The evaluation of radiographs of the nasopharynx. *Clinical Otolaryngology*, **10**, 73–78

DAVIES, D. D. (1964) Re-anaesthetising cases of tonsillectomy and adenoidectomy because of persistent post-operative haemorrhage. *British Journal of Anaesthesia*, **36**, 244–249

DAWES, J. D. K. (1970) The aetiology and sequelae of exudative otitis media. *Journal of Laryngology and Otology*, **84**, 583–610

DENNY, F. W., WANNAMAKER, L. W. and BRINK, W. R. (1950) Prevention of rheumatic fever. *Journal of the American Medical Association*, **143**, 151–153

DHSS (1979–1983) *Hospital Inpatient Enquiry*. London: HMSO

DUNCAN, R. B. (1963) New concept of adenoidectomy haemorrhage. *Archives of Otolaryngology*, **78**, 721–728

EDITORIAL (1965) Bleeding after adenotonsillectomy. *British Medical Journal*, **2**, 1321–1322

ELIASCHAR, I., LAVIE, P., HALPERIN, E., GORDON, G. and ALROY, G. (1980) Sleep apnoeic episodes as indications for adenotonsillectomy. *Archives of Otolaryngology*, **106**, 492–496

EVERETT, M. T. (1979) The cause of tonsillitis. *The Practitioner*, **223**, 253–259

FEINSTEIN, A. R. and LEVITT, M. (1970) The role of tonsils in predisposing to streptococcal infections and recurrences of rheumatic fever. *New England Journal of Medicine*, **282**, 285–291

FIELLAU-NICHOLAJSEN, M., FALBE-HANSEN, J. and KNUDSTRUP, P. (1980) Adenoidectomy for middle ear disorders: a randomised controlled trial. *Clinical Otolaryngology*, **5**, 323–327

GASTAUT, H., TASSINARI, C. and DURON, B. (1966) Polygraphic study of the diurnal and noctural (hypnic and respiratory) manifestations of the Pickwickian syndrome. *Brain Research*, **2**, 167–186

GIBB, A. G. (1958) Hypernasality following tonsil and adenoidal removal. *Journal of Laryngology and Otology*, **72**, 433–451

GIBB, A. G. (1969) Unusual complications of tonsil and adenoid removal. *Journal of Laryngology and Otology*, **83**, 1159–1174

GRANT, H. (1944) Hydrostatic pressure in adenoid haemorrhage. *Annals of Otology, Rhinology and Laryngology*, **53**, 576–577

GUGGENHEIM, P. (1957) Direct adenoidectomy. *Archives of Otolaryngology*, **66**, 26–32

HARMER, D. (1914) Large pulsating vessel in the right portion of the posterior pharyngeal wall partly concealed behind the right tonsil in a boy aged five. *Proceedings of the Royal Society of Medicine*, **7**, 26

HIBBERT, J. and WHITEHOUSE, G. H. (1978) The assessment of adenoidal size by radiological means. *Clinical Otolaryngology*, **3**, 43–47

HOLDEN, H. B. and MAHER, J. J. (1965) Some aspects of blood loss and fluid balance in paediatric adenotonsillectomy. *British Medical Journal*, **2**, 1349–1351

HOLT, G. R. and TINSLEY, P. P. (1981) Peritonsillar abscesses in children. *The Laryngoscope*, **91**, 1226–1230

KAISER, A. D. (1930) A comparative study of twenty two hundred tonsillectomised children with an equal number of controls three and ten years after operation. *Journal of the American Medical Association*, **95**, 837–841

KERR, A. I. G., BASUTTIL, A. A. and MANDELL, C. M. (1977) A study of serum IgA levels in children undergoing tonsillectomy. *Clinical Otolaryngology*, **1**, 85–91

LEVY, A. A., TABAKIN, B. S., HANSON, J. S. and NARKEWICZ, R. M. (1967) Hypertrophied adenoids causing pulmonary hypertension and severe congestive heart failure. *New England Journal of Medicine*, **277**, 506–511

LEVY, D. M. (1945) Psychic trauma of operations in children. *American Journal of Diseases of Children*, **69**, 7–25

LINDER-ARONSON, S. (1970) Effect of adenoids on airflow, facial skeleton and dentition. *Acta Otolaryngologica*, **69**, (suppl. 265), 1–132

LUKE, M. J., MEHRIZI, A., FOLGER, G. M. and ROWE, R. D. (1966) Chronic nasopharyngeal obstruction as a cause of cardiomegaly, cor pulmonale and pulmonary oedema. *Pediatrics*, **37**, 762–768

McKEE, W. J. E. (1963) A controlled study of the effects of tonsillectomy and adenoidectomy in children. *British Journal of Preventive and Social Medicine*, **17**, 133–140

McKENZIE, W. S. and WOOLF, C. I. (1959) Carotid abnormalities and adenoid surgery. *Journal of Laryngology and Otology*, **73**, 596–602

MANGAT, D., ORR, C. W. and SMITH, R. C. (1977) Sleep apnoea hypersomnolence and upper airway obstruction secondary to adenotonsillar enlargement. *Archives of Otolaryngology*, **103**, 383–386

MAUER, K. W., STAATS, B. A. and OLSEN, K. D. (1983) Upper airway obstruction and disordered nocturnal breathing in children. *Mayo Clinic Proceedings*, **58**, 349–353

MAW, A. R. (1983) Chronic otitis media with effusion and adenotonsillectomy: prospective randomised controlled study. *British Medical Journal*, **287**, 1586–1588

MAW, A. R., JEANS, W. D. and FERNANDO, D. J. J. (1981) Interobserver variability in the clinical and radiological assessment of adenoid size and the correlation with adenoid volume. *Clinical Otolaryngology*, **6**, 317–322

MAWSON, S. R., ADLINGTON, P. and EVANS, M. (1968) A controlled study evaluation of adenotonsillectomy in children. *Journal of Laryngology and Otology*, **82**, 963–979

MILLS, R. P. and HIBBERT, J. (1983) The effects of recurrent tonsillitis on growth and cervical lymphadenopathy in children. *International Journal of Paediatric Otolaryngology*, **1**, 77–82

MOFFETT, H. L., SIEGLE, A. C. and DOYLE, H. K. (1968) Non-streptococcal pharyngitis. *Journal of Pediatrics*, **73**, 51–60

MURRAY, A. R. (1972) The appearance of the turbinates and nasal allergy in children. *Annals of Allergy*, **30**, 245–249

PARADISE, J. L. (1983) Tonsillectomy and adenoidectomy. Volume II. *Pediatric Otolaryngology*, pp. 992–1006. Philadelphia: W. B. Saunders

PARADISE, J. L., BLUESTONE, C. D., BACHMAN, R. Z., KARANTONIS, G., SMITH, I. H., SAEY, C. A. *et al.* (1978) History of recurrent sore throat as an indication for tonsillectomy. *New England Journal of Medicine*, **298**, 409–413

POLVOGT, L. M. and CROWE, S. J. (1929) Predominating organisms found in cultures from tonsils and adenoids. *Journal of the American Medical Association*, **92**, 962–964

RASMUS, R. L. and JACOBS, R. M. (1969) Mouth breathing and malocclusion: quantitative technique for measurement of oral and nasal air flow velocities. *Angle Orthodontist*, **39**, 269–299

REILLY, S., TIMMIS, P., BEEDEN, A. G. and WILLIS, A. T. (1981) Possible role of the anaerobe in tonsillitis. *Journal of Clinical Pathology*, **34**, 542–547

ROYDHOUSE, N. (1970) A controlled study of adenotonsillectomy. *Archives of Otolaryngology*, **92**, 611–616

ROYDHOUSE, N. (1980) Adenoidectomy for otitis media with mucoid effusion. *Annals of Otology, Rhinology and Laryngology*, **89**, (suppl. 68), 312–315

RYNNEL-DAGLOO, B., AHLBOM, A. and SCHIRATZKI, H. (1978) Effects of adenoidectomy. *Annals of Otology, Rhinology and Laryngology*, **87**, 1–7

SHALOM, A. S. (1964) Blood loss in ear nose and throat operations. *Journal of Laryngology and Otology*, **78**, 734–756

SHERIDAN, M. R. (1951) Observations on the nasopharynx and removal of adenoids. *Journal of Laryngology and Otology*, **65**, 609–613

SIODLAK, M. Z., GLEESON, M. J. and WENGRAF, C. L. (1985) Post-tonsillectomy secondary haemorrhage. *Annals of the Royal College of Surgeons of England*, **67**, 167–168

SPRINKLE, P. M. and VELTRI, R. W. (1976) The tonsils and adenoids. *Clinical Otolaryngology*, **2**, 153–167

STEARNS, M. P. (1983) The relationship of adenoid weight to tonsillar weight. *Journal of Laryngology and Otology*, **97**, 519–521

TATE, N. (1963) Deaths from tonsillectomy. *The Lancet*, **2**, 1090–1091

TILKIAN, A. C., GUILLEMINAULT, C., SCHRODER, J. S., LOHRMAN, K. L., SIMMONS, F. B. and DEMENT, W. C. (1976) Sleep induced apnoea syndrome: haemodynamic studies during wakefulness and sleep. *Annals of Internal Medicine*, **85**, 714–719

TONER, J. G., STEWART, T. J., CAMPBELL, J. B. and HUNTER, J. (1986) Tonsil flora in the very young tonsillectomy patient. *Clinical Otolaryngology*, **11**, 171–174

TULLEY, W. J. (1964) Malformation of the jaws and teeth in relation to upper respiratory symptoms and certain speech disorders. *Guy's Hospital Reports*, **113**, 261–272

VELTRI, R. W., SPRINKLE, P. M., KELLER, S. A. and CHICKLO, J. M. (1972) Immunoglobulin changes in a paediatric otolaryngologic patient sample subsequent to T and A. *Journal of Laryngology and Otology*, **86**, 905–916

WEIR, N. F. (1972) Clinical interpretation of tonsillar size. *Journal of Laryngology and Otology*, **86**, 1137–1144

WIDEMAR, L., SVENSON, C., RYNNEL-DAGLOO, B. and SCHIRATZKI, H. (1985) The effect of adenoidectomy on secretory otitis media: a two year controlled prospective study. *Clinical Otolaryngology*, **10**, 345–350

YOUNG, I. S. (1962) Adenoidectomy: how often is tonsillectomy necessary later. *Journal of Laryngology and Otology*, **76**, 791–796

25

Tumours of the head and neck

P. N. Plowman and J. Pritchard

Although malignancy is the commonest non-accidental cause of death of children in most 'developed' countries, recent advances in treatment mean that well over 50% of children are now cured. The leukaemias (30–35% of the total), brain tumours (20–25%), lymphomata (10%) and sarcomata (10%) are the most common tumour types. In descending order of frequency, malignant tumours presenting in the head and neck (excluding the brain) are non-Hodgkin's and Hodgkin's lymphomata, rhabdomyosarcoma, neuroblastoma, nasopharyngeal and thyroid carcinomata. Other very rare tumours and two non-malignant conditions usually treated by paediatric oncologists – Langerhans cell histiocytosis and the fibromatoses – are also discussed in this chapter.

The length of the discussion apportioned to the various tumours will not necessarily correspond with their rank order of incidence as this would not be appropriate for an otolaryngological text. For example, children with lymphoma may well present first in the otolaryngology clinic as cervical lymphadenopathy, but they are not subsequently managed there; only the broad staging and treatment strategies will therefore be outlined. Conversely, although much more rare in childhood, salivary tumours and squamous cancer (notably nasopharyngeal carcinoma) have been reviewed more extensively. Ocular and brain primary tumours are omitted but pituitary tumours, craniopharyngiomata and clivus chordomata are reviewed. Angiofibromata are discussed in Chapter 19.

These days, there is general agreement that the management of children with cancer should be coordinated at regional paediatric oncology centres. Here, patients can benefit from the medical, nursing and psychosocial expertise that naturally

develops when relatively large numbers of children are seen and treated. There is now *no* case for treatment of the 'occasional' child in an adult unit. Families usually feel that the inconvenience resulting from long-distance referral is offset by the feeling that their child is receiving the 'best possible' treatment. The inconvenience can be moderated by establishing 'shared care' arrangements with the local paediatric and/or otolaryngology units.

Lymphoma

Non-Hodgkin's lymphoma and Hodgkin's disease

Lymphomata constitute around 10% of malignancy in the 0–14-year-old age group and non-Hodgkin's lymphomata are rather more common than Hodgkin's disease. In both cases, boys are affected more frequently than girls. These and other contrasting features are listed in *Table 25.1*. Of particular clinical importance is that, although Hodgkin's disease usually presents with enlargement of lymph nodes, most often in the cervical or supraclavicular regions, the presentation of non-Hodgkin's lymphoma is more commonly extranodal.

Non-Hodgkin's lymphoma

The histopathological classification of non-Hodgkin's lymphoma in children is a good deal less complicated than in adults. Most tumours have a 'diffuse' (rather than a 'follicular') pattern and, at the cellular level, are 'lymphocytic/lymphoblastic' or 'undifferentiated' (rather than

Table 25.1 Contrasting features of non-Hodgkin's lymphoma and Hodgkin's disease in children

Feature	Non-Hodgkin's lymphoma	Hodgkin's disease
Sex male:female	2.5:1	2:1
Age at presentation (years)	5–10	5–35*
Clinical presentation	Extranodal, e.g. nasopharynx, abdomen, mediastinum, jaw,	Nodal
Spread	Non-contiguous	Contiguous
CNS Bone marrow } involvement	Relatively common	Rare
Cell of origin	Lymphoid	Reed–Sternberg cell, lymphoid? histiocytic?

* Second peak in later adult life

histiocytic). There is so much clinical and laboratory overlap between lymphoblastic non-Hodgkin's lymphoma and acute lymphoblastic leukaemia in children that the convention of distinguishing between the two conditions, based on the percentage of bone marrow blast cells (>25%), is arbitrary and of little real value. Instead, there is an increasing tendency to classify tumours by immunological subtype, for instance 'B-cell disease' or 'T-cell disease'. As *Table 25.2* indicates, sites of presentation correlate with the immunological subtype. Most T-cell lymphomata arise in the mediastinum (30–40% of all non-Hodgkin's lymphomata), probably in the thymus

gland, while gastrointestinal (25–30%) and nasopharyngeal (10–15%) tumours are of B-cell origin. Distinction between T, B and null lymphoid cells is easily made because of the ready availability of panels of specific antibodies which have replaced older techniques such as 'E rosetting' (sheep red cell rosetting). Using these antibodies, 'undifferentiated' cells in fact type as mature immunoglobulin-producing B cells.

The term 'Burkitt's lymphoma' is applied, for historical reasons, to B-cell lymphomata arising in areas of the world where there is holoendemic malaria. The high incidence of jaw tumours is the most striking difference between endemic (Bur-

Table 25.2 Non-Hodgkin's lymphoma subtypes – clinical, immunological and histological features

	T cell	B cell	'Null' ALL (including pre-B cell)
Site	Mediastinum	Nasopharynx Gut and mesentery Jaw	Bone marrow Bone Skin
Histology	Diffuse lymphoblastic	Diffuse 'undifferentiated'	Diffuse lymphoblastic or 'large cell'
Percentage with 'leukaemia'*	30–40	5	95†

* > 25% marrow blasts
† Includes all 'common' acute lymphoblastic leukaemia (ALL)

kitt) and sporadic B-cell lymphoma, but histologically and immunologically the tumours are identical. Studies on Burkitt's lymphoma cell lines and on native tumours consistently show one of three chromosomal translocations within the tumour cells; one break point always involves chromosome 8 while the other variably affects chromosome 2, 22 or 14, precisely at the respective locations of the kappa and lambda light chain and heavy chain genes. In the process, the *c-myc* oncogene is translocated from chromosome 8 to an area of the genome, adjacent to the immunoglobulin (Ig) genes, that is transcriptionally active in B cells. Overproduction of the *c-myc* protein almost certainly contributes to the generation of malignancy.

Around 15% of non-Hodgkin's lymphoma presents with nasopharyngeal symptoms (Traggis *et al.*, 1975). The short history (at most, a few weeks and usually a few days) helps distinguish non-Hodgkin's lymphoma from other nasopharyngeal tumours. Increasing nasal or pharyngeal obstruction, especially at night, is sometimes associated with painless enlargement of nodes in the anterior triangles of the neck (*Figure 25.1*). Endoscopy reveals a pinkish-white fleshy mass arising from one of the structures of Waldeyer's ring, though it

is often impossible (and unimportant) to define the exact site of origin. Since results of haematoxylin and eosin stained sections, as well as confirmatory immunohistological studies, can be available within 24 hours, frozen section studies are particularly not recommended because they can be misleading. Usually, clinical suspicion of tumour is high and, to save further trauma to a child already frightened by a compromised airway, bone marrow and cerebrospinal fluid sampling should be carried out under the same anaesthetic. Chest X-ray and abdominal ultrasonography (to seek evidence of hepatic, splenic and renal involvement) complete the staging procedures.

Nasopharyngeal non-Hodgkin's lymphoma is usually clinically localized. Stage I tumours (Murphy, 1978) are those limited to a single site and stage II those where there is also local node involvement; in 10% (stage IV) the bone marrow and/or central nervous system are infiltrated. Histopathologically, tumours consist of sheets of small or medium-sized round cells containing round or oval-shaped nuclei and interspersed with 'host' histiocytes (the so-called 'starry-sky' appearance, which is *not* specific for Burkitt's lymphoma). Immunohistological studies confirm the B-cell origin of most tumours and, because tumour

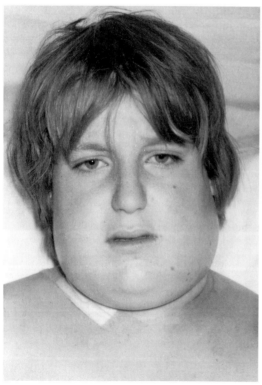 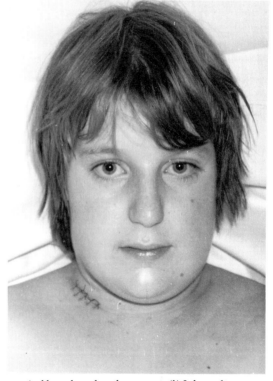

Figure 25.1 Twelve-year-old boy with nasopharyngeal non-Hodgkin's lymphoma (*a*) presenting with massive cervical lymph node enlargement, (*b*) 3 days after commencing chemotherapy. Note node biopsy scar

cells react only with kappa or lambda light chain antisera and not both, the clonal origin can readily be demonstrated.

Lower airway obstruction, when caused by non-Hodgkin's lymphoma, is much more commonly associated with T-cell disease than with other subtypes. Chest X-ray shows an anterior mediastinal mass, sometimes of an alarming size and often associated with pleural fluid. The trachea may be compressed to a diameter of 1–2 mm but, since the obstruction is invariably intrathoracic, tracheostomy is contraindicated. The dangers of anaesthesia or even sedation are such that biopsy is often a hazardous undertaking. Bone marrow or pleural fluid aspiration shows lymphoblasts and yields a diagnosis in 20–30% of cases but sometimes urgent, empirical chemotherapy (vincristine and prednisolone) must be started without delay; patients should be observed, day by day, and mediastinotomy or thoracotomy carried out as soon as acceptable relief of obstruction has been achieved. Hodgkin's disease is the most important differential diagnosis. For 24 hours before and around one week after the start of chemotherapy, patients should receive allopurinol and undergo alkaline diuresis to reduce the risk of urate nephropathy. They should also be monitored carefully for hyperkalaemia and hyperphosphataemia – the other two major features of the life-threatening 'tumour lysis syndrome'.

Since the introduction of combination chemotherapy in the early 1970s, the prognosis for children with non-Hodgkin's lymphoma has improved dramatically. Children with stages I and II (clinically localized) disease have an 80+% expectation of disease-free survival. In an American Children's Cancer Study Group (CCSG) study, the 'COMP' regimen (cyclophosphamide, oncovin, methotrexate and prednisolone) was found to be superior to a more complex multidrug rotating schedule (LSA$_2$L$_2$) (Anderson *et al.*, 1983). Two randomized studies, including one in the UK (Murphy and Hustu, 1980; Mott, Eden and Palmer, 1984) have shown that local irradiation, to the site of initial 'bulk' tumour, does not improve disease-free survival, a finding that is not surprising in view of the fact that local recurrence of non-Hodgkin's lymphoma is the exception rather than the rule. Most current protocols aim at reducing the duration of chemotherapy to around six months and early results (Murphy *et al.*, 1983) are encouraging.

Stage IV B-cell disease is more difficult to eradicate, although some encouragement can be derived from excellent early results using 'massive chemotherapy' (Philip *et al.*, 1984). Autologous bone marrow transplantation is needed to aid haematological recovery after massive therapy and the results of such treatment may, in part, be due to the use of monoclonal antibodies which can be used to 'purge' the reinfused marrow of any residual tumour. Eradication of central nervous system disease is the outstanding problem in the management of non-Hodgkin's lymphoma. Methods of central nervous system 'prophylaxis' that seem successful in 'common' acute lymphoblastic leukaemia are far less successful in B-cell malignancy, perhaps because of the high 'growth fraction' of these tumours.

Recurrences of non-Hodgkin's lymphoma occur relatively early, and the child who reaches 2 years off treatment can almost always be considered cured. Thus a 'typical' patient with head and neck non-Hodgkin's lymphoma is a 7–10-year-old boy with a brief history of pharyngeal obstruction and no clinical evidence of metastatic spread; his symptoms resolve within a few days of starting combination chemotherapy with a COMP-type regimen which continues for 6 months. Between courses he is able to attend school and undertakes almost all normal activities. He has no surgery or radiotherapy. Hair regrows within a few months of stopping treatment and there are no other obvious after effects of therapy although he will probably be subfertile. The chance of disease-free survival is around 90%.

True histiocytic lymphoma ('malignant histiocytosis')

This rare condition, quite distinct from Langerhans cell histiocytosis, most commonly presents with cervical node enlargement. In some cases, 'waxing and waning' of node swelling may induce a false sense of security, by suggesting an infectious aetiology. Liver, spleen, lungs, bones and central nervous system may be involved and bone marrow infiltration is characterized by pancytopenia, because the malignant cells phagocytose normal marrow components. Treatment is with combination chemotherapy and central nervous system 'prophylaxis'. At least 50% of patients are curable.

Hodgkin's disease

Hodgkin's disease accounts for approximately 5% of paediatric cancer, occurring as frequently as non-Hodgkin's lymphoma and with an annual incidence of approximately 7 per 10^6 per year. The disease is rare below the age of 5 years and there is a male predominance (M:F, 1.7:1.0), especially in the younger ages. Supradiaphragmatic, particularly neck, disease is the most common presenting site, as in the adult practice – usually as painless

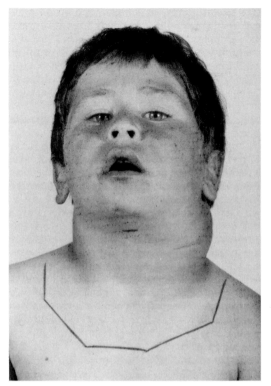

Figure 25.2 Cervical lymphadenopathy due to Hodgkin's disease

lymphadenopathy (*Figure 25.2*). Lymphocyte-predominant histology is more common than in adults although the majority of cases still fall into nodular sclerosing or mixed cellularity subtypes; lymphocyte-depleted Hodgkin's disease is rare in children in the UK.

The Ann Arbor staging system maintains its relevance for paediatric Hodgkin's disease. Staging procedures echo the adult practice, although the 'pick-up rate' from bone marrow trephine biopsy is very low indeed and the interpretation of lymphograms is difficult in children due to the frequent occurrence of lymphoid hyperplasia. The staging laparotomy, with splenectomy, alters staging in approximately 30% of cases and most American groups still consider this an important procedure, accepting the small morbidity and a risk of postsplenectomy sepsis. Standard, megavoltage, extended field radiotherapy (mantle, inverted Y and total nodal irradiation) for stage IA, IIA (IIIA) disease gives high relapse-free survival figures, but significant growth stunting occurs in the axial skeleton. Many UK centres prefer to avoid laparotomy and splenectomy in children, and accept clinical staging.

Childhood Hodgkin's disease has a better overall prognosis than adult Hodgkin's disease and, in recent years, many workers have attempted to decrease the intensity of first therapy. Such workers argue that with very effective modern salvage chemotherapy, relapse after conservative therapy matters less than the infliction of extra morbidity by 'over-treatment' of the majority of patients who would never relapse. This argument runs counter to the 'traditional' approach to cancer management namely the absolute necessity for disease-free survival in order to obtain high overall survival, but the good salvage capacity of chemotherapy in childhood Hodgkin's disease is an exceptional situation. The consequence of these arguments has been moves towards involved field radiotherapy, but usually supplemented by chemotherapy (Sullivan *et al.*, 1982; Tan *et al.*, 1983). In recent years, the St Bartholomew's/Royal Marsden Children's Solid Tumour Group has also explored chemotherapy together with a less than radical dose, involved field radiotherapy for early stage Hodgkin's disease (Robinson *et al.*, 1984), with excellent disease-free and 95% overall survival rates. The logic of systemic therapy is of course greatest in a clinically staged population. However, as chemotherapy has an unquantifiable late morbidity (for example possible infertility and second malignancy), some groups have returned to a therapeutic recommendation from the past, that is for pathologically staged I–IIA disease, involved field radiation and careful follow-up only (Tan *et al.*, 1983; Robinson *et al.*, 1984). This real challenge to the 'traditional' approach to cancer may have more proponents in the future.

Chemotherapy alone is employed for children presenting with more advanced stages of disease and MOPP (mustine, vincristine, procarbazine, prednisolone) remains the most commonly used regimen, although vinblastine substituting vincristine and chlorambucil substituting mustine represent minor variants. Such chemotherapy causes complete remission in 80% of patients of whom two-thirds will enjoy prolonged disease-free remission and probably cure. Relapse after radiotherapy alone is not disastrous as patients can often be 'salvaged' by chemotherapy. Relapse after chemotherapy is more serious but improved 'second-line' regimens such as 'ABVD' or Adriamycin (doxorubicin), bleomycin, vinblastine, dacarbazine, are now available and can cure some patients. In fact, early results of studies in children and in adults indicate that 'ABVD' is very effective in newly diagnosed patients and, because 'ABVD' contains neither an alkylating agent nor procarbazine, it is less likely than 'MOPP' to produce infertility or 'secondary' leukaemia. If these impressions are confirmed, 'ABVD' and variants are likely to replace 'MOPP' as first-line treatment for Hodgkin's disease in children.

Pseudolymphoma

While minor degrees of cervical lymphadenopathy associated with upper respiratory tract and tonsillar infections are accepted as part of the normal childhood spectrum, there are other infections causing greater degrees of cervical lymphadenopathy, for example infectious mononucleosis, or AIDS. Preservation of normal lymph node architecture, albeit with follicular hyperplasia, readily allows distinction from malignant conditions.

Sinus histiocytosis with massive lymphadenopathy (Rosai–Dorfman disease) is a non-malignant disease predominantly of Negro children who develop large, sometimes massive, cervical lymphadenopathy (Rosai and Dorfman, 1972). Other node groups are less frequently involved. Clinically, the condition presents indolently with usually bilateral, painless and often gross cervical node enlargement. Histologically, the involved lymph nodes show pericapsular fibrosis, dilated sinuses, plasma cells (often in abundance) and numerous intrasinusoidal histiocytes containing engulfed lymphocytes and other haemopoietic cells. The cause of this disease is not known and the majority of cases spontaneously remit without treatment. Deaths that occur may be due to progression of the disease locally or distantly or due to complications of a deranged immune system (Foucar, Rosai and Dorfman, 1984).

Rhabdomyosarcoma

Rhabdomyosarcoma is the most common variety of soft tissue sarcoma in childhood and more than one-third of cases arise in the head and neck region. There are no known predisposing factors, although there seems to be a familial association between childhood rhabdomyosarcoma and maternal carcinoma of the breast. Three-quarters of all children with rhabdomyosarcoma are aged less than 10 years at diagnosis, the sex incidence being equal and there being no racial predilection. Surgery, radiotherapy and chemotherapy all have important roles in management but the emphasis on which of the two modalities of 'local' therapy is appropriate depends on site and stage.

Tumours can arise in the orbit (commonest symptoms are proptosis and visual difficulty), anterior facial structures (painless swelling) (*Figure 25.3*), middle ear (deafness, bloody aural discharge) (*Figure 25.4*), nasopharynx (difficulty with phonation, upper airway obstruction), palate (painless swelling), pterygopalatine region and paranasal sinuses. When the tumour arises below a mucus-secreting epithelium, the mass may have a 'botryoid' appearance (*Figures 25.4* and *25.5*) that is almost diagnostic of rhabdomyosarcoma.

The major prognostic factors are: (*a*) the site of the primary tumour, (*b*) whether or not the disease is confined to the tissue of origin and (*c*) its histological subtype. Thus, in one recent study, children with 'confined' primaries, that is no evidence of extensive local, nodal or metastatic spread, had a 5-year survival of 86%, whereas children with tumour extensions outside the tissue of origin had a 5-year survival of 21% (Kingston, McElwain and Malpas, 1983). Within the head and neck region there are well-recognized relatively 'good' prognostic primary sites (orbit, parotid, anterior facial, oral cavity, larynx – all without bone erosion), and 'bad' prognostic primary sites (nasopharynx, nasal cavity, paranasal sinuses, middle ear – mastoid, pterygopalatine region, infratemporal fossae or any other sites with bone erosion). Thus, children presenting to St Bartholomew's Hospital or the Royal Marsden Hospital between 1974 and 1981 with primary orbital rhabdomyosarcoma had a predicted 5-year survival rate of 94%, whereas in the other head and neck sites survival was 50% (Kingston, McElwain and Malpas, 1983). In the same study, children with tumours of embryonal histology (the commonest variant in the head and neck region) had a better prognosis than those whose tumours were of alveolar type, as had previously been reported by others (Sutow *et al.*, 1970; Grosfield *et al.*, 1977). It should be emphasized that prognostic factors may vary with the type of treatment delivered. Thus, in recent studies, chemotherapy has been more intensive and successful and histology is a much less important prognostic variable.

Extension to the meninges and cerebrospinal fluid dissemination is a highly lethal complication. In a comprehensive analysis of 141 patients with tumours in head and neck sites, followed by the American Intergroup Rhabdomyosarcoma Study (IRS – Tefft *et al.*, 1978), 57 children had primaries adjacent to the meninges (parameningeal tumours). Of these 57 children, 20 developed meningeal disease – 10 at diagnosis and 10 later on. Evidence of meningeal involvement was most commonly manifest by cranial nerve palsies and other focal neurological signs including paraparesis. Cerebrospinal fluid cytology and myelography were often diagnostic. Although plain radiology of the skull may show erosion of its base, computerized tomographic (CT) scanning is now an important staging procedure and it is well established that those children with intracranial tumour are very much more likely to develop meningeal involvement than those with little or no skull erosion. More aggressive treatment recommendations have arisen from these observations. Interestingly, none of 17 orbital rhabdomyosarcoma patients studied by Tefft *et al.* (1978) developed meningeal disease, presumably reflecting the fact

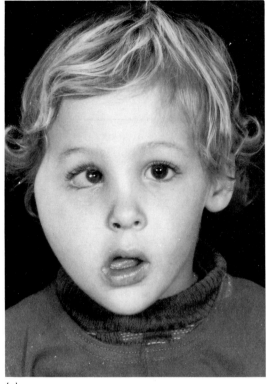

(a)

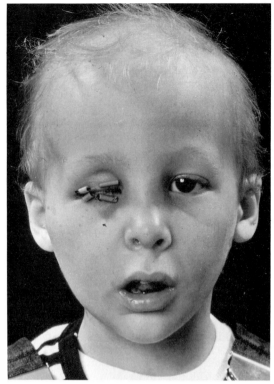

(b)

Figure 25.3 Massive facial rhabdomyosarcoma (initially misdiagnosed as unilateral mumps). (*a*) At diagnosis, age 5 years; (*b*) during therapy (note tarsorrhaphy, needed because of chemotherapy – and radiation-induced corneal ulceration); (*c*) 5 years after diagnosis showing maxillary hypoplasia due to radiation

that these children rarely have evidence of spread into or beyond the optic canal.

Pretreatment staging procedures are essential to define the extent of local and distant spread. Plain X-rays of skull and CT scanning of the head delineate the extent of the primary tumour, including any intracranial extension, and are mandatory. Isotope bone scanning assists in the detection of early skull involvement by the primary tumour and of any bone metastases. Chest X-ray with CT lung scan and bone marrow examination, preferably carried out under the same general anaesthetic as the diagnostic biopsy, supplement the general physical examination for distant metastases. With parameningeal primaries, cerebrospinal fluid cell count and cytocentrifuge are absolutely necessary.

In the absence of distant metastases, a treatment programme with surgery plus or minus radiotherapy for local control, together with chemotherapy,

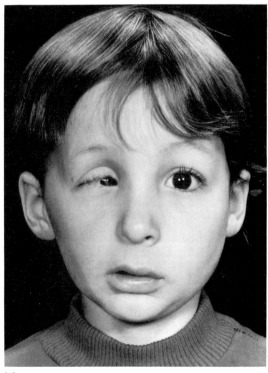

(c)

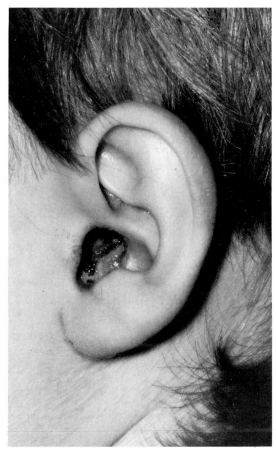

Figure 25.4 Middle ear rhabdomyosarcoma in a 5-year-old boy presenting with a botryoid (grape-like) mass at the external auditory meatus

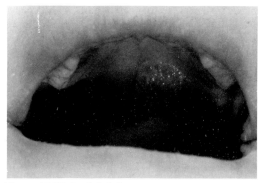

Figure 25.5 Palatal rhabdomyosarcoma: note botryoid appearance

of microscopic disease. Because of the higher normal tissue morbidity, lower doses are used for infants. For sites where local control is known to be particularly difficult, individually planned boosts (which may involve brachytherapy) may be appropriate. Particularly careful radiotherapeutic technique is necessary to minimize normal tissue morbidity. These days, chemotherapy is often used as initial treatment. Responses are often impressive, but the initial radiotherapeutic volume should cover the whole tumour volume as assessed by CT scanning and other imaging procedures carried out at the time of diagnosis. The final 500–1000 cGy are then delivered through reduced portals. Where tumours are superficial, electron therapy is preferred because, compared with photons, normal tissues are relatively 'spared'.

Results of analysis of IRS parameningeal patients, with their high incidence of fatal meningeal relapse (Tefft *et al.*, 1978), led to the recommendation that the skull base should receive higher doses of radiotherapy and that radiation 'neuraxis prophylaxis' was required. (Since the aim is to prevent the growth of occult tumour that is actually present in a proportion of cases, the term 'central nervous system-directed therapy' is preferred.) Indeed, the IRS group have reported that with such 'central nervous system-directed therapy' a meningeal relapse rate of 35% is reduced to 7%. In the UK, meningeal relapse has been relatively uncommon – a paradoxical finding not easily explained (Kingston, McElwain and Malpas, 1983) – although relapse in the primary site around the skull base was much more common. Our current recommendations are for maximal dose radiotherapy by an appropriate and usually individualized technique with whole cranial radiotherapy to a prophylactic dose (25–30 Gy) where there is CT scan evidence of intracranial tumour mass or other evidence of meningeal

is commenced. Although radical surgery (notably orbital exenteration) has great curative potential, orbital rhabdomyosarcoma may now be successfully managed without this mutilating procedure. Similarly, other anterior facial sites may also be managed, with a very high local control rate, without radical surgery. Unfortunately, the poor prognostic sites, where local control is much less easily achieved with chemotherapy and radiotherapy, are also much less easily amenable to surgery, although the opinion of a specialist head and neck cancer surgeon is always relevant.

Local control is achieved by radiotherapy in a high proportion of cases except in those with extensive involvement of the base of skull. Although, following a decade of experience with a broad dose range, conventionally fractionated total doses above 55 Gy have been recommended, it now seems likely with modern chemotherapy that doses of 50–55 Gy are sufficient for local control of bulky disease and 40–50 Gy for control

disease (usually positive cerebrospinal fluid cytology). Though neither agent is particularly active against systemic tumour, intrathecal methotrexate and cytosine arabinoside can reduce the numbers of malignant cells in cerebrospinal fluid, and occasionally eradicate them.

Systemic chemotherapy has greatly improved the overall survival of patients with rhabdomyosarcoma at all sites both because of a reduction in the incidence of distant metastases and an increase in local control rates of the primary tumours. To date, the triple drug regimen 'VAC' (vincristine, actinomycin D and cyclophosphamide), given as bolus injection once every 3 weeks in moderately myelosuppressive doses, has given the best results. The treatment programme for a child with an 'unresectable' tumour often starts with chemotherapy for 6–12 weeks, then radiotherapy to the primary site, followed by more 'VAC' treatment. Although no good studies of the value of 'maintenance' therapy have been carried out, chemotherapy usually continues for at least one year. The addition of doxorubicin (Adriamycin) to 'VAC' has not led to improved survival despite being an active agent in rhabdomyosarcoma. Other agents currently under study include the epipodophyllotoxin VP16, cisplatin and high dose alkylating agents – especially melphalan and isophosphamide. The prognosis for patients with detectable metastatic disease at diagnosis (stage IV) is very poor with 'VAC' alone or 'VAC' plus local irradiation, and experimental approaches similar to those used for stage IV neuroblastoma patients, such as consolidation with high dose melphalan alone or high dose melphalan plus total body irradiation, are currently under study.

The alkylating agents are now known to be relatively potent leukaemogens and are highly likely to produce infertility, especially in males. The early IRS studies showed the efficacy of two-drug (vincristine and actinomycin D) adjuvant therapy for early stage tumours and it is likely that cyclophosphamide will be omitted in future protocols for these 'good risk' patients. By contrast, in 'poor prognosis' parameningeal tumours it seems appropriate to try to find more effective regimens than 'VAC' in an attempt to improve both local and metastatic control. Because of their particularly poor prognosis and evident widespread disease, newer combination regimens are most likely to be tried first on children with stage IV disease. If effective in this context, similar regimens may be used on children with non-metastatic, but 'poor risk', tumours. If high complete response rates can be achieved, it may be possible to reduce the high doses of radiation which, in young children, lead to significant late effects (*see Figure 25.3* and *below*).

The long-term goal of the therapist is to develop more effective therapy regimens that have less short- and long-term effects than those currently in use. In this respect, both alkylating agents and irradiation are under scrutiny.

Neuroblastoma

This tumour, derived from cells of the neural crest, can originate in the sympathetic neural chain, including the cervical portion, or in the adrenal gland. Around 100 new cases per annum are diagnosed in the UK, some 7–8% of all malignant disease in childhood. A closely related tumour – the olfactory neuroblastoma ('aesthesioblastoma') – is of particular concern to otolaryngologists and is discussed separately. Although recent studies showing amplification of an oncogene designated '*n-myc*', may well have a bearing on tumour progression (Schuab *et al.*, 1984), the pathogenesis of neuroblastoma is ill-understood.

Head and neck primaries account for only 5–10% of all neuroblastomata; 60–70% of tumours arise in the abdomen, one-half in the adrenal gland and one-half in the abdominal portion of the sympathetic chain; 15–20% are of cervical or thoracic origin and the remaining 5–10% arise in the pelvis. Boys are more commonly affected than girls; the median age at diagnosis is 3–4 years and some tumours are congenital. Primaries arising from the cervical sympathetic chain usually present when parents note a painless, gradually enlarging mass in the side of the neck. Differential diagnosis includes various causes of lymph node enlargement, cystic hygroma, meningomyelocoele and branchial cyst. Sometimes, there is upper airway obstruction or evidence of spinal cord compression resulting from a 'dumb-bell' intervertebral extension. Rare presentations include ipsilateral Horner's syndrome (*Figure 25.6*) with or without iris heterochromia, opsoclonus–myoclonus (the so-called 'dancing eyes syndrome') and diarrhoea due to hypersecretion of vasoactive intestinal polypeptide. With cervical primaries, regional lymph nodes are rarely enlarged or involved. By contrast, metastatic spread from an abdominal primary to cervical nodes, most characteristically Troisier's node, is relatively common; under these circumstances, airway obstruction rarely occurs. Primary intracranial tumours, now more commonly known as 'primitive neuroectodermal tumours', are almost always localized to one cerebral hemisphere and present with signs of raised intracranial pressure.

Elevated excretion of vanillylmandelic acid and homovanillic acid or their metabolites occurs in the urine of over 90% of patients with neuroblastoma. As a result, sweating is a relatively common symptom and catecholamine-induced hypertension occurs in around 10% of cases. Although

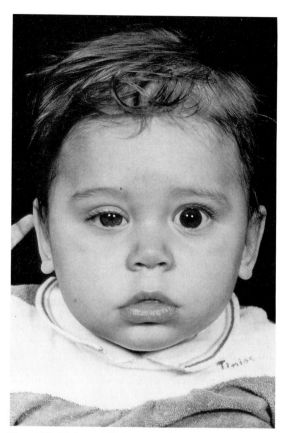

Figure 25.6 Infant with Horner's syndrome due to cervical primary neuroblastoma. The pupil was normally pigmented in this particular patient

usually made by histological examination of material obtained after biopsy or excision of primary or secondary tumour, the diagnosis is virtually assured if significantly elevated levels of urinary vanillylmandelic or homovanillic acids or dopamine are associated with the presence of tumour cells in bone marrow (especially if these cells react with one of several antineural monoclonal antibodies now available) or with characteristic radiological findings (Kemshead and Pritchard, 1984). Histologically, the tumour is classified as a 'small round-cell' tumour which is difficult, without other distinguishing features, to differentiate from lymphoblastic leukaemia/lymphoma or undifferentiated sarcoma. By light microscopy, however, the presence of intercellular fibrillary material and ganglion cells are virtually diagnostic, while at the ultrastructural level the identification of neurosecretory granules clinches the diagnosis.

Investigations at diagnosis relate to possible sites of spread and include multiple bone marrow

aspirates and trephine biopsies, bone scan, penetrated chest X-ray (seeking paraspinal node involvement – parenchymal lung deposits are rare) and abdominal ultrasonography or CT scan (to exclude liver metastases). Because of its simplicity, the Children's Cancer Study Group staging system (*Table 25.3*) (Evans, D'Angio and Randolph, 1971), rather than the TNM classification system is most commonly used. Cervical

Table 25.3 Neuroblastoma – CCSG staging system

Stage	Classification
I	Tumour confined to organ of origin and completely excised
II	Tumour extends outside organ of origin but does not cross midline: lymph nodes may be involved
III	Tumour extends outside organ of origin and crosses midline: lymph nodes may be involved
IV	Metastases
IVS	*See* text

From Evans, D'Angio and Randolph, 1971.

tumours are usually classified as Evans stage I or stage II. The reason for the less aggressive behaviour of supradiaphragmatic tumours compared to their abdominal counterparts, most of which are stage III or IV, is uncertain although a higher proportion of cervicothoracic than abdominal tumours have a more 'mature' histological appearance (ganglioneuroblastoma). Other favourable prognostic features at diagnosis include young age, low levels of serum ferritin and neuron-specific enolase (Zelter *et al.*, 1983), absence of amplification of the oncogene *n-myc* and absence of local lymph node involvement (Kemshead and Pritchard, 1985). Occasionally, an infant under 6 months of age presents with a small primary tumour and metastatic disease in liver and/or bone marrow and/or subcutaneous tissues, but no bone or lymph node deposits. At one time such infants were 'successfully' treated with repeated doses of vitamin B_{12}, but it is now appreciated that this form of neuroblastoma, known as 'stage IVS' (Evans, Chatten and D'Angio, 1980), commonly undergoes spontaneous regression.

Most cervical tumours are localized at diagnosis. Surgery is often indicated first in these cases and should include removal of a representative sample of regional lymph nodes, even if they appear normal. Subsequent management of each patient is individualized and dependent on prognostic variables, but some guidelines can be suggested. If complete macroscopic resection is achieved, no further therapy is given as, ironically, occult micrometastasis is unusual in stage I and II neuroblastoma. If macroscopic disease remains, adjuvant chemotherapy might be advised if the child is over 2 years of age or if the concentrations of serum ferritin or neuron-specific enolase are raised. Lymph node involvement is considered by the authors to be an absolute indication for chemotherapy (Ninane *et al.*, 1982).

When unresectable (stage III) or metastatic (stage IV) disease is present, as is the case in a majority of children with abdominal tumours and occasionally with cervicothoracic primaries, initial treatment is with chemotherapy. The regimen most often used in Europe at the time of writing is known by the acronym 'OPEC' (oncovin, cisplatin, epipodophyllotoxin (VM26) and cyclophosphamide) (Shafford, Rogers and Pritchard, 1984), while in the USA the 'COD' regimen (cyclophosphamide, oncovin, dacarbarine (Finklestein, Klemperer and Evans, 1979) is more commonly used. Most patients respond initially to chemotherapy and, if the response is sufficiently good, delayed surgical excision of the primary tumour is undertaken. Because of the nephrotoxicity, leading to a reduced glomerular filtration rate (GFR), and ototoxicity (high tone hearing loss) of cisplatin, a maximum of 8–12 courses of OPEC can be given. The majority of children with stage III and IV disease are not cured by OPEC and surgery but, nevertheless, treatment seems worthwhile in that remission often lasts over a year (median 15–18 months in one recent UK series, Shafford, Rogers and Pritchard, 1984) with good 'quality of life' and because some 20–30% of children (40–70% of stage III and 10–25% of stage IV) are long-term disease-free survivors.

Although regional radiation therapy has often been used in the past, there is little evidence that it adds to surgery and chemotherapy in the curative treatment of neuroblastoma. However, there is no doubt of its value in the management of bone pain, proptosis and other complications during the terminal phase of metastatic disease.

Currently, major efforts are underway to design more effective 'induction' chemotherapy regimens and to investigate the use of high dose chemotherapy or chemoradiotherapy consolidation (including total body irradiation as a systemic agent), in combination with autologous or allogeneic bone marrow transplantation (August *et al.*, 1985). High dose melphalan therapy, combined with autologous bone marrow transplantation (Pritchard, McElwain and Graham-Pole, 1982) has, for instance, increased the disease-free survival time in a current, randomized clinical trial. Another promising new approach is the use of 'targeted' radiation therapy using *meta*-iodobenzylguanidine (an adrenaline analogue) as a vector for the radioisotope ^{131}I.

For children with stage I and II tumours, the prognosis is reproducibly good (5-year survival of 90+% and 80+%, respectively). Recurrences usually occur within 2 years of diagnosis so follow-up can be relaxed after this time. Survivors of advanced disease with cisplatin-induced hearing loss are greatly helped by the use of high frequency hearing aids (*see below*).

Aesthesioneuroblastoma (olfactory neuroblastoma)

This rare tumour, thought to arise from the embryonal olfactory placode, is clinically distinct from neuroblastoma. It occurs more commonly in males than females, is rare in black races and has a broad peak incidence in the second to fourth decades of life (Bailey and Barton, 1975), although cases have been recorded in children as young as 4 years. Presentation is with nasal obstruction sometimes with epistaxis, rhinorrhoea, epiphora and, rarely, distortion or loss of sense of smell. Because of the slow natural history, symptoms may have been present for several months before diagnosis. If the base of skull is invaded, there may be headache, diplopia or a malar mass (Lewis *et al.*, 1965).

Histopathologically, the tumour shows features similar to neuroblastoma but can, nevertheless, easily be misdiagnosed (Oberman and Rice, 1976). Small round cells are set in a neurofibrillary matrix with pseudo-rosette formation and, rarely, true rosettes. Electron microscopy reveals neurosecretory granules and tumour cells may stain positively for dopamine β-hydroxylase and catecholamines. There is no systematic study of urinary catecholamine excretion but, although increased homovanillic acid/vanillylmandelic acid excretion has been reported in a single case, the frequency is probably lower than in neuroblastoma. Differential diagnosis is from other malignant tumours especially rhabdomyosarcoma, non-Hodgkin's lymphoma, nasopharyngeal carcinoma and glioma, and benign masses such as meningocoele, encephalocoele and hydroencephalocoele.

The staging system suggested by Kadisch, Goodman and Wang (1976) may be helpful for prognosis and treatment planning, but has not yet won general approval. Local invasion is usually too extensive to permit complete surgical removal and metastasis occurs in up to 60% of cases, particularly to cervical lymph nodes, lungs and bones. Tumour extension into the frontal lobes, best delineated by CT scanning, can occur but seeding into the cerebrospinal fluid is rare.

Radiation therapy with or without surgery gives a local control rate of 60–70%. Though no formal dose–response studies have been carried out, doses of at least 60 Gy are usually recommended (Ahmad and Fayos, 1980). There is sufficient evidence of the chemoresponsiveness of aesthesioneuroblastoma (Wade, Smith and Johns, 1984) to justify the use of chemotherapy in every case. Response rates to single agents such as vincristine, cyclophosphamide and dacarbazine are similar to those achieved in neuroblastoma so combinations, such as 'OPEC' or 'COD', are now recommended. With surgery and radiotherapy alone, 5-year survival is around 60–70%, with half of these patients being disease free. There is hope that, with chemotherapy, results will be better although it should be emphasized that at least 10 years follow-up is needed before cure can be assured.

Nasopharyngeal carcinoma

In a series of 248 patients presenting to the Royal Marsden Hospital (London) with nasopharyngeal carcinoma, six patients (2.4%) were less than 15 years of age, 10 (4%) less than 20 and 28 (11%) less than 30 years of age (Lederman, 1961). In North America, the age incidence curve for nasopharyngeal carcinoma is bimodal with a first (albeit smaller) peak incidence between 15 and 25 years (Greene, Fraumeni and Hoover, 1977). This bimodal incidence has also been observed in Puerto Rico (Morales *et al.*, 1984) and several other countries (India, Israel, Tunisia, Greece, Kuwait), but there is no early peak in people of Chinese extraction. The male predominance of nasopharyngeal carcinoma, so obvious in the adult population, is much less apparent in childhood. The very much higher incidence of nasopharyngeal carcinoma in Hong Kong Chinese, southern China and south-east Asian countries, compared with that encountered in the West, is attributed to racial predisposition, smoked and salted dietary fish and Epstein–Barr virus infection (Ho, 1978), but is mainly among adults. Jenkin *et al.* (1981) pointed out that the aetiology of the disease in children and young adults may be different from that encountered in later life. However, Naegele *et al.* (1982) demonstrated Epstein–Barr virus antibody titres suggestive of infection and Epstein–Barr nuclear antigen-positive carcinoma cells in seven American children with nasopharyngeal carcinoma. Furthermore, the pattern of spread and prognosis of nasopharyngeal carcinoma in childhood and adults appear to be similar.

The clinical presentation and pattern of spread is similar in all ages. The primary nasopharyngeal carcinoma may be 'silent' and the disease presents clinically with upper deep cervical neck node masses at a time when mirror examination of the nasopharynx is negative. Indeed, symptoms and signs may appear only when the primary tumour has spread to involve adjacent structures, often at the base of skull. Lesions of the lateral wall may be associated with Trotter's triad of symptoms: (*a*) hypoacusia; (*b*) paresis of the soft palate; (*c*) pain in the territory of the mandibular division of the trigeminal nerve. Larger growths may produce nasal obstruction or bleeding and a 'nasal twang' to the voice. Invasion of the base of the skull leads to severe pain which may presage cranial nerve paresis.

The diagnosis is made by biopsy under general anaesthesia at which time the palpable extent of the primary is assessed. The histological picture is of squamous carcinoma (often poorly differentiated) and tumours previously described as lymphoepithelioma are now recognized to be poorly differentiated squamous carcinomata. Blind adenoidal region biopsy may be positive in occult cases presenting with cervical adenopathy. Nasopharyngeal carcinoma must be distinguished from nasopharyngeal angiofibroma (*see* Chapter 19) and from an anteriorly sited rhabdomyosarcoma arising in the nasopharynx.

The TNM staging system for nasopharyngeal carcinoma is shown in *Table 25.4*. Plain skull

Table 25.4 TNM staging classification of nasopharyngeal carcinoma (UICC)

Stage	Classification
T0	No evidence of primary tumour
T1	Tumour limited to one region
T2	Tumour extending into two regions
T3	Tumour extending beyond the nasopharynx without bone involvement
T4	Tumour extending beyond the nasopharynx with bone involvement, including the cartilaginous portion of the eustachian tube
N0	No palpable cervical nodes
N1	Mobile ipsilateral cervical lymphadenopathy
N2	Mobile bilateral cervical lymphadenopathy
N3	Fixed cervical lymphadenopathy
M0	No metastases
M1	Metastases

radiology, including a submentovertical view, and CT scanning of the head and neck are essential staging procedures (*Figure 25.7*). In the Children's Cancer Study Group (CCSG) analysis, 41 children presented with T1, or T2 lesions, 19 with T3 and 43 with T4 lesions – indicating the high frequency of

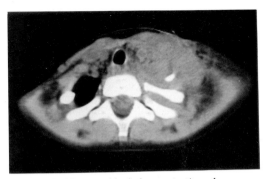

Figure 25.7 CT scan of neck demonstrating a large mass of lymph glands infiltrated by metastatic nasopharyngeal carcinoma. There was no discernible primary in the nasopharynx of this child

skull invasion at presentation (of great prognostic importance). In the same CCSG series, 14 cases were N0, 9 cases N1, 42 N2 and 49 N3 demonstrating the high frequency of clinically obvious node metastases at presentation (Jenkin *et al.*, 1981). Distant metastases are present at diagnosis in only 2–3% of cases, most commonly in bone but also in lung, liver and even bone marrow. Staging investigations should therefore include bone scan, posteroanterior and lateral chest X-rays and abdominal ultrasound.

Nasopharyngeal carcinoma is not amenable to surgical attack, but as the lesion is radiosensitive, treatment is based on high dose, modern megavoltage radiotherapy. Although the world's largest experience and excellent survival results come from Ho's group (Ho, 1978) this group's radiation technique is not ideal. In particular, the dissimilarly canted nasopharyngeal and neck fields produce awkward field junctions in the region of Rouvière's node and the uppermost deep cervical nodes. The radiation technique employed and recommended for children presenting to the Hospital for Sick Children, London, commences with the supine child in an individually made shell with a dental splint keeping the tongue downwards and the floor of the mouth low and outside the radiation portals. The orbitomeatal line (Reid's baseline) is vertical and all planning (including field junctions) is parallel or perpendicular to this plane. Planning and treatment then continue in a fashion similar to a previously published technique (Lederman and Mould, 1968). The recommended tumour dose to the nasopharynx is 55–60 Gy (50 Gy to children less than 4 years, 60 Gy to children over 12 years old), conventionally divided into 175–190 cGy daily fractions. There is no evidence that total doses of more than 50 Gy are more effective, in children and young adults, than doses in the 40–50 Gy range (Jenkin *et al.*, 1981). Therefore, the authors avoid the 70-Gy total

dosage to the nasopharynx recommended for adults by many therapists. By using a three-field boost to the nasopharynx, the incidence of treatment-induced late trismus is low. Even if clinically normal, the neck nodes down to the clavicles receive a conventionally fractionated dose of 50 Gy. A good, reproducible radiation technique for nasopharyngeal carcinoma is a technically demanding exercise.

Recently, several chemotherapeutic agents have been shown to have at least partial efficacy against this tumour. Although single agent data are scanty, there is published evidence of tumour response to the 'VAC' (vincristine, actinomycin D, cyclophosphamide) regimen and personal, albeit anecdotal, experience of response to the 'BEP' (bleomycin, the epipodophyllotoxin VP16, cisplatin) combination. Although a delay to radiotherapy of more than 3 months is not advised, combination chemotherapy is included in the treatment protocol of at least the more advanced cases presenting to the Hospital for Sick Children, London.

The careful study of adults by Ho (1978) established that prognosis related to the stage of the primary tumour (base of skull invasion being a particularly bad prognostic sign), and to neck node status (fixed, bilateral and low cervical neck nodes carrying a worse outlook than high, mobile and unilateral cervical nodes). Distant metastases are almost invariably fatal. For tumours confined to the nasopharynx, the 5-year survival was 84% and for larger primaries (but without base of skull invasion) and/or mobile, high unilateral cervical nodes the survival was 62%, but where there was more extensive nodal involvement the 5-year survival dropped to 40%. Similarly, in a more recent American study, prognosis related directly to stage of disease at presentation, initial performance status and radiation dose received (Petrovich *et al.*, 1985). In this adult series, failure at the primary site was common (88%) when there was invasion of the base of the skull. In the study by Ho (1978) prophylactic neck node irradiation did not add to the survival of that minority of patients with small tumours localized to the nasopharyngeal mucosa. In the study by Petrovich *et al.* (1985), radical neck dissections did not alter the outlook for patients with advanced neck node disease.

Jenkin *et al.* (1981) analysed the results of treatment in 119 Americans under 30 years of age at diagnosis and found overall 5-year relapse-free and overall survival rates of 36% and 51%, respectively. When tumour was confined to the nasopharynx (T1 and T2), 5-year survival was 75%. These figures are similar to those reported for adults (Ho, 1978). Jenkin *et al.* also analysed patterns of relapse in patients whose disease was initially localized. In approximately one-third of patients there was only local recurrence while in the remaining two-thirds of cases, recurrence was outside the irradiation field. Overall, just over one-half of relapses occurred at metastatic sites. Because of this statistic and because further major improvements in irradiation techniques are unlikely, the need for more effective chemotherapy regimens is re-emphasized.

Other carcinomata of the head and neck

Carcinomata in other head and neck sites, for example lip, tongue, oropharynx and larynx (*Figure 25.8*) in childhood are fortunately very rare indeed. When localized they are treated, as in adults, by radical surgery and radiotherapy.

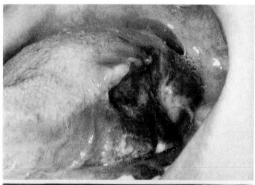
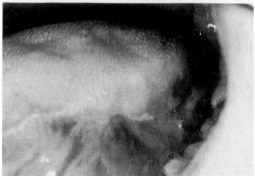

Figure 25.8 Top panel: this 14-year-old boy presented with a T3N0M0 carcinoma of the left lateral tongue border. No predisposing factors were found. Bottom panel: following radiotherapy

Thyroid cancer

Thyroid carcinoma is rare in children and only one or two new cases are seen at the Hospital for Sick Children, London, each year. Of 59 paediatric cases presenting to the Mayo Clinic, 56 were papillary and only three were follicular carcinoma

– a very much higher proportion of papillary to follicular than is encountered in the adult population (Woolner *et al.*, 1961). Of 576 cases of papillary thyroid carcinoma presenting to the United States Armed Forces Institute of Pathology (AFIP), approximately 7% occurred in patients aged 6–19 years (Mazzaferri *et al.*, 1977). Older children are more commonly afflicted and the same female preponderance exists as in adults. Papillary carcinoma usually arises from a thyroid gland with otherwise normal parenchyma but prior exposure of the neck to radiation (mean latency 16 years, Mazzaferri *et al.*, 1977) is a recognized predisposing factor.

Thyroid cancer presents in children, as in adults, as a painless discrete thyroid mass or, less commonly, as a deep cervical chain lymph node mass (the 'lateral aberrant thyroid') (*Figure 25.9*). Treatment recommendations have also been similar to those for adults, here summarized and have been recently and more fully reviewed (Plowman, 1986).

Following histological diagnosis by biopsy, radical thyroidectomy – preserving the recurrent

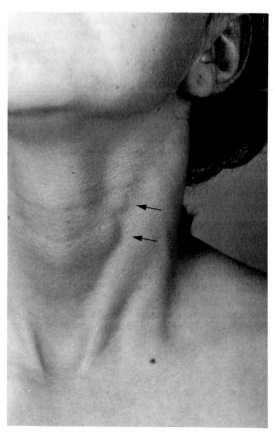

Figure 25.9 Papillary carcinoma of thyroid presenting as a discrete thyroid swelling in a teenage girl

laryngeal nerves and at least one parathyroid gland – is the preferred therapeutic procedure. *All involved lymph nodes must be excised from one or both deep cervical chains and, if CT scan shows that mediastinal nodes are involved, mediastinal exploration to clear such nodes is indicated.* Formal block dissection of the deep cervical chain is not routinely recommended but is occasionally essential.

Following surgery, a normal thyroid remnant is almost invariably demonstrable on radioiodine tracer scanning. This iodine-avid tissue prevents the demonstration of less iodine-avid residual tumour deposits. An ablation dose of radioiodine destroys this high-avidity remnant of normal thyroid tissue and 3 months later a whole body ^{131}I scan should reveal iodine-concentrating metastases, if present.

Papillary thyroid carcinoma in young patients is very slow growing and relapse may occur 10–20 years after diagnosis. The initial site of recurrence is most commonly in the deep cervical node chains, then in the mediastinal nodes followed by lung metastases. The overall incidence of nodal metastases in the Mayo Clinic papillary carcinoma series (all ages) was 39%, but the histological findings in the radical thyroidectomy specimen proved a strong prognosticator for subsequent nodal relapse. Thus, 32% of those patients with intrathyroidal tumours later developed nodal disease, whereas 57% of those with extrathyroidal disease later developed further nodal metastases (Woolner *et al.*, 1961). The vast majority of papillary carcinomata actually exhibit mixed papillary and follicular architecture, although a prominent solid papillary component is more common in younger patients (Woolner *et al.*, 1961). The microscopic architecture (notably the demonstration of a follicular element) is of relevance to subsequent radioiodine tracer studies in the follow-up of these patients and of radioiodine therapy for relapse.

Following radical thyroidectomy and radioiodine ablation of the thyroid remnant, follow-up of the patient is by clinical examination (with particularly careful palpation of the neck), augmented by chest X-rays and iodine profile scans – decreasing in frequency with time. Between radioiodine profile scans the patient is placed on fully TSH suppressive doses of thyroid hormone. Our recommendations for serial radioiodine profile scans in papillary tumour follow-up have been based on the extensive studies of Pochin (1967) who found that over 80% of differentiated thyroid cancer concentrated radioiodine and: '. . . contrary to views sometimes expressed, we have found tumours that were predominantly papillary in structure to be as likely to develop uptake and respond to treatment

as those that were predominantly follicular . . .'. The follicular and colloid component of a papillary tumour allows a prediction concerning iodine concentration.

More recently, serum thyroglobulin estimations have been helpful in the follow-up of patients with differentiated thyroid cancer. Serum thyroglobulin is secreted in small quantities by the cells of many follicular cell origin cancers and Black *et al.* (1981) reported that in radically ablated patients or in those on fully TSH-suppressive doses of thyroid hormone, serum thyroglobulin estimations provided a marker for relapse detection. Since then, it has been shown that positive radioiodine tracer scans may be found in the absence of detectable serum thyroglobulin and also that circulating thyroglobulin autoantibodies may invalidate the thyroglobulin assay (Grant *et al.*, 1984). Thus, while serum thyroglobulin estimations complement radioiodine scans in the follow-up of thyroid cancer patients, they do not reliably substitute.

When a patient with papillary thyroid carcinoma relapses in cervical or mediastinal nodes, a radioiodine tracer study must precede surgical resection of all affected nodal disease. In those cases with a positive preoperative tracer study, a postoperative therapy dose(s) of radioiodine is given. In patients with distant metastases (usually lung), a tracer dose study will demonstrate whether or not the recurrent tumour will concentrate and be amenable to treatment by radioiodine.

The overall prognosis for patients with papillary carcinoma of the thyroid (all ages) is good. In a predominantly young adult population analysed by the AFIP, 10-year survival was 95% (Mazzaferri *et al.*, 1977). In this particular series younger patients clearly had a better prognosis than older patients. Also noteworthy is the apparently paradoxical finding of a higher incidence of neck node recurrences in young patients than in older patients and yet better survival among younger patients. This must be due to the high curability by surgery and radioiodine of neck node recurrences. Mazzaferri *et al.* also demonstrated a significant survival advantage among patients undergoing radical thyroidectomy, radioiodine ablation and receiving fully TSH-suppressive doses of thyroid hormone replacement compared with patients undergoing subtotal thyroidectomy.

In a series of 38 children presenting with differentiated thyroid cancer to the Gustav Roussy institute, Tubiana, Schlumberger and Rougier (1985) found an 88% survival at 15 years. However, it should be noted that there were later two extra deaths from thyroid cancer after more than 20 years of follow-up, demonstrating the long natural history of this disease. Tubiana *et al.* concluded that there was justification for a treatment programme similar to that used in adults. At the Hospital for Sick Children, London, this viewpoint is subscribed to. A policy including radical thyroidectomy, radioiodine ablation and assiduous follow-up has been implemented and is recommended for all patients with extrathyroidal disease.

However, the recommendation for such an aggressive treatment regimen in young patients presenting with papillary cancer limited to the thyroid gland is more contentious and warrants further discussion: if a young patient with an intrathyroidal papillary cancer has the excellent prognosis indicated by Mazzaferri *et al.* (1977), then why is it necessary to perform a radical thyroidectomy and radioiodine ablation – neither of which is without at least potential risk – and then to commit the patient to life-long thyroid hormone tablets? One school of thought argues that the best survival results in the Mazzaferri series were in the radically ablated patients, that papillary thyroid cancer is well recognized to be a multifocal disease, that modern thyroid surgery is relatively safe and lengthy experience has also proved ablative doses of radioiodine to be safe. Added to all this are the late relapses and deaths from thyroid cancer in the long-term follow-up of the less aggressively treated children in the French series (Tubiana, Schlumberger and Rougier, 1985). The recommendations at the Hospital for Sick Children, London, for children with papillary carcinoma limited to the thyroid at presentation can be summarized as follows: after conservative thyroidectomy no radioiodine is administered, but daily TSH-suppressive doses of thyroxine are given to suppress the normal thyroid remnant. Clinical follow-up with careful palpation of the neck may be supplemented with CT scanning of the neck for nodal or thyroid bed recurrence. Thyroglobulin measurements (on thyroid replacement) are made. At the time of any recurrence, normal thyroid gland remnant ablation must usually precede therapeutic radioiodine treatment of disease but the 'pace' of this disease is sufficiently slow for the resultant delay in treatment not to be a practical problem.

Survivors of thyroid carcinoma developing during childhood and treated with radioiodine appear to suffer no discernible infertility or genetic damage (Sarkar *et al.*, 1976).

Bone tumours

Chordoma

Chordomata are rare malignant tumours developing from the vestigial remnants of the notochord. Although they most commonly occur in the sacrococcygeal region, 39% of cases occur in the cranial region – particularly arising from the clivus (Utne and Pugh, 1955). Interestingly, there is a tendency for cranial cases to occur in younger age groups and there is a male predominance.

Macroscopically, chordomata are lobulated, apparently encapsulated growths and of mucoid appearance. Microscopically, large, vacuolated (physaliferous) cells are often arranged in chords in a background of mucus. Mitotic figures are sparse.

Clival chordomata usually present with a lengthy history of headaches or with focal neurological signs. Posterior extension leads to brainstem pressure while anterior extension will lead to obstruction of the nasopharynx or bleeding.

Plain skull X-rays usually show destruction of the clivus perhaps extending rostrally to involve the sella turcica or laterally to involve the sphenoid or petrous temporal bones. Computerized tomographic and magnetic resonance imaging (MR) scanning will delineate the tumour more completely (*Figure 25.10*).

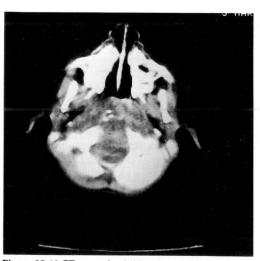

Figure 25.10 CT scan of a child with a clival chordoma. Destruction of bone at a level just rostral to the foramen magnum is clearly demonstrated

While radical surgical resection is the treatment of choice for chordomata, this is rarely possible for intracranial lesions. High dose radiotherapy is certainly palliative and capable of causing tumour regression (Phillips and Newman, 1974).

There does appear to be a radiation dose–effect relationship and, in the series of Phillips and Newman (1974), only those cases receiving high radiation doses remained disease free at 5 years. However, it must be remembered that clivus chordomata abut the central nervous system and meticulous radiation technique is required to achieve the necessary high dosage safely.

The longest survivors of clival primary chordomata are those patients amenable to surgery (including reoperation for recurrences, where possible) as well as high dose radiotherapy (Phillips and Newman, 1974). As metastases occur only in around 10% of cases, local control is of paramount importance.

Ameloblastoma

The ameloblastoma is a rare tumour of the enamel organ stem cells. It usually presents as a cystic mass, much more commonly in the mandible than the maxilla. On section there may be both cystic and solid components. Surgical resection is indicated but incomplete excision frequently leads to local recurrence. Thus wide surgical clearance is optimal treatment with radiotherapy reserved only for failure to achieve microscopically clear margins. Metastatic spread is exceedingly rare.

Osteogenic sarcoma

Osteogenic sarcoma of the craniofacial bones is rare comprising 7% of all cases of the disease. In one series, 45 of 145 cases of craniofacial osteogenic sarcoma occurred in patients below 20 years of age and the mandible followed by the maxilla were the commonest primary sites (Huvos, 1979). Clinically, such lesions present as swellings which may or may not be painful. Radiographically, abnormal areas of osteosclerosis or lysis are present and 'sunray' spiculation, emanating from the cortex (*Figure 25.11*) may be apparent. The

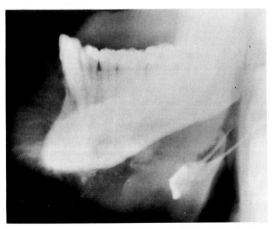

Figure 25.11 Plowman's sign (the radiological bearded chin), pathognomonic of mandibular osteogenic sarcoma

differential diagnosis includes osteomyelitis, reactive osseous lesions (for example ossifying fibroma, fibrous dysplasia) and other bone tumours (*Figure 25.12*). The lungs are the commonest site of metastatic spread and CT lung scanning, as well as ^{99}Tc MDP bone scanning, is important in the staging of all cases.

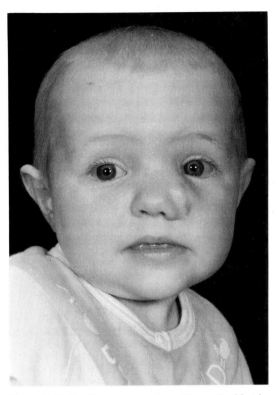

Figure 25.12 Maxillary myxoma in an 18-month-old girl

In general, osteogenic sarcoma arising in craniofacial bones has a very poor prognosis (Caron, Hajdu and Strong, 1971), although for patients with resectable mandibular lesions the 5-year survival approaches 35% (Curtis, Elmore and Sotereanos, 1974) and published series predate the advent of more effective chemotherapy regimens.

Undoubtedly, radical surgical resection is the mainstay of treatment and hemimandibulectomy or radical maxillectomy would be appropriate operations. For unresectable lesions, high dose radiotherapy is delivered with a lesser expectation of local control. Recently, two randomized clinical trials have demonstrated the efficacy of adjuvant chemotherapy in improving the survival in childhood osteogenic sarcoma (Eilber and Eckardt, 1985; Link *et al.*, 1986) and children with this condition would now enter chemotherapy study protocols.

Ewing's sarcoma

This primary bone malignancy is more radio-responsive than osteogenic sarcoma. Although surgical resection is recommended when the bone is 'dispensable', local control rates are high with radical radiotherapy combined with adjuvant chemotherapy (Perez, Tefft and Nesbit, 1981). The most active drugs – vincristine, actinomycin D, doxorubicin (Adriamycin) and cyclophosphamide – are usually given in triple combination ('VAC' or 'VAdriaC') and can be used prior to surgery or irradiation to improve local control. Chemotherapy has also substantially increased the overall survival chance for patients presenting with localized disease (Rosen *et al.*, 1981), but for those with metastases the prognosis, even when there is an initial response, is still poor (10–20% 2-year survival).

Salivary gland tumours

Of all salivary gland tumours 2–4% occur in patients under 16 year of age (Castro *et al.*, 1972; Krolls, Trodahl and Boyers, 1972). Fortunately, the majority of salivary gland swellings in children are not neoplastic and the majority of the true neoplasms are benign.

There were 430 paediatric cases in the series of salivary swellings analysed by the American Armed Forces Institute of Pathology (AFIP), (Krolls, Trodahl and Boyers, 1972). Of these cases 262 were non-neoplastic and, of these, mucocoeles comprised the majority (185 cases). The clinical picture is of a small, smooth, unilocular and painless submucosal swelling. Mucocoeles only occur in the minor salivary glands in the mouth and the lower lip is the most common location. The condition appears to result from an injury to the secretory duct of a minor salivary gland and this tends to occur at the times of teething (both primary and secondary dentition). The other non-neoplastic salivary swellings observed in the AFIP series affected both major and minor salivary glands and were mainly inflammatory lesions – most commonly a non-specific sialadenitis, but also occasionally caused by specific diseases such as tuberculosis or sarcoidosis (Krolls, Trodahl and Boyers, 1972). Mumps is, of course, grossly under-represented in this series from a tertiary referral centre.

In the same analysis, there were 168 true neoplasms of the salivary glands, the majority (124 cases) occurring in the parotid gland (Krolls, Trodahl and Boyers, 1972; Jaques, Krolls and Chambers, 1976). Ninety of 124 parotid neoplasms were benign, including 45 pleomorphic adenomata and 40 vascular tumours.

Pleomorphic adenoma

Pleomorphic adenoma in children, as in adults, occurs predominantly in the parotid gland and more commonly occurs in females, the sex ratio being 2:1 in one series (Malone and Baker, 1984). The tumour occurs in teenagers more commonly than young children. In the experience of Malone and colleagues only 10% of cases occurred in the submandibular gland. As in adults, presentation is usually with a painless and very slowly enlarging mass and conservative surgery is recommended. In the AFIP series of 45 cases, there was local recurrence in six cases and further surgery was needed (Jaques, Krolls and Chambers, 1976). In the Ann Arbor experience, 18 previously untreated patients were treated by conservative parotidectomy with preservation of the facial nerve and all remained disease free at the time of reporting (Malone and Baker, 1984). However, these authors also reported 12 children referred to them with recurrent tumour following surgery elsewhere and only one of these patients had had surgery as major as superficial parotidectomy. Malone and Baker (1984) made the important points that not only is local excision followed by a high rate of local recurrence that is not so easy to cure with nerve sparing 'second-look' surgery, but also that there is a real chance of the later development of true malignancy. In their own series two of the 12 children with local recurrence developed distant metastases as a result of carcinoma ex-pleomorphic adenoma. Local recurrence of pleomorphic adenoma can occur up to 10 or more years after surgery.

The treatment of choice for pleomorphic adenoma of the parotid is parotidectomy with preservation of the facial nerve. Tumours lateral to the facial nerve or in the tail of the parotid gland are managed by a lateral (superficial) parotidectomy, while deep-sited tumours are managed by total parotidectomy with preservation of the nerve. Local excision alone or local excision and radiotherapy are inferior management schemes and wide surgical excision, as outlined above, is the optimal treatment. Similarly, local recurrences are managed by more radical surgical excisions, if necessary with sacrifice of the facial nerve. Radiotherapy is of limited usefulness in this disease and is reserved for the rare instance where radical surgery fails to produce complete microscopic clearance of disease; in this event early postoperative radiotherapy is indicated. An appositional, lateral megavoltage electron source of appropriate energy usually provides the optimal dosimetry and a conventionally fractionated prescription of approximately 50 Gy in 6 weeks is delivered. With this technique later mouth dryness can be avoided, but some late temporomandibular joint dysfunction and mandibular ramus hypoplasia may result.

Benign pleomorphic adenomata of the submandibular gland are managed by complete excision of gland and tumour as a bloc. As with parotid lesions, preoperative incisional biopsy is to be avoided.

Vascular tumours

This group of vascular tumours comprises: juvenile cellular haemangioendotheliomata (in infants), haemangiomata and lymphangiomata. The parotid is the most common site of occurrence and the lesions are much more common in females than males (*Figure 25.13*).

Vascular tumours are usually first noticed at birth or in infancy. They may continue to increase (occasionally rapidly) or fluctuate in size; however, later, many will spontaneously regress. Unless massive, their clinical symptomatology usually relates to their cosmetic effects. The larger ones may require surgery – usually conservative resection of the gland. These vascular tumours, although benign, also respond to low dose radiotherapy but, even with modern treatment

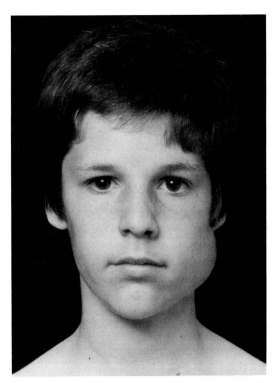

Figure 25.13 Parotid haemangioma presenting in a child with a long history of swelling. (Photograph submitted by courtesy of Professor L. Spitz)

techniques, limiting the dose to adjacent structures, radiotherapy is best avoided unless the tumour is massive (for example preventing feeding, obscuring vision and hence risking amblyopia etc.). Radiotherapy is never indicated for cosmetic reasons and surgery is the preferred definitive treatment unless the operation is likely to be mutilating.

Malignant tumours

Of 168 paediatric true neoplasms of salivary glands assimilated for analysis by the AFIP, 54 were malignant tumours (Krolls, Trodahl and Boyers, 1972). Of these, 35 were malignant epithelial neoplasms and the rest were a heterogeneous collection of primary and secondary tumours with primary sarcomata (rhabdomyosarcomata, fibrosarcomata, anaplastic tumours) most commonly represented. Rhabdomyosarcoma arising in salivary tissue is described elsewhere in this chapter. From the Memorial Hospital series, it seems clear that undiagnosed neoplasms in the submandibular gland are more likely to be malignant than those in the parotid and the albeit rare neoplasms in the sublingual gland were all malignant (Castro *et al.*, 1972).

Mucoepidermoid carcinoma, the commonest carcinoma of salivary tissue, accounted for 20 out of 35 cases in the AFIP series and more frequently occurred in the parotid (14 out of 20 cases; Krolls, Trodahl and Boyers, 1972). The sex incidence is equal and the peak age incidence was 10 years.

In the Memorial Hospital analysis of 288 patients (all ages) with mucoepidermoid carcinoma of the parotid, several points are worth noting (Spiro, Huvos and Strong, 1975). Mucoepidermoid carcinoma is the most common form of carcinoma encountered and usually presents clinically because of swelling; only the minority of patients experienced pain or had facial nerve dysfunction. A histological grading system (grades I–III) was found to be prognostically useful and patients with facial nerve dysfunction or positive cervical nodes were more likely to have high grade (II–III) tumours. Children were more likely to have low grade (I) histology and, although clinically tumours were/are often mobile and discrete, histologically there is no true capsule surrounding the neoplasm. In this large study embracing all age groups, prognosis was clearly better in younger patients (Spiro, Huvos and Strong, 1975).

Treatment recommendations for childhood mucoepidermoid carcinoma are the same as in adult practice and, indeed, these apply to most true salivary neoplasms (with the exception of sarcomata and lymphomata where surgery is usually limited to biopsy). Indeed, for a well-circumscribed salivary gland swelling the histological type will usually not be known prior to definitive surgery, as both incisional or needle aspiration biopsy are to be discouraged. In general, preoperative sialography is of limited usefulness.

The recommended surgical strategy is complete removal of the neoplasm with the minimum normal tissue morbidity. The type of operation depends upon the extent of the lesion. A subtotal parotidectomy with sparing of the facial nerve is optimal if it complies with this strategy but, for more extensive growths, total parotidectomy with nerve sacrifice is necessary. Limited surgery (that is local excision) with postoperative radiotherapy is probably inferior to more radical surgery and is not recommended. Postoperative radiotherapy is indicated only where, following radical surgery, the resection margins are involved or the tumour is of high grade. Under these circumstances, postoperative radiotherapy increases the local control rate (Imperato, Weichselbaum and Ervin, 1984). Mucoepidermoid carcinoma of submandibular or sublingual glands is treated by radical gland resection, also conforming to the above strategy. Block dissection of the cervical lymph nodes is indicated either at presentation or at relapse when these nodes are clinically involved. Overall, the expected survival rate in children with mucoepidermoid carcinoma approximates 95%.

Three very rare malignant epithelial salivary tumours, in order of decreasing incidence and worsening prognosis are: *acinic* cell carcinoma, *adenoid cystic* carcinoma and *adenocarcinoma*. The clinical presentation and treatment recommendations are as described for mucoepidermoid carcinoma.

True neoplasms of the minor salivary glands are extremely rare in childhood but comprise the same tumours with similar relative incidence as discussed above (Budnick, 1982). Treatment principles are also similar.

Craniopharyngioma

Craniopharyngiomata arise from the embryonic remains of the craniopharyngeal duct and are important, albeit uncommon, tumours of childhood. They usually arise in the suprasellar cistern but in rare instances are localized within either the sella or the third ventricle. Histologically, the craniopharyngioma is a well-differentiated tumour with sheets of squamous epithelial cells sometimes in a palisade arrangement. Cyst formation is common.

In very young children, craniopharyngiomata present with hydrocephalus due to raised intracranial pressure. Older children may present with endocrine problems (such as growth failure) or restriction of vision (bitemporal field defects and optic atrophy). Plain X-rays of the skull usually show suprasellar calcification, abnormalities of the sella turcica and/or evidence of raised intracranial pressure. The CT scan is a more sensitive imaging technique.

Although these tumours are benign, they have a propensity to recur locally. Modern neurosurgical techniques which effect total tumour excision give the best survival results, but radical removal is frequently impossible because of the attachment of the tumour or its capsule to central nervous system tissues. Although there has been controversy over its role, there are now compelling data indicating that postoperative radiotherapy decreases the risk of recurrence (Kramer 1974; Sung *et al.*, 1981). This decrease is not dramatic but, considering the substantial mortality from recurring craniopharyngioma over lengthy periods of follow-up and modern radiobiological understanding of the radiation tolerance of the nervous system, postoperative radiotherapy is currently recommended for all patients. For the problematic patient with the recurring cystic craniopharyngioma, β-emitting isotope therapy is now recommended (Strauss *et al.*, 1982; Huk and Mahlstedt, 1983) and effective.

Pituitary tumours

In a series of over 300 pituitary patients presenting to St Bartholomew's Hospital, less than 3% have been in children. Nevertheless, gigantism (due to acidophil adenoma), galactorrhoea or amenorrhoea (due to a prolactin secreting adenoma) or, very rarely indeed, Cushing's disease (due to a basophil adenoma) may occur in childhood. If these patients do not present with the endocrine sequelae of the tumour, then they will present with compressive symptoms from a suprasellar component, and this is how the rare functionless chromophobe adenomata present. The optic pathways are most at risk from the suprasellar growth and bitemporal hemianopia is the classic visual defect.

The investigations vary little from the adult case and high resolution CT and MR imaging techniques are essential. It has been standard teaching for many years that cases with suprasellar extension causing visual field defects require primary surgical decompression. With the greater surgical expertise in the trans-sphenoidal operation, this recommendation has many advocates. With functioning acidophil adenomata and prolactinomata it is current policy at St Bartholomew's Hospital to initiate therapy with the dopamine agonist, bromocriptine, in all patients with less than marked visual field loss, rapidly deteriorating visual fields/acuity or other complicating factors (Besser *et al.*, 1982).

Bromocriptine therapy not only reduces growth hormone or prolactin secretion in the majority of patients but also effects tumour shrinkage, which can be dramatic. However, cure with bromocriptine therapy is very much less certain and rapid, rebound adenoma expansion has been encountered following cessation of bromocriptine (and pregnancy is probably a high risk period for the medically treated prolactinoma patients). Modern megavoltage, external beam radiotherapy is a definitive and effective treatment method which follows initial bromocriptine therapy in both acidophil adenomata (Wass *et al.*, 1985) and prolactinomata (Grossman *et al.*, 1984) at St Bartholomew's Hospital. Any late decline in anterior pituitary function is gradual (compare surgery). Radiotherapy also reduces the recurrence rate following surgery for macroadenomata.

Langerhans cell histiocytosis (histiocytosis X)

Until 1953, eosinophilic granuloma, Hand–Schüller–Christian disease and Letterer–Siwe disease were regarded as separate entities, but in that year Lichtenstein (1953), appreciating that there was much overlap between the three conditions, proposed the unifying rubric 'histiocytosis X'. Although this term is still in common use because it aptly indicates the continuing state of near-ignorance concerning the pathogenesis of the disorder, an international group of clinicians and pathologists has recently recommended that it be replaced by the more informative term 'Langerhans cell histiocytosis'.

Various children's 'tumour' registers suggest an incidence of 30–50 cases per year in the UK, but this is almost certainly an underestimate for the following reasons: (*a*) the disease is almost certainly underdiagnosed, mild skin involvement being mistaken, for instance, for seborrhoeic eczema (*see below*), (*b*) patients present to many 'organ specialists' (otolaryngologists, ophthalmologists, orthopaedic surgeons) and notification is not, of course, obligatory and (*c*) adult cases (probably between 10–20% of the total) are not taken into account. The true incidence is probably well over 100 cases per annum.

Whatever organ is involved, light microscopic appearances of Langerhans cell histiocytosis infiltrates are characterized by the presence of histiocytes and 'small round cells', in differing proportions, together with varying numbers of eosinophils. Langerhans-type histiocytes, which are normally found only in the skin and are

virtually pathognomonic of Langerhans cell histiocytosis when found at other sites, can be identified if electron microscopy reveals characteristic inclusion 'granules' known as Birbeck granules (Nezelof, 1979). Less differentiated cells, however, may contain few or no granules and as normal tissue histiocytes are also found in Langerhans cell histiocytosis lesions, a prolonged search may be necessary. Immunohistochemical studies reveal that Langerhans cells stain positively with the anti-Ia, HTA-1, and OKT6 antibodies. The enzymes α-mannosidase, ATPase and acid phosphatase and the S-100 protein are easily detected by special techniques and can also be helpful in diagnosis. By light microscopy, the appearance of the histiocytes varies but they have no unequivocal features of malignancy and, more important, there appears to be no correlation between the histological grading of a biopsy and the clinical course of the disease.

The cause of Langerhans cell histiocytosis is unknown, but clinical and histopathological features virtually rule out a malignant process, and no infective agent has ever been identified. Some patients have evidence of partial thymic atrophy and a primary immunodeficiency state has been postulated. Though standard immunological tests (serum immunoglobulin levels, phytohaemagglutinin response) are invariably normal, a relative deficiency of suppressor (OKT8 positive) lymphocytes has been demonstrated in the blood of patients with multisystem disease. Despite evidence that suppressor cell numbers increased after incubation *in vitro* of blood with a crude thymic hormone preparation ('thymosin'), neither 'thymosin' nor synthetic thymic hormone preparations have been effective in clinical trials (Broadbent and Pritchard, 1985). Currently, research attention is turning to the Langerhans cells themselves. It seems likely that the underlying abnormality is one of faulty intercellular communication between lymphoid and Langerhans cells, perhaps because of abnormalities in production of lymphokines or other growth factors.

Sites of disease presentation vary enormously and, as a result, symptoms can vary. *Table 25.5* lists the presenting symptoms of 30 children presenting to one large children's hospital over a 3-year period. Clinical features in adults are similar. The disease can present in the newborn period and in the elderly, but the peak age is around 2–4 years. Boys seem to be affected rather more frequently than girls (males:females, 1.5–2:1) but with the same degree of severity. In 75% of patients, many organs are obviously affected at presentation (multisystem disease); in the remainder only one organ or organ system is involved (single-system disease) though detailed investigation may reveal occult multisystem disease.

Table 25.5 Presenting symptoms of 30 children with Langerhans cell histiocytosis

Symptom	Number of children*
Skin rash	15
Recurrent aural discharge	8
Bone pain	5
Scalp lump(s)	5
Proptosis	4
Failure to thrive	3
Breathlessness	3
Lymphadenopathy	2
Hepatosplenomegaly	1
Spinal cord compression	1

Numbers add up to more than 30 as some children had multiple symptoms.

As *Table 25.5* indicates, recurrent or persistent aural discharge is the commonest manifestation of Langerhans cell histiocytosis in the head and neck region. When this is the consequence of otitis externa, there is usually an easily detectable rash, its distribution (scalp, eyelids and postauricular skin) (*Figure 25.14*) being similar to that of seborrhoeic eczema. In other instances there is middle ear disease – frequently in association with mastoid involvement. In either case, secondary infection is frequent and the process is very often chronic.

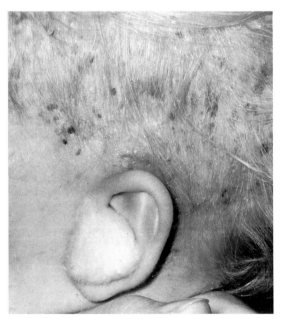

Figure 25.14 Langerhans cell histiocytosis – typical 'seborrhoeic' eczematous rash behind ear. This 2-year-old girl also had chronic aural discharge

Early oral involvement manifests as granularity or thickening of the gingival mucosa (Betts and McNeish, 1972). More extensive involvement may be painful and, exceptionally, a palatal fistula (*Figure 25.15*) may develop. Dental involvement may occur in the absence of lytic lesions in the mandible or maxilla and is then presumably the consequence of direct invasion from involved oral mucosa. In severe cases, erosion of dental alveoli

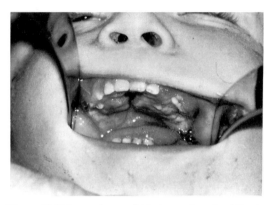

Figure 25.15 Langerhans cell histiocytosis: palatal fistula – a rare complication of oral involvement

and gum retraction may cause premature eruption or loosening of teeth: in these patients, loss of the dental lamina dura is an important radiological sign.

Pulmonary involvement (interstitial infiltrates ± pneumothorax) is relatively common, though often subclinical. Upper airway obstruction, by contrast, is rare and although tracheal obstruction has been described, (Brickman, Nogrady and Wiglesworth, 1973) involvement of Waldeyer's ring has not. Lymph node infiltration, usually painless, is more frequently localized than generalized and cervical nodes are affected more frequently than those at other sites. Occasionally enlargement may be so massive as to cause obstructive symptoms. On occasion, chronic cutaneous fistulae can develop (*Figure 25.16*), but cultures are negative.

Other head and neck manifestations include proptosis, the consequence of retro-orbital deposits (Moore, Pritchard and Taylor, 1985), and skull involvement. Defects in the calvarium can often be palpated and there is sometimes an overlying soft tissue swelling. Radiologically, skull lesions, in common with those in other flat bones, appear to be 'punched out' (*Figure 25.17*). Frequently lesions of varying 'ages' are seen: those in the healing phase have a sclerotic margin. In long bones, lesions may provoke an intense periosteal reaction, sometimes mimicking malignancy.

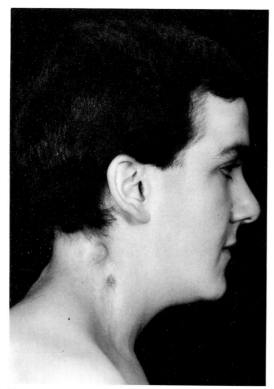

Figure 25.16 Langerhans cell histiocytosis: chronic dermal sinuses the result of chronic underlying lymph node involvement

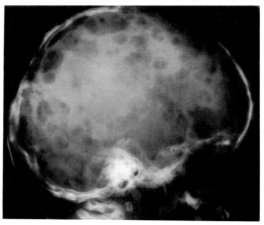

Figure 25.17 Lateral skull X-ray of a child with extensive skull involvement by Langerhans cell histiocytosis

Diabetes insipidus, due to antidiuretic hormone deficiency, occurs in 30–40% of cases (Greenberger *et al.*, 1981): in one-half of these, the complication is manifest at diagnosis, while in the others it develops during the course of the illness. Because lytic bone defects in the region of the pituitary fossa are very uncommon, the pathogenesis was obscure but it is now known, from post-mortem studies, that there are identifiable Langerhans cell histiocytosis deposits in the posterior lobe of the pituitary gland or the infundibulum in most, if not all, of these cases. The larger deposits can be demonstrated by CT scanning (with enhancement); magnetic resonance imaging may be more sensitive. Other manifestations of Langerhans cell histiocytosis include anaemia and thrombocytopenia (due to bone marrow involvement), hepatosplenomegaly, malabsorption, and short stature (due to growth hormone deficiency). By contrast muscles (including the heart), gonads, kidneys and endocrine glands are hardly ever affected.

When several organ systems are involved, the diagnosis is relatively straightforward, but when single system disease dominates the picture or when presentation is atypical, there is often a delay. The diagnosis should certainly be considered in any child with a history of chronic aural discharge, especially if there is no history of otitis media. Distinction from other histiocytic (Groopman and Golde, 1981) disorders and from other malignancies is usually straightforward on clinical and histopathological grounds.

Initial investigation should include full blood count, liver function tests with serum albumin, prothrombin time and partial thromboplastin time, chest radiographs, skeletal survey, bone marrow aspirate and trephine, lung function tests, early morning urine osmolality and water deprivation tests.

A number of elaborate staging systems have been devised. Although such objective criteria may facilitate comparison of treatment results between centres, it is not clear that assignation of a stage is helpful in determining management of a particular patient, or in assessing prognosis. In practice, organ failure seems to be a more important prognostic factor than organ involvement; bone marrow failure, manifested by pancytopenia and liver failure, are particularly ominous.

Because the nature of the disorder is obscure there can be no scientifically rational approach to treatment, but clinical observation and clinical trials have led to development of moderately effective measures. Now that the disease is no longer regarded as a malignancy, the therapeutic strategy is a good deal more conservative than in the past; 'aggressive' chemotherapy, because of its immediate and delayed toxicity, is contraindicated (Broadbent and Pritchard, 1985).

When Langerhans cell histiocytosis is apparently limited to one system (single system disease), it is the skeleton that is most often involved. Spontaneous resolution often occurs and a period of observation is appropriate unless the function of a vital structure (for example optic nerve or spinal cord) is threatened or if there is pain that cannot be controlled by simple analgesics. Intralesional corticosteroid injections (50–100 mg hydrocortisone (Solu-Cortef)), repeated two or three times at 2–3 weekly intervals if necessary, are often effective when active intervention is needed. Because aural disease is usually adjacent to an open cavity it is difficult, in practice, to ensure that the steroid solution remains within the lesion but an attempt is worthwhile. Because of the risk of induction of 'second tumours', radiation therapy should be used only when a site of disease is inaccessible to the needle or when vital organs (for example optic nerve or spinal cord) are threatened, and the dose should not exceed 10 Gy (Smith *et al.*, 1973).

Spontaneous resolution can occur and an initial period of observation may be appropriate (Broadbent *et al.*, 1984). Indications for systemic therapy are (*a*) systemic symptoms (fever, failure to thrive), (*b*) discomfort, especially from multiple sources, (*c*) organ 'failure'. Agents active against cancer are generally used and responses are often impressive. Published data suggest that steroids alone are as effective as 'cytotoxic' drugs, even when these are used in combination (Broadbent and Pritchard, 1985). By contrast there is strong evidence that 'aggressive' combination drug regimens are associated with a higher complication rate. Thus a relatively conservative approach is indicated. In most patients, there is response to daily prednisolone 2 mg/kg; after an arbitrary 4 weeks' induction therapy, and depending on the quality of the response, the regimen can be modified with the intent of controlling disease by the smallest possible dose of steroids, and preferably none at all. If maintenance treatment is needed, alternate day administration is preferable so that there is less-than-complete suppression of adrenal function. In children, growth failure and immunosuppression are the most worrying features of chronic steroid therapy and diabetes mellitus, osteoporosis and hypertension are uncommon.

When response to corticosteroids is unsatisfactory, a vinca alkaloid (vincristine or vinblastine) or an epipodophyllotoxin (VP16) can be added. Claims that methotrexate, cyclophosphamide and 6-mercaptopurine are active agents in steroid-resistant Langerhans cell histiocytosis have not yet been substantiated, and cyclophosphamide may be leukaemogenic.

Other measures may be helpful where specific organ systems are involved. Steroid eardrops (Predsol) can reduce the volume of discharge from otitis externa and antibiotics are indicated when secondary infection of the middle or external ear is suspected or proven. If gingival involvement is severe, surgical curettage can be helpful and may also reduce the incidence of later dental complications. The symptoms of diabetes insipidus are completely reversed by administration of DDAVP (a synthetic form of antidiuretic hormone) intranasally 5 µg twice or three times daily. Potassium permanganate soaks are helpful topically in the management of an ulcerated skin rash. Ung. coco oil, followed by washing with a keratolytic shampoo, can be helpful in the removal of crusted lesions from the scalp; topical steroid lotion is then applied to inflamed areas. Topical nitrogen mustard can be very effective where other methods have failed to control skin rash, but expert dermatological advice is needed. Where the lungs are involved, and the patient is immunosuppressed, regular co-trimoxazole (Septrin) should be considered as prophylaxis against *Pneumocystis carinii*.

The prognosis for patients with single-system disease is uniformly good. Progression to multisystem involvement is rare and mortality is close to zero. Some 10–20% of patients develop chronic problems but there is a tendency for disease to 'burn itself out' over 1–5 years. Patients with multisystem Langerhans cell histiocytosis fare less well, but the prognosis is better than some publications suggest. In a few patients spontaneous regression occurs. Almost all those receiving systemic therapy show some response. In most patients symptomatic and objective improvement is marked, sometimes with reversal of organ failure. Infections, including those with opportunistic organisms, are common treatment-related complications, especially with the more aggressive chemotherapy regimens.

Overall, 20–30% of patients enter sustained complete remission and about 10%, especially those who present with or develop organ failure, die. The remaining 60–70% enter a chronic disease phase, with involvement of new organ systems in some cases. During this phase, problems include chronic discharging ears, deafness (in 15–20% of survivors), lymph node 'suppuration' (Smith and Evans, 1984), recurrent pneumothorax and dental and orthopaedic problems (Sims, 1977; Komp, 1981). Diabetes insipidus is usually permanent and growth hormone deficiency can occur.

Fibromatosis

The fibromatoses are a heterogeneous collection of clinical conditions, with similar histopathological appearances, that are difficult to distinguish from fibrosarcoma (Stout and Lattes, 1967). Tumours can appear at any age, from birth onwards, and at a number of sites, including the head and neck.

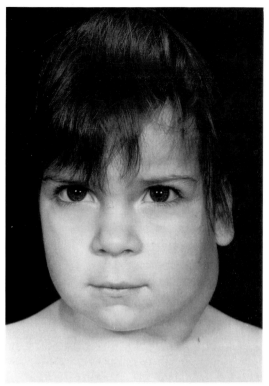

Figure 25.18 Cervical fibromatosis in a 4-year-old boy. There was slow spontaneous resolution over 2 years

Patients with Gardner's syndrome (intestinal polyposis, sebaceous cysts and osteomata) are predisposed to fibromatosis, although the pathogenic link is not understood. Tumours develop slowly, and are usually firm and lobulated and can become very large. By reason of location, head and neck fibromatosis is often unresectable; anecdotal responses to 'VAC'-type chemotherapy and to irradiation have been reported (Stein, 1977) and seen by the authors (*Figure 25.18*) and are worth considering in these cases. Sometimes, despite all efforts progression is remorseless and the condition proves fatal.

Unwanted effects of chemotherapy and radiotherapy

Unwanted effects of chemotherapy can be grouped into those that are non-specific and the inevitable result of the cytotoxic action of individual drugs and those that are specific to one agent or group of agents. Bone marrow and immune suppression are almost invariable, but the duration and severity depends upon the type of regimen that is used. In general, intermittent chemotherapy is less immunosuppressive than continuous treatment, while there is a direct relationship between dose and the degree of marrow damage. Thus high-dose treatments are associated with prolonged periods of myelo- and immunosuppression. Several drugs cause mucosal damage, which is aggravated because epithelial cell repopulation is prevented. Thus oropharyngeal ulceration is a common side-effect of treatment with methotrexate, actinomycin D and doxorubicin. Mucosal damage opens the way to invasion by bacterial, fungal, and viral pathogens so careful oral toilet is necessary in all such patients. If a severely neutropenic ($<0.5 \times 10^9$/l) child develops fever, an urgent clinical search should be made for a focus of infection – including careful examination of ears, nose and throat – and cultures taken from any suspicious site as well as from nose, throat, urine, stool, vagina and blood. Broad-spectrum antibiotics should be started without delay and continued for at least 5 days even if the patient becomes afebrile and cultures are negative. Frequent (at least daily) clinical re-examination is necessary as signs may develop and progress alarmingly fast. It is critically important to be aware that, in the absence of circulating neutrophils, pus forms slowly or not at all and that signs of inflammation may be minimal. White blood cell transfusions are only indicated when the neutrophil count shows no signs of recovery and certain organisms, especially *Pseudomonas* spp., have been isolated.

There are relatively few otolaryngology-related drug-specific side-effects. The 'glove-stocking' peripheral neuropathy of vincristine is usually less severe in children than in adults but mononeuropathy can sometimes occur. Facial (seventh nerve), phrenic and recurrent laryngeal palsies have all been described and recovery is usually spontaneous, albeit over several weeks or months. Jaw pain, sometimes referred to the ear, is another relatively common and unpredictable side-effect of vinca alkaloids, especially vincristine: its onset is usually within 24 hours of administration of the drug and it lasts no longer than 48 hours. Older patients are more commonly affected than infants. More persistent pain should arouse suspicion of herpes zoster infection. Cisplatin is a relatively new but important addition to the chemotherapeutic arsenal and now has an established role in the management of neuroblastoma, malignant germ cell and liver tumours and osteogenic sarcoma. However, its usefulness is limited by dose-dependent nephrotoxicity and ototoxicity. Hearing loss (McHaney *et al.*, 1983) is unusual at an accumulative dose less than 400 mg/m^2 but above this dose a degree of deafness is almost invariable and appears irreversible. Hearing loss is initially in the high-tone range but extends to lower frequencies as the accumulative dose of the drug rises. Patients receiving cisplatin should not be prescribed gentamicin or other ototoxic antibiotics unless absolutely necessary. High-tone hearing aids are often invaluable to children with hearing loss. Newer cisplatin analogues (for example carboplatin) cause less inner ear and kidney damage but their efficacy in the treatment of childhood cancers is, as yet, uncertain.

Both radiotherapy and cytotoxic chemicals have mutagenic capability and an increased incidence of second cancers has been documented in patients treated with each of these anticancer therapies. Rarely should this lead to a reduction in the chance of cure in a child with a malignancy, but the indications for any such treatment must always be carefully reviewed. In addition, radiotherapy will cause dose-dependent retardation in the growth of irradiated bone (*see Figure 25.3*) and viscera, especially in young children and consideration of the late sequelae must always be made before a radical treatment programme is initiated.

Conclusion

The striking improvement in prognosis for children with cancer has been one of the most exciting advances in paediatrics during the last 15–20 years. Improvements in chemotherapy have been central to this progress but side-effects are of major and continuing concern. Thus, attempts are underway to phase out alkylating agents, procarbazine and radiation therapy – all of which are tumorigenic and cause sterility – with agents that lack these side-effects. Exciting, though preliminary, efforts are underway to 'target' tumour deposits selectively with ^{131}I and other tumoricidal radioisotopes and drugs, using monoclonal antibodies and other vectors. The longer the duration of chemotherapy, the greater the risk of infective complications resulting from bone marrow and immunological suppression. Therefore, there is a trend towards 'short, sharp' courses of chemotherapy rather than protracted maintenance programmes. In summary, the current objective of most paediatric oncology teams is to provide 'cure at least cost' rather than 'cure at any cost'.

References

AHMAD, K. and FAYOS, J. V. (1980) Role of radiation therapy in the treatment of olfactory neuroblastoma. *International Journal of Radiation, Oncology, Biology and Physics*, **6**, 349–352

ANDERSON, J. R., WILSON, J. F., JENKINS, O. T. et al. (1983) Childhood non-Hodgkin's lymphoma. The results of a randomized therapeutic trial comparing a 4-drug regimen (COMP) with a 10-drug regimen (LSA$_2$L$_2$). *New England Journal of Medicine*, **308**, 559–565

AUGUST, C. S., SEROTA, F. T., KOCK, P. A., BURKEY, E., SCHLESINGER, H., ELKINS, W. L. et al. (1984) Treatment of advanced neuroblastoma with supralethal chemotherapy radiation and allogeneic or autologous marrow reconstitution. *Journal of Clinical Oncology*, **2**, 609–616

BAILEY, B. J. and BARTON, S. (1975) Olfactory neuroblastoma: management and prognosis. *Archives of Otolaryngology*, **101**, 1–5

BESSER, G. M., WASS, J. A. H., GROSSMAN, A., PLOWMAN, P. N., SCHWANDER, J. and LYTRAS, N. (1982) The medical management of pituitary tumours. In *Endocrinology*. International Congress Series No. 598. Proceedings of the 7th Asia and Oceania Congress of Endocrinology, Tokyo, edited by K. Shizume, H. Imura and N. Shizumu, pp. 62–72. Amsterdam: Excerpta Medica

BETTS, P. R. and McNEISH, A. S. (1972) Oral manifestations of Letterer-Siwe disease. *Archives of Disease in Childhood*, **47**, 463–464

BLACK, E. G., CASSONI, A., GIMLETTE, T. M. D., HARMER, C. L., MAISEY, M. N., OATES, G. D. et al. (1981) Serum thyroglobulin in thyroid cancer. *The Lancet*, **2**, 443–445

BRICKMAN, H. F., NOGRADY, M. B. and WIGLESWORTH, F. W. (1973) Scrofula and tracheal obstruction. *American Journal of Respiratory Disease*, **108**, 1208–1211

BROADBENT, V. and PRITCHARD, J. (1985) Histiocytosis X current controversies. *Archives of Disease in Childhood*, **60**, 605–607

BROADBENT, V., PRITCHARD, J., DAVIES, E. G., LEVINSKY, R. J., HEAF, D., ATHERTON, D. J. et al. (1984) Spontaneous remission of multi-system histiocytosis X. *The Lancet*, **1**, 253–254

BUDNICK, S. D. (1982) Minor salivary gland tumours in children. *Journal of Dentistry for Children*, **49**, 44–47

CARON, A. S., HAJDU, S. I. and STRONG, E. W. (1971) Osteogenic sarcoma of the facial and cranial bones. A review of 43 cases. *American Journal of Surgery*, **122**, 719–725

CASTRO, E. B., HUROS, A. G., STRONG, E. W. and FOOTE, F. W. (1972) Tumours of the major salivary glands in children. *Cancer*, **29**, 312–317

CURTIS, M. L., ELMORE, J. S. and SOTEREANOS, C. (1974) Osteosarcoma of the jaws: report of case and review of the literature. *Journal of Oral Surgery*, **32**, 125–130

EILBER, F. R. and ECKARDT, J. (1985) Adjuvant therapy for osteosarcoma: a randomized prospective trial. *Proceedings of American Society of Clinical Oncology*, **4**, 144, C-561

EVANS, A. E., CHATTEN, J. and D'ANGIO, G. (1980) A review of 17 IVs neuroblastoma patients at the Children's Hospital of Philadelphia. *Cancer*, **45**, 833–839

EVANS, A. E., D'ANGIO, G. and RANDOLPH, J. (1971) A proposed staging for children with neuroblastoma. *Cancer*, **27**, 374–378

FINKLESTEIN, J. Z., KLEMPERER, M. R. and EVANS, A. E. (1979) Multiagent chemotherapy for children with metastatic neuroblastoma: a report from the Children's Cancer Study Group. *Medica and Pediatric Oncology*, **6**, 179–188

FOUCAR, E., ROSAI, J. and DORFMAN, R. F. (1984) Sinus histiocytosis with massive lymphadenopathy. *Cancer*, **54**, 1834–1840

GRANT, S., LUTTRELL, B., REEVE, T., WISEMAN, J., WILMSHURST, E., STIEL, J. et al. (1984) Thyroglobulin may be undetectable in the serum of patients with metastatic disease secondary to differentiated thyroid carcinoma. *Cancer*, **54**, 1625–1628

GREENBERGER, J. S., CROCKER, A. C., VAWTER, G., JAFFE, N. and CASSADY, J. R. (1981) Results of treatment of 127 patients with systemic histiocytosis (Letterer–Siwe syndrome, Schüller–Christian syndrome and multifocal eosinophilic granuloma). *Medicine*, **60**, 311–338

GREENE, M. H., FRAUMENI, J. F. and HOOVER, R. (1971) Nasopharyngeal cancer among young people in the United States: racial variations in cell type. *Journal of National Cancer Institute*, **58**, 1267–1270

GROOPMAN, J. E. and GOLDE, D. W. (1981) The histiocytic disorders – pathophysiologic analysis. *Annals of Internal Medicine*, **94**, 95–107

GROSFELD, J. L., WEBER, T. R., WEETMAN, R. M. and BAEHNER, R. L. (1977) Rhabdomyosarcoma in childhood: analysis of survival in 98 cases. *Journal of Pediatric Surgery*, **18**, 141–146

GROSSMAN, A., COHEN, B. L., CHARLESWORTH, M., PLOWMAN, P. N., REES, L. H., WASS, J. A. H. *et al.* (1984) Treatment of prolactinomas with megavoltage radiotherapy. *British Medical Journal*, **288**, 1105–1109

HO, J. H. C. (1978) An epidemiologic and clinical study of nasopharyngeal carcinoma. *International Journal of Radiation Oncology, Biology and Physics*, **4**, 183–198

HUK, W. J. and MAHLSTEDT, J. (1983) Intracystic radiotherapy (^{90}Y) of craniopharyngiomas: CT-guided stereotaxic implantation of indwelling drainage system. *American Journal of Neuroradiology*, **4**, 803–806

HUVOS, A. G. (1979) *Bone tumours. Diagnosis, Treatment and Prognosis*. Philadelphia: Saunders

IMPERATO, J. P., WEICHSELBAUM, R. R. and ERVIN, T. J. (1984) The role of post-operative radiation therapy in the treatment of malignant tumours of the parotid gland. *Journal of Surgical Oncology*, **27**, 163–167

JAQUES, D. A., KROLLS, S. O. and CHAMBERS, R. G. (1976) Parotid tumours in children. *American Journal of Surgery*, **132**, 469–471

JENKIN, R. D. T., ANDERSON, J. R., JEREB, B., THOMPSON, J. C., PYESMANY, A., WARA, W. M. *et al.* (1981) Nasopharyngeal carcinoma – a retrospective review of patients less than thirty years of age. *Cancer*, **47**, 360–366

KADISCH, S., GOODMAN, M. and WANG, C. C. (1976) Olfactory neuroblastoma: a clinical analysis of 17 cases. *Cancer*, **35**, 1571–1576

KEMSHEAD, J. T. and PRITCHARD, J. (1984) Neuroblastoma: Recent developments and current challenges. *Cancer Surveys*, **3**, 691–708

KINGSTON, J. E., McELWAIN, T. J. and MALPAS, J. S. (1983) Childhood rhabdomyosarcoma: experience of the Children's Solid Tumour Group. *British Journal of Cancer*, **48**, 195–207

KOMP, D. M. (1981) Long-term sequelae of histiocytosis X. *American Journal of Pediatric Hematology and Oncology*, **3**, 165–168

KRAMER, S. (1974) Radiation therapy in the management of craniopharyngiomas. In *Modern Radiotherapy and Oncology. Central Nervous System Tumours*, edited by T. J. Deeley, pp. 204–223. London: Butterworths

KROLLS, S. O., TRODAHL, J. N. and BOYERS, R. C. (1972) Salivary gland lesions in children. *Cancer*, **30**, 459–469

LEDERMAN, M. (1961) *Cancer of the Nasopharynx: Its Natural History and Treatment*. Springfield, Illinois: C. C. Thomas

LEDERMAN, M. and MOULD, R. F. (1968) Radiation treatment of cancer of the pharynx: with special

reference to telecobalt therapy. *British Journal of Radiology*, **41**, 251–274

LEWIS, J. S., HUTTER, R. V. P., TOLLEFSEN, H. R. and FOOTE, F. W. JR. (1965) Nasal tumours of olfactory origin. *Archives of Otolaryngology*, **81**, 169–173

LICHTENSTEIN, L. (1953) Integration of eosinophilic granuloma of bone, Letterer–Siwe disease and Schüller–Christian disease as related in manifestations of a single nosologic entity. *Archives of Pathology*, **56**, 84–102

LINK, M., GOORIN, A., MISER, A., GREEN, A. A., PRATT, C. B., BELASCO, J. B. *et al.* (1986) The effect of adjuvant chemotherapy on relapse-free survival in patients with osteosarcoma of the extremity. *New England Journal of Medicine*, **314**, 1600–1606

McHANEY, V. A., THIBADOUX, M. A., HAYES, F. A. and GREEN, A. A. (1983) Hearing loss in children receiving cisplatin chemotherapy. *Journal of Pediatrics*, **102**, 314–316

MALONE, B. and BAKER, S. R. (1984) Benign pleomorphic adenomas in children. *Annals of Otology, Rhinology and Laryngology*, **93**, 210–214

MAZZAFERRI, E. L., YOUNG, R. L., OERTEL, J. E., KEMMERER, W. T. and PAGE, C. P. (1977) Papillary thyroid carcinoma: the impact of therapy in 576 patients. *Medicine (Baltimore)*, **56**, 171–196

MOORE, A. T., PRITCHARD, J. and TAYLOR, D. S. I. (1985) Histiocytosis X, an ophthalmological review. *British Journal of Ophthalmology*, **69**, 7–14

MORALES, P., BOSCH, A., SALAVERRY, S., CORREA, J. N. and MARTINEZ, I. (1984) Cancer of the nasopharynx in young patients. *Journal of Surgical Oncology*, **27**, 181–185

MOTT, M. G., EDEN, O. B. and PALMER, M. K. (1984) Adjuvant low dose radiation in childhood non-Hodgkin's lymphoma. (Report from the UKCCSG). *British Journal of Cancer*, **50**, 463–469

MURPHY, S. B. (1978) Childhood non-Hodgkin's lymphoma. *New England Journal of Medicine*, **299**, 1446–1448

MURPHY, S. B. and HUSTU, H. O. (1980) A randomized trial of combined modality therapy of childhood non-Hodgkin's lymphoma. *Cancer*, **45**, 630–637

MURPHY, S. B., HUSTU, H. O., RIVERA, G. and BERARD, C. W. (1983) End results of treating children with localized non-Hodgkin's lymphomas with a combined modality approach of lessened intensity. *Journal of Clinical Oncology*, **50**, 326–330

NAEGELE, R. F., CHAMPION, J., MURPHY, S., HENLE, G. and HENLE, W. (1982) Nasopharyngeal carcinoma in American children Epstein–Barr virus specific antibody titers and prognosis. *International Journal of Cancer*, **29**, 209–212

NEZELOF, C. (1979) Histiocytosis X: a histological and histogenetic study. *Paediatric Pathology*, 153–173

NINANE, J., PRITCHARD, J., MORRIS-JONES, P., MANN, J. R. and MALPAS, J. S. (1982) Stage II neuroblastoma: adverse prognostic significance of lymph node involvement. *Archives of Disease in Childhood*, **57**, 438–442

OBERMAN, H. A. and RICE, D. H. (1976) Olfactory neuroblastoma: a clinicopathologic study. *Cancer*, **38**, 2494–2502

PEREZ, C. A., TEFFT, M. and NESBIT, M. (1981) The role of radiation therapy in the management of non-metastatic Ewing's sarcoma of bone. Report of the Intergroup Ewing's Sarcoma Study. *International Journal of Radiation Oncology, Biology and Physics*, **7**, 141–149

PETROVICH, Z., COX, J. D., MIDDLETON, R., OHANIAN, M., PAIG, C. and JEPSON, J. (1985) Advanced carcinoma of the nasopharynx. Pattern of failure in 256 patients. *Radiotherapy and Oncology*, **4**, 15–20

PHILIP, T., BIRON, P., MARANINCHI, D., GASTAUT, J. A., HERVÉ, P. *et al.* (1984) Role of massive chemotherapy and autologous bone-marrow transplantation in non-Hodgkin's malignant lymphoma. *The Lancet*, **1**, 391

PHILLIPS, T. L. and NEWMAN, H. (1974) Chordomas. In *Modern Radiotherapy and Oncology. Central Nervous System Tumours*, edited by T. J. Deeley, pp. 184–203. London: Butterworths

PLOWMAN, P. N. (1986) Endocrine cancer. In *Radiotherapy in Clinical Practice*, edited by H. Hope-Stone, chap. 13, pp. 300–315. London: Butterworths

POCHIN, E. E. (1967) Prospects for the treatment of thyroid carcinoma with radio-iodine. *Clinical Radiology*, **18**, 113–135

PRITCHARD, J., McELWAIN, T. J. and GRAHAM-POLE, J. (1982) High-dose melphalan with autologous bone marrow for treatment of advanced neuroblastoma. *British Journal of Cancer*, **45**, 86–98

ROBINSON, B., KINGSTON, J. K., COSTA, R. N., MALPAS, J. S., BARRETT, A. and McELWAIN, T. J. (1984) Chemotherapy and irradiation in childhood Hodgkin's disease. *Archives of Disease in Childhood*, **59**, 1162–1167

ROSAI, J. and DORFMAN, R. F. (1972) Sinus histiocytosis with massive lymphadenopathy: a pseudolymphomatous benign disorder. *Cancer*, **30**, 1174–1188

ROSEN, G., CAPARROS, B., NIRENBERG, A., MARCOVE, R. C., HUVOS, A. G., KOSLOFF, C. *et al.* (1981) Ewing's sarcoma – ten year experience with adjuvant chemotherapy. *Cancer*, **47**, 2204–2213

SARKAR, S. D., BEIERWALTES, W. H., GILL, S. P. and COWLEY, P. J. (1976) Subsequent fertility and birth histories of children and adolescents treated with ^{131}I for thyroid cancer. *Journal of Nuclear Medicine*, **17**, 460–464

SCHUAB, M., ELLISON, J., BUSCH, M., ROSENAU, W., VARMUS, H. E. and BISHOP, J. H. (1984) Enhanced expression of the human gene N-myc consequent to amplification of DNA may contribute to malignant progression of neuroblastoma. *Proceedings of the National Academy of Sciences of the USA*, **15**, 4940–4944

SHAFFORD, E. A., ROGERS, D. W. and PRITCHARD, J. (1984) Improved response rate using a multiagent regime (OPEC) including sequential cisplatinum and VM-26. *Journal of Clinical Oncology*, **2**, 742–747

SIMS, D. G. (1977) Histiocytosis X: follow up of 43 cases. *Archives of Disease in Childhood*, **52**, 433–440

SMITH, D. G., NESBIT, M. E. JR., D'ANGIO, G. J. and LEVITT, S. H. (1973) Histiocytosis X: role of radiation therapy in management with special reference to dose levels employed. *Radiology*, **106**, 419–422

SMITH, R. J. H. and EVANS, J. N. G. (1984) Head and neck manifestations of histiocytosis X. *The Laryngoscope*, **94**, 395–399

SPIRO, R. H., HUVOS, A. G. and STRONG, E. W. (1975) Cancer of the parotid gland. A clinicopathologic study of 288 primary cases. *American Journal of Surgery*, **130**, 452–459

STEIN, R. (1977) Chemotherapeutic response in fibromatosis of the neck. *Journal of Pediatrics*, **90**, 482–483

STOUT, A. P. and LATTES, R. (1967) Tumours of the soft tissues. *Atlas of Tumour Pathology*, 2nd series. Armed Forces Institute of Pathology. Fascicle, **1**, 17–30

STRAUSS, L., STURM, V., GEORGI, P., SCHLEGEL, W., OSTERTAG, H., CLORIUS, J. H. *et al.* (1982) Radioisotope therapy of cystic craniopharyngiomas. *International Journal of Radiation Oncology, Biology and Physics*, **8**, 1581–1585

SULLIVAN, M. P., FULLER, L. M., CHEN, T. *et al.* (1982) Intergroup Hodgkin's disease in children study of stages I and II. A preliminary report. *Cancer Treatment Reports*, **66**, 937–947

SUNG, D. O., CHANG, C. H., HARISIADIS, L. and CARMEL, P. W. (1981) Treatment results of craniopharyngiomas. *Cancer*, **47**, 847–852

SUTOW, W. W., SULLIVAN, M. P., REID, H. I. and TAYLOR, H. G. (1970) Prognosis in childhood rhabdomyosarcoma. *Cancer*, **25**, 1384–1390

TAN, C., JEREB, B., CHAN, K. W., LESSER, M., MANDORA, A. and EXELBY, P. (1983) Hodgkin's disease in children. *Cancer*, **51**, 1720–1725

TEFFT, M., FERNANDEZ, C., DONALDSON, M., NEWTON, W. and MOON, T. E. (1978) Incidence of meningeal involvement by rhabdomyosarcoma of the head and neck in children. *Cancer*, **42**, 253–258

TRAGGIS, D., JAFFE, N., VAWTER, G. *et al.* (1975) Non-Hodgkin's lymphoma of the head and neck in childhood. *Journal of Pediatrics*, **87**, 933–936

TUBIANA, M., SCHLUMBERGER, M. and ROUGIER, P. (1985) Long-term results and prognostic factors in patients with differentiated thyroid carcinoma. *Cancer*, **55**, 794–804

UTNE, J. R. and PUGH, D. G. (1955) The roentgenologic aspects of chordoma. *American Journal of Roentgenology*, **74**, 595–602

WADE, P. M., SMITH, R. E. and JOHNS, M. E. (1984) Response of esthesioneuroblastoma to chemotherapy: report of 5 cases and review of the literature. *Cancer*, **53**, 1036–1041

WASS, J. A. H., PLOWMAN, P. N., JONES, A. W. and BESSER, G. M. (1985) The effects of radiotherapy in acromegaly – results of long term follow-up in 80 patients. *Proceedings of the 2nd European Neuroendocrine Association Meeting*, Milan. Abstract

WOOLNER, L. B., BEAHRS, O. H., BLACK, B. M., McCONAHEY, W. M. and KEATING, F. R. (1961) Classification and prognosis of thyroid carcinoma. *American Journal of Surgery*, **102**, 354–388

ZELTZER, P. M., MARANGOS, P. J., PARMA, A. M., SATTRER, H., DALTON, A., HAMMOND, D. *et al.* (1983) Raised neurone-specific enolase in serum of children with metastatic neuroblastoma. *The Lancet*, **2**, 361–363

26

Congenital disorders of the larynx, trachea and bronchi

Michael J. Cinnamond

The true incidence of congenital deformities of the upper airway is not known for certain, but van den Broek and Brinkman (1979) quoted an incidence for congenital laryngeal defects of between 1:10 000 and 1:50 000 births. Of 219 children with stridor who underwent endoscopic examination, Holinger (1980) found 81% to have evidence of congenital abnormalities of the larynx, trachea or bronchi. Of the total, 60% had abnormalities of the larynx, 16% had tracheal abnormalities and 5% had congenital anomalies of the bronchi. Significantly, 45% of the patients had more than one congenital abnormality; it is thus mandatory that a full endoscopic examination be carried out in all children presenting with congenital stridor (Shugar and Healy, 1980).

Larynx

Supraglottis

Laryngomalacia

The term 'laryngomalacia' (malacia is derived from a Greek word, μαλακια, indicating morbid softening of a part), was introduced by Jackson and Jackson (1942), to describe a form of congenital laryngeal stridor characterized by flaccidity of the supraglottic structures.

Although the exact pathophysiological correlates of the condition are not known for certain, the following features have been noted (Sutherland and Lack, 1897; Kelemen, 1953):

(1) softness, flabbiness or lack of consistency of the laryngeal tissues
(2) thinning and hypocellularity of the laryngeal cartilages

(3) wrinkled, loose or redundant mucosa, especially over the arytenoid cartilages.

Laryngomalacia is by far the most common cause of congenital stridor, accounting for 60–70% of all cases (Fearon and Ellis, 1971; Holinger, 1980). The male to female ratio is approximately equal (McSwiney, Cavanagh and Languth, 1977).

In the vast majority of patients, inspiratory stridor is the only symptom. Characteristically, the stridor is high pitched, crowing and fluttering. It is usually first noticed within a few days of birth, but in some patients it may not become obvious until the child begins to be more active or develops an acute upper respiratory tract infection. The stridor tends to increase in severity during the first 8 months of life, reaching a maximum between 9 and 12 months, thereafter beginning to resolve (Lane et al., 1984). The stridor is often intermittent, appearing only while the child is feeding or crying and may be much more pronounced during sleep, especially if the child lies on its back. Hyperextension of the head sometimes results in significant lessening of the stridor.

The diagnosis can only be established for certain by direct observation of the appearance and movement of the laryngeal structures. Four significant findings are consistently noted, either separately or in combination:

(1) a tall, tubular, in-rolled epiglottis, with a tendency to prolapse backwards and which is often likened to the Greek letter omega (Ω); it should be noted, however, that this is a common finding in otherwise normal neonates and, almost certainly, merely represents an exaggeration of the infantile form (Lane et al., 1984)

(2) short, sometimes almost non-existent, flaccid, medially prolapsing aryepiglottic folds

(3) prominent, elongated arytenoid cartilages, often covered by loose, redundant mucosa and separated by a deep interarytenoid cleft. On inspiration, the arytenoids will be seen to be sucked inwards, often crossing one over the other, obstructing the airway and giving rise to the typical stridor

(4) the whole supraglottic larynx is deepened and narrowed with the result that the vocal cords are often quite difficult to see.

In order to observe these features properly, it is not only essential that the child is breathing spontaneously but that the respiratory efforts should be deep and vigorous. These conditions are, perhaps, best achieved during recovery from anaesthesia. It is likewise important to avoid splinting of the laryngeal inlet; the beak of the laryngoscope must be kept in the vallecula with as little disturbance as possible to the supraglottic structures. Insertion of the tip of the laryngoscope between the aryepiglottic folds will usually result in cessation of the stridor.

One important feature of this condition is that the stridor will often become more noticeable during the early stages of anaesthesia, especially the phase of excitation; this might be explained, perhaps, by the supine position of the child under anaesthesia and the increased respiratory effort.

In most cases, laryngomalacia is otherwise asymptomatic. Occasionally, however, there may be associated feeding difficulties, sometimes severe enough to produce failure to thrive. Rarely, the child will have respiratory distress of such a degree as to require active treatment – this may take the form of tracheostomy, excision of redundant mucosa (Lane *et al.*, 1984) or laser division of the aryepiglottic folds (Seid *et al.*, 1985).

Although the stridor will, in most cases, have disappeared spontaneously by 18 months to 2 years, this is not invariably the case (Smith and Cooper, 1981). The author has seen children in whom both the stridor and the characteristic appearance of the larynx persisted into late childhood and adolescence.

Laryngeal cyst

A laryngeal (saccular) cyst is a mucus-filled dilatation of the laryngeal saccule which may distort the aryepiglottic fold, the false cord or the laryngeal ventricle (Suhonen *et al.*, 1984). Saccular cysts may sometimes be confused with laryngocoeles. In the former, however, there is no communication with the airway and the contents are fluid rather than gaseous.

Generally, such cysts are asymptomatic and are only noted, incidentally, during endotracheal intubation. Occasionally, however, the cysts enlarge or become infected, resulting in a rather hoarse stridor and rapidly increasing airway obstruction. Endoscopic examination reveals a large bluish swelling, in the region of the aryepiglottic fold, sometimes totally obscuring the vocal cords. Treatment is aimed at endolaryngeal excision of the cyst or, if this proves impossible, wide marsupialization. Very occasionally, tracheostomy may be required if the respiratory distress becomes severe.

Extensive cystic hygromata (lymphangiomata) can involve the posterior part of the tongue, the vallecula and the epiglottis, resulting in airway obstruction. The most satisfactory method of dealing with this problem is wide excision of the cystic masses using the CO_2 gas laser, but recurrence is common and tracheostomy may prove necessary.

Congenital laryngocoele

A laryngocoele is an air-filled dilatation of the ventricular sinus of Morgagni. If the sac extends beyond the limits of the thyroid cartilage, piercing the thyrohyoid membrane, the laryngocoele is classified as being external, the internal variety remaining deep to the laryngeal cartilages. Clinically, the condition is recognized by intermittent hoarseness or respiratory distress which increases on crying or straining. Rarely, the external variety may be diagnosed by palpation of a soft, fluctuant swelling in the neck, presenting above the thyroid cartilage. Plain X-rays of the neck may demonstrate the air-filled sac.

Glottis

Laryngeal web

Formation of a normal laryngeal lumen depends upon complete canalization of the epithelial lamina between the vestibulotracheal canal above and the pharyngotracheal canal below, a process which begins at about the fifth week of intrauterine development. Total failure of this process will produce a complete laryngeal atresia but, more commonly, partial canalization occurs, resulting in the formation of a laryngeal web. Such webs may involve the supraglottis, or subglottis, but by far the greatest number (over 75%) are sited in the glottis (McHugh and Loch, 1942).

Most glottic webs are located anteriorly, involving a variable length of the vocal cords, but occasionally the membrane lies at the posterior commissure. They may be thin and membranous or, rather more frequently, thick and fibrotic, often extending downwards to involve the subglottis.

The symptoms produced depend, to a degree, upon the extent and thickness of the web but stridor, which may be biphasic in timing, hoarseness of the voice or cry and respiratory distress, may all occur.

Thin webs can be lysed endoscopically using scissors, knife or laser. Thick, fibrotic webs, however, are much more difficult to treat successfully. Some authors advocate the formation, as an initial stage, of an anteriorly sited, epithelial-lined tract (Lynch and Le Jeune, 1960); others recommend insertion of a keel, either endoscopically or via a laryngofissure approach (van den Broek and Brinkman, 1979). In many cases, however, where the web is small and causing little in the way of symptoms, the best approach is to leave well alone.

Cri-du-chat syndrome

The most striking feature of this relatively uncommon condition is the characteristic high-pitched 'mewing' stridor. At endoscopy, the rima glottis is observed to be diamond shaped, the vocal cords are narrow and the supraglottis is curved and elongated. Respiratory distress is uncommon and tracheostomy rarely required (Ward, Engel and Nance, 1968). Chromosomal investigation confirms the diagnosis, showing partial deletion of the short arm of the fifth chromosome in group B (Cotton and Reilly, 1983).

Vocal cord paralysis

Congenital paralysis of the vocal cord is the third most common cause of congenital stridor, accounting for between 6% and 13% of all cases (Fearon and Ellis, 1971; Holinger, 1980). It may be unilateral or bilateral, the former occurring four times more frequently than the latter (Emery and Fearon, 1984).

In unilateral paralysis, the cry is often breathy or weak, stridor is uncommon and there is little tendency to airway obstruction. In contrast, bilateral paresis is associated with a normal cry, and stridor and significant respiratory distress are almost invariable, though these may not appear until the child becomes more active.

The diagnosis is confirmed at laryngoscopy with direct observation of vocal cord movement but this can be difficult, particularly in the small child and, undoubtedly, many cases are missed. Problems may arise from incorrectly placing the tip of the laryngoscope posterior to the epiglottis, causing distortion of the glottis or from too deep an anaesthetic causing inhibition of laryngeal reflexes. The best opportunity to observe vocal cord movement is during recovery from anaesthesia. Care must also be taken to distinguish between true paresis of the vocal cord and fixation of the cricoarytenoid joint – this may be achieved by gentle palpation of the arytenoid cartilage.

Many of these infants exhibit other congenital defects involving the central or peripheral nervous systems, the heart and great vessels or the respiratory tract. Thus neonates with hydrocephalus, meningoencephalocoele, meningocoele, meningomyelocoele, or the Arnold–Chiari malformation, who present with stridor or abnormality of the cry, should have their vocal cords inspected. Congenital myasthenia gravis, which is characterized in the child by drooping of the eyelids (ptosis), inability to suck or intermittent facial paralysis, may present with progressive weakness of the cry and stridor. Cardiomegaly or abnormalities of the great vessels may result in stretching of the left recurrent laryngeal nerve. Either recurrent laryngeal nerve may be involved in abnormalities of the tracheobronchial tree or oesophagus.

Benign congenital hypotonia, Werdnig–Hoffman syndrome, leucodystrophy, Charcot–Marie–Tooth disease and other progressive congenital muscular disorders may demonstrate paralysis of the vocal cords (Dedo and Dedo, 1983).

Most cases of unilateral vocal cord paralysis can be treated expectantly. In the author's opinion there is no justification for the use of Teflon paste injection in the management of this condition in childhood. Bilateral paralysis will almost always necessitate tracheostomy to protect the airway, at least initially. Late recovery of one or both vocal cords has been noted – in one case this occurred at the age of 9 years (Emery and Fearon, 1984). Attempts at improving the airway by lateralization of the vocal cord should, therefore, be postponed. Reduction of one cord using the laser, with or without arytenoidectomy, may be an effective alternative.

Subglottis

Subglottic stenosis

If is often difficult to distinguish between the congenital and acquired varieties of this condition; indeed the two frequently coexist. Stenosis may be considered to be present if the diameter of the subglottic space is less than 3.5 mm, as measured by failure to achieve the unforced passage of a bronchoscope of this size (Fearon and Cotton, 1972). The abnormality lies in the cricoid cartilage which is thickened and oval in shape. There is also a concomitant increase in the thickness of the submucosa, giving rise to the characteristic crescentic narrowing of the anterior subglottic space, maximal 2–3 mm below the true vocal cords. Occasionally, this submucosal thickening extends upwards to involve the cords at the anterior commissure.

Congenital subglottic stenosis demonstrates a wide variation, both in severity and in symptomatology. Airways resistance changes as the fourth power of the radius (Poiseuille's law); as a consequence, even minor degrees of subglottic oedema will produce a disproportionately large increase in airways resistance. Thus, in mild cases of subglottic stenosis, there may be no stridor until the child develops an upper respiratory tract infection or the subglottis is traumatized by endotracheal intubation. In such patients, the stridor is usually inspiratory in nature, whereas, in the more severe case, it is often biphasic. Every once in a while, a child will present with such severe stenosis that the subglottic airway is reduced to pinhole dimensions. Remarkably, a few of these children, while noted to be stridorous, do not appear to get into respiratory difficulty until infancy has passed and the ambulatory phase of childhood has begun.

Demonstration of the characteristic endoscopic findings, referred to above, and the absence of a history of previous prolonged endotracheal intubation, provide the mainstays of diagnosis. Plain X-rays of the neck and thoracic inlet are notoriously unreliable, with many instances of both false-positive and false-negative findings being reported. Considerable care and gentleness must be employed during bronchoscopy in these patients, in order to avoid damage to the subglottic area, otherwise the airway may be further compromised, precipitating the need for tracheostomy. It is the author's practice to record the diagnosis clearly on the front of the patient's chart to warn anaesthetic personnel should the child require endotracheal intubation in the future.

There is a tendency towards spontaneous improvement in congenital subglottic stenosis and, in mild cases, it is often sufficient to advise the parents that problems are only likely to arise during upper respiratory tract infections or following intubation for anaesthesia. In more severe cases tracheostomy may be required and should be performed earlier rather than later. Treatment consists of either serial dilatation or laryngotracheoplasty, although the former method is of much less value in congenital stenosis than in the acquired form of the disease. For further details on management, the reader is referred to Chapter 34.

Subglottic haemangioma

Congenital haemangiomata are hamartomata of blood-vessel origin. The association between skin haemangiomata and vascular tumours affecting internal organs is well recognized (Garfinkel and Handler, 1980). The best known of these symptom complexes is the Sturge–Weber syndrome, in which 'port wine stains' in the area of distribution of one trigeminal nerve are coupled with angiomata of the cerebral cortex.

Similarly, laryngeal haemangiomata, almost always affecting the subglottis, may appear in conjunction with capillary naevi of the face or neck. Symptomatically, the affected child presents with inspiratory or biphasic stridor, dyspnoea and a rather harsh cry. On direct laryngoscopy, the distinctive appearance of the subglottis is almost diagnostic. There is a bluish, pear-shaped swelling arising from the lateral wall of the subglottic space often extending upwards to involve the undersurface of the vocal cord. In most cases the subglottis is affected on one side only, but occasionally there are bilateral tumours. Although often associated with facial lesions, subglottic haemangiomata may also be present in isolation. The tumours are soft and compressible and can be easily bypassed with the bronchoscope. In the author's experience, the angiomata are always of the capillary type, do not bleed and may, therefore, be safely biopsied to provide a tissue diagnosis.

Like the facial haemangiomata, the subglottic lesions often rapidly increase in size during the first few years, thereafter spontaneously regressing. A tracheostomy is usually necessary, at least initially, though some authors have claimed that this can be avoided by using steroid therapy (Cohen and Wang, 1972; Sadan, Sade and Grunebaum, 1982); others, however, disagree (Leikensohn, Benton and Cotton, 1976). Laser excision, unfortunately, has not proved to be efficacious (Healy *et al.*, 1980).

Laryngotracheal cleft

The respiratory primordium is derived from the foregut at about day 20 of embryonic life by the development of the median pharyngeal groove. Subsequently, the groove deepens to form the pharyngotracheal canal, becoming separated from the oesophagus by development of a tracheo-oesophageal septum which starts caudally and grows in a cephalad direction. Failure in the formation of this septum, or arrest of its rostral advancement, will result in open communication between the laryngotracheal airway and the oesophageal lumen (van den Broek and Brinkman, 1979).

Pettersson (1955) has classified these clefts into three types:

(1) laryngotracheal cleft
(2) partial laryngotracheo-oesophageal cleft
(3) total laryngotracheo-oesophageal cleft.

The hallmark of this condition is persistent aspiration, sometimes accompanied by stridor, respiratory distress and a toneless cry. Diagnosis is difficult and is frequently missed; in one series, 42% were diagnosed at autopsy (Burroughs and Leape, 1974). Screening of the swallow using Gastrografin or dilute barium will demonstrate aspiration, although the precise site of occurrence may be difficult to determine and is, of course, found in other conditions, such as H-type tracheo-oesophageal fistula. Any patient in whom the possibility of a cleft is considered should be examined, using the laryngeal microscope, and the interarytenoid cleft palpated using a blunt hook or similar instrument. The defect between the larynx and oesophagus may be repaired via a lateral pharyngotomy (Kauten, Konrad and Wichterman, 1984).

Laryngotracheal clefts occur in isolation, but may also be associated with other congenital abnormalities as in the 'G' or Opitz–Frias syndrome (Opitz *et al.*, 1969). This is an autosomally dominant disease with male predominance, characterized by craniofacial, aerodigestive and urogenital anomalies. The head and neck manifestations are related to midline defects, including cleft lip and palate, laryngotracheal cleft and neuromuscular dysfunction of the pharynx and oesophagus (Kimmelman and Denneny, 1982).

Anterior clefts of the larynx, due to failure of fusion of the laminae of the thyroid cartilage, creating an anterior midline defect, have also been described (Montgomery and Smith, 1976). It should be noted, however, that these are glottic rather than subglottic.

Trachea and bronchi

Abnormalities of the tracheobronchial tree account for about 26% of congenital causes of stridor (Holinger, 1980).

Agenesis

Complete or partial agenesis of the trachea is incompatible with life. Short-term survival may be possible, however, if there is a fistulous connection between the oesophagus and bronchus, but utilization of the oesophagus as a tracheal replacement has proved unsuccessful (Peison, Levitsky and Sprowls, 1970). Agenesis of one main bronchus and its associated lung is, however, survivable, although most affected infants are weakly and tend to succumb to chest infections. In the majority of cases, there are other severe, associated congenital abnormalities which further diminish the chances of survival of these patients beyond the neonatal period.

Stenosis

Congenital narrowing of the tracheal or bronchial lumen may take the form of membranous webs, segmental or whole organ stenosis. Where the obstruction is sited in the lower trachea or main bronchi, treatment is confined to attempts at gentle dilatation using bronchoscopes of increasing diameter. Rather surprisingly, such management is often successful and should certainly be tried. Stenosis of the upper trachea may be managed in the same way or recourse may be had to tracheoplasty where the lumen is increased by making a vertical incision in the anterior tracheal wall and inserting an elliptical wedge of costal cartilage. Where the stenosis is affecting a long segment of the trachea, an attempt may be made to increase the lumen by separation of one side of the trachea from the oesophagus and reattachment more laterally.

Tracheomalacia

Tracheomalacia exists in both generalized and localized forms, of which the latter is much more common. Although there are some pathological correlates between tracheomalacia and laryngomalacia and, occasionally, they may coexist, there is no proven relationship between the two. The characteristic stridor, which is high pitched and expiratory is said to resemble the expiratory wheeze of asthma (Baxter and Dunbar, 1963). In the localized form, cough is a frequently associated symptom and is harsh and barking in quality, rather like that of viral croup. At bronchoscopy, the trachea is seen to be compressed in its anteroposterior diameter due to a flattening of the anterior aspect of the cartilaginous rings. This abnormal appearance is accentuated by expiration and even more so by coughing, when the anterior and posterior walls may come in contact. Care must be taken, however, to distinguish between this anomaly and that produced by laxity of the trachealis muscle with forward ballooning of the posterior wall – an almost universal finding in the neonate.

As with laryngomalacia, complete spontaneous recovery is the rule. In a few cases, however, where approximation of the anterior and posterior walls is marked, severe obstruction to the airway may be present and a tracheostomy found to be necessary. In these circumstances, it is often imperative to use a longer than usual tracheostomy tube, one which will reach to just above the carina, otherwise the infalling anterior wall may block the end of the tube (Cinnamond, 1977). Suspension of the anterior tracheal wall from the inner surface of the sternum has also been recommended.

In a high proportion of cases of the generalized type, the malacic process will be found to be also affecting the main bronchi. In about 10% of cases, additional abnormalities of the trachea will be present, especially tracheo-oesophageal fistulae, which are considered in Chapter 37. In every case, a careful search should be made for the tracheal opening of an H-type tracheo-oesophageal fistula as this condition may otherwise be missed.

The localized form of the disease is almost always due to compression of the affected portion of the anterior tracheal wall from without. The most probable causes are vascular rings or abnormal vessels, congenital mediastinal or cervical tumours or bronchogenic cysts.

Vascular compression

The primary cause of anomalies of the great vessels of the neck and thorax is faulty embryonic development and the only adequate way to classify them is embryologically. Desnos *et al.* (1980), however, have produced a simplified but satisfactory classification based on endoscopic findings.

Vascular ring

(1) Double aortic arch, in which the ascending aorta divides into two arches, one passing to the right of the trachea and the other to the left, rejoining posterior to the oesophagus to form the descending aorta. The trachea and oesophagus are thus confined within a compressing ring of vascular structures. There is considerable variation in the morphology of these rings, the arches may be of equal or unequal size and different configurations of the main branches may occur.
(2) Neuhauser's anomaly, where the aorta is single but passes to the *right* of the trachea. In this case the ring is only partly vascular, the component to the left of the trachea being formed by the ligamentum arteriosum, the remnant of the ductus arteriosus which, in the fetus, connects the pulmonary artery to the descending aorta.

Vascular sling

Here, the left pulmonary artery, instead of passing anterior to the trachea, passes between it and the oesophagus, compressing the trachea from behind and the oesophagus from in front.

Anterior compression

(1) Compression of the anterior tracheal wall by an anomalous innominate artery, the origin of which from the aortic arch is more posteriorly sited and more to the left than normal. This produces a characteristic sloping compression of the lower trachea 1–2 cm above the carina, more marked on the right anterolateral aspect. Further confirmation is afforded by noting diminution or absence of the patient's right radial or right carotid pulses, using the tip of the bronchoscope to collapse the vessel against the sternum. On rare occasions, the anomalous innominate artery may be associated with an aberrant right subclavian artery, which passes posterior to the oesophagus (Macdonald and Fearon, 1971).
(2) A larger than normal pulmonary artery may compress the trachea and bronchi at or just below the carina.

Posterior compression

This is usually due to an aberrant right or, more rarely, left subclavian artery, passing posterior to the oesophagus. The oesophagus, alone, is compressed in this case.

In those instances where both trachea and oesophagus are involved, the patient may present with symptoms that can be referred to either; in practice, however, the tracheal symptoms of stridor, dyspnoea and a harsh, brassy cough tend to dominate the picture. Similar symptoms are found where the trachea alone is affected. In about one-third of those children in whom there is significant airway obstruction due to innominate artery compression, stimulation of the area of compression with the tip of the bronchoscope may initiate reflex apnoea (Moes, Izukawa and Trusler, 1975). It has been suggested that activation of this reflex may explain some cases of sudden infant death syndrome.

Barium swallow may show indentation of the oesophagus – this will be bilateral when the abnormality is a double aortic arch or Neuhauser's anomaly, anteriorly in vascular sling or posteriorly with an aberrant subclavian artery. High-resolution ultrasound scanning is often helpful and computerized tomography may give additional information, but the conclusive investigation, in all cases, is aortography.

In those patients in whom the symptoms are severe and, especially, when the tracheal airway is judged to be inadequate, as demonstrated by an inability to see the carina from a position proximal to the compression, surgical decompression should be undertaken. In almost all cases of vascular ring, surgery will be necessary, the definitive management being division of the lesser component of the ring. Where the compression is due to an anomalous innominate artery, the vessel may be slung anteriorly away from the trachea by suturing the adventitia to the undersurface of the sternum (Gross and Neuhauser, 1948; Mustard *et al.*, 1969). This, however, is seldom necessary and indeed, in the neonate, some degree of innominate artery compression of the trachea is so common as to be the rule rather than the exception.

In all types of vascular compression, tracheostomy should be avoided as bypassing the obstruction may result in intubation of the right main bronchus and, in addition, there is significant, and usually fatal, risk of erosion of the vessel by the tip of the tracheostomy tube. In all cases where surgical correction of the deformity has been undertaken, it should be borne in mind that the localized area of tracheomalacia, which invariably accompanies compression, may remain for many months postoperatively.

Anomalous bronchial bifurcations

Origin of the right upper lobe bronchus from the right lateral wall of the trachea above the carina is relatively common. In almost every case this is an incidental finding and is entirely asymptomatic. Bronchography may be required to delineate the exact morphology. Other minor variations in the bronchial tree also occur and are, likewise, symptom free.

Congenital cysts and tumours

These cause *non-pulsatile* compression of the trachea and main bronchi but their presentation and appearance on endoscopy is otherwise similar to vascular compression.

Tracheogenic and bronchogenic cysts are thought to originate from evaginations of the primitive tracheal bud. They are lined with respiratory epithelium and may contain thick, inspissated mucus. In contrast to bronchogenic cysts, those arising from the trachea do not usually communicate with the lumen. Infection may occur, with resulting increased compression of surrounding structures. Thoracotomy and excision of the cyst will often be required.

Cervical and mediastinal cysts or tumours, including thymomata and teratomata may compress the trachea or bronchi from without (Mills and Hussain, 1984). Teratomata affecting the anterior neck present particular difficulties as the tumour may intimately involve the anterior wall of the trachea. Complete excision of the mass is likely to entail removal of part of the tracheal wall with the possibility of long-term airway stenosis.

References

BAXTER, J. D. and DUNBAR, J. S. (1963) Tracheomalacia. *Annals of Otology, Rhinology and Laryngology*, **72**, 1013–1023

BURROUGHS, N. and LEAPE, L. L. (1974) Laryngotracheoesophageal cleft: report of a case successfully treated and review of the literature. *Pediatrics*, **53**, 516–522

CINNAMOND, M. J. (1977) Tracheomalacia – or is it? *Proceedings of the Irish Otolaryngological Society*, **18**, 33–35

COHEN, S. R. and WANG, C. (1972) Steroid treatment of hemangiomas of the head and neck in children. *Annals of Otology, Rhinology and Laryngology*, **81**, 584–590

COTTON, R. and REILLY, J. S. (1983) Stridor and airway obstruction. In *Pediatric Otolaryngology*, edited by C. H. Bluestone and S. E. Stool, pp. 1190–1204. Philadelphia: W. B. Saunders

DEDO, D. D. and DEDO, H. H. (1983) Neurogenic diseases of the larynx. In *Pediatric Otolaryngology*, edited by C. H. Bluestone and S. E. Stool, pp. 1278–1284. Philadelphia: W. B. Saunders

DESNOS, J., ANDRIEU-GUITRANCOURT, J., DEHESDIN, D. and DUBIN, J. (1980) Vascular strictures of the respiratory tract in children. *International Journal of Pediatric Otorhinolaryngology*, **2**, 269–285

EMERY, P. J. and FEARON, B. (1984) Vocal cord palsy in pediatric practice: a review of 71 cases. *International Journal of Pediatric Otorhinolaryngology*, **8**, 147–154

FEARON, B. and COTTON, R. B. (1972) Subglottic stenosis in infants and children. The clinical problem and experimental surgical correction. *Canadian Journal of Otolaryngology*, **1**, 281–289

FEARON, B. and ELLIS, D. (1971) The management of long term airway problems in infants and children. *Annals of Otology, Rhinology and Laryngology*, **80**, 669–677

GARFINKEL, T. J. and HANDLER, S. D. (1980) Hemangioma of the head and neck. *Journal of Otolaryngology*, **9**, 435–450

GROSS, R. E. and NEUHAUSER, E. D. B. (1948) Compression of the trachea by an anomalous innominate artery. An operation for its relief. *American Journal of Diseases of Childhood*, **75**, 570–574

HEALY, G. B., FEARON, B., FRENCH, B. and MAGILL, T. (1980) Treatment of subglottic hemangioma. *The Laryngoscope*, **90**, 809–813

HOLINGER, L. D. (1980) Etiology of stridor in the neonate, infant and child. *Annals of Otology, Rhinology and Laryngology*, **89**, 397–400

JACKSON, C. and JACKSON, C. (1942) *Diseases and Injuries of the Larynx*, pp. 63–68. New York: McMillan Publishing Co. Inc.

KAUTEN, J. R., KONRAD, H. R. AND WICHTERMAN, K. A. (1984) Laryngotracheoesophageal cleft in a newborn. *International Journal of Pediatric Otorhinolaryngology*, **8**, 61–71

KELEMEN, G. (1953) Congenital laryngeal stridor. *Archives of Otolaryngology*, **58**, 245–268

KIMMELMAN, C. P. and DENNENY, J. C. (1982) Opitz (G) syndrome. *International Journal of Pediatric Otorhinolaryngology*, **4**, 343–347

LANE, R. W., WEIDER, D. J., STEINEM, C. and MARIN-PADILLA, M. (1984) Laryngomalacia. A review and case report of surgical treatment with resolution of pectus excavatum. *Archives of Otolaryngology*, **110**, 546–555

LEIKENSOHN, J. R., BENTON, C. and COTTON, R. (1976) Subglottic hemangioma. *Journal of Otolaryngology*, **5**, 487–491

LYNCH, M. G. and LE JEUNE, F. E. (1960) Laryngeal stenosis. *The Laryngoscope*, **70**, 315–317

MACDONALD, R. E. and FEARON, B. (1971) Innominate artery compression syndrome in children. *Annals of Otology, Rhinology and Laryngology*, **80**, 535–540

McHUGH, H. E. and LOCH, W. E. (1942) Congenital webs of the larynx. *The Laryngoscope*, **52**, 43–65

McSWINEY, P. F., CAVANAGH, N. P. C. and LANGUTH, P. (1977) Outcome in congenital stridor. *Archives of Disease in Childhood*, **52**, 215–218

MILLS, R. P. and HUSSAIN, S. S. M. (1984) Teratomas of the head and neck in infancy and childhood. *International Journal of Pediatric Otorhinolaryngology*, **8**, 177–180

MOES, C. A. F., IZUKAWA, T. and TRUSLER, G. A. (1975) Innominate artery compression of the trachea. *Archives of Otolaryngology*, **101**, 733–738

MONTGOMERY, W. W. and SMITH, S. A. (1976) Congenital laryngeal defect in the adult. *Annals of Otology, Rhinology and Laryngology*, **85**, 491–497

MUSTARD, W. T., BAYLISS, C. E., FEARON, B., PELTON, D. and TRUSLER, G. A. (1969) Tracheal compression by the innominate artery in children. *Annals of Thoracic Surgery*, **8**, 312–319

OPITZ, J. M., FRIAS, J. L., GUTENBERGER, J. E. and PELLETT, J. R. (1969) The G syndrome of multiple congenital anomalies. In *Malformation Syndromes, Birth Defects: Original Article Series*, edited by D. Bergsma, pp. 95–101. White Plains: The National Foundation – March of Dimes

PEISON, B., LEVITSKY, E. and SPROWLS, J. J. (1970) Tracheoesophageal fistula associated with tracheal atresia and malformation of the larynx. *Journal of Pediatric Surgery*, **5**, 464–467

PETTERSSON, G. (1955) Inhibited separation of the larynx and upper part of the trachea from the esophagus in the newborn: report of a case successfully operated on. *Acta Chirurgica Scandinavica*, **110**, 250–254

SADAN, N., SADE, J. and GRUNEBAUM, M. (1982) The treatment of subglottic hemangiomas of infants with prednisone. *International Journal of Pediatric Otorhinolaryngology*, **4**, 7–14

SEID, A. B., PARK, S. M., KEARNS, M. J. and GUGENHEIM, S. (1985) Laser division of the aryepiglottic folds for severe laryngomalacia. *International Journal of Pediatric Otorhinolaryngology*, **10**, 153–158

SHUGAR, M. A. and HEALY, G. B. (1980) Coexistent lesions of the pediatric airway. *International Journal of Pediatric Otorhinolaryngology*, **2**, 323–327

SMITH, G. J. and COOPER, D. M. (1981) Laryngomalacia and inspiratory obstruction in late childhood. *Archives of Disease in Childhood*, **56**, 345–349

SUHONEN, H., KERO, P. O., PUHAKKA, H. and VILKKI, P. (1984) Saccular cyst of the larynx in infants. *International Journal of Pediatric Otorhinolaryngology*, **8**, 73–78

SUTHERLAND, G. A. and LACK, H. L. (1897) Congenital laryngeal obstruction. *The Lancet*, **2**, 653–655

VAN DEN BROEK, P. and BRINKMAN, W. F. B. (1979) Congenital laryngeal defects. *International Journal of Pediatric Otorhinolaryngology*, **1**, 71–78

WARD, P. H., ENGEL, E. and NANCE, W. E. (1968) The larynx in the cri du chat syndrome. *The Laryngoscope*, **78**, 1716–1733

27

Stridor

Michael J. Cinnamond

Definitions

Stridor is an auditory manifestation of disordered respiratory function due to air-flow changes within the larynx, trachea or bronchi, and as such merits investigation in every case. Despite its derivation from the Latin, *stridere*, meaning a harsh, creaking or grating sound (Onions, 1978), stridor is not always discordant but is, in fact, more often musical or sibilant in character. The frequency of the sound produced also varies, from low-pitched and sonorous to high-pitched squeaking or whistling. Not all sounds emanating from the respiratory tract are, however, stridorous: voluntary or involuntary vocalizations (stertor), moist sounds, such as rattling or bubbling of secretions in the pharynx or larynx, and rales or crepitations arising in the distal portions of the bronchial tree or alveoli, should be excluded. Conditions producing stertor are dealt with in Chapter 23.

Aerodynamic considerations

Stridor is due to turbulence of the air flow within a partially obstructed respiratory tract. In order to understand the mechanisms by which stridor is produced, it is necessary first to review a few of the basic physical principles pertaining to contained gases at rest and in motion. Pascal's principle states that

'in a fluid (whether liquid or gaseous) at rest, a pressure change in one part is transmitted, without loss, to every portion of the fluid and to the walls of the container' (adapted from Encyclopaedia Britannica, 1981, by courtesy of the Publisher).

In other words, the pressure exerted by the gas is the same at every point on the containing walls. Steady gas flow, along a tube, is described by Bernoulli's equation which, in simple terms, relates velocity of the gas to the pressure which it exerts. If the tube is constricted or throttled, the gas velocity increases through the narrowed portion and, in order to preserve the law of conservation of energy, the local gas pressure falls.

Application of Bernoulli's equation to air flow through the tracheobronchial tree, especially the flaccid, compressible airway of the child, demonstrates that an increased transmural pressure gradient will occur at sites of constriction, resulting in collapse of the airway and temporary cessation of air flow (Forgacs, 1978). Pascal's principle and the resilience of the cartilaginous support causes the airway to spring open again and the cycle is repeated. The fluttering vibrations thus created are amplified by the resonators of the vocal tract and chest cavity, giving rise to the audible sounds which are known as stridor.

Stridor can be described in terms of its relationship to the phases of the respiratory cycle, its component frequencies and its tonal qualities. To a certain extent, some categories of stridor so defined can be assigned to specific causes of respiratory obstruction, although considerable overlap occurs and caution should be exercised in the application of such diagnostic criteria to individual patients.

The following points should be noted:

(1) during inspiration, the relatively mobile, poorly supported structures of the infantile supraglottis tend to be drawn into the glottic aperture, as a result of the pressure differential

between pharynx and trachea; expiration, on the other hand, forces the prolapsing tissues out of the laryngeal inlet. The inspiratory stridor thus produced is often low-pitched and harsh in character

(2) in the smaller bronchi and bronchioles, accentuation of the normal physiological contraction, which occurs during expiration, combined with high velocity gas flow, results in collapse of the airway; this type of stridor is exemplified by the expiratory wheeze of asthma but may also be caused by retained bronchial foreign bodies

(3) the relatively rigid walls of the rima glottis, subglottis and trachea prevent collapse and stridor arising in these areas is presumably due to turbulence of the air flow alone. In severe obstruction, biphasic or to-and-fro stridor may result.

Associated signs and symptoms

A variety of other signs and symptoms may be found in association with stridor.

Cough

Cough is usually harsh and barking in nature and is particularly associated with subglottic inflammation and tracheal compression.

Hoarseness

Hoarseness, whether of speech or the cry, reflects changes in the structure and/or function of the vocal cords and suggests laryngeal inflammation, trauma, tumours or vocal cord immobility.

Deglutition and respiration

Deglutition and respiration share a common pathway, namely the oropharynx. It is not surprising, therefore, that disorders of swallowing may interfere with breathing and vice versa; thus stridor is often observed to increase during feeding. Conversely, and especially in the suckling infant, tachypnoea and prolongation of inspiration conspire to impede or even prevent normal swallowing activity. Stridorous infants, even in the absence of overt respiratory distress, are frequently noted to be poor or slow feeders; in some cases this may lead to failure of growth, due both to lack of nutrition and to the increased expenditure of energy on respiration. Choking, caused by accidental inhalation of ingested liquids or solids, may further compound the difficulties.

Stridor and dyspnoea

Stridor and dyspnoea are both manifestations of airway obstruction; severity of one tends to reflect severity of the other. Thus, loud raucous stridor, audible at a distance from the patient, generally occurs in the presence of other signs of respiratory embarrassment, such as flaring of the alae nasi, suprasternal, intercostal or substernal recession, use of the accessory muscles of respiration, or, in extreme cases, actual cyanosis.

There are, however, pitfalls for the unwary in relation to the detection of dyspnoea in the neonate and small infant. In many normal, non-airway-obstructed infants, the soft, compliant nature of the chest wall may give rise to a false impression of intercostal or sternal recession; this may become extreme with relatively minor degrees of obstruction. In contrast, cases of severe, chronic airway obstruction are seen in which signs of respiratory distress are minimal – the author has observed this in children with congenital subglottic stenosis in whom the airway was reduced to pinhole size. It is difficult to explain the exact mechanism by which this perplexing phenomenon occurs but it is presumably, in part, one of necessary adaptation. A rather similar picture, though for different reasons, occurs in acute epiglottitis: in the early stages of the disease, the child may learn that increased respiratory effort serves only to exacerbate 'corking' of the glottic aperture by the swollen supraglottic structures; at a later stage, simple exhaustion may account for the decreased respiratory effort.

General features

Stridor is always a symptom or a sign, never a diagnosis or a disease. Although it may often appear innocuous, fleeting and of little import, it is well to remember that stridor is *always* indicative of obstruction of the airway. This does not, of course, imply that every child with stridor must be regarded as an emergency but, rather, that a search for the cause should always be made.

Although endoscopy will be the final arbiter in most instances, time spent on a careful history and a thorough physical examination is time well spent. This is particularly true for the inexperienced or occasional endoscopist, as the information thus obtained will often direct the attention to areas which might otherwise have been overlooked.

History

Character

Stridor is often described by the parents as 'noisy breathing'. Others, perhaps of a more perspicacious nature, will characterize the noise as wheezing, crowing, whistling, croaking, sighing, rattling or snoring. These latter terms may be useful in evoking a mental image of the sound when it is absent at the time of examination.

Stridor may be continuous or intermittent; the former suggests a more serious cause than the latter.

Severity

The loudness of the stridor, as measured by the distance from the patient at which it can be heard, may provide information about its severity. The parents should also be asked specifically about features of obstructed respiration such as shortness of breath, difficult or laboured breathing, cyanosis and periods of apnoea.

Age at onset

It is a curious feature of congenital stridor that the symptom may not make an appearance for some considerable time after birth. This may reflect the increasing activity of the older infant or the stridor may not become manifest until the child suffers from his/her first upper respiratory tract infection.

Relationship to feeding, crying and exercise

Many patients with stridor will exhibit alteration in severity of the sound in relation to changes in position. This tends to be rather variable. Shallower, slower breathing during sleep will often result in diminution of the stridor while increased respiration during crying, feeding or when the child is active, all tend to increase the sound. In some children, the stridor will only be noticeable during such activity.

Related diseases

Enquiry should also be made about other known congenital or acquired disorders particularly in relation to the respiratory, cardiovascular and neurological systems. It is essential to ask about problems associated with previous endotracheal intubation and whether the child has undergone any prolonged periods of assisted ventilation.

Physical examination

General appearance

An alert, active, happy and well-fed infant is unlikely to have any serious pathology. In some children there may be pectus excavatum (Lane *et al.*, 1984), although the significance of this finding in relation to airway obstruction is not clear.

Marked head retraction is a feature of some types of upper respiratory obstruction; extension of the neck will often reduce the stridor in laryngomalacia (Cotton and Reilly, 1983). Signs of increased airways resistance to be looked for are: flaring of the nostrils, intercostal, suprasternal or substernal recession, tachypnoea and cyanosis. In the acutely obstructed child, a rising pulse rate is the most reliable sign of increasing distress. The pattern of respiration is important; in neonates especially, the increased effort of breathing through an obstructed airway may lead to periods of apnoea, sometimes prolonged. Reflex apnoea, after coughing or during feeding, may indicate the presence of innominate artery compression of the trachea (Macdonald and Fearon, 1971).

Nutritional status

Overweight children are more likely to develop croup or airway obstruction, perhaps due to increased effort of breathing and higher oxygen requirements. Poor nutrition, in stridorous infants, may be ascribed to the slow, laboured feeding, marked by frequent, and often prolonged, pauses for breath and, perhaps also, to the higher energy expenditure consequent upon increased airways resistance. Anaemia, from deficient nutrition, may further add to the child's respiratory difficulties.

Auscultation

The importance of listening to the stridor cannot be overstressed. Attention should be paid to the timing of the sound in relation to the respiratory cycle, its quality and pitch. Listening, with the child lying on his back, front and side and while sitting up, may yield valuable clues; if possible, the child should also be observed during feeding, sleeping and crying. Very quiet stridor is, sometimes, only audible when the examiner's ear is held close to the child's open mouth. When heard through a stethoscope placed over the trachea or upper chest, the sound is often 'purer' in pitch due to the filtering action of the chest cavity (Forgacs, 1978).

Tape recording

Magnetic recording of the sound can be a valuable method of detecting change in the quality of stridor over a period of time. On occasions, it may also be useful as a means of convincing worried parents that their child's condition is improving.

Palpation

In some low-pitched stridors, palpable vibrations are transmitted through the chest wall. Palpation of the neck may reveal congenital thyroid enlargement, thymic tumours or cysts extending upwards from the superior mediastinum or teratomata involving the anterior wall of the trachea.

Related organ systems

Congenital causes of stridor are frequently associated with other congenital disorders; special attention should be paid to the state of the lungs, heart and central nervous system. Bronchopneumonia often supervenes in the child with an obstructed airway and atelectasis may follow impaired coughing ability. In the acute phase of foreign body impaction in the bronchial tree, there may be signs of air trapping, while prolonged retention of a foreign body can lead to the development of bronchiectasis. In severe cases of chronic obstruction of the respiratory tract, there may be evidence of right heart failure with pulmonary congestion.

Investigations
Laboratory

Malnutrition, particularly in the neonate, is a frequent concomitant to respiratory difficulty. Blood chemistry analysis may reveal evidence of dehydration or depleted serum proteins, while haematological investigations will be of value in the detection and management of anaemia. Ampicillin-resistant strains of *Haemophilus influenzae* are being increasingly reported (Schwartz et al., 1978); it is, therefore, imperative that all children with acute epiglottitis should have blood culture studies, to ensure that the correct antibiotic therapy is instituted. In the patient with an acutely obstructed airway, arterial blood gas estimation can give an accurate, dynamic analysis of the respiratory state. Incompetence of the immunological system is occasionally found in children with repeated episodes of viral croup and may be a factor in some cases of persistent laryngeal papillomatosis.

Radiology

Plain lateral soft-tissue X-rays of the head, neck and upper thorax will often reveal a surprising amount of detail of the functional anatomy of the airway, providing the films are of good quality (Dunbar, 1970). Even small degrees of rotation in either the sagittal or coronal planes, however, will obscure detail by superimposing other structures on the airway shadow; this is especially true in the infant. Owing to the laxity of the soft tissues and the flexible nature of the cartilaginous structures of

the child's larynx, care must be taken in the interpretation of such X-rays (Valvassori et al., 1984). Thus, during inspiration, the subglottic region may collapse, giving rise to the mistaken view that stenosis is present; a film taken during expiration will demonstrate the error. Anteroposterior and lateral plain X-rays of the chest may show up distortion of the tracheobronchial air shadow in cases of vascular anomaly or mediastinal cysts. Lobar atelectasis and areas of consolidation, related to a foreign body or other causes of airway obstruction, may be demonstrated.

Xeroradiography gives enhanced soft tissue differentiation allowing detailed visualization of stenoses, granulomata and other lesions, but at the cost of greatly increased radiation exposure; the technique should, therefore, be used sparingly.

Although computerized tomographic scanning has dramatically enhanced the visualization of many parts of the body, it has proved to be something of a disappointment in the elucidation of upper airway disease in small children. There are two reasons for this: first, the avoidance of motion artefact, consequent upon the long scan times needed, is difficult to achieve in children (Valvassori et al., 1984), and second, there is a lack of deep body fat in babies, an essential requirement for obtaining good differentiation between tissue layers. Magnetic resonance imaging may prove to be more valuable in this area but the author has no experience of its use.

Contrast studies, using barium or Gastrografin, with fluoroscopic screening, enable the surgeon to obtain valuable information about the dynamic relationships between the air and food passages; they may also demonstrate encroachment on the oesophageal lumen by aortic arch anomalies or distortion of the tracheo-oesophageal complex by mediastinal masses. Aortography with videotaping is an essential tool in the investigation of great vessel anomalies causing tracheal or bronchial compression. Where possible, the surgeon should attend contrast screening sessions in person, in order to obtain first-hand knowledge of the altered anatomical and physiological relationships.

Future trends

A number of recent studies have suggested the possibility of characterization of stridor and other airway sounds using Fourier analysis techniques (Hirschberg, 1980; Mori et al., 1980). The hope has been expressed that further development of the method could provide matching of specific spectral patterns with individual pathological causes for stridor, enabling diagnosis without the need for endoscopic examination (Gray et al., 1985).

Comparison of preoperative and postoperative spectral analyses could be useful in evaluating treatment. Should the early promise shown by such techniques be confirmed, the paediatric laryngologist might be provided with a tool equivalent to evoked response audiometry.

Endoscopy

All children with stridor should be endoscoped. Where the onset has been recent or sudden this must be carried out as a matter of urgency; in well established cases, however, provided there is no respiratory distress, laryngoscopy and bronchoscopy may be delayed.

The larynx and tracheobronchial tree continue to grow throughout childhood. In order to allow for this, a minimum set of paediatric laryngoscopes, bronchoscopes, oesophagoscopes and endoscopic instruments, as outlined in *Table 27.1*, should be available. Refinements to the basic list of instruments might include additional sizes of bronchoscopes, a selection of Hopkin's rod telescopes, fibreoptic endoscopes or facilities for photographic or video recording.

The author has found the Storz instruments to

Table 27.1 Instrumentation

Instruments	Diameter (mm)	Length (cm)
Intubating laryngoscopes		11
		9.5
		8.5
Anterior commissure laryngoscope		11
Ventilating bronchoscope	2.5	20
	3	20
	3.5	20
	3.5	30
	4	30
	5	30
	6	30
Oesophagoscopes	3	20
	3.5	20
	4	30
	5	30
	6	30
Metal suction tubes		35
(with and without rubber tips)		25
Bronchoscopic instruments:	2	35
	1.5	25
Alligator		
Sharp-pointed rotating		
Peanut		
Circular cup		
Retroangle cup		

be the most satisfactory. Older, non-ventilating bronchoscopes, such as the Negus instruments, make the task not only more difficult but less safe; whenever possible these endoscopes should be replaced. A good light source and carefully maintained fibreoptic light cords are essential. For lesions affecting the larynx, and especially where biopsy or removal of tissues is contemplated, an operating microscope fitted with a 350 mm or 400 mm focal length objective lens, is essential.

Technique

Development of a good technique demands practice and patience. A well-performed endoscopy is characterized by skill, gentleness and thoroughness; it should be unhurried and safe. Particular care should be taken to avoid trauma to the subglottis, especially when there is pre-existing oedema or inflammation.

Laryngoscopy

The instrument is inserted into the right-hand corner of the mouth, with the tip of the middle finger resting on the hard palate; the thumb is placed beneath the instrument and is used to protect the upper teeth by acting as a fulcrum. The tongue is displaced to the left hand side to minimize its tendency to flop over the laryngoscope, causing obstruction to the view. At the same time, the laryngoscope is pushed forwards against the base of the tongue, opening up the pharyngeal lumen and allowing the epiglottis to be visualized. Once this has been achieved, the beak of the instrument is moved to the midline and, by a combination of caudal displacement of the laryngoscope into the vallecula and anterior pressure on the base of the tongue, the epiglottis is persuaded to ride forwards away from the laryngeal inlet thus uncovering the vocal cords and rima glottis. This affords the best view of the larynx and allows thorough inspection of the supraglottic and glottic larynx, at the same time causing the least interference with vocal cord movement.

Where the larynx is difficult or impossible to visualize in this way, the tip of the standard laryngoscope can be placed posterior to the epiglottis allowing it to be held forwards more positively, or an anterior commissure laryngoscope may be used. In exceptional cases, and particularly in children with the Pierre Robin or Hunter–Hurler syndromes, it may prove to be completely impossible to gain any view of the larynx by these means. In such circumstances a tracheoscope or flexible laryngoscope, if available, can be very helpful; as an alternative, the forward view Hopkin's rod telescope may be used on its own.

Bronchoscopy

The correct size of bronchoscope to be used in any individual child is a function of that child's weight and maturity. A rough guide is given in *Table 27.2*; where significant narrowing of the airway is suspected and, particularly if the subglottis is involved, a size smaller bronchoscope than that which would normally be employed should be tried first. While intubation of the airway should

Table 27.2 Selection of bronchoscopes by age

Bronchoscope size		Age of child
External diameter (mm)	Length (cm)	
2.5 or 3	20	Preterm (<2.5 kg)
3.5	20 or 30	0–6 months
3.5	30	6–18 months
4	30	18 months–3 years
5	30	3–12 years
6	30	>12 years

be performed in as calm and unhurried a fashion as possible, access should be given back immediately to the anaesthetist if there is cause for alarm.

Intubation may be achieved either using the intubating laryngoscope or by direct insertion of the bronchoscope. Inexperienced or casual bronchoscopists are strongly advised to use the former method, especially in cases of acute obstruction; no credit is given for an apparently slick approach when the end result is a traumatized larynx or a dead child.

Before inserting the laryngoscope, it is wise to ascertain that the chosen bronchoscope will pass easily through the lateral opening of the laryngoscope blade; if not, a straight bladed Magill laryngoscope may be used instead. The bronchoscope is then inserted, through the laryngoscope, under direct visual control, until the tip lies at the level of the false cords. From this point onwards, passage of the instrument is achieved by looking through the bronchoscope itself.

The major problem that occurs at this stage is displacement of the tip of the bronchoscope posterior to the arytenoids with subsequent passage of the scope into the oesophagus; failure

to identify any tracheal rings should alert the operator to the possibility that this has happened.

The bronchoscope should now be rotated through 90° so that the 'handle' points directly to the right. The tip is moved laterally until the right vocal cord can be identified and is then moved medially until the left cord appears. At this point, the tip of the scope should lie directly in line with the glottic aperture. The bronchoscope is advanced through the glottis and subglottis with a 'screwing' motion returning the 'handle' to its original straight ahead position. This manoeuvre ensures that the cords are gently separated and reduces the possibility of trauma to the vulnerable subglottic region. If the cords are in spasm, the tip of the scope may become accidentally displaced into the right laryngeal ventricle with the possibility of penetration into the neck. No advancement of the scope should be attempted unless the airway can be seen. The arytenoids are also at risk during this manoeuvre and care must be taken to avoid engaging the superior process of the arytenoid (especially the left one) with the bronchoscope, otherwise accidental dislocation at the cricoarytenoid joint may occur. The laryngoscope can now be removed.

Having achieved passage of the bronchoscope through the subglottis, it should be advanced to the carina and the anaesthetic gas supply connected to the side arm. The more experienced endoscopist will have taken the opportunity to form an impression of the state of the subglottis and trachea during this part of the procedure, but once the child's blood oxygen level has been replenished the scope should be gently and carefully withdrawn again to the subglottis to allow for a more detailed examination. Next, the bronchoscope is passed into each main bronchus in turn and the various segmental bronchial orifices identified and inspected. It should be noted that, unlike the situation in the adult, it is usually possible to get a direct and satisfactory view of the upper lobe bronchi in the small child by suitable positioning of the head and neck.

Particular care is required, when using rigid metal suckers, to avoid traumatizing the bronchial mucosa. Any bleeding which occurs may seriously impair the view obtained and, especially during attempted removal of a bronchial foreign body, this is likely to have profound consequences. Because of the small lumen of the paediatric bronchoscopes, only uniocular vision is possible; use of the bronchoscopic forceps is, therefore, difficult and success depends more on gentle touch and experience than on good eyesight. Practice in the use of the instruments is essential; clumsy, inexperienced snatching at an impacted peanut may turn a difficult problem into an impossible one.

Microlaryngoscopy

The small adult-sized operating laryngoscope may be used for older children, but for babies and small children a paediatric model is necessary (the Storz or Holinger instruments are recommended). For preference, a suspension system such as Vaughan's modification of the Boston University holder should be used, rather than the more commonly available Loewy's jack. The former reduces the likelihood of damage to the upper teeth and helps also in stabilizing the head, especially in dolichocephalic patients.

The endoscope is inserted in the midline of the mouth, although, when the larynx lies very anteriorly, it is sometimes better to introduce the instrument from the right side. Unlike the beaked, intubating laryngoscope, the operating laryngoscope should be placed posterior to the epiglottis holding it forwards to expose the glottic aperture. The operating microscope must be fitted with either a 400 mm or 350 mm focal length objective lens; the latter is better with the paediatric scope as it brings the operator slightly closer to the patient, making the use of the long shanked instruments somewhat easier. A padded Mayo table or some similar support, placed between the surgeon and patient's head, upon which the operator may rest the forearms, makes prolonged endolaryngeal microsurgery somewhat less tiring. Placing the patient in a partial reverse Trendelenburg position will often result in a more comfortable operating stance.

Flexible endoscopy

In difficult cases, where a rigid endoscope cannot be passed or where a satisfactory view is not obtained, flexible laryngoscopes, bronchoscopes or oesophagoscopes may be invaluable. These instruments, however, are not only costly and easily damaged but are much less versatile than their rigid counterparts and are, generally, more difficult to use. The flexible bronchoscope, in particular, creates problems in the maintenance of a satisfactory airway in the infant.

Documentation

A simple line drawing of the larynx, trachea and bronchi, indicating the pathology, is always much more informative than a few terse sentences and should be used in every case. This is especially true where repeated endoscopic examination proves necessary, both in reminding the surgeon of the circumstances found on the previous occasion and how the situation has changed since.

The shape, position and distribution of nodules, papillomata and similar lesions can be documented with considerable accuracy by this method.

Estimation of the size of the airway is often useful and is mandatory when subglottic stenosis is present. In its simplest form this may be merely a note to the effect that, for example, while a 3.0 mm bronchoscope could be inserted easily, a 3.5 mm one could not. For more accurate measurement, a graduated series of endotracheal tubes (Pracy, 1979) or gum elastic oesophageal dilators may be used.

Table 27.3 Classification of causes of stridor in childhood

Congenital
Larynx
  supraglottis
    laryngomalacia
    web
    saccular cyst
    cystic hygroma
    laryngocoele
  glottis
    web
    cri-du-chat syndrome
    vocal cord paralysis
  subglottis
    web
    stenosis
    haemangioma
    cleft larynx
Trachea and bronchi
  web
  stenosis
  tracheomalacia
  vascular compression
  tracheogenic cyst
  bronchogenic cyst
Mediastinal tumours
Acquired
Trauma
  thermal and chemical
  external
  intubation
  surgical
Foreign body
  laryngeal
  tracheal
  bronchial
  oesophageal
Inflammatory
  acute laryngitis
  laryngotracheobronchitis
  acute epiglottitis
  diphtheria
Allergy
Neoplasms
  papilloma

Still photography, cine photography and video techniques are very useful for teaching purposes but are difficult to use routinely. The interested reader is advised to study the methods and equipment described by Benjamin (1981).

Classification

The causes of childhood stridor and upper airway obstruction may be classified according to aetiology, pathology, anatomical site of origin or individual characteristics of the stridor itself, such as pitch or timing.

The subject is a complex one and several authors have produced extensive lists of possible causes (Kelemen, 1953; Cotton and Reilly, 1983). In practice, however, the actual number of different causes commonly met with is relatively small, as reference to *Table 27.3* will show. What the classification used here lacks in refinement, it makes up for in simplicity.

References

BENJAMIN, B. (1981) Documentation in paediatric laryngology. *Annals of Otology, Rhinology and Laryngology,* **90,** 478–482

COTTON, R. and REILLY, J. S. (1983) Stridor and airway obstruction. In *Pediatric Otolaryngology,* edited by C. H. Bluestone and S. E. Stool, pp. 1190–1204. Philadelphia: W. B. Saunders

DUNBAR, J. S. (1970) Upper respiratory tract obstruction in infants and children. *American Journal of Roentgenology,* **109,** 227–246

ENCYCLOPAEDIA BRITANNICA (1981) 15th edn. Pascal's principle, **VII,** 780. Chicago: Encyclopaedia Britannica Inc

FORGACS, P. (1978) *Lung Sounds.* London: Ballière Tindall

GRAY, L., DENNENY, J. C., CARVAJAL, H. and JAHRSDOERFER, R. (1985) Fourier analysis of infantile stridor: preliminary data. *International Journal of Pediatric Otorhinolaryngology,* **10,** 191–199

HIRSCHBERG, J. (1980) Acoustic analysis of pathological cries, stridors and coughing sounds in infancy. *International Journal of Pediatric Otorhinolaryngology,* **2,** 287–300

KELEMEN, G. (1953) Congenital laryngeal stridor. *Archives of Otolaryngology,* **58,** 245–268

LANE, R. W., WEIDER, D. J., STEINEM, C. and MARIN-PADILLA, M. (1984) Laryngomalacia. A review and case report of surgical treatment with resolution of pectus excavatum. *Archives of Otolaryngology,* **110,** 546–555

MACDONALD, R. E. and FEARON, B. (1971) Innominate artery compression syndrome in children. *Annals of Otology, Rhinology and Laryngology,* **80,** 535–540

MORI, M., KINOSHITA, K., MORINARI, H., SHIRAISHI, T., KOIKE, S. and MURAO, S. (1980) Waveform and spectral analysis of crackles. *Thorax,* **35,** 843–850

ONIONS, C. T. (1978) Editor. *The Oxford Dictionary of English Etymology.* Oxford: Clarendon Press

PRACY, R. (1965) Stridor in children. *Proceedings of the Royal Society of Medicine,* **58,** 267–270

PRACY, R. (1979) Congenital diseases of the larynx. In *Scott-Brown's Diseases of the Ear, Nose and Throat,* 4th edn, edited by J. Ballantyne and J. Groves, vol. 4, pp. 309–328. London: Butterworths

SCHWARTZ, R., RODRIGUEZ, W., KAHN, W. and ROSS, S. (1978) The increasing incidence of ampicillin resistant *Haemophilus influenzae.* A cause of otitis media. *Journal of the American Medical Association,* **239,** 320–323

VALVASSORI, G. E., POTTER, G. D., HANAFEE, W. N., CARTER, B. L. and BUCKINGHAM, R. A. (1984) *Radiography of the Ear, Nose and Throat.* Philadelphia: W. B. Saunders

28

Neonatal pulmonary disorders

R. Dinwiddie

The establishment of breathing and the adaptation of the neonatal circulation to extrauterine life are two of the most important events which occur at the time of birth. These physiological changes are mediated by a number of factors acting both systemically and locally, but the major control of these events is via the respiratory centres in the brainstem. It is thus vital that these are present in an intact and functional state if the adaptation to extrauterine life is to occur uneventfully. Most of the diseases seen in the neonatal period are a consequence of adverse factors affecting these normal physiological processes, such as immaturity, infection, damage at the time of birth, or congenital malformation.

Onset of breathing

The onset of breathing is brought about by the responses to a number of complex reflexes which stimulate the respiratory centres. These include thermal stimulation such as cold, external sensory stimulation, particularly tactile, and intrinsic reflexes within the rib cage as the chest changes in shape secondary to the pressure applied during and immediately after the birth process itself. Biochemical changes, such as hypoxaemia and hypercarbia also have an important stimulatory effect on the central nervous system, as do the acute pressure changes within the cardiovascular system which occur secondary to clamping of the umbilical cord. The inspiratory pressures required to open the lungs are thought to be relatively low, of the order of 10–20 cmH$_2$O, which is sufficient to overcome the resistive forces of the lungs, the residual fluid within them and the chest wall (Milner and Vyas, 1982). A functional residual capacity (FRC) is established within the first few breaths and a positive expiratory force is exerted during the later part of each breath in order to aid the clearance of lung liquid. The normal functional residual capacity of the newborn is approximately 30 ml/kg and this lung volume is stabilized during the first 30–60 minutes of life (Klaus *et al.*, 1962).

The lungs are normally filled with surfactant rich fluid *in utero* at the same volume as the subsequent functional residual capacity after birth. This liquid is emptied from the lungs during and after the birth process, partly by external compression of the chest as it passes through the vagina, or the uterine wall in the case of caesarean section. This accounts for approximately one-third of the lung liquid, the remaining fluid is absorbed directly across the pulmonary lymphatics or into the pulmonary capillaries during the first minutes after birth (Strang, 1977).

These changes in lung volume and compliance are matched by major circulatory adaptation which occurs simultaneously. Before birth only about 10% of the cardiac output passes through the lungs because of the high pulmonary vascular resistance and the fact that the lungs are not being used to sustain oxygenation. After birth the aeration of the lungs produces a rapid reduction in pulmonary vascular resistance and this is accompanied by a rise in $P_{a}O_2$ from the intrauterine levels of 4 kPa (30 mmHg) to the postnatal level of 8–12 kPa (50–90 mmHg); these changes stimulate the closure of the ductus arteriosus and foramen ovale, thus closing off the large right to left intracardiac shunts which are present before birth. These fetal channels are not, however, irreversibly closed at this stage and may re-open during periods of stress and hypoxia.

Central control of breathing is vital to the

maintenance of life and the respiratory centres must be maintained intact throughout this period. They are particularly sensitive to asphyxial insult, including hypoxia and hypercarbia associated with respiratory and metabolic acidosis. They may be damaged by trauma or by localized areas of haemorrhage during a difficult or protracted delivery. They are also sensitive to the effects of drugs such as pethidine given to the mother before birth for sedation or analgesia. Any interruption to these normal physiological processes will result in birth asphyxia.

Birth asphyxia

Asphyxia at birth may be acute of chronic. Some babies suffer from acute lack of oxygen during the birth process, for example as a consequence of cord prolapse, while others may have had chronic intrauterine asphyxia as a result of postmaturity or placental dysfunction secondary to hypertensive changes.

The major groups of conditions leading to birth asphyxia may be divided into three categories, maternal, placental/cord related and fetal. Maternal predisposing factors include hypertension, diabetes, underlying cardiac or renal disease, abuse of drugs or alcohol, hypotension, or anaesthetic complications such as aspiration. Other causes include multiple births, abnormal presentation, cephalopelvic disproportion and prolonged labour. Placental problems will include abruption, placenta praevia, early separation and cord prolapse. Fetal conditions include pulmonary hypoplasia, anaemia secondary to Rhesus disease, intrauterine meconium aspiration and congenital malformations, particularly of the lungs or heart.

The events which occur during an asphyxial episode have been well described by Dawes *et al.* (1963). The asphyxiated infant gasps initially and this is followed by a period of primary apnoea during which there is a decrease in heart rate, but maintenance of blood pressure and peripheral circulation; hypoxaemia results in profound cyanosis. Resuscitation during this period will be effective by the use of external stimulation and the application of oxygen which will be inhaled during the next phase of breathing, beginning 1–2 minutes later. This secondary gasping period lasts for a further 4–5 minutes following which terminal apnoea occurs. At this stage there is profound hypoxia, hypercarbia, acidosis and circulatory collapse. After 7–8 minutes of significant hypoxia cerebral damage will begin (*Figure 28.1*). Resuscitation at this stage requires positive pressure ventilation, usually following endotracheal intubation utilizing pressures of up to 20–30 cm with an initial breath of 3–5 seconds (Vyas *et al.*, 1981). Bag

and mask ventilation may also be effective in the absence of personnel skilled in intubation. Circulatory support by external cardiac massage is essential in those with profound bradycardia or cardiac arrest. Drugs such as glucose, sodium bicarbonate and calcium gluconate may also be required. Adrenaline may be given via the endotracheal tube in those with profound circulatory depression (Greenberg, Roberts and Baskin, 1981). Reversal of maternal sedative drugs such as pethidine, which prolongs the period of primary apnoea, may also be achieved by the use of parenteral naloxone.

After acute resuscitation severely asphyxiated infants may require extensive support including ventilation, maintenance of blood pressure and stimulation of cardiac output, control of renal failure and acid–base balance. Neurological outcome also depends on the control of seizures and cerebral oedema in the perinatal period. The

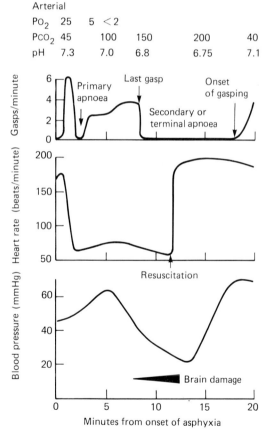

Figure 28.1 Changes in Rhesus monkeys during asphyxia and on resuscitation by positive-pressure ventilation. Brain damage was assessed by histological examination some weeks or months later. (From Dawes 1968 with kind permission of the author and publisher Year Book Medical Publishers, Chicago)

outcome is extremely variable, although a very significant proportion of those who survive the initial neonatal period may turn out to be normal (Thompson, Searle, and Russell, 1977).

Hyaline membrane disease

Hyaline membrane disease (HMD) is the commonest cause of respiratory difficulty in this age group and remains the major cause of mortality and morbidity in the neonatal period. Its incidence is inversely proportional to birth weight and it is particularly prevalent in babies who weigh less than 1.5 kg at birth and whose gestation is less than 32 weeks. The illness is caused primarily by surfactant deficiency (Avery and Mead, 1959). Other predisposing factors include birth asphyxia, caesarean section without labour, maternal haemorrhage, maternal diabetes and multiple pregnancy.

The infant typically develops signs of respiratory difficulty within the first 2 hours after birth. These include indrawing of respiratory muscles, rapid respiratory rate, sternal recession and the classical grunt heard on expiration – a mechanism used to maintain oxygen levels (Harrison, Heese and Klein, 1968). The chest X-ray typically shows a ground glass appearance secondary to alveolar hypoventilation and air bronchogram due to maintenance of large airway patency of the cartilage content. The differential diagnosis must include group B streptococcal pneumonia (Pyati *et al.*, 1981), persistent fetal circulation (Fox and Duara, 1983), and underlying cardiac abnormalities such as transposition of the great arteries.

Treatment

Treatment of hyaline membrane disease is complex. Prevention of preterm delivery is desirable wherever possible, antenatal steroids may stimulate lung maturity in selected patients (Liggins and Howie, 1972). More recently, the replacement of surfactant artificially has begun to achieve some success, although the benefits remain short lived (Morley, 1984). Standard treatment for hyaline membrane disease is shown in *Table 28.1*.

The use of mechanical ventilation in conjunction with positive end expiratory pressure (PEEP) has been the mainstay of respiratory support for infants with hyaline membrane disease over the last 20 years. However, this treatment carries a significant risk of side-effects such as induction of pneumothorax or subsequent bronchopulmonary dysplasia and should therefore not be instituted unless significant respiratory failure is present. Indications for its introduction include significant

Table 28.1 Treatment of hyaline membrane disease

Neutral thermal environment
Maintenance of fluid balance
Oxygen P_aO_2 7–12 kPa (70–90 mmHg)
Correction of acid–base imbalance
Continuous positive airway pressure (CPAP)
Artificial ventilation
Paralysis
Pulmonary vasodilators (tolazoline)
Antibiotics for other causes (group B streptococci)

apnoea or impending exhaustion of the infant, inability to maintain P_aO_2 above 8 kPa (60 mmHg) in 60% oxygen or P_aCO_2 below 8 kPa (60 mmHg). Most neonatal ventilators available at present are pressure limited, time cycled, constant flow generators, which produce a square wave input and which are applied at peak inspiratory pressures of less than 20 cmH$_2$O, initially at rates of 30–35 breaths per minute, inspiratory time 0.3–0.5 seconds and with positive end expiratory pressure of 3–4 cmH$_2$O. More recently, rapid rate ventilation of 60–120 breaths per minute has been under investigation (Field, Milner and Hopkin, 1984). High frequency ventilation, utilizing jet ventilators or an oscillator pump circuit, has also been evaluated in this condition (Frantz, Werthammer and Stark, 1983). Treatment is not without hazard to the infant, and a number of important complications are commonly seen including pneumothorax (Greenhough *et al.*, 1984) – this may be prevented by selective paralysis – subglottic stenosis from prolonged endotracheal intubation, secondary infection and subsequent bronchopulmonary dysplasia (Northway, Rosan and Porter, 1967). Nowadays, with adequate support, 95% of infants suffering from significant hyaline membrane disease may expect to survive (Greenhough and Roberton, 1985), although the mortality rate remains significantly greater in those infants weighing less than 1 kg (Yu, Zhao and Bajuk, 1982). The ultimate prognosis for lung function is good providing that there has not been significant associated bronchopulmonary dysplasia.

Transient tachypnoea of the newborn

This condition is seen in a number of infants who show signs of respiratory distress, including tachypnoea, indrawing and cyanosis, lasting from 12 to 24 hours and sometimes longer. The chest X-ray shows mild bilateral haziness secondary to persistent interstitial lung fluid. These infants have a good prognosis and require basic supportive care and oxygen therapy with adequate control of blood gases. Very few require ventilation. The recovery is usually fairly rapid and the long-term outlook is excellent (Yu, 1986a). This disease is more common in infants born after caesarean section, probably because less fluid is squeezed from the lungs during the birth process itself so some of these infants may have a lower initial functional residual capacity (Milner, Saunders and Hopkin, 1978).

Patent ductus arteriosus

Patent ductus arteriosus is uncommon among normal term infants. It is, however, extremely common in infants with hyaline membrane disease, reaching levels of over 40% in those under 1 kg and 20% in those between 1.0 and 1.5 kg at birth (Ellison *et al.*, 1983). It is more common in those who have higher fluid intakes (Bell *et al.*, 1980).

Many preterm infants, especially those with hyaline membrane disease, develop classical signs of patent ductus arteriosus during the first 3 or 4 days of life, these include tachycardia, bounding peripheral pulses, a murmur below the mid-clavicular region, which gradually becomes continuous, and a palpable systolic thrill over the precordium. During the latter part of the first week of life the shunt in these babies becomes increasingly left to right in nature and this leads to pulmonary oedema and decreased lung compliance. The infant commonly has an associated increase in ventilatory requirements as this process occurs and often develops secondary infection in the lungs at this stage. The liver is also frequently enlarged and this indicates the onset of cardiac failure. Diagnosis may be confirmed utilizing echocardiography which will also exclude other underlying cardiac lesions. Chest X-ray shows cardiomegaly and plethoric lung fields in addition to the background pulmonary shadowing present from the hyaline membrane disease.

Management initially includes restriction of fluid intake to 60–70% of daily requirement, diuretic therapy and increased end expiratory pressure to reduce pulmonary oedema. If these measures fail to produce significant reduction in ductal shunting within 24–48 hours then indomethacin, a prostaglandin synthetase inhibitor, is given in a dose of 0.2 mg/kg per day in two divided doses over 2–3 days. This has been shown to produce a satisfactory response in most infants in a large multicentre trial (Gersony *et al.*, 1983). A significant proportion will re-open subsequently but, in many cases, a satisfactory response is produced which allows weaning of the infant from the ventilator. If these measures fail then surgical ligation, preferably undertaken in the neonatal unit, is performed.

Persistent pulmonary hypertension (persistent fetal circulation)

Persistent fetal circulation occurs when the normal reduction in pulmonary vascular resistance fails to occur after birth. The normal stimuli for this process include the increased oxygen levels after breathing starts and the changes in circulatory pressures which occur with clamping of the cord. Increased tone of the pulmonary arterioles may be brought about by persistent hypoxia, especially in the presence of acidosis, and this results in an attempt by the newborn to revert to the fetal circulatory pattern. This complication may occur in babies with hyaline membrane disease, but is particularly likely to happen in those who have had intrauterine asphyxia. It is also seen in infants with meconium aspiration syndrome (Fox *et al.*, 1977) and in those with group B streptococcal septicaemia. It is difficult in some cases to distinguish this from cyanotic congenital heart disease and echocardiography is required to exclude underlying cardiac lesions.

Treatment consists of ventilatory support and an attempt to increase the pH to more than 7.48. At this level pulmonary vasodilatation is more likely to occur. Hyperventilation reducing the P_aCO_2 to 3.5–4 kPa (25–30 mmHg) may assist this process (Drummond *et al.*, 1981). Administration of sodium bicarbonate may also improve the pH. If hyperventilation fails to produce an adequate response infusion of tolazoline in a dose of 1–2 mg/kg may produce an improvement in P_aO_2 and this should be followed with a continuous infusion at the same dosage/kg per hour if a satisfactory response occurs.

Tolazoline may also produce systemic hypotension and in this situation the baby will need to be supported with colloids in the form of plasma or blood transfusion and some may require dopamine in addition to maintain blood pressure.

Meconium aspiration syndrome

The passage of meconium before birth may be present in 8–15% of deliveries. In a study of 1000 consecutive births Gregory *et al.* (1974) demonstrated the wide variability of X-ray changes and disease, with an overall incidence of 1.6% of neonates producing symptoms. The disease is most commonly seen in term or postmature infants and is much less common in preterm infants (Ting and Brady, 1975). The most dangerous consequence of the passage of meconium is its aspiration into the lower respiratory tract. Since it is usually a response to intrauterine asphyxia it is not uncommonly associated with the presence of fetal gasping and meconium may readily be aspirated into the trachea or even into the peripheral parts of the lung before or during birth itself. The results of this process may produce profound effects on the respiratory system. Large plugs can obstruct the main airway, leading to acute asphyxia, smaller amounts aspirated into the peripheral airways will cause partial obstruction secondary to chemical pneumonitis and lead to significant overinflation, or collapse and atelectasis of adjacent lung tissue. This results in a high functional residual capacity with generalized overinflation and areas of marked ventilation–perfusion abnormality. Air leak with pneumothorax and pneumomediastinum is common and may be seen in as many as 40–50% of severely affected cases. There is also frequently an associated persistent pulmonary hypertension secondary to the asphyxial insult and this further contributes to the profound hypoxia which is present in those with the worst disease (Fox *et al.*, 1977).

The disease is preventable with adequate antenatal care and the rapid delivery of infants who show signs of intrauterine distress. At birth it is vital to clear the airway by adequate suction of the trachea (Ting and Brady, 1975). After this procedure the infant should be observed for signs of respiratory distress. A chest X-ray should be performed in all who show any signs of respiratory difficulty. Treatment thereafter is supportive and includes correction of acid–base imbalance, antibiotics because of possible secondary bacterial infection and ventilatory support when indicated. Those who fail to respond to ventilation by the demonstration of persistent hypoxia have a very poor prognosis (Vidyasagar *et al.*, 1975). Paralysis may be helpful (Runkle and Bancalari, 1984) and tolazoline should be given to those who have evidence of significant pulmonary hypertension. This condition continues to carry a significant mortality and a number of survivors have chronic lung disease secondary to the pressures required to ventilate them, these result in bronchopulmonary dysplasia. The long-term prognosis, in the vast majority of cases, is however, for normal lung function.

Infections

Neonatal pneumonia

Pneumonia in the neonatal period is extremely common particularly in babies who have other respiratory problems. It may be acquired before, during or after birth. The causative organisms may be bacterial or viral. The most serious bacterial pneumonia at present is due to the group B β-haemolytic streptococcus. Up to 15% of mothers may harbour this organism in the birth canal and the infants will be in contact with this during normal birth. Less than 1% of such infants become significantly ill (Pyati *et al.*, 1981), but the mortality in this group is extremely high. Predisposing factors include preterm delivery, prolonged rupture of the membranes and birth asphyxia. Presenting features are identical to hyaline membrane disease, with tachypnoea, indrawing, respiratory distress and cyanosis. Chest X-ray shows a ground glass appearance with bilateral generalized opacity present indistinguishable from hyaline membrane disease. In these cases the condition may be rapidly fatal unless early and appropriate antibiotics are given. Most babies at this stage are septicaemic and may show other complicating features such as disseminated intravascular coagulation.

Treatment consists of circulatory support and antibiotics, usually penicillin and gentamicin, or a third generation cephalosporin such as cefotaxime or ceftazidime. Other management consists of full intensive care including ventilation, maintenance of cardiovascular stability and the prevention of hypoxia and acidosis. Despite early and aggressive therapy the mortality for those with rapidly progressive disease remains extremely high and is of the order of 60%.

A number of other bacteria may cause neonatal pneumonia including staphylococci. *Staphylococcus aureus* or *Staph. epidermidis* may be found in respiratory secretions among babies who are being ventilated, also *Pneumococcus* and *Listeria monocytogenes*. Gram-negative organisms, such as *Escherichia coli*, *Klebsiella* and particularly *Pseudomonas aeruginosa* are more commonly found in infants who have chronic lung disease and are often acquired via the ventilator and its humidification system.

Chlamydia and fungi

Chlamydia trachomatis has recently been shown to cause pneumonia in neonates and should be sought in those who have persistent symptoms or those who do not respond to usual antibiotic therapy (Frommell *et al.*, 1979). Fungi, including *Candida albicans*, have recently been seen more frequently, particularly among debilitated neonates who have required repeated courses of antibacterial agents to control chronic chest infections. Extended treatment with appropriate parenteral antifungal agents is necessary.

Viral pneumonia

Viral pneumonia, particularly due to organisms such as cytomegalovirus, is also being increasingly recognized in the neonatal period. Recent surveys have shown that as many as 0.3–1% of neonates have passively acquired cytomegalovirus in the upper airway at the time of birth (Peckham *et al.*, 1983). These infants may develop persistent pneumonitis, which can lead to recurrent episodes of wheezing and clinically evident respiratory infection. The organism is also readily cultured from the urine in such cases. Another important virus is rubella which may cause interstitial pneumonitis (Boner *et al.*, 1983). Herpes simplex types 1 and 2 are other causes of generalized infection and fatal lung disease in a small number of neonates, although this may be amenable to antiviral agents such as acyclovir.

Bronchopulmonary dysplasia

Bronchopulmonary dysplasia (BPD) is a chronic lung condition which has become increasingly frequent as more small babies have survived after intensive support with extended periods of oxygen therapy and mechanical ventilation. The incidence of the condition varies between 6 and 25% and is more common among those under 1 kg (Yu *et al.*, 1983a). The aetiology is multifactorial and the classical changes were originally described by Northway, Rosan and Porter in 1967. Contributory factors include inhibition of mucociliary clearance secondary to endotracheal intubation, barotrauma from extended ventilatory support especially at high pressures, oxygen toxicity, chronic infection of the lower respiratory tract and hypersecretion secondary to the chronic respiratory disease. Other contributory factors may include pulmonary oedema and patent ductus arteriosus (O'Brodovich and Mellins, 1985). Vitamin deficiencies, including vitamins A and D and phosphate deficiency resulting in rickets and vitamin E deficiency have also been proposed as contributory factors. Infants developing bronchopulmonary dysplasia remain ventilator dependent after the first 3–4 weeks of life. In the most severe cases they may be ventilator dependent and subsequently oxygen dependent for many months.

Chest X-ray shows widespread overinflation, particularly in the lower zones, with fibrosis and loss of lung volume present throughout the lungs, but particularly in the upper zones. In the most severe cases these changes worsen with time and with intercurrent infections cardiac failure supervenes. Feeding, weight gain and growth may be extremely difficult to achieve in those who remain persistently hypoxic despite intensive support (Yu *et al.*, 1983b).

Treatment consists of adequate oxygenation, diuretics, theophylline and other bronchodilators where indicated, adequate vitamins including vitamins A, D and E and antibiotics for intercurrent infections. Steroids may be helpful (Mammell *et al.*, 1983) and their role is currently under further investigation. Those who survive show gradual improvement in lung function. There is also a considerably higher incidence of sudden infant death syndrome in this group. Those with milder disease may have virtually normal lung function after recovery and particularly after the first 2 years of life, during which time respiratory infections appear to be especially common.

Recurrent apnoea

This is an extremely common condition of preterm babies and is a variation from the normal pattern of periodic breathing which is seen at this age. Significant apnoea may be defined as episodes of cessation of breathing lasting 20 seconds or more, or less than 20 seconds if accompanied by bradycardia of significance (American Academy of Pediatrics, 1978). They occur for a variety of reasons including infections, for example pneumonia, meningitis or septicaemia, metabolic acidosis, hypoglycaemia, secondary to seizures or intracranial haemorrhage, respiratory depression from drugs and as a result of exhaustion in relation to respiratory or cardiac failure. They may be of central origin indicating immaturity of the respiratory centres. Upper airway obstruction such as cleft palate, choanal atresia or micrognathia will also contribute to such symptoms. Prior to treatment babies should receive full investigation for underlying disorders. These should be corrected whenever possible.

Those for whom no underlying pathology is found, except for immaturity of the respiratory centres, may respond to the administration of theophylline which is more effective than continuous positive airway pressure (Jones, 1982). It is important to ensure that the baby is not anaemic or chronically hypoxic or acidotic, as correction of these abnormalities will reduce the incidence of the apnoeic attacks. Those who have severe apnoea may require ventilation until such time as the respiratory system has matured and they are able to sustain an adequate breathing pattern spontaneously.

Congenital anomalies of the respiratory tract

These include abnormalities of the nose, palate, pharynx, larynx, trachea and major bronchi, lungs, ribcage and neuromuscular disorders. The range of lesions seen is shown in *Table 28.2*.

Table 28.2 Congenital anomalies of the respiratory tract

Upper respiratory
Choanal atresia
Cleft lip and/or palate
Pierre Robin syndrome

Larynx
Laryngomalacia
Stenosis
Cleft
Web
Vocal cord paralysis
Atresia

Obstructive lesions of larynx
Haemangioma
Cysts
Papilloma

Tracheobronchial lesions
Tracheo-oesophageal fistula with or without
    oesophageal atresia
Tracheal pouch
Tracheomalacia
Tracheal stenosis
Tracheal agenesis
Bronchial stenosis
Bronchial agenesis

Extrinsic lesions
Vascular ring
Aberrant innominate artery
Duplication cyst

Intrapulmonary lesions
Congenital lobar emphysema
Congenital lung cysts
Cystic adenomatoid malformation
Pulmonary sequestration
Pulmonary hypoplasia
Pulmonary agenesis

Diaphragm
Diaphragmatic hernia
Eventration of diaphragm
Paralysis of diaphragm

Rib cage
Asphyxiating thoracic dystrophy
Camptomelic dwarfism
Hypophosphatasia
Osteogenesis imperfecta

Neuromuscular disease
Congenital spinal muscular atrophy (Werdnig-Hoffman)
Neonatal myotonic dystrophy
Congenital myasthenia gravis

Diseases of the upper respiratory tract and larynx are considered elsewhere in this volume and will not be discussed further at this stage. Disorders of the lower respiratory tree, below the larynx, are discussed in the following sections.

Trachea

Tracheal stenosis may be congenital or acquired. These infants present with biphasic stridor and respiratory difficulty, which is not always present at birth but which may become evident during an intercurrent respiratory infection. Wheezing is another common presenting feature due to retention of lung secretions below the level of the obstruction. Tracheal stenosis is more commonly caused by scarring secondary to prolonged endotracheal intubation. Direct tracheal surgery is an extremely high risk procedure and most children will be treated with a tracheostomy until subsequent tracheal enlargement, either spontaneous or surgically induced, occurs as age increases. Tracheal atresia is an extremely rare lesion and not usually compatible with life. It is commonly associated with congenital malformations of the oesophagus since the two structures have a common embryological origin. Tracheomalacia is due to weakening of the tracheal wall, either spontaneously or in association with an extrinsic compressive lesion such as an aberrant blood vessel or vascular ring. It is also commonly found at the site of a tracheo-oesophageal fistula. Infants with tracheomalacia may suffer from respiratory difficulties, particularly during intercurrent infection, and during expiration when positive expiratory pressure in the lungs compresses the tracheal wall and causes collapse of the airway. If major apnoeic attacks are occurring as a consequence of this then aortopexy may be necessary (Filler, Rossello and Lebnowitz, 1976).

Extrinsic lesions

Lesions outside the trachea or major bronchi may produce respiratory obstruction by pressure on the airway, these include aberrant blood vessels (Westaby *et al.*, 1984), hyperdynamic arteries in association with a cardiac lesion causing large left to right shunt, and bronchogenic cysts. Cystic hygroma may also produce tracheal compression if it lies in the upper mediastinum and particularly if there is sudden haemorrhage into it which can occasionally occur.

Vascular rings occur in various types and may produce localized pressure on the trachea and oesophagus. This may result in secondary tracheomalacia, which may be persistent postoperatively (Roesler *et al.*, 1983). Vascular rings take various forms including double aortic arch 54%, right aortic arch and left ligamentum arteriosum 16%, anomalous subclavian artery 12%, pulmonary artery sling 12%, anomalous innominate artery 6%. Treatment is operative to re-route the aberrant vessels and to allow natural growth of the trachea and recovery of the tracheomalacia.

Lung abnormalities

Congenital lung cysts

Congenital lung cysts may be found incidentally on the chest X-ray when it is taken for other reasons, but are more commonly noticed when they become infected. They may be difficult to differentiate from pneumatocoeles, particularly in staphylococcal infection. After the acute phase they are persistent whereas infective pneumatocoeles usually disappear with time. They may also be seen in a sequestered lobe of the lung which has become infected and this too must be excluded by subsequent investigation using ventilation perfusion lung scan. Treatment is by surgical removal since there is a high risk of recurrent infection for these children in the future.

Cystic adenomatoid malformation

This abnormality is often found in the neonatal period when it may be associated with inability to establish normal breathing. It is also seen as a persistent shadowing on the chest X-ray, either as an area of apparent non-aeration or with multicystic lesions present. These are most commonly found in the right middle lobe, although the upper lobes may also be affected (Yu, 1986b). Treatment is surgical in all cases after resolution of any underlying infection. The prognosis after the removal of the cyst is usually extremely good and the rest of the lung compensates well for the area which has been removed.

Congenital lobar emphysema

This condition is thought to be due to an abnormality of the bronchial or mucosal lining of the associated airway. It is most frequently due to abnormal development of the cartilage within the airway, but may be secondary to extrinsic airway compression by a cyst, tumour or a blood vessel. The lobe progressively overinflates and presses on the surrounding lung. This will result in respiratory distress, wheezing and reduced air entry over the affected lobe. Most cases present in infancy, but a few are found incidentally in later childhood and are relatively asymptomatic at this time. The lobes are affected with the following frequency, left upper, right middle, right upper, and rarely the lower lobes. A significant proportion of patients have associated cardiac disease and this should be excluded by echocardiography.

Treatment consists of lobectomy in those who have significant symptoms, particularly in the younger child. Those with few symptoms may be treated conservatively and a number will improve with natural growth and development. The long-term lung function after surgery is good (McBride *et al.*, 1980).

Lobar sequestration

These are areas of non-functioning lung tissue derived from abnormal embryonic development. They have aberrant connections to the tracheobronchial tree and an abnormal blood supply. They may be divided into two major groups – extralobar and intralobar. The extralobar type, which has its own separate pleura and an arterial blood supply usually from the aorta, may communicate with the trachea or bronchi or occasionally with the gut. Intralobar sequestrations lie within the visceral pleura and are intimately associated with normal lung tissue. They may have tracheobronchial communication, but usually ventilate extremely poorly, they also have a systemic blood supply. Repeated infection in these lobes is not uncommon. On dynamic imaging they show extremely poor ventilation and no perfusion because they are not supplied from the pulmonary vascular bed. Treatment is by surgical removal, since repeated infections commonly occur in these lesions.

Pulmonary agenesis

Unilateral pulmonary agenesis may be asymptomatic and found on incidental chest X-ray. There is, however, a significant incidence of related congenital malformations particularly affecting the vertebral column and the cardiovascular system. Chest X-rays show an opaque hemithorax with the heart shifted to the affected side. There is no specific treatment and the prognosis for lung function is good since the unaffected lung usually compensates to a very significant degree.

Bilateral pulmonary hypoplasia occurs in relation to a number of neonatal problems including renal agenesis (Potter's syndrome). It is also seen after prolonged amniotic fluid leak, intrauterine hydrops and skeletal abnormalities such as asphyxiating thoracic dystrophy. The outlook in this condition depends to a great extent on the degree of hypoplasia that is present. Severe cases are incompatible with life. Unilateral pulmonary hypoplasia occurs in association with diaphragmatic hernia.

Rib cage abnormalities

Abnormalities of the rib cage occur in a number of neonatal syndromes, including asphyxiating thoracic dystrophy, camptomelic dwarfism, hypophosphatasia and osteogenesis imperfecta. Many of these are lethal in the neonatal period, although a number of cases have survived beyond this time with intensive respiratory support and surgery to enlarge the chest cavity.

Neuromuscular disease

A number of infants are born with congenital neuromuscular disease which may be present at birth. Some infants have similar symptoms following severe birth asphyxia. The most common disease of this type is congenital spinal muscular atrophy (Werdnig-Hoffman disease), which presents with weakness, poor respiratory effort, feeding problems and often a history of poor intrauterine fetal movements. Most infants die of respiratory failure secondary to associated swallowing difficulties and recurrent aspiration. Other conditions producing similar problems include neonatal myotonic dystrophy and congenital myasthenia gravis.

References

AMERICAN ACADEMY OF PEDIATRICS (1978) Task force on prolonged apnea. *Pediatrics*, **61**, 651–652

AVERY, N. E. and MEAD, J. (1959) Surface properties in relation to atelactasis and hyaline membrane disease. *American Journal of Diseases in Children*, **97**, 517–523

BELL, E., WARBURTON, D., STONESTREET, B. S. and OH, W. (1980) Effect of fluid administration on the development of symptomatic PDA and congestive heart failure in premature infants. *New England Journal of Medicine*, **302**, 598–604

BONER, A., WILMOTT, R. W., DINWIDDIE, R., JEFFRIES, J. G., MATTHEW, D. J., MARSHALL, W. C. *et al.*, (1983) Desquamative interstitial pneumonia and antigen-antibody complexes in two infants with congenital rubella. *Pediatrics*, **72**, 835–839

DAWES, G. S. (1968) *Foetal and Neonatal Physiology; a Comparative Study of Changes at Birth*, pp. 141–159. Chicago: Year Book Medical Publishers

DAWES, G. S., JACOBSON, H. N., MOTT, J. C., SHELLEY, H. J. and STAFFORD, A. (1963) Treatment of asphyxia in newborn lambs and monkeys. *Journal of Physiology*, **169**, 167–184

DRUMMOND, W. H., GREGORY, G. A., HEYMANN, N. A. and PHIBBS, R. A. (1981) The independent effects of hyperventilation, tolazoline and dopamine on infants with persistent pulmonary hypertension. *Journal of Pediatrics*, **98**, 603–611

ELLISON, R. C., PECKHAM, G. J., LANG, P., TALNER, N. S., LENER, T. J., LIN, L. *et al.* (1983) Evaluation of the preterm infant for patent ductus arteriosus. *Pediatrics*, **71**, 364–372

FIELD, D. J., MILNER, A. D. and HOPKIN, I. E. (1984) High and conventional rates of positive pressure ventilation. *Archives of Disease in Childhood*, **59**, 1151–1154

FILLER, R. M., ROSSELLO, P. J. and LEBNOWITZ, R. L. (1976) Life threatening anoxic spells caused by tracheal compression after repair of esophageal atresia: correction by surgery. *Journal of Pediatric Surgery*, **11**, 739–748

FOX, W. W. and DUARA, S. (1983) Persistent pulmonary hypertension in the neonate – diagnosis and management. *Journal of Pediatrics*, **103**, 505–514

FOX, W. W., GEWITZ, M. H., DINWIDDIE, R., DRUMMOND, W. H. and PECKHAM, G. J. (1977) Pulmonary hypertension in the perinatal aspiration syndromes. *Pediatrics*, **59**, 205–209

FRANTZ, I. D., WERTHAMMER, J. and STARK, A. R. (1983) High frequency ventilation in premature infants with lung disease, adequate gas exchange at lower tracheal pressure. *Pediatrics*, **71**, 483–488

FROMMELL, G. J., ROTHENBERG, R., WANG, S. and MacINTOSH, K. (1979) Chlamydial infection of mothers and their infants. *Journal of Pediatrics*, **95**, 28–32

GERSONY, W. M., PECKHAM, G. J., ELLISON, R. S., MIETTINEN, O. S. and NADAS, A. S. (1983) Effects of indomethacin in premature infants with patent ductus arteriosus: results of a national collaborative study. *Journal of Pediatrics*, **102**, 895–906

GREENBERG, M. I., ROBERTS, J. R. and BASKIN, S. I. (1981) Use of endotracheally administered epinephrine on a pediatric patient. *American Journal of Diseases of Children*, **135**, 767–768

GREENHOUGH, A. and ROBERTON, N. R. C. (1985) Morbidity and survival of neonates ventilated for the respiratory distress syndrome. *British Medical Journal*, **290**, 597–600

GREENHOUGH, A., MORLEY, C. J., WOOD, S. and DAVIES, J. A. (1984) Pancuronium prevents pneumothoraces in ventilated premature babies who actively expire against positive pressure inflation. *The Lancet*, **1**, 1–3

GREGORY, G. A., GOODING, C. A., PHIBBS, R. H. and TOOLEY, W. H. (1974) Meconium aspiration in infants – a prospective study. *Journal of Pediatrics*, **85**, 848–852

HARRISON, V. C., HEESE, H. de V. and KLEIN, M. (1968) The significance of grunting in hyaline membrane disease. *Pediatrics*, **41**, 549–559

JONES, R. A. K. (1982) Apneoa of prematurity – 1: a controlled trial of theophylline and face mask continuous positive airway pressure. *Archives of Disease in Childhood*, **57**, 761–764

KLAUS, M., TOOLEY, W. H., WEAVER, K. J. and CLEMENTS, J. A. (1962) Lung volume in the newborn infant. *Pediatrics*, **30**, 111–116

LIGGINS, G. C. and HOWIE, R. N. (1972) A controlled trial of antepartum glucocorticoid treatment for the prevention of respiratory distress syndrome in premature infants. *Pediatrics*, **50**, 515–525

McBRIDE, J. T., WOHL, M. E., STRIEDER, D. J., JACKSON, A. C., MORTON, J. R., ZWERDLING, R. G. *et al.* (1980) Lung growth and airway function after lobectomy in infancy for congenital lobar emphysema. *Journal of Clinical Investigation*, **66**, 962–970

MAMMEL, M. C., GREEN, T. P., JOHNSON, D. E. and THOMPSON, T. R. (1983) Controlled trial of dexamethasone therapy in infants with bronchopulmonary dysplasia. *The Lancet*, **1**, 1356–1358

MILNER, A. D. and VYAS, H. (1982) Lung expansion at birth. *Journal of Pediatrics*, **101**, 879–886

MILNER, A. D., SAUNDERS, R. A. and HOPKIN, I. E. (1978) Effect of delivery by caesarean section of lung mechanics and lung volume on the human neonate. *Archives of Disease in Childhood*, **53**, 545–548

MORLEY, C. J. (1984) Surfactant treatment for respiratory distress syndrome – a review. *Journal of the Royal Society of Medicine,* **77,** 788–792

NORTHWAY, W. H., ROSAN, R. C. and PORTER, D. Y. (1967) Pulmonary disease following respirator therapy of hyaline membrane disease. Bronchopulmonary dysplasia. *New England Journal of Medicine,* **276,** 357–368

O'BRODOVICH, H. M. and MELLINS, R. B. (1985) Bronchopulmonary dysplasia – state of the art. *American Review of Respiratory Diseases,* **132,** 694–700

PECKHAM, C. S., CHIN, K. S., COLEMAN, J. C., HENDERSON, K., HURLEY, R. and PREECE, P. M. (1983) Cytomegalovirus infection in pregnancy: preliminary findings from a prospective study. *The Lancet,* **1,** 1352–1355

PYATI, S. P., PILDES, R. S., RAMAMURTHY, R. S. and JACOBS, N. (1981) Decreasing mortality in neonates with early onset group B streptococcal infection: reality or artifact. *Journal of Pediatrics,* **98,** 625–627

ROESLER, N., DE LEVAL, M., CHRISPIN, A. and STARK, J. (1983) Surgical management of vascular ring. *Annals of Surgery,* **197,** 139–146

RUNKLE, B. and BANCALARI, E. (1984) Acute cardiopulmonary effects of pancuronium bromide in mechanically ventilated newborn infants. *Journal of Pediatrics,* **104,** 614–617

STRANG, L. B. (1977) Editor. Lung liquid absorption. In *Neonatal Respiration, Physiological and Clinical Studies,* pp. 73–80. Oxford: Blackwell Scientific Publications

THOMPSON, A. J., SEARLE, N. and RUSSELL, G. (1977) Quality of survival after severe birth asphyxia. *Archives of Disease in Childhood,* **52,** 620–626

TING, P. and BRADY, J. (1975) Tracheal suction in meconium aspiration. *American Journal of Obstetrics and Gynecology,* **122,** 767–771

VIDYASAGAR, D., YEH, T. F., HARRIS, V. and PILDES, R. S. (1975) Assisted ventilation in infants with meconium aspiration syndrome. *Pediatrics,* **56,** 208–213

VYAS, H., MILNER, A. D., HOPKIN, I. E. and BOON, A. W. (1981) Physiologic responses to prolonged and slow rise inflation in the resuscitation of the asphyxiated newborn infant. *Journal of Pediatrics,* **99,** 635–639

WESTABY, S., DINWIDDIE, R., CHRISPIN, A. R. and STARK, J. (1984) Pulmonary artery sling in identical twins. *Thoracic and Cardiovascular Surgery,* **32,** 182–183

YU, V. Y. H. (1986a) Editor. Transient tachypneoa of the newborn. In *Respiratory Disorders of the Newborn,* pp. 74–76. London: Churchill Livingstone

YU, V. Y. H. (1986b) Editor. Congenital respiratory anomalies. In *Respiratory Disorders in the Newborn,* pp. 140–141. London: Churchill Livingstone

YU, V. Y. H., ZHAO, S. M. and BAJUK, B. (1982) Results of intensive care for 375 very low birthweight infants. *Australian Paediatric Journal,* **18,** 188–192

YU, V. Y. H., ORGIL, A. A., LIM, S. V., BAJUK, B. and ASTBURY, J. (1983a) Bronchopulmonary dysplasia in very low birthweight infants. *Australian Paediatric Journal,* **19,** 233–236

YU, V. Y. H., ORGILL, A. A., LIM, S. B., BAJUK, B. and ASTBURY, J. (1983b) Growth and development of very low birthweight infants recovering from bronchopulmonary dysplasia. *Archives of Disease in Childhood,* **58,** 791–794

29

Foreign bodies in the larynx and trachea

J. N. G. Evans

Even the most experienced of endoscopists would agree that the prospect of having to deal with a very young child with a history of possible inhalation of a foreign body, fills them with some trepidation – not only because of the demands that the removal of a foreign body makes on their skill as an endoscopist, but also on account of the fact of the unpredictability in the degree of difficulty of the procedure. The degree of difficulty will depend on a number of factors: the age of the patient, the type of foreign body inhaled, the interval between inhalation and removal, the skill of the anaesthetist and the equipment available.

A strong case can be made for every 6-month-old child with a suspected peanut in the bronchus, which has been there for 3–4 weeks, being referred to a specialist centre for its removal.

Modern techniques of endoscopic removal of bronchial foreign bodies stem from the advances made in the early part of the century by Chevalier Jackson, who reduced the mortality of removal of foreign bodies from over 20% to approximately 2%. He achieved a 98% success rate of bronchoscopic removal of foreign bodies, all the procedures being performed under local anaesthesia.

Since then, improvement in the illumination provided by the Hopkins rod lens system and the advent of the ventilating bronchoscope (Hopkins, 1976), coupled with the advances in anaesthesia, have further reduced the mortality and greatly facilitated the task of the endoscopist (Tucker, 1985), and most paediatric endoscopists use these instruments and perform the removal of the foreign body under general anaesthesia (Gans and Berci, 1971).

Other techniques such as postural drainage (Burrington and Cotton, 1972; Campbell, Cotton and Lilly, 1982), the Heimlich (1975) manoeuvre

and the introduction of fingers into the pharynx in an attempt to remove the foreign body, are to be deprecated, since these manipulations may dislodge the foreign body and cause total respiratory obstruction and hypoxic cardiac arrest.

Incidence

The maximum incidence of inhalation of foreign bodies occurs between the age of one and three years: 74% of 115 patients (Brown and Clark, 1983) and 77% of 225 patients (Rothman and Boeckman, 1980); 74% in a much larger series (Jackson and Jackson, 1936). Holinger (1962) found that children under 4 years old constituted 55% of their series of foreign bodies, but their cases included adults.

The most common cause of accidental death in the home in children under 6 years of age, is the inhalation of a foreign body (National Safety Council of America, 1980). It is estimated that almost 600 children under 15 years old die per year in the USA from asphyxia following the aspiration or ingestion of large foreign bodies. The peak incidence of inhalation of foreign bodies in early childhood is of course related to the fact that children have a habit of putting objects into their mouths to determine their texture and taste, and to chew on when teething. It is extremely important, therefore, where possible to keep objects which might be inhaled out of the reach of small children. *Table 29.1* shows the types of foreign body removed in Rothman's series (Rothman and Boeckman, 1980). Boys are more likely to inhale foreign bodies than girls by almost 2:1 (Rothman and Boeckman, 1980; Brown and Clark, 1983; O'Neill, Holcomb and Neblett, 1983; Schloss,

Table 29.1 Type of foreign body

Type	Number
Portion of nut	86
Food	32
Carrot	18
Popcorn	8
Fruit (stem/seed)	5
Bone	8
Plastic	27
Metal	19
Tooth	4
Stone	4
Timothy hay	4
Bead	2
Mucus	2
Balloon	1
Crayon	1
Wood	1
Paper	1
Acorn	1
Pine needle	1

From Rothmann and Boeckman (1980)

Table 29.2 Duration of enlodgement

Duration	Number
2–8 hours	24
8–24 hours	35
1–5 days	14
5–10 days	14
10–30 days	19
1–6 months	9
6 months–1 year	2
Longer	1

From Cohen *et al.* (1980)

Pham-Dang and Rosales, 1983). The reasons for this are not clear!

A minority of these objects impact the larynx; 4% in Cohen's series (Cohen *et al.*, 1980) were removed from the larynx. Foreign bodies lodge in the larynx if they are too large to pass through or if they are of an irregular shape or have sharp edges which can catch on the laryngeal mucosa. Egg shells and fragments of glass or plastic are not infrequent offenders.

History

In most cases of inhaled foreign body, there is a definite history of choking followed by paroxysmal coughing which then subsides. In 85% of the patients in Rothman's series (Rothman and Boeckman, 1980), a positive history of aspiration was obtained but in some patients this positive history is only obtained retrospectively, after removal of the foreign body.

After the initial paroxysm of coughing the tracheobronchial mucosa becomes tolerant of the foreign body and coughing ceases. This feature is often responsible for delays in diagnosis – 18% of cases of foreign body were diagnosed one week and 8% one month after the event (Rothman and Boeckman, 1980). In Cohen's series, 50% of the cases were recognized and treated within 24 hours and, by 10 days, 74% of the cases had been treated, 26% of the cases being diagnosed between

10 days and one month (Cohen *et al.*, 1980) (*Table 29.2*). In a series of 51 cases of foreign body reported by Ross and McCormick (1980) there was no history of aspiration in 8%. One symptom of the triad – coughing, choking and wheeze – was present in 91% of patients with foreign body aspiration (Black *et al.*, 1984).

A history of wheeze, often diagnosed and treated as asthma, is the next most common symptom. Sudden onset of a wheeze in a child not previously known to have asthma, should alert one to the possibility of a foreign body being the cause – especially if the wheeze is predominantly unilateral. Unexplained persistent fever, a fever associated with persistent respiratory symptoms which continues in spite of treatment, and persistent or recurrent lobar pneumonia demand a diagnostic bronchoscopy to exclude a foreign body.

Most endoscopists have on some occasion found an unsuspected foreign body at routine endoscopy for other reasons. The author has removed the horizontal limb of a Montgomery 'T' tube from the trachea of a child with laryngeal stenosis. There was no history of any previous treatment of his stenosis and the plastic tube was found quite by chance at routine endoscopy.

Acute respiratory distress is, fortunately, an uncommon but most alarming presentation of an inhaled foreign body. Fourteen or 6% of the patients in Rothman's series (Rothman and Boeckman, 1980) presented with respiratory distress, five of these patients having had a laryngeal foreign body. Pain at the root of the neck or over the larynx also suggests the presence of a laryngeal foreign body. Large oesophageal foreign bodies may compress the trachea and cause symptoms of respiratory obstruction. Sharp and long-standing oesophageal foreign bodies may produce a fistula between the oesophagus and trachea and cause respiratory symptoms (Yee, Schild and Holinger, 1975).

Clinical examination

A general examination of the child is essential. Respiratory distress or cyanosis demands immediate action; special care should be taken during the induction of anaesthesia in these patients since the foreign body may change position and completely obstruct the airway.

Inhaled foreign bodies are more common in children with upper respiratory tract infections, caused presumably by mouth breathing and the presence of a cough – inhalation of food particles may easily occur with the sharp intake of breath which follows a cough.

If there is a change in the child's cry or if the cry becomes hoarse or stridulous, a laryngeal foreign body should be suspected. Excessive salivation may also occur.

In the first few hours after aspiration the signs in the chest are due to changes in air flow through the tracheobronchial tree. These changes may be detected with a stethoscope on auscultation of the chest. An audible click may be heard due to movement of the foreign body up and down the trachea; a fluttering noise may also be detected due to rapid oscillation of the object in the air stream in the trachea or main bronchi. A unilateral expiratory wheeze and reduced air entry may indicate a foreign body in the bronchus.

Obstructive emphysema may be detected by mediastinal shifts but is most easily detected radiologically and will be discussed more fully later in the chapter.

If the foreign body is not removed within 24 hours, pneumonic signs supervene. The severity of these signs will depend on the reaction of the bronchial mucosa to and the size of the foreign body (Strome, 1977). If the foreign body is of vegetable origin an intense inflammatory reaction of the bronchial mucosa occurs, ultimately with the production of granulation tissue. The mucosal swelling and inflammatory exudate may then obstruct the bronchial lumen, causing atelectasis of the distal lung. A lung abscess may then supervene but this takes several months. An unusual complication of a foreign body in the bronchus, namely a brain abscess, was reported by Spencer *et al.* (1981) – a child inhaled a grass head which entered the bronchus, stem first. This enabled the grass head to migrate peripherally, causing pneumonia and a lung abscess, which in turn caused a cerebral abscess. The time interval between inhalation and development of the brain abscess was 3 months.

Dry vegetable foreign bodies, for example a bean, cause very rapid obstructive changes due to a combination of mucosal irritation and swelling of the bean itself by hygroscopic action. Atelectasis of the occluded segment of lung occurs with the utmost rapidity in this type of foreign body.

The presence of florid granulation tissue around the inhaled foreign body may also cause haemoptysis. It occurred in 6% of cases in a series reported by Ross and McCormick (1980). Haemoptysis itself is a rather uncommon symptom in the paediatric age group. Tom, Weisman and Handler (1980) investigated 40 patients who presented with this symptom and found 15% of the cases were due to a foreign body.

If the foreign body is made of ferrous metal or it has a particularly rough surface, some bronchial irritation will occur, but the process of bronchial occlusion will, however, take much longer.

If the foreign body is inert and has a smooth surface, very little mucosal reaction takes place and pneumonic changes may never supervene.

Radiological findings

X-ray examination of the patient must be performed and should include all the structures from the nasopharynx to the tuberosities of the ischia, otherwise a foreign body may be overlooked (Jackson and Jackson, 1936). X-rays should be taken with the neck extended with anteroposterior and lateral views. Anteroposterior views in expiration and inspiration should be obtained, although these views are sometimes difficult to obtain in very young children. A lateral chest X-ray completes the examination.

Screening may also help but standard X-rays are usually sufficient (Gaafar *et al.*, 1982). Computerized tomographic studies may help to show a foreign body not seen with conventional studies (Berger, Kuhn and Kuhns, 1980). Isotope scans will demonstrate changes in ventilation and perfusion of lung tissues. These more sophisticated radiographic techniques are rarely necessary in obvious cases of inhaled foreign bodies. They should not be ordered if they delay the definitive endoscopic assessment of the patient.

Obstructive emphysema

Obstructive emphysema is produced by a valvular obstruction to the expiratory air stream due to the presence of a foreign body in the lumen of the air passage. It also occurs in endogenous extrinsic compression of the intrathoracic air passages. The action of the valve is due to the fact that the air passages dilate on inspiration and contract on expiration. Thus, on each respiration, a small volume of air is trapped beyond the obstruction and the lung is literally pumped up with air during each phase of the respiratory cycle (*Figure 29.1*). There is mediastinal shift during expiration to the

EXPIRATION   INSPIRATION

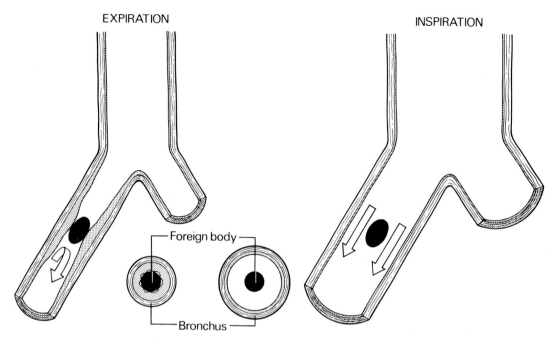

Figure 29.1 Demonstrating the mechanism by which obstructive emphysema occurs with a foreign body in the right main bronchus

unobstructed side of the chest; in inspiration the mediastinum may be in the midline (*Figures 29.2 and 29.3*). In atelectasis of the lung, mediastinal shift occurs towards the obstructed side of the chest, the mediastinum remaining deviated during inspiration and expiration. *Tables 29.3 and 29.4* show the relative incidence of radiological findings in the Rothman (Rothman and Boeckman, 1980) and Black (Black *et al.*, 1984) series.

Positive plain X-ray evidence suggestive of a foreign body was obtained in 81% of patients in a review by Black *et al.* (1984), who also reported 88% of radiographic screening to be positive. Normal radiographs were noted in approximately 10% of the patients in whom foreign bodies were found at bronchoscopy. The time interval between inhalation and abnormal radiological findings was noted by Baraka (1974) and he found negative X-ray evidence of a foreign body within 24 hours of inhalation in his paediatric patients; this figure altered dramatically after 24 hours when abnormal X-rays were noted in 90% of the patients.

Site of foreign body

The majority of foreign bodies come to rest in the right bronchial tree, since the right main bronchus is wider than the left and the interbronchial

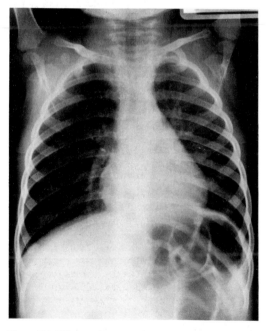

Figure 29.2 X-rays showing obstructive emphysema of the right lung due to the presence of a cashew nut in the right main bronchus, which had been present for one month. Note the radiolucency of the right lung compared with the left

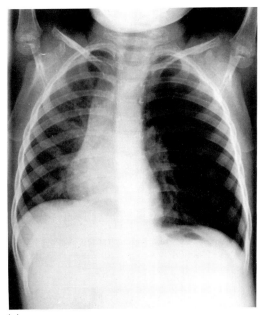

(a)

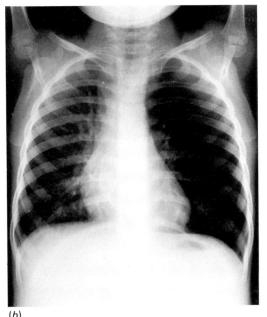

(b)

Figure 29.3 The two X-rays demonstrate mediastinal shift due to obstructive emphysema of the left main bronchus. The mediastinal shift is to the right and is maximal on expiration (a), since the unobstructed right lung can empty more easily. On inspiration (b) the mediastinum moves back towards the midline

Table 29.3 X-ray findings

Radiographic signs	Patient nos.
Obstructive emphysema	135
Foreign body visualized	31
Atelectasis	27
Pneumonia	18
Normal	17
Mediastinal emphysema	4

From Rothmann and Boeckman (1980)

Table 29.4 Radiographic findings in patients with airway foreign bodies

Radiographic signs	Patients	
	No.	%
Air tapping	91	41
Atelectasis	27	12
Perihilar infiltrates	24	11
Opaque foreign body	24	11
Lobar collapse	4	2
Other	9	4
Normal radiograph	29	13
Radiograph not obtained	31	14

From Black *et al.* (1984)

septum projects to the left. The effect of the inspiratory air currents also determines the site of final impaction and the anatomical differences between the right and left bronchial septum are of less significance than might be supposed (Moazamn, Talbert and Rodgers, 1983). In Jackson's series (Jackson and Jackson, 1936), 588 foreign bodies were on the right and 322 on the left, a ratio of 1.82:1.

In young children, where the difference is less pronounced, there is a more equal distribution of foreign bodies between the right and left bronchial tree. In Svensson's (1985) series of children only, there were 59 foreign bodies in the right bronchial tree and 46 in the left, a ratio of 1.28:1.

Management

If a foreign body in the respiratory tract is suspected or diagnosed radiologically, endoscopic examination and removal, under general anaesthesia, is the method of choice. In the case of laryngeal or large tracheal foreign bodies this should be performed as an emergency procedure. If the airway is compromised, the endoscopy must be performed immediately with the facilities for performing an emergency tracheostomy. Large tracheal foreign bodies may have to be delivered through a tracheostomy (Swensson *et al.*, 1985). Bowdler and Emery (1985) recorded two cases of unusual foreign bodies in the trachea. In both cases silver tracheostomy tubes became detached from their neck plates – due to failure of the braising material. The tubes had been in use for a number of years, and the inhaled tubes were removed from the tracheostome with some difficulty! If the airway is not compromised the procedure should be performed within hours, allowing a suitable time to elapse for the stomach to be empty.

Laryngeal foreign bodies are removed by direct laryngoscopy. In the majority of cases this is accomplished without difficulty, often indeed in the anaesthetic room much to the delight of anaesthetic colleagues. Rarely, large foreign bodies may cause total respiratory obstruction during induction of anaesthesia and an emergency tracheostomy will then be necessary. A commonly encountered difficulty in cases of laryngeal foreign body is delay in diagnosis (Moskowitz, Gardiner and Sasaki, 1982).

Tracheal and bronchial foreign bodies are best removed using a rigid bronchoscope. In the absence of respiratory distress the operation should be performed as an elective procedure, by the 'surgical team' that are used to working together in their accustomed operating theatre. Under these 'ideal' circumstances, a 99% success rate for removal of foreign bodies should be achieved. There is no place for endoscopy for a foreign body being performed in an infant by inexperienced personnel in unfamiliar surroundings (Bush and Vivori, 1981).

In the author's opinion the efficiency and safety of rigid bronchoscopy completely supersedes any form of conservative approach using bronchodilators, thoracic percussion and postural drainage (Burrington and Cotton, 1972). Indeed this technique of inhalation and postural drainage may be the cause of severe respiratory obstruction and even hypoxic cardiac arrest, if the foreign body is moved and impacts in the subglottis (Kosloske, 1980). Preoperative physiotherapy, together with the administration of antibiotics is, however, useful in patients with a peripherally situated, usually organic, foreign body of long standing, in which there is considerable atelectasis of the lung with pneumonia or a lung abscess. Postoperative physiotherapy is also helpful in expanding areas of atelectatic lung (*Figure 29.4*).

In the rare event of being unable to remove a foreign body endoscopically, in spite of satisfactory operating conditions, it must be removed by thoracotomy and bronchotomy. In practice this generally has to be organized as a separate procedure, since the decision to abandon the bronchoscopic attempt at removal is only made after an already prolonged struggle to remove it bronchoscopically. The author recalls having to

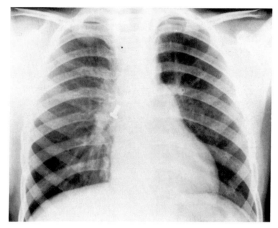

Figure 29.4 X-ray of foreign body spontaneously expelled by coughing

abandon a bronchoscopy in a 2-year-old child who had choked on a pebble, after his father in attempting to remove it with his finger, had pushed it through the laryngeal inlet. The pebble was oval in shape and almost exactly fitted the glottis. Once in the trachea sufficient air was able to pass around it to maintain respiration, but the author was unable, however, to exert sufficient traction with a pair of forceps to pull it back through the larynx. It was successfully removed at thoracotomy the following day.

Technique of removal

In most cases removal of the foreign body is undertaken as an elective procedure – in this instance the surgical anaesthetic and nursing personnel know each other and the 'team' are able to perform their allotted tasks efficiently and peacefully. These factors increase the chances of a successful removal of the foreign body and reduce the operative morbidity.

Instruments

A complete set of ventilating bronchoscopes with a Hopkins rod lens system, such as manufactured by Karl Storz (*Figure 29.5*), is used by many paediatric endoscopists (*Table 29.5*). These instruments, by virtue of their superior illumination and optics, which magnify the image nine times improve the visualization of the foreign body in the infant and young child. The bronchoscopes are equipped with two side channels, one for ventilation and the other for instrumentation and suction. The disadvantage of these instruments is that the side channel will only permit the

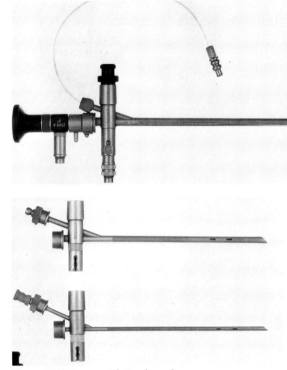

Figure 29.5 Storz ventilating bronchoscope

introduction of very small forceps, and the author finds that the removal of soft foreign bodies (for example peanuts) is made easier by using the larger Chevalier Jackson instruments through an open bronchoscope.

For this reason the author also has available a set of Negus bronchoscopes in the following sizes: suckling, infant, child, adolescent and small adult. A swing-arm magnifier (*Figure 29.6*) is available for use with these instruments and provides a magnification × 4. This enables assessment of the forceps space between the foreign body and the bronchial wall so the best position for insertion of the instrument can be determined. The irregular

shape of most foreign bodies will allow the forceps to be inserted in the gap between the foreign body and the bronchial wall, thus reducing the risk of pushing the foreign body distally and jamming it in the bronchus.

In older children, the combined bronchoscope and grasping forceps overcome the difficulty of removing soft foreign bodies because the jaws of the grasping forceps are larger and prevent the fragmentation of soft vegetable foreign bodies, which occurs with smaller 'side-arm forceps' (*Figures 29.7* and *29.8*).

In some centres (Kosloske, 1980), Fogarty balloon catheters designed for arterial

Table 29.5 Recommended set of Storz bronchoscopes

Diameter (mm)	Length (cm)
2.5 3.0	20
3.0 3.5	25
4.0 5.0 6.0	30

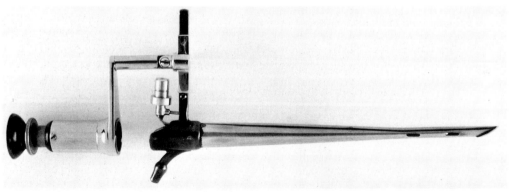

Figure 29.6 Swing-arm magnifier for Negus bronchoscope

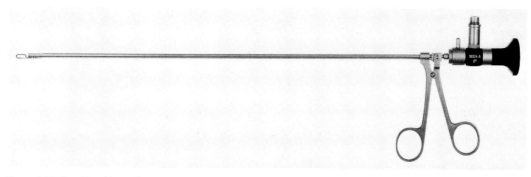

Figure 29.7 Combined bronchoscope and grasping forceps

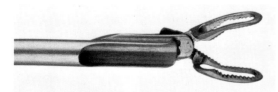

Figure 29.8 Enlarged view of forceps of combined bronchoscope and grasping forceps

embolectomy are used particularly in the removal of peanuts (Stein, 1970). The catheter size 3 or 4 is passed down the side-arm of the Storz broncho-scope. The tip of the catheter is passed beyond the foreign body and the balloon is inflated with saline (Wiesel *et al.*, 1982; Bannerjee, Khanna and Narayanan, 1984). The telescope is withdrawn approximately 1 cm to allow space for the present-ing part of the peanut to be accommodated within the lumen of the bronchoscope as traction is exerted on the Fogarty catheter. The catheter, bronchoscope and foreign body are removed together (*Figure 29.9*).

The Fogarty catheter is also useful for removing foreign bodies with holes, for example beads: the catheter can be threaded through the hole, inflated and the foreign body removed. A Dormia basket used by urologists to remove ureteric calculi may also be used in a similar manner (Dajani, 1971) (*Figure 29.10*).

Before commencing endoscopy, the surgeon must be satisfied that all the equipment is in working order. This applies particularly to the

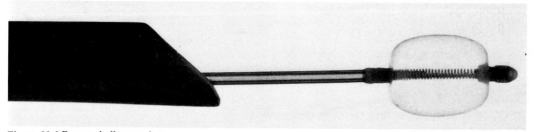

Figure 29.9 Fogarty balloon catheter

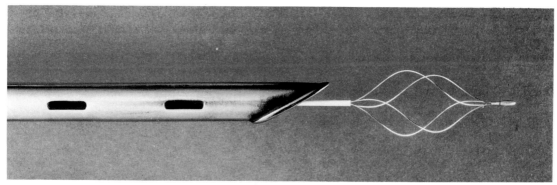

Figure 29.10 Dormia basket

jaws of the Jackson forceps – these are made of spring steel which tends to rust and, therefore, may jam in the outer casing of the forceps. Suckers must be checked for patency and also that they are long enough to protrude beyond the end of the bronchoscope.

Bronchoscopes and forceps, suitable in size and shape for the case in hand, are selected (*Figures 29.11–29.14*). Practice passes of the forceps

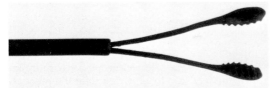

Figure 29.11 Typical Chevalier Jackson grasping forceps

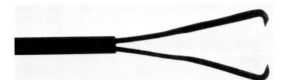

Figure 29.12 Rotation forceps

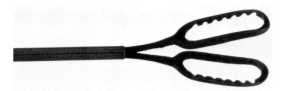

Figure 29.13 Fenestrated forceps – useful for removing peanuts

Figure 29.14 Ball forceps for removal of small hard round objects such as ball-bearings

through the chosen bronchoscope are made, the blades of the forceps are inserted into the bronchoscope and then opened, and the emergence of the opened forceps beyond the tip of the bronchoscope is felt rather than seen, because of the lack of stereoscopic vision down the bronchoscope. This manoeuvre is practised, while the patient is being anaesthetized, until the surgeon is confident that he will know when the tip of the forceps is just protruding beyond the end of the bronchoscope. This is the correct position for grasping the foreign body (*Figure 29.15*).

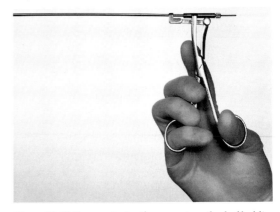

Figure 29.15 Demonstrates the correct method of holding the Chevalier Jackson forceps – traction is made with the index finger in the deviation of the long axis of the forceps

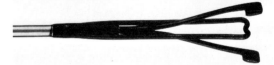

Figure 29.16 Clerf–Arrowsmith safety-pin closing forceps

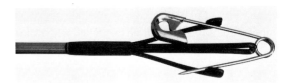

Figure 29.17 Clerf–Arrowsmith safety-pin closing forceps, closing safety pin

In cases where a particular difficulty is likely to be encountered, for example open safety pins or other sharp foreign bodies (*Figures 29.16* and *29.17*), the use of a dummy tracheobronchial tree and a duplicate foreign body (*Figure 29.18*) will enable the surgeon to practise the manoeuvre necessary to remove the foreign body safely. Time spent in practice will be amply rewarded by reducing the time spent during the actual endoscopy.

The actual technique of bronchoscopy is described in Volume 5. Special care must be taken in young children to keep the bronchoscope in line with the trachea to ensure adequate ventilation of the patient. Ventilation may be difficult when the bronchoscope is passed deeply into the obstructed bronchus; adequate ventilation will be maintained if the holes in the side of the bronchoscope remain unobstructed, and direct towards the normal main bronchus.

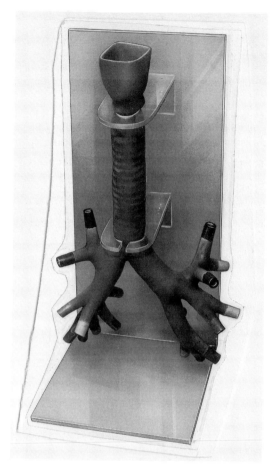

Figure 29.18 Bronchial tree – Manikin (Richard Wolf UK Ltd)

When the precautions mentioned above are taken, a successful removal of a foreign body can be achieved in the majority of cases.

Following removal

It is very important after removal of the foreign body, while the child is still anaesthetized, that a *second look* is taken to ensure that a second foreign body has not been overlooked, and to remove any remaining small fragments particularly in the case of peanuts. Pus and mucus can be aspirated from the distal bronchus – speeding the resolution of atelectasis or pneumonia. It is also important to make sure that all major bronchopulmonary segments including the upper lobe orifices are inspected.

If the bronchoscopy is prolonged, or if the bronchoscope was noted to be a tight fit in the subglottic larynx, the use of a systemic corticosteroid, dexamethasone 0.5 mg/kg, is advised to reduce the incidence of laryngeal oedema post-operatively.

Prevention

The vast majority of cases of inhaled or ingested foreign bodies occur as a result of carelessness either in the preparation or ingestion of food or drinks, or as a result of placing inedible or unsuitable objects in the mouth. The accidental inhalation or ingestion of foreign bodies is therefore almost entirely preventable. Infants and children under the age of two should not be allowed to eat peanuts, and their play areas should be cleared of small objects that could be inhaled. Adults should set a good example by never placing pins or tacks in their mouths. The long-term deleterious effects of a foreign body on the lung parenchyma, such as lung abscesses or bronchiectasis, are also preventable provided that the medical attendant of the child always considers the possibility that a foreign body may be present (Clerf, 1952), even in a case where a good history of inhalation has not been obtained, in a patient who develops a wheeze where asthma has not been previously diagnosed, or when pneumonic signs persist for a longer period than one would expect. In such cases a bronchoscopy should always be performed.

References

BANERJEE, A., KHANNA, S. K. and NARAYANAN, P. S. (1984) Use of Fogarty catheters for removal of tracheobronchial foreign bodies (letter). *Chest*, **85**, 452

BARAKA, A. (1974) Bronchoscopic removal of inhaled foreign bodies in children. *British Journal of Anaesthesia*, **46**, 124–126

BERGER, P. E., KUHN, J. P. and KUHNS, L. R. (1980) Computed tomography and the occult tracheobronchial foreign body. *Radiology*, **134**, 133–135

BLACK, R. E., CHOI, K. J., SYME, W. C., JOHNSON, D. G. and MATLAK, M. E. (1984) Bronchoscopic removal of aspirated foreign bodies in children. *American Journal of Surgery*, **148**, 778–781

BOWDLER, D. A. and EMERY, P. J. (1985) Tracheostomy tube fatigue. An unusual cause of inhaled foreign body. *Journal of Laryngology and Otology*, **99**, 517–521

BROWN, T. C. and CLARK, C. M. (1983) Inhaled foreign bodies in children. *Medical Journal of Australia*, **2**, 322–326

BURRINGTON, J. D. and COTTON, E. K. (1972) Removal of foreign bodies from the tracheobronchial tree. *Journal of Pediatric Surgery*, **7**, 119–122

BUSH, G. H. and VIVORI, E. (1981) How to remove a foreign body from the trachea and bronchial tree (letter). *British Journal of Hospital Medicine*, **26**, 102

CAMPBELL, D. N., COTTON, E. K. and LILLY, J. R. (1982) A dual approach to tracheobronchial foreign bodies in children. *Surgery*, **91**, 178–182

CLERF, L. H. (1952) Historical aspects of foreign bodies in the air and food passages. *Annals of Otology, Rhinology and Laryngology*, **61**, 5–17

COHEN, S. R. (1981) Unusual presentations and problems created by mismanagement of foreign bodies in the aerodigestive tract of the pediatric patient. *Annals of Otology, Rhinology and Laryngology*, **90**, 316–322

COHEN, S. R., HERBERT, W. I., LEWIS, G. B. JR and GELLER, K. A. (1980) Foreign bodies in the airway. Five-year retrospective study with special reference to management. *Annals of Otology, Rhinology and Laryngology*, **89**, 437–442

DAJANI, A. M. (1971) 'Bronchial foreign body' removed with a Dormia basket. *The Lancet*, **1**, 1076–1077

GAAFAR, H., ABDEL-DAYEM, M., TALAAT, M. and MANDOUR, M. (1982) The value of X-ray examination in the diagnosis of tracheobronchial foreign bodies in infants and children. *Journal of Otorhinolaryngology and its Related Specialties*, **44**, 340–348

GANS, S. L. and BERCI, G. (1971) Advances in endoscopy of infants and children. *Journal of Pediatric Surgery*, **6**, 199–234

HEIMLICH, H. J. (1975) A life saving manoeuvre to prevent food choking. *Journal of the American Medical Association*, **234**, 398–401

HOLINGER, P. H. (1962) Foreign bodies in the food and air passages. *Transactions of the American Academy of Ophthalmology and Otolaryngology*, **66**, 193–210

HOPKINS, H. H. (1976) *Endoscopy*, p. 17. New York: Appleton Century Crofts

JACKSON, C. and JACKSON, C. L. (1936) *Diseases of the Air and Food Passages of Foreign Body Origin*. Philadelphia: W. B. Saunders

KOSLOSKE, A. M. (1980) Tracheobronchial foreign bodies in children: back to the bronchoscope and a balloon. *Pediatrics*, **66**, 321–323

KOSLOSKE, A. M. (1982) Bronchoscopic extraction of aspirated foreign bodies in children. *American Journal of Diseases of Children*, **136**, 924–927

MOAZAMN, F., TALBERT, J. L. and RODGERS, B. M. (1983) Foreign bodies in the pediatric tracheobronchial tree. *Clinical Pediatrics*, **22**, 148–150

MOSKOWITZ, D., GARDINER, L. J. and SASAKI, C. T. (1982) Foreign-body aspiration. Potential misdiagnosis. *Archives of Otolaryngology*, **108**, 806–807

NATIONAL SAFETY COUNCIL OF AMERICA (1980) *Accident Facts*, 7

O'NEILL, J. A. JR, HOLCOMB, G. W. JR and NEBLETT, W. W. (1983) Management of tracheobronchial and esophageal foreign bodies in childhood. *Journal of Pediatric Surgery*, **18**, 475–479

ROSS, A. H. and McCORMICK, R. J. (1980) Foreign body inhalation. *Journal of the Royal College of Surgeons of Edinburgh*, **25**, 104–109

ROTHMANN, B. F. and BOECKMAN, C. R. (1980) Foreign bodies in the larynx and tracheobronchial tree in children. A review of 225 cases. *Annals of Otology, Rhinology and Laryngology*, **89**, 434–436

SCHLOSS, M. D., PHAM-DANG, H. and ROSALES, J. K. (1983) Foreign bodies in the tracheobronchial tree – a retrospective study of 217 cases. *Journal of Otolaryngology*, **12**, 212–216

SPENCER, M. J., MILLET, V. E., DUDLEY, J. P., SHERROD, J. L. and BRYSON, Y. J. (1981) Grassheads in the tracheobronchial tree: two different outcomes. *Annals of Otology, Rhinology and Laryngology*, **90**, 406–408

STEIN, L. (1970) Foreign bodies of the tracheobronchial tree and oesophagus – a new approach to therapy. *Annals of Thoracic Surgery*, **9**, 382–383

STROME, M. (1977) Tracheobronchial foreign bodies: an updated approach. *Annals of Otology, Rhinology and Laryngology*, **86**, 649–654

SVENSSON, G. (1985) Foreign bodies in the tracheobronchial tree. Special reference to experience in 97 children. *International Journal of Pediatric Otorhinolaryngology*, **61**, 5–17

SWENSSON, E. E., RAH, K. H., KIM, M. C., BROOKS, J. W. and SALZBERG, A. M. (1985) Extraction of large tracheal foreign bodies through a tracheostoma under bronchoscopic control. *Annals of Thoracic Surgery*, **39**, 251–253

TOM, L. W. C., WEISMAN, R. A. and HANDLER, S. D. (1980) Haemoptysis in children. *Annals of Otology, Rhinology and Laryngology*, **89**, 419–424

TUCKER, G. JR (1985) Instrumentarium for foreign body removal. *New Dimensions in Otorhinolaryngology – Head and Neck Surgery*, **1**, 585–588

WIESEL, J. M., CHISIN, R., FEINMESSER, R. and GAY, I. (1982) Use of a Fogarty catheter for bronchoscopic removal of a foreign body (letter). *Chest*, **81**, 524

YEE, K. F., SCHILD, J. A. and HOLINGER, P. H. (1975) Extraluminal foreign bodies (coins) in the food and air passages. *Annals of Otology, Rhinology and Laryngology*, **84**, 619–623

30

Acute laryngeal infections in childhood

Andrew P. Freeland

Laryngeal infections in childhood result in airway obstruction, the prime symptom of which is stridor. This chapter discusses the various causes of laryngeal infection and their management so that a safe course of action is followed, resulting in a favourable outcome.

The first aim in management is to establish a diagnosis rapidly and this is dependent on a good knowledge of the various possibilities. From a practical point of view it is vital to distinguish inflammation *above the glottis* (epiglottitis or supraglottitis) from inflammation at or *below the glottis* (laryngotracheobronchitis). A variety of organisms, both bacterial and viral, have replaced *Corynebacterium diphtheriae* as the commonest cause of acute laryngeal infection. Diphtheria, however, still needs to be considered, as do conditions which may mimic laryngeal infections, such as acute retropharyngeal abscesses and foreign bodies.

Stridor is the noise caused by obstruction of airflow due to narrowing in the respiratory tract. It may be inspiratory, biphasic or expiratory, but in most cases of acute laryngeal infection, inspiratory stridor dominates. An expiratory phase is very common when the tracheal lumen is also narrowed by oedema or inflammation. Inspiratory stridor alone usually indicates that the lesion is at vocal cord level or above. Tucker (1979) has pointed out that in a full-term baby's larynx measuring 7×4 mm, 1 mm of oedema reduces the lumen to 35% of normal. It is therefore not surprising that the child with laryngeal infection develops airway obstruction, whereas the adult with similar disease does not.

Croup, as defined by the Shorter Oxford English Dictionary (1973) is 'an inflammatory disease of the larynx and trachea of children marked by a peculiar, sharp, ringing cough'. An alternative definition is 'to cry hoarsely, or to make the hoarse, ringing cough of croup'. There is tremendous variation in the diseases included in the literature under the term 'croup'. It appears to be more of a lay term rather than a pathological entity and parents seem to adhere more to the dictionary definition by referring to their children as having 'croupy coughs' than do the medical profession who usually imply it to mean airway obstruction. Since it is an imprecise term, it would seem more acceptable to classify all children as having an acute inflammatory stridor until a more specific diagnosis can be established. Margolis (1980) pointed out that there is a major problem in deciding whether drug therapy is effective if the definition of the disease is inaccurate in the first place. There is even confusion as to whether croup includes epiglottitis. Since there is no generally agreed classification of this group of diseases, the author feels that epiglottitis is a separate entity and that 'croup' includes acute viral laryngotracheobronchitis, bacterial laryngotracheobronchitis (pseudomembranous croup), spasmodic croup, and diphtheria.

Anatomy of the larynx

The larynx is relatively and absolutely smaller than in the adult (Pracy, 1979) and is higher in the neck and more difficult to see. The coronal (*Figure 30.1*) and sagittal (*Figure 30.2*) whole organ laryngeal sections show two important points in relation to childhood infections. The epiglottis is surrounded by loose connective tissue – the pre-epiglottic and paraglottic spaces – and inflammation may spread quickly from the epiglottis within these spaces.

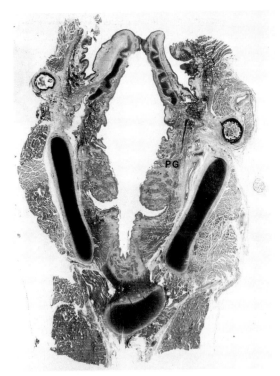

Figure 30.1 Coronal section through an infant larynx. Note the loose connective tissue in the paraglottic space (PG) into which inflammation from the epiglottis may quickly spread

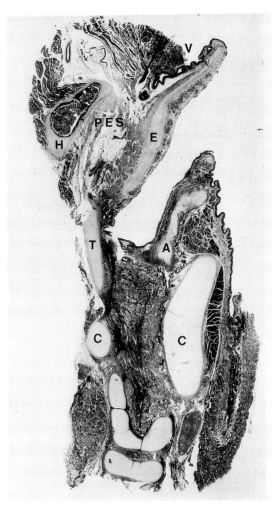

Figure 30.2 Sagittal section through an infant larynx. Note the pre-epiglottic space (PES) bounded by the hyoid (H) anteriorly, the vallecula (V) superiorly and the epiglottis (E) posteriorly into which epiglottitis can quickly spread. This space is continuous with the paraglottic space shown in *Figure 30.1.* T = thyroid cartilage; A = arytenoid cartilage; C = cricoid cartilage

Rough instrumentation or even tongue depression, may encourage the inflammatory oedema to surround the laryngeal inlet completely. This is a hazard referred to in the section on management of epiglottitis. Secondly, the mucosa in the subglottis (within the cricoid ring) is lax and full of mucous glands, and easily becomes oedematous. If it does so, a biphasic stridor occurs since this is the only part of the laryngotracheobronchial tree that is completely surrounded by cartilage; it is therefore rigid and the airflow is restricted in both inspiratory and expiratory phases. It is also worth noting that laryngeal spasm occurs more easily in the child than in the adult. The childhood larynx seems to be physiologically more brittle.

Causes of laryngeal infection in childhood

The causes of acute laryngeal infection in childhood will be considered first, in isolation. Their management, however, will be discussed together since in most cases the child will present in the casualty department as an acute infective airway

obstruction of unknown cause. The correct management depends on a logical sequence of events leading to an accurate diagnosis and a successful outcome for each condition.

Acute epiglottitis (acute supraglottic laryngitis, acute supraglottitis)

Acute epiglottitis is the most frightening of paediatric emergencies; if unrecognised, it can kill and all medical practitioners should be aware of its existence and significance. It is rare, occurring 43 times less frequently than laryngotracheobronchitis, but the mortality even in experienced hands is 3–4% (Fearon, 1975). *Haemophilus influenzae* type B is, in the vast majority of cases, the causative organism. The β-haemolytic streptococcus, Pneumococcus and Staphylococcus have also been reported as causal agents (Schwartz *et al.*, 1982). *H. influenzae* type B epiglottitis may present at any time during the year, although it is more common in the winter months. Drake-Lee, Broughton and Grace (1984) found no cases in the months of July, August or September over a 7-year-period.

The disease is concentrated maximally on the epiglottis, but it is common to find inflammation involving the whole supraglottic compartment of the larynx. The infection spreads in the loose connective tissue anterior and posterolateral to the epiglottis (*see Figures 30.1 and 30.2*). The laryngeal surface of the epiglottis is largely spared from the inflammation.

Most cases are seen in children between the ages of one and 6 years with the peak incidence occurring between the ages of 3 and 4. This is in contrast to laryngotracheobronchitis which usually affects younger children, the peak incidence being 18 months of age. Epiglottitis is occasionally seen in adults but most children over the age of six have protective antibodies against *H. influenzae* type B and it also seems that some immunity exists below the age of 2 years. However, in this younger age group, haemophilus meningitis is more common. Why the organism spares the epiglottis in preference to the meninges is not clear. It has been suggested that previous contact with *H. influenzae* in early childhood may later be followed by a type III Arthus hypersensitivity reaction which would account for the rapid onset of epiglottitis (Broniatowski, 1985).

Clinical features

The sudden transformation of a fit child into one who is desperately ill, often within a period of only a few hours, is the most striking feature of this disease. However, not all cases present in this classical manner and Welch and Price (1983) found that one-third of their patients with epiglottitis had a history of an upper respiratory tract infection during the previous 24 hours and some had a surprisingly long history of stridor prior to admission. The classical picture is described below.

A fit child, aged about 3 years, complains of a sore throat which intensifies and within half an hour dysphagia is reported. Inspiratory stridor then occurs and within 2 hours a critically ill child presents to the casualty department. The child will be sitting up and leaning forward, as if he lies back, suffocation may occur as a result of the

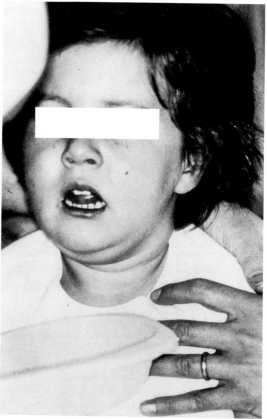

Figure 30.3 Epiglottitis illustrating a frightened child, sitting up, dribbling with cervical lymphadenopathy

epiglottis occluding the laryngeal inlet (*Figure 30.3*). Dribbling of saliva will be profuse since dysphagia is total. His voice, if he is strong enough to speak, will not be hoarse but muffled. Inspiratory stridor is usually present but, as time goes by, the child will become quiet and floppy and respiratory distress seems to lessen. This is an ominous sign caused by extreme fatigue and indicates that respiratory and cardiac arrest are imminent.

Unlike laryngotracheobronchitis where children are restless and pink, most children with epiglottitis are quiet, pale and look terrified. This is a systemic infection and the bacteraemia causes shock which gives rise to the pallor. Pyrexia is always present, although the degree is variable. Some authors feel that marked cervical lymphadenopathy is always present and in the casualty department this is the only physical sign, other than observation from a distance, that it is safe to elicit. On no account should the pharynx be examined since immediate asphyxia may occur.

Radiology of this condition is discussed in the section on management, but it is the author's view that, although X-rays of the epiglottis in this condition are frequently to be found in articles and textbooks, the taking of an X-ray may be a dangerous practice. This is due to the delay and distress caused in aligning a child for an X-ray which is usually quite unnecessary for the diagnosis to be made.

The above picture is enough to be highly suspicious that the child has epiglottitis and no investigations should be carried out until an alternative airway has been established. Throat swabs, taking of blood for cultures, and needling for blood gases are liable to agitate the child and increase the likelihood of airway obstruction.

The only time to confirm the suspected diagnosis is as the child is being provided with an alternative airway. The further management of epiglottitis is considered later.

Laryngotracheobronchitis (croup, acute subglottic laryngitis, non-diphtheritic croup, acute laryngotracheitis)

As the name implies, laryngotracheobronchitis involves a larger proportion of the respiratory tract than epiglottitis and the maximum effect is in the subglottic area. In most cases the causative organism is parainfluenza virus type I, but parainfluenza virus types II and III, influenza virus type A, respiratory syncytial and rhinoviruses may also occur. Laryngotracheobronchitis may also follow measles. It is not uncommon for secondary bacterial infection to supervene.

The vocal cords are inflamed and may be ulcerated, but it is the subglottis that seems to take the brunt of the disease. Here there is gross oedema and occasionally ulceration. As the name implies, the rest of the tracheobronchial tree may also be affected.

As mentioned previously the incidence of hospital admissions for laryngotracheobronchitis is about 40 times more frequent than for epiglottitis (Fearon, 1975). *Figures 30.4* and *30.5* show that

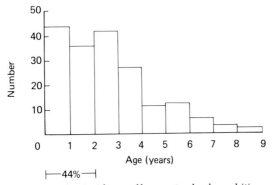

Figure 30.4 Age incidence of laryngotracheobronchitis

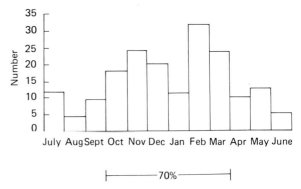

Figure 30.5 Seasonal incidence of laryngotracheobronchitis. Total = 183; 128 male (70%); 55 female (30%)

experience in Oxford with age and seasonal incidence is very much the same as in other reports. The mean age is about 18 months and boys are more frequently affected than girls. Denny *et al.* (1983) reported that boys are affected 1.43 times more commonly as girls and also state that November is the peak month for the disease in North Carolina. It is certainly more common in the winter months in temperate climates, particularly in October, November and December, and there is often another peak in early spring (*Figure 30.5*).

Clinical features

Unlike epiglottitis, laryngotracheobronchitis is always preceded by an upper respiratory tract infection, usually of at least 48 hours' duration. It is not uncommon for the child to have had a previous history of inflammatory stridor. The initial symptom is hoarseness and this is followed by a 'croupy' cough which is described as a 'musical cough of crowing quality', or 'the bark of a seal'. Signs of respiratory distress then appear, often at night. The temperature is usually raised, but not unduly so. Although stridor is initially inspiratory, it soon becomes biphasic as subglottic oedema develops. Flaring of the ala nasae, and suprasternal and intercostal recession develop as respiratory distress increases. At this stage, the child becomes very restless and prefers to lie down. Crying and coughing occur, which make the stridor worse and give rise to the physician's natural inclination to sedate the child. The safety of this will be discussed later. Very careful assessment is needed if the child's stridor and chest retraction diminish; it may mean there is genuine improvement, but occasionally it represents exhaustion with imminent respiratory failure.

It is unknown how many children are managed at home, usually with some form of moist inhalation administered by their parents and family doctors, and how many are admitted to hospital. It is therefore difficult to know the true incidence of this disease. According to Mitchell and Thomas (1980), only 5–10% of all croup cases need hospital admission and, in the USA, an overall incidence of 5–10/1000 preschool children is quoted (Hall and Hall, 1975). A rough estimate from 10 Oxford general practitioners suggests that they request hospital admission for one in every six cases they are called to see. The management in hospital will be discussed later, approximately one out of 20 of these admissions needs an alternative airway. Milner (1984) quoted an even lower incidence of 1% requiring intubation. This is in contrast to epiglottitis where all patients need an alternative airway.

Bacterial laryngotracheobronchitis (pseudomembranous croup)

This condition may be a separate disease or be caused by a secondary bacterial infection of viral laryngotracheobronchitis. Some authors call this disease bacterial tracheitis (Broniatowski, 1985) since it seems to involve the trachea predominantly. It is a much more severe illness than laryngotracheobronchitis, but very much less common. Henry (1983), over a 2-year period, reported seven children who had this condition and exhibited severe sloughing of the respiratory epithelium. The children were older than is normally associated with laryngotracheobronchitis and they had more severe obstruction. An artificial airway is often needed and this may easily obstruct with thick crusts of sloughed epithelium. The causative organism is, in most cases, *Staphylococcus aureus*. A similar experience with this condition was reported by Friedman *et al.* (1985), who quoted 10 patients ranging in age from 3 months to 12 years, three of whom required intubation and seven needed bronchoscopy for diagnosis and treatment.

Clinical features

Bacterial laryngotracheobronchitis begins in a fairly insidious way with a history of an upper respiratory tract infection. It progresses, however, and is accompanied by a brassy cough and high fever. The child becomes toxic and the white blood cell count is greatly elevated. It is likely, on admission, that the child will be diagnosed as having severe laryngotracheobronchitis and, because of the respiratory distress, an alternative airway will be considered. If a bronchoscopy is performed at this stage, the trachea will be seen to be ulcerated and sloughed epithelium will be aspirated. This should be sent for bacterial culture since, if bacterial laryngotracheobronchitis is suspected, appropriate antibiotic therapy is essential.

This condition poses major problems for intensive care nurses because of a strong tendency to endotracheal tube obstruction. Very efficient humidity and expert nursing care are necessary to manage these patients successfully. A tracheostomy may be safer, since there is less risk of obstruction of the tube, from inspissated secretions.

Spasmodic laryngitis (spasmodic croup, acute subglottic oedema, laryngismus stridulus)

This condition is not universally recognized in all classifications but it has the following characteristics. Recurrent attacks are common. The bouts usually begin very suddenly at night without any prodromal features and, equally, disappear just as rapidly, often in the morning. The attacks respond to mist therapy or even vomiting (Davis *et al.*, 1981). If the child is bronchoscoped for any reason, subglottic oedema is the only abnormal feature. Most cases, however, do not require an alternative airway.

Zach (1983) studied immunoglobulin levels in recurrent croup and demonstrated low IgA levels in spasmodic laryngitis and showed that an association existed between the disease activity and the IgA levels. Some children seem to grow out of these attacks only to develop asthma or other allergic states.

There may be a place for treating spasmodic laryngitis with anti-asthma inhalants such as topical steroids or sodium cromoglycate. Systemic corticosteroids also relieve this condition (Koren *et al.*, 1983). These authors found that dexamethasone 0.6 mg/kg as a single dose was useful in spasmodic laryngitis but had no effect in laryngotracheobronchitis.

Diphtheria

Diphtheria is extremely rare in countries where routine immunization is the rule. In 1984 there were only 70 cases in the USA (Broniatowski, 1985), but it is still an important differential diagnosis of airway obstruction in children, especially in immigrants who may not always be immunized. Laryngeal diphtheria nearly always follows pharyngeal infection.

The causative organism is *Corynebacterium diphtheriae* and of the three strains – gravis, intermedius and mitis – it is nearly always the gravis strain that has been responsible for the major epidemics and high mortality rates. Clinical variants are being reported as causing membranous pharyngitis. It is rare to see diphtheria in children over the age of 10 years.

It is not only the laryngeal obstruction that causes mortality in this condition, but also the production of an endotoxin with the risk of myocarditis and peripheral neuritis. The initial lesion is usually in the region of the tonsil where necrosis is seen and the characteristic grey membrane is formed – a mixture of necrotic tissue, a rich fibrinous exudate and a large number of bacteria. Attempts to remove the membrane often produce bleeding. The membrane appears to become thicker later in the disease process and is easier to separate from underlying mucosa. The characteristic bull neck appearance is due to cellulitis and regional lymphadenopathy.

Clinical features

The onset is insidious and begins with a barking cough, followed by inspiratory stridor with chest wall recession as the disease spreads from the pharynx to the larynx. General symptoms of malaise, pyrexia and sore throat are often present early in the disease but, occasionally, a membrane over the faucial pillars is the only sign during the early stages. General signs of toxaemia then occur and dysphagia increases prior to laryngeal involvement which is evidenced by a barking cough and stridor. The cough comes in paroxysms, and exhaustion from coughing and toxaemia soon occur unless an alternative airway is provided. Many children die, however, from acute toxic myocarditis occurring during the second week of the illness. Palatal paralysis is the most common of the peripheral neuropathies to occur and presents with nasal regurgitation of food and 'nasal escape' to the voice.

Management

The main problem nowadays is to remember that laryngeal diphtheria still exists. *Corynebacterium diphtheriae* is penicillin sensitive and penicillin therapy is therefore a mainstay in treatment but, because of the danger of diphtheritic toxins, antitoxin treatment is also essential and both should be used early in the management. Intravenous benzyl penicillin 600 mg 6-hourly, should be used and the dose of antitoxin, which may also be given intravenously, varies from 10 000 –100 000 units, dependent on the severity of the infection.

It may also be necessary to remove the membrane from the larynx and insert an endo-tracheal tube for airway support. The decision to do this will depend entirely on the clinical situation and will probably be reserved for failed conservative treatment which should include humidification and oxygen therapy. Extubation (if intubation has been necessary) can be commenced early since the disease responds very well to medical therapy. Once the airway obstruction has been successfully managed, the child will need careful assessment and possibly total bed rest for 2–4 weeks until the danger of myocarditis is past.

Conditions which mimic laryngeal infections in childhood

Conditions that must be eliminated as mimics of acute laryngeal infections are foreign bodies, infectious mononucleosis (glandular fever), peritonsillar abscess, retropharyngeal abscess and paraquat poisoning.

Foreign bodies

This subject is beyond the scope of this chapter since it appears elsewhere in this volume (*see* Chapter 29) but a history of a child who is apyrexial, who has been playing with small objects and who then begins to have paroxysms of coughing suggests an inhaled foreign body and removal via endoscopy is obviously essential. Absence of pyrexia is the most obvious way to distinguish foreign body impaction from acute inflammatory disease of the childhood larynx.

Infectious mononucleosis (glandular fever)

Airway obstruction may occasionally occur in glandular fever. The membrane is less adherent than in diphtheria but tonsillar hypertrophy may be massive and may result in inspiratory stridor. Glandular fever is more common in young adults, but is not infrequently found in children. If the airway is becoming embarrassed and the stridor increasing, large doses of intravenous hydrocortisone often alleviate the need for an alternative airway. Ampicillin and amoxycillin should be avoided.

Peritonsillar abscess (quinsy)

Peritonsillar abscess occurs more commonly in adolescence than retropharyngeal abscess, but the reverse is true in infancy (White, 1985). The clinical features are of trismus, dribbling and airway obstruction which occurs as a result of the tonsils being displaced medially to threaten the oropharyngeal airway. There may be a history of antecedent recurrent tonsillitis.

It may be difficult to decide whether frank pus is present or whether the disease is in the cellulitic stage. If the airway is in jeopardy, it is recommended that surgical drainage of the abscess is carried out. The usual site of the incision for the evacuation of pus is at a point which is transected by a line drawn horizontally from the base of the uvula with one drawn vertically from the anterior pillar of the tonsil. Release of pus by open drainage results in rapid improvement of the symptoms and of the child's well-being.

Retropharyngeal abscess

Retropharyngeal abscess is the commonest of the deep neck space infections occurring in infancy and may well mimic laryngotracheobronchitis by presenting with airway embarrassment. Young children have many retropharyngeal lymph nodes and these may become infected via lymphatics from the tonsils, teeth, nasopharynx or paranasal sinuses. Most children will have a history of a previous upper respiratory tract infection. Unsuspected foreign bodies are another important cause. Syphilis and tuberculosis affecting the cervical spine may also present with a retropharyngeal abscess. Children over the age of 4 years have far fewer nodes in the retropharyngeal space, hence this infection is more common in very young children (Grodinski and Holyoke, 1938).

Once necrosis of a retropharyngeal lymph node takes place or there is direct extension from tuberculosis of the cervical spine, an abscess is formed which bulges anteriorly into the pharynx. The child becomes toxic, has dysphagia and may dribble. His head is held stiffly and is eventually hyperextended. Prominent cervical glands are present. Inspiratory stridor may occur from associated laryngeal oedema or forward displacement of the laryngopharynx.

Examination is difficult, for apart from the signs referred to above, the oropharynx is not easy to see in an infant, especially with unswallowed secretions pooling in the throat. The retropharyngeal space is in direct continuity with the posterior mediastinum and palpation of the pharynx may well strip the abscess inferiorly or else cause it to be inadvertently ruptured with a consequent risk of inhalation of pus.

The management of this condition is considered later but by far the most reliable way of diagnosing a retropharyngeal abscess is with a lateral soft tissue neck X-ray (*Figure 30.6*).

Paraquat poisoning

Paraquat (1,1'-dimethyl 4,4'-bipyridyldiylium dichloride) is a herbicide which is occasionally

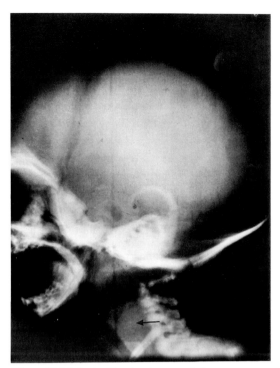

Figure 30.6 Infant with retropharyngeal abscess (arrowed). Note the width of the cervical spine compared with the width of the retropharyngeal space. The trachea is displaced anteriorly

ingested and gives rise to a pseudo-diphtheritic picture (Broniatowski, 1985). It causes a marked pharyngeal membrane which is less adherent to underlying tissues than that in diphtheria. The tongue, characteristically, is more heavily involved with membrane than are the tonsils (Stevens, Walker, Schaffner, 1981). Systemic signs of shock and sepsis are also present.

The management of acute laryngeal infections in childhood

The two aims in management are to arrive swiftly at the correct diagnosis and to treat safely the child's airway obstruction. In order that this may be achieved, there must be a laid down admissions policy in each district which all family doctors are aware of and adhere to. The ambulance crew must also know of the arrangements and the hospital staff from different specialities must cooperate smoothly together. There is a necessity for frequent reminders in the form of postgraduate seminars to all grades of staff to keep those that may have only just joined a general practice or hospital department informed as to the local procedures.

It is only by adhering to a rigid protocol that safety in the management of airway obstruction in the child will be maintained. Each hospital receiving such children should work out their own arrangements, but cooperation between anaesthetists, otolaryngologists and paediatricians (alphabetical order only!) is essential. Ideally, there should be a special resuscitation room near the main emergency department and adjacent to an operating theatre suite where children may be revived. Personnel involved in the management should be as senior as possible. It is not the situation for the newly appointed anaesthetist or otolaryngology resident.

The equipment in the resuscitation room needs to be checked daily to make sure it is complete and in working order – particularly bulbs, fibre light cables and suction equipment. The room must have enough space to house the mother and child, an anaesthetist, nurse, an otolaryngologist, theatre nurse, and a paediatrician. In practice, other personnel frequently swell the numbers.

The resuscitation trolley requirements include a full range of naso- and orotracheal tubes ranging from 2.5 mm upwards. Introducers for the endotracheal tubes are essential. Two laryngoscopes with straight blades should be available in case one fails. A complete anaesthetic machine is also in the room with all necessary anaesthetic drugs and intravenous equipment. There will also need to be bronchoscopy equipment and the Storz, rigid fibre light bronchoscopes are a personal preference, six sizes being available ranging from 2.5 mm to 5 mm. These need to be equipped with side arms for anaesthetic ventilation. Venturi systems are dangerous, since there may be little room for escape of gases around a tightly fitting bronchoscope and pneumothoraces may occur with their use. Various foreign body forceps for use down the bronchoscope need to be at hand, as do the correct lengths of suction cannulae. A paediatric tracheostomy set is also available, although rarely used in the author's practice.

One of the most important pieces of equipment

Table 30.1 Summary of differential diagnosis

	Epiglottitis	Laryngotracheobronchitis	Laryngeal foreign body	Retropharyngeal abscess
Pathology	Bacterial, usually *Haemophilus influenzae* type B	Viral, Parainfluenza virus type I		Bacterial, *Staphylococcus aureus*
Age	2–6 years	Under 3 years	Any	1–4 years
History				
onset	Rapid – less than 6 hours	Slow – usually 48 hours	Rapid	Slow – usually history of tonsillitis or upper respiratory tract infection
previous attacks	Not reported	Quite often	Occasional	Not reported
Symptoms				
cough	Absent	Barking cough	Paroxysms of coughing	Absent
dysphagia	Severe	None	Occasional	Severe
stridor	Inspiratory	Biphasic	Inspiratory	Inspiratory
Signs				
temperature	Elevated	Elevated	Apyrexial	Elevated
posture	Sitting, leaning forward	Lying on back	Variable	Sitting, stiff neck
drooling	Marked	None	Occasional	Marked
cervical glands	Large	Small	None	Large
behaviour	Quiet and terrified	Struggling	Variable	Restless
colour	Pale or grey	Pink – cyanotic in late stages	Usually normal	Flushed
voice	Muffled	Hoarse	Hoarse	Hoarse
X-ray	'Thumb sign' dangerous to perform	'Steeple sign'	Foreign body is visible if opaque	Marked widening of retropharyngeal space

is the suction apparatus. There need to be two separate units, one, a large pharyngeal sucker such as a Yankauer, for pharyngeal secretions and occasional sudden vomits, and the other for fine catheters or rigid fine metal suction tubes required for the bronchoscope.

The first stage of management is to arrive at a sensible diagnosis in a short space of time. Unnecessary questioning of parents for irrelevant information causes a waste of precious time. The most important consideration is to distinguish epiglottitis and laryngeal foreign body from laryngotracheobronchitis and its mimics, since the former need immediate attention, whereas the latter can usually be managed in a more leisurely fashion. Although not all cases are typical, the boundary between the supraglottic compartment, the rest of the larynx and the tracheobronchial tree is crossed in both directions by both groups of infections. *Table 30.1* may help to summarize the usual distinguishing features.

If all cases were typical, as in *Table 30.1*, which sadly they are not, there would be no difficulty distinguishing one disease from another! The signs of retropharyngeal abscess and epiglottitis appear to be much the same, except that the former is usually accompanied by a history of a previous upper respiratory tract infection and is of a much slower onset. A laryngeal foreign body can be excluded from epiglottitis, despite its rapid onset, by the absence of pyrexia and the common history of a foreign body being actually inhaled. The most important decision to be made in the emergency department is whether the child has epiglottitis or, if his airway is immediately threatened by one of the other causes. In either event, an alternative airway must be secured without delay and no further investigations or radiology should be carried out.

Management of epiglottitis

If it is thought the child is suffering from epiglottitis, the following is considered a safe protocol.

The terrified child is comforted and his mother allowed to hold him upright (*see Figure 30.3*). No attempt should be made to restrain or undress him, carry out venepuncture, X-ray or examine him further since all these procedures may cause crying and precipitate immediate respiratory arrest (Goel, 1984; Tarnow-Mordi *et al.*, 1985; Williams *et al.*, 1985). Radiology is not advised but a lateral neck X-ray may show the classical 'thumb' sign of the swollen epiglottis (*Figure 30.7*). If radiological services are present in the emergency room and the child's condition is so stable as to throw some doubt on the diagnosis of epiglottitis,

then there may be justification for radiology. If the clinical situation suggests that the diagnosis is epiglottitis, there is no point in confirming it with what might turn out to be a fatal X-ray.

Examination of the throat by tongue depression is particularly dangerous and in no circumstances should be carried out since respiratory obstruction may occur suddenly – possibly from increase and spread of the swelling in the pre-epiglottic space or from vagal stimulation.

The child is carried by his mother to the resuscitation room, described above, where experienced anaesthetic, otolaryngologic and paediatric staff will prepare to secure an alternative airway. Since the airway may obstruct completely if the child is supine, he should be anaesthetized in the upright position. Occasionally, the child collapses prior to anaesthesia, in which case, intubation or bronchoscopy is required without delay and without induction of anaesthesia.

The otolaryngologist is present in case intubation fails, in which case rigid bronchoscopy is necessary followed, possibly, by tracheostomy onto the bronchoscope through which anaesthesia is maintained. However, in most cases, the anaesthetist will perform the intubation. The author prefers inhalation anaesthesia with halothane plus 100% oxygen delivered to the child in the sitting position.

If a mask is too frightening, the gases are applied as near to the child's face as possible using

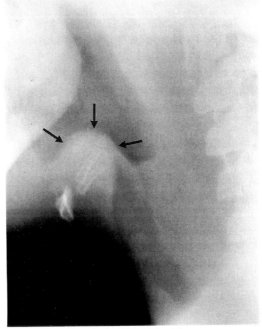

Figure 30.7 'Thumb sign' in epiglottitis

the anaesthetist's hand as a mask. Muscle relaxants are not used as there is a risk of producing an apnoeic patient with a mechanically obstructed airway. Intravenous induction is also avoided since obstruction may occur if the child cries as the needle is inserted.

As soon as the child loses consciousness, the mother is shown from the room and the child laid on his back ready to be intubated. A laryngoscope is inserted and the diagnosis of epiglottitis is confirmed. The usual description is of a cherry red, swollen epiglottis, but very often the aryepiglottic folds are grossly oedematous and the picture is more one of *supraglottitis* rather than inflammation being confined to the epiglottis. It is at this stage that a powerful pharyngeal sucker may be necessary to clear all the secretions. If the entrance to the laryngeal inlet is not apparent, sudden compression of the child's chest will often produce a bubble of air in the mucus to indicate the position of the glottis. An appropriately sized orotracheal tube is inserted and hopefully the airway is fully and suddenly restored.

If the first attempt at intubation fails, further manipulation may increase soft tissue oedema and obscure the airway as well as causing marked vagal stimulation resulting in severe bradycardia or cardiac arrest. Further attempts at intubation with floppy plastic tubes will probably also fail. The patient should be handed over to the otolaryngologist who should be able to insert a rigid bronchoscope behind the epiglottis and into the trachea. Experience has shown that if a bronchoscope is not available, intubation can often be achieved using a metal, round-tipped, female urethral cannula which has the advantage of being rigid. Once the airway is secured, by whichever method, the immediate danger is over and at this stage an intravenous cannula is inserted to allow the anaesthetist better control.

The decision now has to be made about the type of airway to stay in place for the next 48 hours. The author prefers nasotracheal intubation, but if the orotracheal tube was only inserted with great difficulty, then it would seem unwise to remove it. Usually, however, a nasotracheal tube can be inserted via the nose to a position adjacent to the oral tube behind the epiglottis and then the latter removed with immediate replacement of the former. If bronchoscopy has been necessary, it is probably safer to perform a tracheostomy onto the bronchoscope, although recent personal experience has not required this, the bronchoscope being replaced with a nasotracheal tube as described above.

At this stage culture swabs are taken from the epiglottis, and a blood culture performed. A good intravenous infusion line is inserted for fluid replacement and for antibiotic therapy. A nasogastric tube should also be inserted for feeding since the child will have to be heavily sedated to avoid swallowing and struggling against the endotracheal tube, which would otherwise cause it to abrade the inflamed epiglottis. One advantage of a tracheostomy is that it allows the child to be ambulant and swallow normally. Cantrell, Bell and Morioka (1978) reviewed 19 series, totalling 738 cases of epiglottitis, and found that the mortality rate if tracheostomy was performed was 0.86% compared with 0.92% if endotracheal intubation had been utilized. However, this rate rose to 6.1% if an artificial airway of some sort was not used in the treatment of epiglottitis. It seems clear, therefore, that whether a tracheostomy or an endotracheal tube is used, there is little change for the outcome of the patient, but there is a significant difference if the child is treated without an alternative airway. The morbidity of tracheostomy and endotracheal intubation will be considered later.

The child is now transferred from the emergency room to a paediatric intensive care unit. If he has been intubated, sedation is necessary prior to transfer to avoid the risk of extubation during the move. Intravenous diazepam 0.1 mg/kg as a bolus followed by a continuous infusion of approximately 0.1 mg/kg per hour is an effective method. The choice of antibiotic is difficult since the emergence of ampicillin and occasionally chloramphenicol resistant strains of *Haemophilus influenzae* type B has been reported (Philpott-Howard and Williams, 1982). It has been suggested that one of the newer cephalosporins–cefotaxime (Claforan) – is highly effective against both ampicillin- and chloramphenicol-resistant strains (Drake-Lee, Broughton and Grace, 1984). Other organisms, such as β-haemolytic streptococcus, pneumococcus and staphylococcus, causing epiglottitis require appropriate treatment once blood cultures and epiglottic swabs are available. The current choice of antibiotic is chloramphenicol, 100 mg/kg of body weight per 24 hours.

Steroids are not indicated for the treatment of epiglottitis, although Cantrell, Bell and Morioka (1978) reported their widespread use.

The most important feature about the care of nasotracheal tubes is the personnel who look after the airway. It requires highly trained nurses, and enough of them, to care for these patients and it is only in an intensive care situation that these criteria are likely to be met. If an alternative airway has had to be secured in a hospital without intensive care facilities, then a tracheostomy is likely to be safest, since it requires less intense nursing skills in the immediate postoperative period.

Intravenous fluids are necessary to keep the child hydrated. The nasogastric tube is used more for aspiration of stomach contents to prevent vomiting than for feeding.

Extubation is usually possible within 48 hours. Corticosteroids may be given just before extubation to help reduce oedema by the tube. The airway will need to be carefully observed after extubation. It is also advisable to keep the child in a humidified atmosphere for a few hours.

One of the rewarding features about managing this most frightening of paediatric emergencies is that, if cared for correctly, most children with epiglottitis are extubated within 48 hours – having been transformed from a moribund to a fully active, apparently healthy child within that time.

Deaths still occur (Welch and Price, 1983) but with a protocol such as suggested above the outcome should be favourable. Since it is the observed cases that die, it is essential that every practitioner is aware of this condition. If there is the slightest suspicion that a child may have epiglottitis, then immediate transference to hospital is mandatory, if necessary in the practitioner's car, so that an alternative airway can be secured as soon as possible.

Management of laryngotracheobronchitis

Some children with acute laryngotracheobronchitis will need an alternative airway on admission, especially if the diagnosis is bacterial laryngotracheobronchitis (pseudomembranous croup), in which case, the preceding protocol for epiglottitis will serve as the management. However, since only approximately 1% of laryngotracheobronchitis will need intubation (Milner, 1984), a different approach is adopted.

Provided epiglottitis is unlikely, then conservative management with careful observation is usually all that is required while the disease settles. There are many controversial aspects of the management of laryngotracheobronchitis and these will be discussed.

Radiology

While in the emergency department lateral, anteroposterior neck, and chest X-rays are performed. The lateral neck X-ray is the only reliable way to exclude a retropharyngeal abscess (*see Figure 30.6*) and hopefully will not demonstrate a swollen epiglottis which should have been excluded clinically. Foreign bodies may also be seen. The neck X-ray may show a narrowed subglottis (*Figure 30.8*), with the so-called 'steeple' sign typical of laryngotracheobronchitis and may also show 'ballooning' of the hypopharynx. The chest X-ray is a helpful baseline to exclude collapsed lobes and mediastinal shift or obstructive

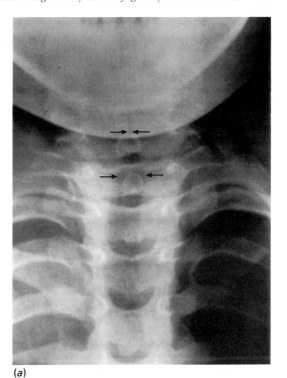

(a)

(b)

Figure 30.8 (a) Anteroposterior neck X-ray of laryngotracheobronchitis showing 'steeple sign'. (b) Lateral neck X-ray of laryngotracheobronchitis showing 'steeple sign' and 'ballooning of hypopharynx'. Lower arrows show normal trachea and upper arrows narrowed area ('steeple')

emphysema as may occur with bronchial foreign bodies. Pulmonary oedema and pneumonia are also occasionally seen.

Once the X-ray has been taken, the child is admitted to the appropriate ward for observation.

Observation

Croup scoring systems are used in some hospitals (Davis *et al.*, 1981) but a numerical score has not been found to influence the clinical management of patients. It is hoped that observations will show the stridor lessening, the restlessness settling, the colour remaining pink and the respiration and cardiac rates reducing. These parameters will not improve readily if the child is frightened and to remove a child from his mother, place him in a cold fog in a dripping plastic tent (Henry, 1983) where he cannot see his surroundings and subject him to frequent pulse readings and painful blood gas estimations does not help the situation.

Reassurance

Most of the treatments suggested for laryngotracheobronchitis are controversial, but the one aspect on which all authors agree is that the child needs strong reassurance, as does the mother. It is a recommended practice not to separate mother and child and once in a calm, confident, reassuring atmosphere both seem to relax. Sedation is rarely necessary and there are serious dangers of suppressing the central drive to respiration with some drugs. If sedation seems essential, then chloral hydrate 30 mg/kg is the safest choice.

Humidification

Most authors agree that warm, moist air does little harm (Henry, 1983) and others suggest it should be delivered via a head box in very young children or in a tent in those who are older (Davis *et al.*, 1981). Most parents whose children have had recurrent problems will report the beneficial effects of a steam kettle at home, but there has been no controlled trial giving evidence that humidity is efficacious, although there seems to be evidence that spasmodic laryngitis responds to mist therapy (Fogel *et al.*, 1982). However, since it does no harm and probably helps to prevent drying of secretions from the respiratory tract, some form of humidity should be given. There is no place for cold mist. Jet nebulizers have no effect on humidifying the larynx and ultrasonically generated mist increases airway obstruction in children with abnormally labile airways (Henry, 1983).

The ideal situation is to have a 'croup room' where the relative humidity of the atmosphere in the whole room can be kept high. Placing the child in a plastic humidified tent, may increase his anxiety and make careful observation more difficult through the fog, and is not recommended. If a 'croup room' is not available a nebulizer, blowing warm, wet air as near as possible to the face of the child is of some help. Hydration is also essential with oral fluids if possible, but if the child is not willing to drink, then intravenous fluids are necessary.

Oxygen

Oxygen therapy is also controversial. If a decision is made that the child needs an alternative airway, then obviously it is used until the airway is secured. In less severe cases, there is one view (Welch and Price, 1983) that its use may mask early signs of hypoxia but, on the other hand, Broniatowski (1985) feels that oxygen is mandatory since hypoxia is the most important blood gas abnormality. It is also suggested that supplemental humidified oxygen in the presence of diffuse bronchial involvement will help to prevent reflex bronchoconstriction, sputum retention and pulmonary oedema (Levison, Tabachnik and Newth, 1982). If oxygen is not used for fear of missing cyanosis, it should be pointed out that this is a late clinical sign, when arterial oxygen saturation is less than 40%. The problem with oxygen therapy is in its mode of application. Unless it is given via a face mask, the inspired percentage is variable and certainly the concentration of oxygen in an average plastic tent when 100% is delivered is only 35%. Unless there is evidence of severe bronchial involvement, or a decision has been made to intubate, the routine use of oxygen is not advised because of the fear induced by a face mask.

Steroids

The place of steroids is not settled, probably because response has not been related to the cause of the airway obstruction. A recent double-blind trial (Koren *et al.*, 1983) using dexamethasone 0.6 mg/kg as a single dose against placebo, found the steroid to be helpful in spasmodic laryngitis, but not in laryngotracheobronchitis. Severe cases of laryngotracheobronchitis were not accepted into the study and the difficulty in clinically distinguishing spasmodic laryngitis from laryngotracheobronchitis was pointed out. A totally opposite opinion was expressed in another report (Asher and Beaudry, 1981), where steroids were found to have a dramatic effect on laryngotracheobronchitis but not on spasmodic laryngitis. A previous study showed no significant benefit from steroid usage (Eden, Kaufman and Yu, 1967).

Since there is confusion the routine use of steroids is not recommended except possibly as a last resort to resuscitate a child in the hope of avoiding intubation, and occasionally to reduce oedema prior to extubation if this has previously failed.

Antibiotics

There is no evidence that antibiotics are of benefit in viral laryngotracheobronchitis except when a secondary bacterial bronchitis supervenes. Bacterial laryngotracheitis (pseudomembranous croup) is probably a separate disease and since *Staphylococcus aureus* is normally the causative organism, flucloxacillin is given. In practice, most children who are intubated for laryngotracheobronchitis receive antibiotics which are changed depending on clinical response and the culture sensitivities from aspirates.

Racemic adrenaline (epinephrine)

There has been enthusiasm for this form of treatment in the USA, Canada, Australia and more recently in the UK. According to Fogel *et al.* (1982) racemic adrenaline, nebulized and delivered by intermittent positive pressure breathing in uncontrolled studies seems effective, but in other controlled studies it has been shown to be no more beneficial than nebulized saline. Fogel *et al.* (1982) designed a randomized trial whereby nebulized racemic adrenaline was compared with its delivery via intermittent positive pressure breathing. They included only patients who failed to respond to nebulized saline. The results show that delivery via intermittent positive pressure breathing was not necessary for the effect and that it did reduce obstruction for up to 30 minutes in laryngotracheobronchitis. Spasmodic laryngitis responded to normal saline mist alone. These authors used 0.25 ml of 2.25% racemic adrenaline diluted with isotonic saline, nebulized and given via a tight fitting face mask. Continuous ECG monitoring is necessary and there are dangers of a rebound effect. It is therefore only appropriate as a hospital management. The use of a tight fitting mask is controversial and because of its uncertain value, the application of this treatment as a routine form of therapy is not recommended.

Summary of management of laryngotracheobronchitis

Since only 1% of children with laryngotracheobronchitis fail to respond to conservative management, however controversial, the main reason for admission to hospital is to observe and secure safely an airway should that be necessary.

Recommended management includes effective reassurance and possibly efficient humidification. It does not include routine use of oxygen, steroids, antibiotics or racemic adrenaline. Careful monitoring of the progress of the child is the most important aspect.

Monitoring of laryngotracheobronchitis

As mentioned previously, croup scoring systems have been suggested. They are useful as an initial baseline measurement but need to be continuously updated by the same nurses and the same medical staff, since they are very subjective. Objective methods of monitoring include pulse and respiration rates and blood gas estimation. Blood gas anslysis is only used on rare occasions because it is a disturbing and painful procedure. It is necessary when there is significant bronchial involvement. Unfortunately, transcutaneous oxygen and carbon dioxide probes are not easy to use in restless children as the transducers move and their readings are unreliable.

A quarter-hourly pulse rate charted from a monitor is of most value. Respiration rates can also be used and, according to Newth, Levison and Brown (1972), they correlate best with arterial oxygen tension. In practice, it is often a combination of a falling pulse rate, relaxation of a restless child, quietening of stridor and maintenance of a good colour that suggest favourable progress. There is no substitute for experience in assessing this condition and a good deal can be learnt by trainee doctors and nurses sitting for 2 or 3 hours with the child and observing progress. If a decision is made that a child needs an alternative airway, the same anaesthetic care is required as was described for epiglottitis.

Management of retropharyngeal abscess

As mentioned in the description of the clinical features of this infection, a lateral neck X-ray (*see Figure 30.6*) is the most reliable method of establishing the diagnosis. Computerized tomographic scanning has also been shown to be of value, especially in assessing the extent of the abscess cavity (White, 1985). This makes it easier to decide which route to use for drainage. X-rays, however, must be interpreted correctly and a true lateral X-ray is necessary (Seid, Dunbar, Cotton, 1979).

Normal variance must not be confused with disease, for instance neck flexion causes a widening of the retropharyngeal space and a reversed lordosis of the cervical spine can be caused by any condition that gives rise to muscle spasm and not just by infection. A useful rule is that the anteroposterior diameter of the prevertebral soft tissues should not exceed the diameter of the vertebral bodies. Pathological lesions of the vertebral bodies and discs must also be assessed. A chest X-ray needs to be performed to exclude spread from the neck into the posterior mediastinum. Providing that the child is not in immediate danger of serious airway embarrassment and if the X-rays suggest a retropharyngeal abscess, intravenous antibiotics should be the first line of treatment. *Staphylococcus aureus, Streptococcus pyogenes* and anaerobic bacteria are the most common organisms in deep neck space infections (White, 1985). It is personal practice to use a combination of penicillin, flucloxacillin and metronidazole in appropriate doses for the weight of the child.

If the airway is compromised, or if there is no response to antibiotic therapy, drainage will be necessary. The safety of modern anaesthesia is such that, with an experienced anaesthetist, intubation is possible without trauma. The danger exists, however, of rupturing the abscess before the airway is secured or stripping the abscess into the posterior mediastinum.

Once the child is safely intubated, the posterior pharyngeal wall can be examined using a standard tonsillectomy gag. The abscess can then be aspirated or incised through the pharynx. External approaches, either anterior or posterior to the sternomastoid muscle have been suggested (Levitt, 1976) and are appropriate if extension of the abscess has occurred into the parapharyngeal space or posterior mediastinum. Cultures of the pus evacuated can now be obtained and the antibiotic therapy adjusted depending on the bacteria found.

It is recommended that intubation is continued for at least 24 hours after aspiration or incision of the abscess or until there is an obvious clinical improvement in the child's condition as judged by radiology and a settling of the pyrexia.

Choice and care of an alternative airway in inflammatory laryngeal obstruction

Tracheostomy is discussed in Chapter 32 and only brief comments relevant to the infected airway will be made here.

The choice as to whether endotracheal intubation or tracheostomy is performed may be a personal one or may be dependent upon local nursing services. There is no doubt that specialized intensive care facilities are necessary for the management of endotracheal tubes, whereas tracheostomy care needs less specialized personnel. Therefore, individual hospitals will have different criteria depending on local circum-

stances. The mortality rates between the two modalities of intubation and tracheostomy for epiglottitis are said to be very similar at 0.92% and 0.86% respectively (Cantrell, Bell and Morioka, 1978). However, Friedberg and Morrison (1974) demonstrated a 3% mortality rate due to childhood tracheostomy from pneumothoraces, displacement or obstruction of the tube.

The differences in morbidity rates are more striking. Mitchell and Thomas (1980) reporting a series of 2567 patients with laryngotracheobronchitis admitted to the Hospital for Sick Children, Toronto, stated that 2.5% required airway support. When they used tracheostomy, the tubes were in place for a mean time of 11 days, whereas endotracheal tubes stayed *in situ* for only 6 days. There were no deaths in the tracheostomy group, but there was one fatality caused by tube obstruction among the children treated with endotracheal tubes. Despite this, their management has changed from tracheostomy to endotracheal tubes, but they do emphasize the need for experienced nursing care in the management of the intubated patient.

Endotracheal intubation

Whether intubation is via naso- or oroendotracheal routes, the major complication is tube obstruction. Occasionally multiple intubations are necessary to replace blocked tubes or because of failed trials of extubation. Mitchell and Thomas (1980) found that there were no cases of subglottic stenosis from intubation, but it did occur four times in 30 tracheostomies.

It must be emphasized that an endotracheal tube used in an inflammatory disease of the larynx will pass through the affected site. It is therefore essential that good fixation of the tube is achieved and that the child is sedated enough to avoid struggling which might cause movements of the tube which would further damage the inflamed larynx. The vocal cords are, of course, splinted apart by the tube and this prevents the child from being able to cough or talk. A nasogastric tube is also necessary for feeding. Expert nursing care is obviously required not only to manage the above problems, but also to provide adequate humidity and regular aspiration of the tube to prevent obstruction.

The type of tube is a matter of preference. Most units use polyvinyl chloride (PVC) endotracheal tubes. It may be sensible to spray these with a silicone compound to increase the lubrication of the tube. Silastic tubes are available but are expensive and have a thicker wall which tends to increase the size of the tube necessary to maintain adequate ventilation. The size of tube is extremely important. It should be as small as possible to prevent traumatizing already damaged tissue. A rough guide to the size of tube needed in normal patients without inflammatory airway disease can be worked out by the formula of dividing the child's age by four and adding 4.5 mm. It is recommended that a tube one size smaller than would be required for the normal child is selected for the inflamed larynx.

Fixation of a nasotracheal tube is easier than an orotracheal tube and requires a brace onto the forehead. Regular aspiration with suction catheters is necessary to prevent accumulation of secretions. Humidification is vital to prevent the secretions becoming too tenacious. This may take the form of a warm nebulizer attached by a T-tube to the endotracheal tube with or without added oxygen depending on the child's blood gases. Humidification may be supplemented by the installation of 2 ml of normal saline immediately prior to aspiration. The suction catheters used should be graduated and measured against the known length of the endotracheal tube. It is important that the catheter goes beyond the endotracheal tube to clear it, but not so far that it

continually abrades the carina of the trachea, thereby causing a granuloma. Regular physiotherapy is essential to prevent bronchopneumonia.

Extubation is usually possible within 48 hours with epiglottitis but, as mentioned previously, 6 days seems an average length of time in laryngotracheobronchitis (Mitchell and Thomas, 1980). Every child will be different but it would seem reasonable to attempt extubation when there is no evidence of any chest infection and the secretions are less tenacious. There should be an obvious leak around the tube indicating that the oedema has lessened. It may be worth using corticosteroids for 6 hours prior to extubation to reduce any postintubation oedema. Racemic adrenaline can also be used via a nebulizer prior to extubation for similar purposes. Once the child has been extubated, then efficient humidification is necessary as is very careful observation for the first few hours. It is usually obvious within an hour or two whether the child will be able to cope without the need for re-intubation. The parents will need to be reassured about the very weak, husky voice that often follows prolonged intubation, but this is usually nearly back to normal within 24 hours.

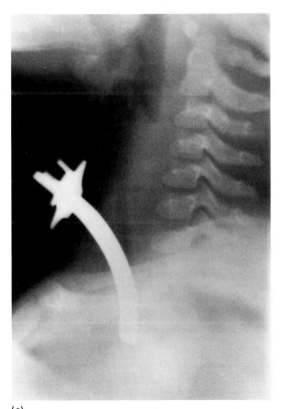

(a)

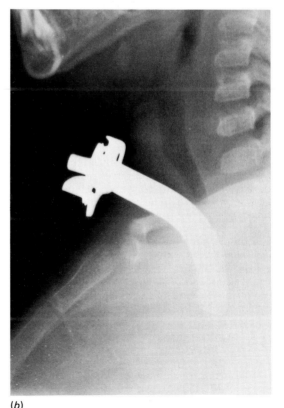

(b)

Figure 30.9 (*a*) Tracheostomy tube in good position without tracheal wall distortion. (*b*) Tracheostomy tube which is too large and which causes posterior displacement of the anterior wall of the trachea above the tracheostomy site

Tracheostomy

The main advantages of tracheostomy are that the disease process is bypassed, the child does not need sedating and normal feeding is usually possible. Occlusion of the tube with a finger on expiration or with the use of a valve allows talking and coughing to occur. However, tracheostomy has major disadvantages. The mortality rate and increased length of time before extubation is possible, have already been mentioned. The operation of tracheostomy leaves a scar which, in some instances, can be quite unsightly. Although tracheostomy on the whole requires less skilled nursing care, there is a risk of accidental extubation, especially on return from the operating theatre. It may be extremely difficult to replace the tube in this situation, with disastrous consequences.

A less serious complication but, nevertheless, a well recognized one, is pneumothorax and air tracking in the neck. It is recommended that immediately after a tracheostomy has been performed a chest X-ray is carried out to make sure there is no pneumothorax present. It is also recommended that, on the first postoperative day a lateral neck X-ray is taken to make sure that the tracheostomy tube is in line with the trachea and not causing backward displacement of the anterior wall of the trachea immediately above the tracheostomy site (*Figure 30.9*). If this complication is seen on X-ray it is worth changing the tracheostomy tube for one with a different shape which hopefully will not produce this deformity. If it is unrecognized, then there may be a permanent tracheal stenosis which will cause difficulties in extubation.

A personal preference in design of tracheostomy tube is the Great Ormond Street pattern which is usually made from polyvinyl chloride (PVC). Silastic may be a preferable material. Although this does not have the advantage of an inner tube, or a fenestra and valve to aid in extubation, it becomes soft at body temperature and moulds itself well to the correct shape of the trachea.

In ideal situations, it would seem that endotracheal intubation is preferable to tracheostomy as an alternative airway in acute laryngeal inflammatory obstruction in childhood.

References

ASHER, M. I. and BEAUDRY, P. H. (1981) Croup and corticosteroid therapy. *Journal of Pediatrics*, **97**, 506–507

BRONIATOWSKI, M. (1985) Epiglottitis. *Ear, Nose and Throat Journal*, **64**, 22–27

CANTRELL, R. W., BELL, R. A. and MORIOKA, W. T. (1978) Acute epiglottitis: intubation versus tracheostomy. *The Laryngoscope*, **88**, 994–1005

DAVIS, H. W., GARTNER, J. C., GALVIS, A. G., MICHAELS, R. H. and MESTAD, P. H. (1981) Acute upper airway obstruction: croup and epiglottitis. *Pediatric Clinics of North America*, **28**, 859–880

DENNY, F. W., MURPHY, T. F., CLYDE, W. A., COLLIER, A. M. and HENDERSON, F. W. (1983) Croup: an 11-year study in paediatric practice. *Pediatrics*, **71**, 871–876

DRAKE-LEE, A. B., BROUGHTON, S. J. and GRACE, A. (1984) Children with epiglottitis. *British Journal of Clinical Practice*, **38**, 218–220

EDEN, A. N., KAUFMAN, A. and YU, R. (1967) Corticosteroids and croup. *Journal of the American Medical Association*, **200**, 133

FEARON, B. (1975) Acute epiglottitis: a potential killer. *Canadian Medical Association Journal*, **112**, 760

FOGEL, J. M., BERG, I. J., GERBER, M. A. and SCHERTER, C. B. (1982) Racemic epinephrine in the treatment of croup: nebulization alone versus nebulization with intermittent positive pressure breathing. *Journal of Pediatrics*, **101**, 1028–1031

FRIEDBERG, J. and MORRISON, M. D. (1974) Pediatric tracheotomy. *Canadian Journal of Otolaryngology*, **3**, 147–155

FRIEDMAN, E. M., JORGENSEN, K., HEALY, G. B. and McGILL, T. J. I. (1985) Bacterial tracheitis – 2 year experience. *The Laryngoscope*, **95**, 9–11

GOEL, K. M. (1984) Are neck radiographs necessary in the management of croup syndrome? *Archives of Disease in Childhood*, **59**, 908

GRODINSKI, M. and HOLYOKE, E. A. (1938) The fascia and fascial spaces of the head, neck and adjacent regions. *American Journal of Anatomy*, **63**, 367–408

HALL, C. B. and HALL, W. J. (1975) Viral croup: acute laryngotracheobronchitis. *Update*, **10**, 561

HENRY, R. (1983) Moist air in the treatment of laryngotracheitis. *Archives of Disease in Childhood*, **58**, 577

KOREN, G., FRAND, M., BARZILAY, Z. and MacLEOD, S. M. (1983) Corticosteroid treatment of laryngotracheitis v spasmodic croup in children. *American Journal of Diseases of Children*, **137**, 941–944

LEVISON, H., TABACHNIK, E. and NEWTH, C. J. L. (1982) Wheezing in infancy, croup and epiglottitis. *Current Problems in Paediatrics*, **12**, 38–60

LEVITT, G. W. (1976) Cervical fascia and deep neck infections. *Otolaryngologic Clinics of North America*, **9**, 703–716

MARGOLIS, C. Z. (1980) Definition of croup. *Journal of Pediatrics*, **96**, 1123–1124

MILNER, A. D. (1984) Acute stridor in the pre-school child. *British Medical Journal*, **288**, 811–812

MITCHELL, D. P. and THOMAS, R. L. (1980) Secondary airway support in the management of croup. *Journal of Otolaryngology*, **9**, 419–422

NEWTH, C. J. L., LEVISON, H. and BROWN, A. C. (1972) The respiratory status of children with croup. *Journal of Pediatrics*, **84**, 1068

PHILPOTT-HOWARD, J. and WILLIAMS, J. D. (1982) Increase in antibiotic resistance in *Haemophilus influenzae* in the UK since 1977: report of a study group. *British Medical Journal*, **284**, 1597–1599

PRACY, R. (1979) Congenital diseases of the larynx. In *Scott-Brown's Diseases of the Ear, Nose and Throat*, 4th edn, edited by J. Ballantyne and J. Groves, pp. 309–328. London: Butterworths

SCHWARTZ, R. H., KNERR, R. J., HERMANSEN, K. and

WIENTZEN, R. L. (1982) Acute epiglottitis caused by beta-haemolytic group C streptococci. *American Journal of Diseases of Children*, **136**, 558–559

SEID, A. B., DUNBAR, J. S. and COTTON, R. T. (1979) Retropharyngeal abscesses in children revisited. *The Laryngoscope*, **89**, 1717–1724

STEVENS, D. L., WALKER, D. H. and SCHAFFNER, W. (1981) Pseudodiphtheria: prominent pharyngeal membrane associated with fatal paraquat ingestion. *Annals of Internal Medicine*, **94**, 202–204

TARNOW-MORDI, W. D., BERRILL, A. M., DARBY, C. W., DAVIS, P. and POOK, J. (1985) Precipitation of laryngeal obstruction in acute epiglottitis. *British Medical Journal*, **290**, 629

TUCKER, J. A. (1979) Obstruction of the major pediatric airway. *Otolaryngologic Clinics of North America*, **12**, 329–341

WELCH, D. B. and PRICE, D. G. (1983) Acute epiglottitis and severe croup. Experience in two English regions. *Anaesthesia*, **38**, 754–759

WHITE, B. (1985) Deep neck infections and respiratory distress in children. *Ear, Nose and Throat Journal*, **64**, 30–38

WILLIAMS, P. A., ARMITAGE, E. N., FISHER, N. G. and HATCHER, G. W. (1985) Precipitation of laryngeal obstruction in acute epiglottitis. *British Medical Journal*, **290**, 1007

ZACH, M. S. (1983) Airway reactivity in recurrent croup. *European Journal of Respiratory Disease*, **128**, (suppl.), 81–88

31

Recurrent respiratory papillomatosis

M. Stuart Strong

It is over 100 years since Mackenzie described what was thought to be an entity – juvenile laryngeal papillomata (Mackenzie, 1880). The implication was that papillomata were common only in children and that the only site of involvement was the larynx. This notion prevailed until the 1960s when it became apparent that the disease is not confined to the laryngeal mucosa and does occur in other areas of the respiratory tract. Furthermore, it became obvious that the disease was notoriously recurrent and that it persisted into adult life and, on other occasions, presented initially in adult life. This being the case, it appeared that a more descriptive term would be recurrent respiratory papillomatosis.

Background

The purpose of this chapter is to describe the characteristics of the disease, its behaviour and its management in children. The author's experience is based on 258 patients who were followed at University Hospital, Boston, USA, between 1971 and 1985. Of these patients, 150 were followed for one year or more and 81 patients were under the age of 15 years. Patients who could not be followed for more than one year are not included in the quoted statistics.

Presenting symptoms

The majority of children with recurrent respiratory papillomatosis present before the age of 4 years, although a not insignificant number may present during the first 6 months of life.

The initial symptom is hoarseness of voice or an abnormal cry. Increasing stridor and acute respiratory obstruction may occur but are usually late manifestations of the disease process. Papillomata form initially on the vocal cords themselves so interference with laryngeal function occurs early in the disease and hoarseness in a child should not be dismissed as being the result of vocal abuse: an endoscopy must be performed to establish the diagnosis.

There is a tendency for papillomata to occur at the anterior aspect of the glottis and the anterior commisure itself is frequently involved. It is uncommon for the interarytenoid mucosa to be involved in early cases; perhaps the thickness of the mucus blanket and the more rapid rate of its movement exerts a protective role in this situation. When the larynx is extensively involved the normal flow of the mucus blanket is disrupted and the papillomata then invade the whole of the larynx with equal facility. The disruption of the tracheal mucus blanket that occurs after tracheostomy may also be a factor in the often explosive increase in tracheal papillomata that is seen after a tracheostomy has been performed. It is for this reason that a tracheostomy should be avoided if it is possible to establish a normal airway by endoscopic removal of the papillomata.

Characteristics of the disease

The papillomata of recurrent respiratory papillomatosis are benign squamous papillomata that occur in clusters on the involved mucosa (*Figure 31.1*); the fronds of papilloma may be sessile and spread over a wide area of mucosa or they may be pedunculated and localized. The lesions are characteristically non-keratinizing (*Figure 31.2*).

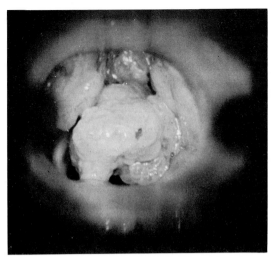

Figure 31.1 Fronds of papillomata filling the laryngeal lumen: the patient was tracheostomy dependent

It is characteristic that the lesions are multiple; occasionally at the onset of the disease or if the disease is about to become quiescent, only a single lesion may be manifest.

The lesions are notoriously recurrent even after the most radical extirpation. Recurrence may become an airway problem within 2 weeks or nothing may be visible for perhaps 5 or 20 years. The reason for this is that the lesions do not recur from the depth of the wound, but rather from the apparently normal mucosa adjacent to the original lesion. On some occasions it appears that removal of the papillomata has an enhancing effect on the growth rate of the lesions, so that the recurrence may be larger than the original lesion.

Recurrent respiratory papillomatosis is a diffuse diathesis of the mucous membrane of the upper air and food passages; the papillomata may be encountered in the nostrils at the mucocutaneous junction, on the gingiva and lips (*Figure 31.3*), on both surfaces of the soft palate and the adjacent tonsillar pillars, in the larynx, in the tracheobronchial tree and occasionally in the pulmonary parenchyma and at the oesophageal inlet. The lesions have a predilection for points of airway constriction, where there is increased air flow, drying, crusting and irritation; this is particularly evident around the tracheostomy site and at the tip of the tracheostomy tube. Most commonly the larynx is the site of greatest involvement and is often the only site (Strong *et al.*, 1976).

Aetiology

The aetiology of recurrent respiratory papillomatosis is now known to be infection of the epithelial cells with human papilloma virus. Although electron microscopy has only rarely demonstrated viral particles in papilloma specimens (Incze *et al.*, 1977), immunofluorescent techniques have shown incontrovertible evidence of the footprints of human papilloma virus DNA having been incorporated into the cellular DNA (Steinberg *et al.*,

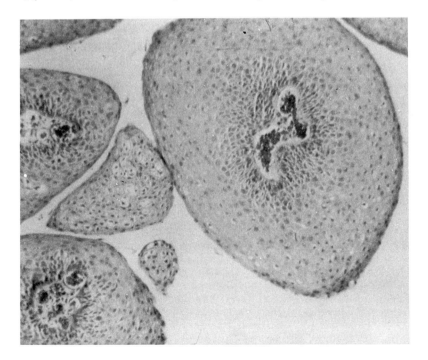

Figure 31.2 In each frond of papilloma, the hyperplastic squamous epithelium is supported by a thin vascular core of connective tissue. Maturation takes place but ceases prior to keratinization unless the lesion is otherwise irritated or stimulated

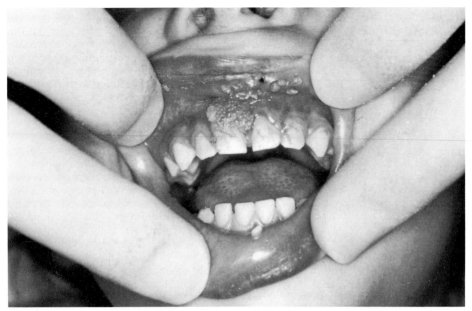

Figure 31.3 Papillomata on the gingiva and lips of a 5-year-old girl who habitually breathes through her mouth

1983). Furthermore, it has been shown by electron microscopy and immunofluorescence that apparently normal mucosa adjacent to the papillomata contains intracellular viral DNA of human papilloma virus. After removal of the lesions, these infected cells may become activated, leading to the formation of another lesion – a recurrence. This of course explains the difficulty in affecting 'a cure' of the disease by using mechanical means of removal alone. This phenomenon has been duplicated in the finding of latent human papilloma virus in the normal skin surrounding genital warts (Ferenczy *et al.*, 1985). So far it has not been possible to isolate and propagate the virus.

Epidemiology

Recurrent respiratory papillomatosis has a worldwide distribution, although in some countries and areas it is more prevalent than in others. The incidence in the USA was 7/1 000 000 per year in 1976 (Strong *et al.*, 1976); this suggests an incidence of approximately 1500 or more new cases per year. These cases were distributed between children and adults; slightly more cases being diagnosed before the age of 16 years than after. Furthermore, recurrent respiratory papillomatosis is found in all socio-economic segments of society and is not confined to disadvantaged patients as was previously thought. At the present time there is a suspicion that the incidence of the disease starting in early adult life is increasing.

The natural history of recurrent respiratory papillomatosis

Transmission

The transmissibility of recurrent respiratory papillomatosis must be very low because, as yet, it has not been recorded in siblings. There is considerable circumstantial evidence that, in some patients, the disease is transmitted at the time of delivery from a mother infected with genital warts. If a child contracts a disease before 5 years of age, there is a 60% probability that the mother had genital warts at the time of delivery (Strong *et al.*, 1976). Because of this worrisome association, some thought was given to advising the mother of a child with recurrent respiratory papillomatosis who is infected with genital warts, to consider having the delivery of her next child by caesarean section. However, since the disease has not been demonstrated in siblings, this precaution seems to be unnecessary.

Remission

Remission of recurrent respiratory papillomatosis can take place at any age and at any time; whether remission occurs or not appears to be unrelated to the thoroughness of the removal or to the method of removal of the disease. The use of the CO_2 laser allows removal of all visible disease while causing minimal damage to the laryngeal musculature and function. *Table 31.1* shows that the chance of remission is greatest if the disease presents between the ages of 6 and 10 years ($P = 0.01$). The

Table 31.1 Age of patients at time of remission

Age (years)	No. in remission (%)
1–5	15/46 (33)
6–10	16/23 (70)
11–13	6/12 (50)
Total	37/81 (46)

overall chance of achieving remission in patients less than 16 years of age at the time of presentation is 46% if they are followed for one year and treated by appropriate endoscopy and laser destruction; this can be compared with a 26% chance of remission if the disease becomes manifest at 16 year of age or later. Furthermore, the disease is more likely to undergo remission in the larynx (48%), than in the tracheobronchial tree (27%) or in the lungs (0%).

Duration of remission

The duration of remission varies from 2 years to life long; relapses may occur at any time and for no apparent reason. Since a relapse may occur in any patient at any time, the best we can hope for at present is prolonged remission rather than cure.

Recurrent respiratory papillomatosis does have the potential to spread. In 34 patients who had disease confined to the larynx and required tracheostomy for airway control prior to being seen by the author's team, 29 patients had developed tracheobronchial lesions that frequently were more difficult to keep under control than the original laryngeal lesions; in seven patients the disease progressed to involve the pulmonary parenchyma. In the lungs, the squamous epithelium of recurrent respiratory papillomatosis produces cystic spaces that are clearly visible on X-ray; the cysts are lined with squamous epithelium and are filled with fluid and sometimes air (*Figure 31.4*). Because the pulmonary spread is usually multicentric, it is relentlessly progressive and eventually fatal.

Malignant degeneration

The risk of malignant degeneration is extremely low unless radiotherapy had been used in an attempt to control the disease; thus radiotherapy is contraindicated in recurrent respiratory papillomatosis. In adults who smoke, malignant degeneration is not unusual; in this series two cases of squamous cell carcinoma and three of verrucous carcinoma were encountered. A few cases have been documented in the literature (Matsula *et al.*, 1985).

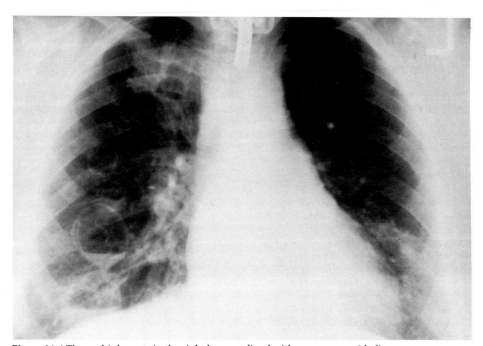

Figure 31.4 The multiple cysts in the right lung are lined with squamous epithelium; some contain air

Management

Surgery

The only satisfactory treatment of this condition is surgical, and this is usually carried out endoscopically. Endoscopy is carried out after the airway has been secured by the passage of an endotracheal tube. On occasions, the tube is withdrawn and ventilation continued with the Venturi apparatus to allow complete removal of papillomata on the arytenoids and elsewhere. The patient is then reintubated prior to the termination of anaesthesia.

Biopsy and total destruction of the papillomata with the CO_2 laser are carried out with complete removal of all visible papillomata on at least one occasion. If disease is found to involve the anterior commissure, two operations, 4 weeks apart, are required to avoid web formation, first treating one cord and then the other. In the event of recurrence, laryngoscopy and CO_2 laser destruction are repeated as often as necessary to preserve the airway and the voice; a purposeful attempt is made during these repeated operations to avoid exposing muscle.

Current adjuvant therapy trials

Because surgical removal with or without the laser does not eradicate the disease but merely preserves the airway and voice until such a time as a spontaneous remission occurs, the need for an effective adjuvant therapy is self evident.

Topical 5-fluorouracil was used after surgical removal in 11 patients; there was no question that the drug had a therapeutic effect on the residual lesions, but unfortunately after 8–10 months the disease would 'break through' the treatment. Topical 5-fluorouracil was therefore abandoned.

Systemic cisretinoic acid has been used in a controlled series of patients. The recurrence rate appeared to be slowed in some patients while in others there was no effect. One patient went into remission for 3 years – it is of interest that she had received the placebo! The side-effects of cisretinoic acid were significant. Elevation of liver enzymes and skin excoriation were most troublesome. Systemic cisretinoic acid is of no value in the treatment of recurrent respiratory papilloma.

Initially interferon held promise as an adjuvant therapy; the early reports from Scandinavia, Houston and Iowa were encouraging (Haglund *et al.*, 1981; Goepfert *et al.*, 1982; McCabe and Clark, 1983). However, in the cold light of day, it was apparent that in using currently available varieties of interferon, the most that can be anticipated is a slowing of the rate of recurrence or a temporary remission of the disease; the incidence of prolonged remission appears to be no greater than that accounted for by chance and spontaneous remission. Because frequent and prolonged remissions are not to be expected, the cost and morbidity of interferon are not warranted at this time.

Conclusions

Recurrent respiratory papillomatosis is a diffuse diathesis that affects the mucosa of the upper air and food passages in children. Spontaneous remissions of one year's duration occur in about 50% of patients, followed-up for one year. Dependable adjuvant therapy is not yet available. Treatment should be directed towards maintaining the airway and voice, and avoiding tracheostomy. Thus far, adjuvant therapy has not been shown to be of value. We must await the outcome of future clinical trials.

References

FERENCZY, A., MITAO, M., NAGAI, N. and SILVERSTEIN, S. J. (1985) Latent papilloma virus and recurring genital warts. *New England Journal of Medicine*, **313**, 784–788

GOEPFERT, H., GUTTERMAN, J. U., DICHTEL, W. J., SESSIONS, R. B., CANGIR, A. and SULEK, M. (1982) Leukocyte interferon in patients with juvenile laryngeal papillomatosis. *Annals of Otology, Rhinology and Laryngology*, **91**, 431–436

HAGLUND, S., LUNDQUIST, P., CANTELL, K. and STANDER, H. (1981) Interferon therapy in juvenile laryngeal papillomatosis. *Archives of Otolaryngology*, **107**, 327–332

INCZE, J. S., LUI, P. S., STRONG, M. S., VAUGHAN, C. W. and CLEMENTE, M. P. (1977) The morphology of human papillomas of the upper respiratory tract. *Cancer*, **39**, 1634–1646

McCABE, B. F. and CLARK, K. F. (1983) Interferon and laryngeal papillomatosis – the Iowa experience. *Annals of Otology, Rhinology and Laryngology*, **92**, 2–7

MACKENZIE, M. (1880) *A Manual of Diseases of the Throat and Nose, vol. 1. Diseases of the Pharynx, Larynx and Trachea*, p. 305. New York: William Wood and Company

MATSULA, H. M., THAWLEY, S. E., SPECTOR, G. J., MAUNCY, M. and PIKUL, F. J. (1985) Laryngeal epidermoid carcinoma associated with juvenile laryngeal papillomatosis. *The Laryngoscope*, **95**, 1264–1271

STEINBERG, B., TOPP, W. C., SCHNEIDER, O. and ABRAMSON, A. (1983) Laryngeal papilloma virus infection during clinical remission. *New England Journal of Medicine*, **308**, 1262–1264

STRONG, M., VAUGHAN, C. W., HEALY, B., COOPERBAND, S. and CLEMENTE, M. (1976) Recurrent respiratory papillomatosis. *Annals of Otology, Rhinology and Laryngology*, **85**, 508–516

32

Tracheostomy and decannulation

J. H. Rogers

A tracheostomy involves the construction of a channel between the trachea and the skin surface of the neck in the midline. With time, this channel may acquire an epithelial lining and may then qualify in pathological parlance as a 'fistula'. The alternative spelling of 'tracheotomy' is often employed but etymological discussion is best avoided and in this chapter the more traditional 'tracheostomy' is preferred. The operation is performed at all ages but there are significant differences between children and adults because of the smaller structures involved and the degree of immaturity which may be present in children. With medical progress, the emphasis on these differences becomes greater as the operation is performed on the infant, the neonate and now the preterm neonate.

Historical

Historical accounts of this operation vie with each other in plumbing the depths of antiquity for plausible evidence (Goodall, 1934; Salmon, 1957; Nelson, 1958; Frost, 1976). The operation has been attributed to various oriental potentates who employed the sword as scalpel and hazy descriptions have been given by certain medico-philosophers. No doubt, some fossil-find, decorated potsherd or deciphered hieroglyphic will eventually push its origins even further into prehistory.

Since the Renaissance, this life-saving operation has been better described and certain trends become apparent. Initially, it was performed for choking, caused either by an inhaled foreign body, drowning or trauma to the upper respiratory tract. Indeed, the first successful tracheostomy in a child

was reported in 1766 by Caron, a French surgeon who removed an inhaled bean from a 7-year-old boy. Later a common indication was 'croup', a label given by a Scottish physician, Francis Home (Home, 1765) to the combination of sore throat and stridor. Some of these patients would probably have suffered from laryngotracheobron-chitis, but more probably from 'diphtheria', a term coined later by a French physician, Pierre Breton-neau. Indeed, the term 'croup' is still reserved exclusively for diphtheria in many parts of western Europe. In the nineteenth century, tracheostomy became widely used in the treat-ment of diphtheria in children, and by 1887, some 20 000 such operations had been reported in western Europe and the USA. About this time, intubation became a feasible alternative with the appearance of the O'Dwyer tube and the discov-ery of diphtheria antitoxin in 1895 hastened the demise of diphtheria as the pre-eminent indication for childhood tracheostomy. However, the opera-tion continued to be carried out for various forms of upper respiratory obstruction, although the notoriety resulting from a 30% survival rate caused many parents to refuse the operation. The employment of tracheostomy for the removal of bronchial secretions is a relatively recent innova-tion and it was first described by Galloway in patients with bulbar poliomyelitis. Subsequently a similar approach was taken for chronic chest disease. The poliomyelitis epidemics of the early 1950s stimulated the use of tracheostomy for positive pressure respiration and this opened the doors for similar treatment in tetanus, cardiac surgery, severe burns and, most recently, the care of the preterm infant. The introduction of active immunization against diphtheria in 1940 and poliomyelitis in 1956 almost eliminated these diseases and left epiglottitis and laryngotracheo-bronchitis as the principal indications for tracheostomy in children. Over the last 20 years, intubation has taken over as the treatment of choice in these conditions and the frequency of tracheostomy has, therefore, decreased dramatically in the developed world. In the last decade, the increased skills of the neonatologists have permitted the increased survival of the very preterm infant with its concomitant multiple problems. These infants require prolonged ventilation and the resulting subglottic stenosis and failure of extubation necessitates tracheostomy. However, even in these infants, the need has again decreased as the neonatologists have become more adept in avoiding subglottic trauma.

The historical vista of tracheostomy depicts a life-saving operation which becomes superseded as some less traumatic treatment becomes available. It remains a life-saving operation, but with the associated improvements in anaesthesia, antibiotics and surgical technique, the morbidity and mortality of the operation have been greatly reduced.

Anatomy and physiology

In the child, the air passages are both absolutely and relatively smaller than in the adult (Tucker and Tucker, 1979). The cervical trachea usually lies in the midline of the neck and its length varies with body build and the degree of extension. The distance from the cricoid to the suprasternal notch varies from 2.5 cm in neonates to 6.0 cm in the 10-year-old child, but in short, heavy individuals, the cricoid cartilage may be sited almost within the suprasternal notch. The larynx is higher in the child and the cricoid cartilage lies at the level of the third cervical vertebra in the infant and descends to the sixth cervical vertebra at puberty. Since the thyroid cartilage does not take on its adult configuration until adolescence, the larynx is not easily palpable in the infant and the cricoid may be the easiest landmark to identify. The trachea is softer and lies nearest the skin at the cricoid, but it becomes deeper as it approaches the thoracic inlet. The thyroid isthmus varies in size but crosses the trachea at the second, third and fourth tracheal rings (*Figure 32.1*). The recurrent laryngeal nerves lie laterally and a pretracheal pad of fat is generally present in the suprasternal notch in infants. In extension, the mediastinal contents may enter the neck so that the surgeon may encounter a high pleural dome, large vessels crossing the midline and, rarely, the thymus. The articulation between the head and neck is considerably more mobile in infants and the chin may easily deviate from the midline during surgery.

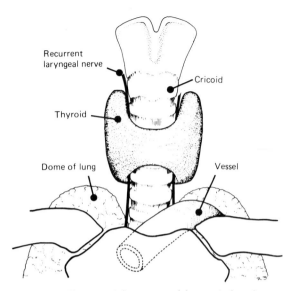

Figure 32.1 The essential anatomy of the cervical trachea

The trachea provides an air passage between the larynx and the lungs. Since it needs to maintain its lumen and to remain flexible, it is constructed of incomplete cartilaginous rings. It is lined by respiratory mucosa which continues the process of warming and humidifying the inspired air, and the cilia waft the mucous blanket upwards towards the larynx. The larynx is a valvular mechanism which allows the passage of air but normally denies access to solids and fluids. It also provides a defence mechanism in the form of the cough reflex and it has been adapted to a sophisticated degree for the production of sound.

Indications for tracheostomy

The indications for tracheostomy in the past have been largely usurped by the indications for intubation and a tracheostomy may only become necessary when intubation is no longer feasible. In general the indications are conveniently placed in three groups as in the adult, although the specific details are different in the child.

Airway obstruction

Obstruction or the threat of obstruction to the upper respiratory tract is an indication for tracheostomy. Apart from laryngeal and subglottic lesions, indications include physical trauma to the face, jaws, oral and pharyngeal cavities as well as burns by corrosive chemicals or the inhalation of smoke or gases.

Dead space and secretions

Tracheostomy is indicated for improved respiration where a reduction in dead space or the removal of bronchial secretions is considered to be advantageous. This situation is found in chronic lung disease and in certain neonatal chest conditions.

Ventilation

The provision of prolonged positive pressure ventilation where voluntary or spontaneous respiration is not possible indicates tracheostomy. The patient with poliomyelitis, tetanus or brain damage may require such assistance, as also will the child with a damaged chest wall. Positive pressure ventilation is also employed as an adjunct to cardiac surgery or in the cases of severe burns and the preterm neonate.

In the first and last groups, intubation may be employed in the short term but, for prolonged treatment, the tracheostomy becomes easier to manage. Until recently, intubation was only employed for periods of up to 3 weeks, but improvements in technique now permit intubation for periods of several months. A tracheostomy, therefore, becomes a necessity whenever prolonged endotracheal intubation poses the threat of laryngotracheal injury.

Several authors have recently reviewed their indications for tracheostomy over the last 10–15 years (Cohen *et al.*, 1977; Rodgers, Rooks and Talbert, 1979; Tepas *et al.*, 1981; Gerson and Tucker, 1982; Wetmore, Handler and Potsic, 1982; Carter and Benjamin, 1983; Line *et al.*, 1986; Swift and Rogers, 1987). There is no purpose in quoting the precise statistics from these reviews because they reflect the different patterns of referral to the centres concerned. Rapid changes have also occurred over the last 15 years and the indications will vary with the precise period under review. The specific indications are, therefore, described below in general terms and in order of decreasing frequency.

Congenital laryngeal abnormalities

Although there are variations as described above, this group now accounts for the largest proportion of tracheostomies. In one series, (Carter and Benjamin, 1983) laryngeal webs and subglottic haemangiomata account for most cases within this group, but this is unusual and the unit in question attracts these cases from a large area. Bilateral vocal cord paralysis is generally found to be the most common single indication, while congenital subglottic stenosis and cysts come next in frequency. Laryngomalacia or supraglottic floppiness is by far the most common laryngeal abnormality, but tracheostomy is very rarely required for its treatment.

Prolonged ventilation

Trauma to the head or chest continues to be common and is even increasing. Eventually it may, therefore, be the most common indication for tracheostomy. Tetanus occurs intermittently and is still very common in some large rural areas (Mukherjee, 1979). Poliomyelitis has largely been eliminated in the developed world, but continues to be a threat elsewhere.

Supralaryngeal obstruction

This may be present or threatened and is commonly seen in conditions such as the Pierre Robin syndrome, severe sleep apnoea and craniofacial surgery. Advances in the surgical treatment of congenital facial abnormalities are making tracheostomy more common in this latter group.

Acquired laryngeal abnormalities

Ten years ago, acquired subglottic stenosis would have been one of the most common indications for tracheostomy because of the increased resuscitative skills of the neonatologist. Although it is still a very significant problem in those units which attract the worst problems of this nature (Black, Baldwin and Johns, 1984; Quiney *et al.*, 1986), improved intubation skills have in general reduced the necessity for tracheostomy. Indeed, in one series, (Carter and Benjamin, 1983), no tracheostomies were performed for acquired subglottic stenosis over a period of 10 years, although some 300 infants were intubated annually in the associated neonatal and intensive care units. Those authors attributed this remarkable success to the use of small-diameter (2.5 or even 2.0 mm) polyvinylchloride (PVC) nasotracheal tubes. Other centres receive patients from areas where such expertise may not be available.

Laryngeal papillomatosis as a cause of tracheostomy is also on the decline. The need in this condition is dictated not only by the virulence of the causative agent but by the degree of oedema and scarring following treatment. The use of the laser has reduced the postoperative oedema and the frequency of removal and has consequently obviated the need for an alternative airway.

Acute infections

Fifteen years ago, infections of the respiratory tract were the most common indication for tracheostomy, but oro- and nasotracheal intubation has changed all that. Intubation is now widely used for acute epiglottitis and laryngotracheobronchitis, although it makes great demands on medical and nursing facilities and is, therefore, not so available in less developed countries (Mukherjee, 1979; Okafor, 1983; Soni, Chatterji and Thind, 1984), where tracheostomy is still widely employed.

Miscellaneous

This review is necessarily based on trends in the developed world but indications differ elsewhere. Diphtheria is an important acute infection and inhaled foreign bodies are a common indication, particularly where patients may take several days to reach hospital and, if still alive, will, therefore, have considerable oedema around the impacted object.

The operation of tracheostomy

The operation is more common in males because of their increased susceptibility to congenital and acquired disorders. The aim of the operation is to construct an airway into the trachea as safely as possible.

Since the emphasis is on safety, the operation should be carried out in an environment where there is complete control of the airway at all times. There are rare occasions when an emergency tracheostomy is life saving but in the hospital environment, intubation or cricothyroidotomy is preferable when that urgent need arises. The technique of emergency tracheostomy will not be described here since, by definition, the facilities available are unknown, but the aim is to provide an airway as rapidly as possible by whatever means possible.

Since more than half of all paediatric tracheostomies are performed on children below the age of one year, it is essential that the operation is carried out in a paediatric unit or hospital where the nursing and medical staff are accustomed to the care of infants and neonates. Details of the anaesthetic and general care of a neonate will not be included here, although these are obviously of the greatest import.

The operation should be performed electively in a sterile environment under a general anaesthetic administered through an endotracheal tube. The anaesthetic should be given by an experienced paediatric anaesthetist and the operation should be performed by, or supervised by, an experienced paediatric otolaryngologist.

Preparation

Antibiotics are not needed prophylactically but they should be given if there is some medical reason to do so. A sample of sputum should be taken for culture and antibiotic sensitivity in readiness for a possible postoperative infection. Blood loss is minimal during the operation, but since the blood volume of a neonate may be very small it is wise for a sample of blood to be grouped and kept for cross-matching.

The infant, suitably warmed, is laid supine on

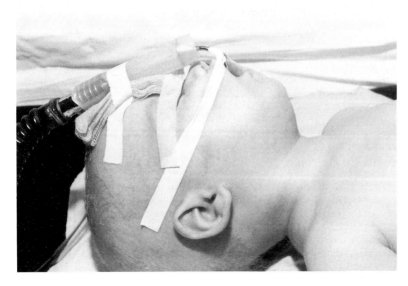

Figure 32.2 An infant in the tracheostomy position. Note the partial extension of the neck

the operating table. The head is extended to increase the distance between the chin and sternal notch, to smooth out the redundant folds of skin in the neck and to bring the trachea and larynx closer to the skin surface (*Figure 32.2*). This is achieved by placing a suitable roll of soft material under the neck and the head is prevented from lolling by using a small head ring. It is important not to overdo the extension as this draws the lower trachea and mediastinal contents into the neck. Not only does this place the lung apices and mediastinal vessels at risk but it may tempt a low tracheal incision, which retreats into the chest on flexion.

The skin of the chin, neck and upper chest is cleaned with a suitable disinfectant and the surrounding area is draped with sterile towels. The chin is left uncovered in order that the surgeon can check the midline and some anaesthetists like to keep the face uncovered. Before the towels are positioned a little adrenaline (1:80 000 or 1:200 000 if halothane is being used) and local anaesthetic are infiltrated subcutaneously between the cricoid and the sternal notch. This allows the adrenaline to disperse and to exert its vasoconstrictive effect before the incision is made a few minutes later. The local anaesthetic reduces postoperative discomfort. At this stage it is also wise to check that the intended tracheostomy tube is available and that the proper connections are at hand.

Surgical technique

Both the vertical and horizontal skin incisions are employed, but there are theoretical and practical reasons for preferring the vertical incision. The horizontal skin crease incision has its supporters in the adult because of the better cosmetic result, but in the infant both incisions are so small that they produce similar scars. The main advantage of the vertical incision is that it runs in the line of the trachea. This is important in the infant since it is often difficult to judge the precise level of the proposed tracheostomy externally and the improved access gives a greater freedom of choice. The midline is also less vascular and for both these reasons the vertical incision is best used by the inexperienced surgeon.

The cricoid cartilage is palpated, often with some difficulty, and a vertical midline skin incision of 1.5 cm is made with the upper end at the level of the cricoid. If a horizontal incision is to be employed, it should be of similar length and sited in a skin crease midway between the cricoid and the suprasternal notch. It is important that the chin and sternal notch are in line when the skin is incised. The bleeding is usually minimal but

diathermy should be employed if necessary. An assistant retracts the edges of the incision with a skin hook or small retractor and blunt dissection is carried out in the midline with artery forceps or small scissors. It is important not to open up tissue planes unnecessarily as this encourages surgical emphysema later. As the dissection probes deeper, the assistant repositions the retractors and in this way the strap muscles are separated and the trachea approached. If the surgeon stays in the midline, this procedure can usually be completed without any bleeding, but the degree of difficulty in exposing the trachea varies greatly. Even in the more difficult cases, patient persistence is rewarded as long as the midline is sought and the level of the cricoid checked.

It is difficult to mistake the trachea when it is reached, although the tracheal rings are softer and less obvious than in the adult. It is, however, sometimes a problem to identify an individual tracheal ring and this may be facilitated by exposing the cricoid cartilage and its attached cricothyroid muscle and numbering the rings from that level. The identification of the thyroid isthmus also provides a landmark for the tracheal rings. Although the isthmus varies in width from a tenuous sliver of connective tissue to a more substantial mass, it consistently overlies the second, third and fourth tracheal rings (*see Figure 32.1*). Some authorities feel that the isthmus should always be cut and sutured (Gerson and Tucker, 1982) in order to facilitate recannulation later, but this is rarely necessary. It is usually simple to free the isthmus from the underlying trachea and to retract it superiorly or inferiorly for the exposure of the relevant tracheal rings. Good access to the trachea is obtained by clearing the fascia from its anterior surface, although care must be taken not to disturb the recurrent laryngeal nerves which lie posterolaterally. The trachea should now be exposed in a small but bloodless field and, after rechecking the tracheostomy tube and its attachments, the anaesthetist is alerted to the imminent incision of the trachea itself.

The tracheal incision

In the adult, there has always been considerable discussion about the best form of tracheal incision but in the infant it is generally agreed that the vertical incision is simplest and best. This is given support by a recent attempt (Fry *et al.*, 1985) to evaluate the relative merits of the vertical slit, the inferiorly based trapdoor and the horizontal H. Using young ferrets as a paediatric model, the authors assessed the tracheal airway after decannulation and healing and demonstrated that the vertical slit resulted in less stenosis and less airway resistance.

It is important that the vertical incision is made at the correct level. If it is too near to the cricoid, it will predispose to subglottic stenosis and the surgeon should, therefore, aim at keeping the upper two tracheal rings intact. Conversely, if the incision is made too low, the tip of the tracheostomy tube may enter the right main bronchus and the tube is more likely to come out accidentally. The tracheal rings are identified again and a vertical incision is made through the second, third and fourth rings. A larger incision should be extended to include the fifth ring. The slit is made from below upwards to avoid damage to the mediastinal contents and it should be made in a controlled manner because a slip will extend the incision into the cricoid. Even in the infant, the tracheal wall is rather thicker than one would suspect but care must be taken not to damage the posterior wall of the trachea with the point of the scalpel. In practice this is most unlikely since the anaesthetist's endotracheal tube lies in the tracheal lumen unless it has become displaced superiorly. There is sometimes a little bleeding from the tracheal mucosa and the perichondrium of the ring, but this is rarely significant.

Some surgeons feel that the procedure is assisted by the insertion of a silk suture, to either side of the midline. Before the vertical incision is made, a black silk suture is introduced to circle the third and fourth tracheal rings on either side. These are left long and initially are held laterally in artery forceps. After the vertical incision has been made between them these sutures are retracted to assist cannulation. Later they are taped to the chest wall for up to one week and may be used for recannulation if necessary. In the author's experience, these sutures are not mandatory since there is rarely any problem in introducing the tracheostomy tube at operation and decannulation is prevented by other means described below. In addition, there is a possibility that the sutures will weaken the anterior tracheal wall and the threads become sodden and something of an obstacle during subsequent care of the tracheostomy.

The anaesthetist now withdraws the endotracheal tube just proximal to the upper end of the incision under the guidance of the surgeon. The trachea is sucked out and a tracheostomy tube of suitable design and size is inserted under direct vision. This is done in a calm, unhurried way since the anaesthetist still has full control of the airway. If any difficulty is experienced in introducing the tube the following points may be helpful. It should be checked that the incision is long enough and stay sutures should be retracted if they are available. If the tube is a metal one then the introducer should be properly in place while, if it is plastic, the ends can be compressed in an artery forceps and inserted through the incision (Pracy, 1979) (*Figure 32.3*). The tracheostomy tube can also be 'railroaded' down a fine catheter which has been passed through the tube and the tracheal incision.

Unless there is some good reason, a synthetic plastic or silicone tube should be used for the initial intubation. The standard tube used by the

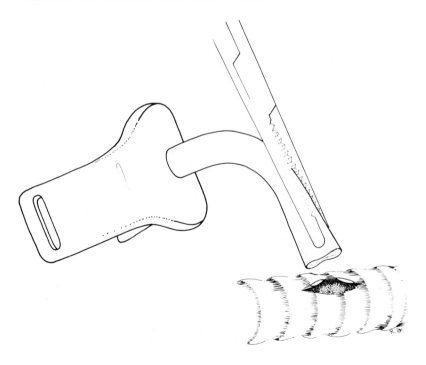

Figure 32.3 The tip of the tracheostomy tube is compressed by artery forceps to facilitate insertion

author is the Great Ormond Street pattern of the Aberdeen tube made by Franklin, but other models are available and are described below. The standard size used for a 3-month-old baby is the 3.5 mm (internal diameter), but the tube should obviously be measured for the patient in terms of its lumen and length.

The correct position of the tube in the tracheal lumen is checked and the anaesthetist makes the attachments for continued ventilation. Once the anaesthetist is satisfied that both lungs are being ventilated, the endotracheal tube is withdrawn. No sutures are placed in the edges of the skin incision which usually fits comfortably around the tube and a tight fit is to be avoided since it predisposes to surgical emphysema.

The tube is now held in place by suturing the flange to the neck skin and by tying tapes around the neck (*Figure 32.4*). The importance of securing the tube cannot be overestimated since accidental decannulation is avoided if it is done properly. Silk sutures are placed through the flange and adjacent skin just lateral to the opening of the tube. This positioning prevents the substantial tube movement which can occur if the sutures are placed towards the tip of the flange. A tape is then tied from one side of the flange to the other around the back of the neck. One end of the tape is knotted to one side of the flange while the other is passed through a piece of tubing of suitable length. This tubing conforms to the convexity of the baby's neck and protects the skin from the rubbing of the tape. The free end of the tape is then knotted to the other end of the flange and is adjusted so that the tube is held firmly, but not tightly, in place. It is most important that these adjustments to the tape are carried out while the neck is in slight flexion. If they are done while the neck is extended, the tube will loosen on subsequent flexion and accidental decannulation will be encouraged. It is, therefore, important that the tape adjustments are made by the surgeon or the anaesthetist and the task should not be delegated to an inexperienced member of the team. Children above the age of 6 months are given sedation, but those younger babies are best left without to discourage apnoeic attacks. The child is now moved from the operating table and care is taken to avoid traction on the tube while this is being carried out.

Postoperative care

For the first few days, the child should be in an intensive care unit where there are adequate trained nursing and medical staff on duty for 24 hours of the day. As soon as the infant arrives on the ward, an X-ray of the chest and neck is taken to confirm that the tip of the tracheostomy tube is

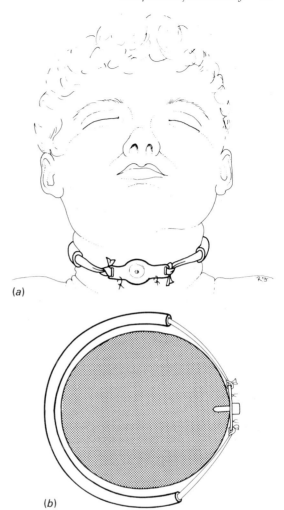

(*a*)

(*b*)

Figure 32.4 (*a*) The flanges are secured to the neck skin by a tape and by sutures adjacent to the collar of the tube. (*b*) A cross-section of the neck demonstrating the tape passing through protective tubing

not so low that it impinges on the carina or enters the right main bronchus. The X-ray may also demonstrate surgical emphysema in the superficial tissues or in the mediastinum. Initially feeding is via the intravenous drip which is established during the operation, but within a few hours, the baby is able to feed by mouth. The maintenance of adequate hydration is important since it contributes to the prevention of tracheal crusting.

If the baby has previously suffered from chronic airway obstruction, the sudden relief may produce apnoea and it may be wise initially to increase the dead space by a suitable attachment. In the preterm baby, positive end expiration pressure may be necessary to maintain lung stability. The chin may also obstruct the stomal opening in the small baby, but this can be avoided by choosing a suitable tube (as described below), or by inserting a segment of plastic tubing into the opening of the tracheostomy.

Since the tracheostomy has bypassed the nose, it is essential that humidified air is supplied to the infant, but care must be taken to avoid over-humidification. Particle size is not as important as was previously thought but cold humidity is probably best and an ultrasonic humidifier may be necessary to provide a sufficient volume. The glottis is also bypassed by the operation and the cough reflex is therefore lost. The trachea and bronchi respond to the surgical insult by an increase in mucus secretion and, because the cough reflex is lost, suction is essential. Regular aseptic suction is required but the frequency varies and must be assessed by the experienced attendant staff. The suction catheter is inserted without suction and the negative pressure is exerted as the catheter is withdrawn. The size of the catheter is most important. The external diameter of the catheter should be less than half the internal diameter of the tracheostomy tube because, if not, hypoxia or, at worst, lung collapse may occur.

At first a careful watch must be kept for surgical emphysema or pneumothorax but these are unlikely to occur after 12 hours. It is not usually necessary to place a dressing between the peristomal skin and the tubal flanges, but a barrier cream is helpful if skin excoriation threatens.

The parents of the child are encouraged to take an active role in the routine care from the outset. In the neonate, this is important for bonding, but it is particularly important in the older child because speech will now be impossible and a parent must be immediately available for reassurance and communication. Both parents should initially observe the routine procedures of tracheostomy care and should then be supervised in doing it themselves to overcome their natural fear. At this stage they should also be introduced to the idea of contacting one of the relevant parental organizations such as 'Aid for children with tracheostomies'.

One week after the tracheostomy, the track will be well formed. The tube can now be changed although this is not mandatory and it can be left longer if it is clean and well positioned. The first change is best done in the intensive care unit or in the operating theatre where emergency facilities are available. An endotracheal tube, spare tracheostomy tube and tracheal dilators are essential and the change is done after cutting the flange sutures by an experienced doctor, whether surgeon or anaesthetist. The tapes are again tied with great care and the position of the tube is checked. The baby can now be returned to a normal ward but only if the staff are accustomed to

dealing with a patient with a tracheostomy and are capable of continuing with the training of the parents. Regular aseptic suction and humidification are continued and the necessary equipment is ordered for the home care of the child. Before a return home is contemplated, both parents should be able to change the tracheostomy tube and the surgeon must be happy that they are confident about the routine daily care.

Later, if decannulation has not been achieved, questions will arise concerning the development of speech and the proposed nature of future education. The problem of speech is linked to the type of tracheostomy tube to be used and this is discussed in a separate section below. It is imperative to seek the aid of an experienced speech therapist and every effort must be made to enrol the, otherwise normal, child in a normal school although this may prove to be difficult.

Complications

Since the tracheostomy is now the main route for respiration, any complication which interferes with this route may be fatal. The mortality and morbidity following the tracheostomy itself (as opposed to the associated disease) is now much less than it was 10 years ago (Fearon and Cotton, 1974), although results still vary from different centres. The improvement is attributed to the avoidance of emergency tracheostomies where possible and to the emphasis on basic surgical technique as described above. If these guidelines are followed, complications are infrequent although the vulnerability of the tracheostomized child must never be forgotten. Complications are conveniently considered as being early or late, the dividing line being about one week into the postoperative period. Some problems such as crusting and granulation formation are so common that they may be regarded as the normal consequences of the operation, but if these are exaggerated, they qualify as complications.

Early complications

Apnoea

Apnoeic attacks are more likely to occur in the small infant with chronic airway obstruction. Such a child should not be given postoperative sedation and the dead space can be increased temporarily by a suitable attachment to the tracheostomy tube.

Air in the tissues

A little surgical emphysema is commonly seen immediately after the operation and it may only be recognized on the postoperative X-ray. Usually the emphysema resolves without any treatment but the position of the tube and the tightness of the skin around the stoma should be checked. *Pneumomediastinum* presents in a similar manner and should be treated in the same way but a *pneumothorax* is more serious and is treated on its merits. A low tracheostomy predisposes to a pneumothorax and a tight stoma aggravates the situation. Prevention is, therefore, the best form of treatment. The neck should not be over-extended during the operation and blunt dissection in the midline will avoid the opening-up of lateral tissue planes.

Accidental decannulation

This can be a serious complication in the first 2 or 3 days after surgery because the fistula track will not have formed and the slit incision in the trachea will make recannulation difficult. If the tracheostomy has been performed at the right level and the tube has been sutured and taped accurately, it should not occur. In this situation, stay sutures come into their own, but, even in their absence, the experienced staff of an intensive care unit should be able to recannulate or pass an endotracheal tube and the necessary instruments should always be immediately available.

Creation of a false passage

The changing of the tube or its reinsertion following accidental decannulation may lead to the creation of a false passage. It is particularly likely to occur before the track is well formed and the tube should not normally be changed until this has occurred. The false passage may lead to obstruction or to a pneumothorax and the position of the tube should always be carefully checked after recannulation.

Obstruction

This is obviously a potentially fatal complication. If the tube is the correct length and is positioned correctly, the most common cause is the accumulation of mucus and crusts in the tube or the tracheal lumen and it is best prevented by adequate humidification and suction. Intermittent obstruction by the baby's chin is prevented by a suitable restraining attachment to the tube and this is discussed below.

Haemorrhage

Blunt dissection in the midline during the operation will often result in a bloodless field but a little bleeding may occur from the skin edges, the tracheal perichondrium and the tracheal mucosa. Such bleeding is usually trivial and will stop after an hour or two. Serious haemorrhage from the erosion of a large vessel is often fatal but rarely occurs in the first week since the most common cause is secondary infection.

Chest infections

Even with strict attention to aseptic technique during suction, pulmonary infections occur, particularly in the infant with previous lung problems. In this latter group, prophylactic antibiotics should be given preoperatively and in all cases the appropriate medical treatment is commenced. The choice of antibiotic is aided by taking a sample of sputum or tracheal aspirate at operation and sending it for culture and sensitivity.

Late complications

All the complications mentioned above may occur later but their importance varies. The most common and, therefore, the most important fatal complications, are accidental decannulation and obstruction and these are particularly likely to happen at home.

Accidental decannulation

Accidental decannulation at this later stage is less dangerous because the tube can be easily replaced into the established track within a few minutes of decannulation. However, the track can stenose rapidly and tracheal dilators may be required even within 10 minutes of the decannulation. The avoidance of decannulation at home is most important and the parents must be instructed to tie the securing tapes firmly. To counteract the efforts of an active child, it may be necessary to have tapes which are tight enough to mark the neck, but a marked neck is preferable to a decannulated child.

Obstruction

This may be caused by a granuloma or by a mucus plug. Granulations almost always appear at the site of the stoma, particularly within the tracheal lumen above the stoma (*Figure 32.5*). They may obstruct the tracheal lumen following elective or accidental decannulation, but may also block the tube or cause bleeding during recannulation. Granulations are very likely to occur when a metal tube is used and this tendency has led the metal tube into disrepute. The characteristics of the various tubes and the management of granulations are discussed below. Obstruction of the tube

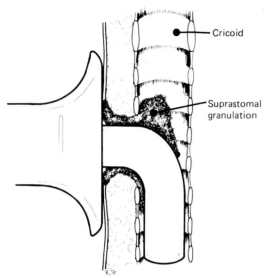

Figure 32.5 Granulations from around the tracheostomy tube. The suprastomal granulation is seen above the tube on the anterior wall

or the tracheal lumen by a mucus plug is best prevented by adequate humidification and suction. Such humidification is provided by a plastic humidifier in the home but also by a heat–moist exchanger (of which there are several models), which is easily connected to the tube. This latter device allows freedom in the open air without the encumbrance of a standard humidifier and may even permit the child to play in sand under supervision.

Haemorrhage due to the erosion of a large vessel is usually fatal and can only be prevented by the proper positioning of the tracheostomy and by attention to operative technique and the prompt treatment of infection. Haemorrhage and mediastinitis have also been caused by an erosion of the tracheal wall by the tip of a badly positioned tube. Chest infections continue to be more frequent than in the normal child and are treated symptomatically.

Tracheostomy tubes

Every otolaryngologist must have wished many times that an available tracheostomy tube could be modified to suit the problem of the patient in hand. The perfect tube does not exist but successive modifications have occurred with advances in medical knowledge and in the science of materials (Pracy, 1976).

The early tracheostomy tubes were made of bone, rubber or metal and the paediatric tube was a smaller version of the adult model. The tubes were of varying curvature with a flange around the external opening for the attachment of stabilizing tapes. Latterly, these tubes were made of silver and incorporated an inner tube, which was longer than the outer and could be easily removed when blockage occurred. Later a valve was fitted to the tube by Negus to allow inspiration through the tube and expiration through the glottis for phonation. Thirty years ago, Wilson introduced a silver tube for children with a funnel-shaped projection, which could be easily attached to a respirator. This tube also had a window in the shoulder of the outer tube to allow transglottic breathing prior to decannulation. The addition of a window and a valve to the inner tube produced the Alder Hey tube, which has been widely used in the UK for many years.

A great advance was made with the discovery of flexible plastics such as polyvinylchloride and silicone rubber. Since several of these are thermoplastic, the initial curvature of the tube is not so important because the shaft conforms to the shape of the track as the material warms. Unfortunately, the wall of these tubes needs to be thicker in order to preserve sufficient rigidity. This reduces the size of the lumen and makes the use of an inner tube impracticable in the smaller, paediatric models. The theoretical characteristics of an ideal tube are discussed in detail elsewhere (Pracy, 1976), but a few factors are summarized here. The design of the tube should permit an optimum flow of air, a situation which is favoured by a shorter shaft, a greater radius of curvature and a smooth inner surface (Yung and Snowdon, 1984). The material should be non-toxic and should possess minimal tissue reactivity demonstrated by implantation tests. It is probable that various chemicals are leached out from these plastic tubes while they are in use and that their tissue reactivity changes. However, it is not known if, or how rapidly, this occurs and, therefore, how long to leave a tube in place before disposing of it (G. H. Bush, 1986, personal communication).

There are also desirable practical considerations. The tube should be comfortable, easy to clean and easy to change. It must be easily connected to ventilation equipment and attachments should fulfil standard international requirements. At present it is agreed that the external opening of the tube, known as the collar, should have an internal diameter of 15 mm. In babies and small children it is helpful to have a projection from the opening of the tube, a chin restrainer, which will prevent the chubby chin of the baby from occluding the tube. It would also be most desirable if the measurements of the tubes were easily accessible and expressed clearly. The choice of an ideal tube would be facilitated by a knowledge of the internal and external diameters of the tube and the length of the shaft. In practice there are two groups of tubes: the metal tubes and the synthetic tubes. The characteristics of those in common use are described.

Metal tubes

The Alder Hey tube is typical of this group and is described above. It has an inner tube which means that it is easily cleaned and it inspires confidence in the inexperienced parent who, initially, does not need to change the complete tube. It has a large radius of curvature and its smooth surface encourages laminar air flow (Yung and Snowdon, 1984). Both the inner and outer tubes are fenestrated and a valve is available to allow transglottic expiration and speech. Similar, but not identical, paediatric metal tubes are those of Jackson and Holinger, but all are durable and may last for several years.

There are also disadvantages. They are said to be less comfortable than the synthetic tubes and cosmetically they are less satisfying. The edges of the fenestra and the shaft-tip are sharp and it is the impression of the author and others (Quiney *et al.*, 1986) that granulations are more likely to occur in the trachea and around the stomal skin. The tracheal granulations are sited above the stoma, at the level of the tube tip and at the level of the fenestra on the posterior wall. The fenestrated tube was designed for transglottic air flow. This was thought to be of major importance for the continued development of the child's larynx, as a prelude to decannulation (Pracy, 1976) and in the production of speech. This theory of laryngeal development is no longer thought to be true and it is now known that an adequate air flow through the glottis can be achieved by employing a smaller tube. In addition, it has proved difficult to site the

fenestra at a suitable point on the curvature. The tube sits differently in different patients and the opening of the fenestra often impinges on the posterior tracheal wall.

Synthetic tubes

Those commonly used in the UK are the Franklin tube of Great Ormond Street pattern, the Portex paediatric tube and the Shiley paediatric or neonatal tube. The Great Ormond Street tube is a winged tube which sits comfortably on the infant neck. Its external opening does not project and lies flush with the winged flanges. The outer section of the lumen expands to an opening of constant size and this is convenient for the attachment of anaesthetic or ventilation equipment. An attachment is now available which provides a projecting connector of international standard diameter. This projecting connection doubles as a chin restrainer but, if no such attachment is available, a suitable length of tubing can be inserted to achieve the same effect.

The Portex tube is not winged but it has square-ended flanges and a projecting collar connector of international standard dimensions. This connector is sometimes found to be rather bulky. Unlike the Great Ormond Street tube it does not have a bevelled tip and it is, therefore, a little more difficult to introduce through a vertical slit in the trachea. The quoted size of this and the Great Ormond Street tube refers to their internal diameter.

The Shiley tube comes in a paediatric or neonatal size. It has a large winged flange with a standard projecting connector and both structures make an effective chin restrainer. A recent investigation (Yung and Snowdon, 1984) into the respiratory resistance of these tubes showed that

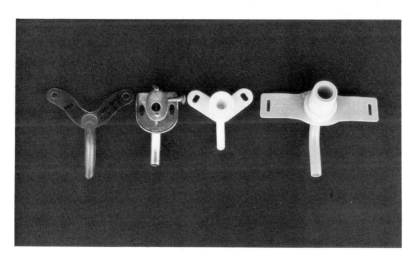

Figure 32.6 A selection of paediatric tracheostomy tubes in common use. From left to right: the Great Ormond Street tube (Franklin), the silver Alder Hey tube, the Shiley tube, and the Portex tube. Note the standardized collars on the latter two tubes

resistance to air flow was greater in the Shiley tube owing to the rougher inner surface. However, it is doubtful whether this is of practical importance (*Figure 32.6*).

Although the metal tubes still have their use, many practitioners (Line *et al.*, 1986; Quiney *et al.*, 1986) including the author have virtually ceased to use them routinely over the last 2 years. The synthetic tubes are cosmetically better and parents seem to have little trouble in cleaning them and changing them. Obstruction of the tube at home is the most common fatal complication, but it does not appear to be more common with the use of synthetic tubes. Indeed, the standard connectors now available for the synthetic tubes allow the attachment of a heat-moist exchanger with consequent avoidance of dry mucoid plugs. Until recently the metal tubes were valuable in the provision of speech by means of the fenestra and the valved inner tube. However, an effective phonation valve as made by Rusch is now available and can be simply attached to a standard connector (*Figure 32.7*). The use of a tube of lesser diameter provides an adequate expiratory flow through the cords.

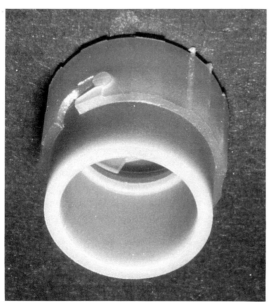

Figure 32.7 Phonation valve (Rusch) which can be attached to any tube with a standardized collar

Decannulation

It is always hoped that any child with a tracheostomy will eventually be decannulated. The outcome obviously depends upon the original lesion, but fortunately many resolve either spontaneously or with medical and surgical treatment.

The time comes when the airway appears to be adequate and it is felt that the patient will manage without the tracheostomy. However, it is well established that the removal of the tracheostomy tube in these circumstances may still result in problems and it is these which are discussed below.

Assessment before decannulation

Children with tracheostomies may be in hospital or at home but in both situations they are seen at regular intervals and assessed clinically. The child should appear to be well and show no sign of aspiration during eating and drinking. It should be noted that he has a good voice or cry in the absence of a valved tube and the temporary occlusion of the tube with the finger permits respiration to continue adequately through the glottis. Radiography and particularly xerography of the larynx and trachea will demonstrate any narrowing of the airway and a picture taken during temporary extubation may be particularly helpful. A method for physiological assessment has been described (Mallory *et al.*, 1985) whereby the peak inspiratory flow through the tracheostomy tube is compared with that through the mouth and the authors considered this to be useful. Lastly, endoscopy is carried out and the larynx, trachea and bronchi are examined with special attention to the sites of the original lesion and the tracheal stoma. The lumen of the subglottis is also measured by the passage of an endotracheal tube of known diameter and the vocal cords are observed for normal movement towards the end of the anaesthetic.

It is advisable to carry out such endoscopic examinations at least every 6 months because a tracheostomy carries a morbidity and mortality rate which justifies decannulation as soon as it is feasible.

In most cases, this assessment will lead to a definite decision with regard to decannulation but there will be some where considerable doubt will remain. The child may suffer from recurrent chest infections or the lumen of the subglottis may be smaller than was expected. There are occasions when the presence of a tracheostomy predisposes to chest infections and to adjacent subglottic oedema. This latter finding is more significant when there is a mild congenital subglottic narrowing which had not previously been diagnosed. In these borderline cases, a trial of decannulation may be necessary.

When the endoscopy is carried out, a suprastomal granulation of varying size is nearly always seen on the anterior tracheal wall. Indeed, this finding is so common that it should be regarded as a normal consequence of tracheostomy rather than as a complication. The suprastomal granulation, which may be mixed with fibrous tissue, is more likely to be present with a long-standing tracheostomy but a substantial granulation can be present after only one week. In the infant, even a small granulation causes a significant blockage of the lumen and it should be removed endoscopically or surgically through the stoma. Endoscopically, the granulation is removed with microscopic cup forceps, diathermy, cryosurgery or the laser. Through the stoma, the granulation is removed at the time of the endoscopy (Reilly and Myer, 1985) or during surgical decannulation as described below. Varying degrees of anterior tracheal wall collapse may also be noted above the stoma at endoscopy.

The decannulation procedure

Broadly speaking, decannulation may be performed in two ways. The most common method is to remove the tube and to allow the track to close down and heal. The alternative is to excise the track and allow it to heal by first intention. In both methods, the final decannulation is preceded by various manoeuvres which constitute a trial decannulation and are aimed at ensuring the safety of the final extubation.

The child is brought into hospital for a period of observation, which need not exceed 2 or 3 days. If there is any choice in the timing, then it is preferable to do it in the early summer when there is a low incidence of respiratory infection. The general health is checked, chest physiotherapy is arranged and a sample of sputum is taken for culture and sensitivity. Although the tube may already have been blocked for a trial period, this period should be repeated and the child should be watched carefully by the ward staff while he/she carries out normal physical activities. Some advocate the use of a fenestrated metal tube such as the Alder Hey tube (Black, Baldwin and Johns, 1984) for this procedure, but a small plastic tube allows an adequate airway around it. Indeed, this latter method is preferable, since the partial blockage of the tracheal lumen by the tube makes the trial more stringent and, if it is well tolerated, then the final decannulation is even more likely to be successful. If the blocking is well tolerated during the day, then it should be continued at night as long as there are enough qualified nursing staff to provide a constant watch. If there are still no problems, the tube is removed and the stoma is covered by a sterile dressing. The child is then kept under observation as an in-patient for at least one week before being allowed home. Various other pre-decannulation procedures are practised

but they are all variations on a theme of progressive tube blockage with an increase in the dead space.

During the whole of the decannulation and pre-decannulation period, essential emergency equipment must be at the bedside and humidification must be continued. The equipment should include a tracheostomy tube, an endotracheal tube, a laryngoscope, suitable retractors or skin hooks and tracheal dilators. Antibiotics are only given if there is a medical reason for doing so and there is no indication for routine mucolytics or steroids.

Decannulation problems

Although the airway is deemed to be adequate or near adequate before the decannulation trial is commenced, significant numbers still have problems. In one recent report (Black, Baldwin and Johns, 1984), 30% had some initial problem with chest infections and respiratory distress but this large percentage is unusual and can be attributed to the large numbers of problem patients with subglottic stenosis who are referred to that centre. Others (Carter and Benjamin, 1983; Line *et al.*, 1986) reported very few problems and the present author shares this experience. When respiratory distress does occur, the causative factors are thought to be as described below.

Dead space

An increase in the dead space occurs when the tracheostomy is closed. In addition, the infant's air passages are absolutely and relatively smaller than those of the adult and the airway resistance will, therefore, be relatively increased. An increased oxygen requirement in children will emphasize any airway resistance and further compromise a previously diseased lung. However, these factors should have manifested their effects in the early assessment prior to decannulation and it is doubtful whether they would be very significant after decannulation.

Tracheal narrowing above the stoma

This is the most probable cause of decannulation problems and there is more than one aetiology. First, a significant granuloma may have been misjudged at the endoscopic assessment, or it may have increased in size or reappeared in the interval between assessment and decannulation. A failed decannulation should, therefore, be followed by a repeated endoscopic assessment and a removal of the granulation if necessary. Second, there may be a flap of fibrous tissue or a displaced anterior tracheal wall above the stoma, which may not be immediately obvious to the uninitiated. In the author's experience, a flap of fibrous tissue is much more common. It has been claimed that the flap can be repositioned by inserting a naso-tracheal tube for 72 hours (Carter and Benjamin, 1983), but it can also be sutured forwards or removed surgically through the stoma (Rogers, 1980). Third, the trachea may be weakened in the vicinity of the stoma by a low-grade chondritis and this may cause collapse of the trachea during inspiration. Lastly, the repeated interference with the larynx, which occurs during the period of assessment and decannulation, may cause oede-ma in the subglottis where the lumen is critical for decannulation. This is particularly likely to occur where there was previously some congenital narrowing or where the original problem was one of acquired subglottic stenosis.

Reduced movement of vocal cords

It has been reported (Sasaki, Fukuda and Kir-chner, 1973) that the reflex abduction of the vocal cords with inspiration is dependent on airway resistance and that this reflex disappears in the presence of a long-standing tracheostomy. Although this had been demonstrated electromyo-graphically and is a possible source of trouble, practical experience shows that it is not of real clinical significance.

All the above may combine to cause trouble but the most likely problems are those of *suprastomal granulations* and *tracheal narrowing* due to tracheal weakness or a displaced anterior tracheal wall. Both these common problems are well treated by surgical decannulation.

Surgical decannulation

In this operation, the tracheostomy track is excised and the tracheal stoma is examined under direct vision. A pre-decannulation assessment is carried out as described above and endoscopy is per-formed immediately prior to the operation to confirm the presence or otherwise of granulations or a displaced anterior tracheal wall flap. A suitable orotracheal tube is introduced for general anaesthesia.

A horizontal elliptical skin incision is made around the external stoma and the resulting island of skin is grasped in an Allis forceps. The track with its surrounding cuff of fibrous tissue is freed down to the trachea with cutting diathermy. It is important not to pull too hard on the fibrous track as the weakened trachea may be tented upwards and damaged when the track is incised horizontal-ly at the tracheal stoma. The tracheal opening and the intraluminal orotracheal tube can now be

clearly seen and any visible granulations or excessive fibrous tissue are excised. A small triangular piece of anterior tracheal wall tissue, about 2 mm long, is now excised from the superior border of the tracheal stoma. This piece of tracheal wall is made up of fibrous tissue which may have been displaced posteriorly into the tracheal lumen and it often carries on its internal surface the suprastomal granuloma (*Figure 32.8*). One hori-zontal Vicryl suture is now placed in the stoma to

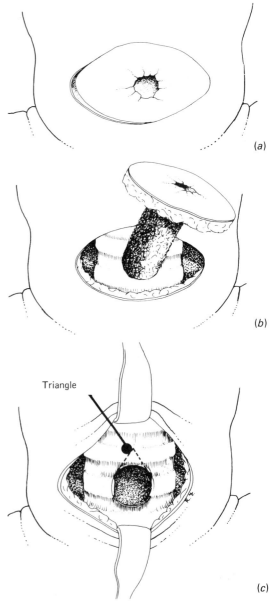

Figure 32.8 Surgical closure of the stoma: (*a*) the elliptical skin incision; (*b*) ellipse of skin with fibrous track around the stoma is freed by cutting diathermy; (*c*) a suprastomal triangle of anterior tracheal wall is excised

reconstruct the tubular structure of the trachea at this level and a repeat endoscopy is performed to ensure that there is no residual granuloma or displaced anterior wall flap. It should also be checked that there is no excessive narrowing of the tracheal lumen as a result of the suture, although this has never been the case. The orotracheal tube is reinserted and two more Vicryl sutures are placed in the tracheal incision to prevent the leakage of air into the neck tissues. After achieving haemostasis, the strap muscles, the subcutaneous tissues and skin are closed in layers. The child is sedated and taken back to the intensive care unit with the endotracheal tube still in place. Adequate humidification is maintained and the endotracheal tube is removed after about 2 hours when the child has sufficiently recovered from the anaesthesia and sedation. Initially, the child sleeps peacefully since he is partially sedated but normal activity is gradually regained and a return to the otolaryngology department is usually possible within 48 hours. Humidification is continued as required and the child is observed for a further 5 days before the skin sutures are removed. The child can then return home if the domestic arrangements are suitable.

There are several advantages in this approach which has been employed by the author for the majority of decannulations:

(1) it allows direct access to the tracheal stoma and permits the removal of any possible obstruction under direct vision
(2) the suturing of the tracheal stoma reconstitutes the cylindrical wall of the trachea and, therefore, increases the strength of the trachea at this weakened point. In practice, the closure does not produce narrowing of the lumen, which is prevented in any case by the presence of the endotracheal tube
(3) the removal of the tough fibrous track hastens the healing in the soft tissues and the horizontal elliptical incision produces a better cosmetic result.

An obvious disadvantage of this surgical decannulation is that an operation is required, but other disadvantages encountered have been relatively infrequent. In the author's experience, re-opening of the tracheostomy was necessary on two occasions within 3 days of the closure. In one, there was a residual granuloma and the other developed marked surgical emphysema following inadequate suturing of the trachea. This resolved spontaneously.

This surgical method of decannulation was originally employed by the author to decannulate three children who had resisted all other attempts at decannulation (Rogers, 1980). It was so successful that it is still employed in most cases.

However, it is not suggested that others should use this form of closure in all cases, but it is certainly a most useful addition to the methods available for treating difficult decannulation.

Summary and conclusion

Tracheostomy in children is no longer the fearsome operation of the last century. There are still occasions when it is the primary treatment of choice, but its position has been largely usurped by intubation, particularly in inflammatory disease. The operation has become much safer by treating it as an elective operation and emphasizing basic principles of surgical technique and aftercare. The mortality as a result of the tracheostomy itself is still around 5% even in the best of hands and the main cause of death is obstruction of the tube at home. Decannulation is no longer a significant problem except in the worst cases of acquired subglottic stenosis and the scar on the neck is often unnoticeable by adulthood.

In the future, the aim should be to eliminate the need for tracheostomy but, with the advances in neonatal medicine, cranial and thoracic surgery and the increase in the numbers and speeds of motor vehicles, this is unlikely. There will gradually be changes in the types of tubes and their attachments and the operation itself may change as the age-old cricothyroidotomy and its successor, the minitracheostomy, are assessed more thoroughly.

References

BLACK, R. J., BALDWIN, D. C. and JOHNS, A. N. (1984) 'Decannulation panic' in children: fact or fiction? *Journal of Laryngology and Otology*, **98**, 297–304

CARTER, P. and BENJAMIN, B. (1983) Ten year review of pediatric tracheotomy. *Annals of Otology, Rhinology and Laryngology*, **92**, 398–400

COHEN, S. R., DESMOND, M. S., EAVEY, R. D. and MAY, B. C. (1977) Endoscopy and tracheostomy in the neonatal period. A 10-year review. *Annals of Otology, Rhinology and Laryngology*, **86**, 577–583

FEARON, B. and COTTON, R. (1974) Surgical correction of sub-glottic stenosis of the larynx in infants and children. A progress report. *Annals of Otology, Rhinology and Laryngology*, **83**, 428–431

FROST, E. A. M. (1976) Tracing the tracheostomy. *Annals of Otology, Rhinology and Laryngology*, **85**, 618–624

FRY, T. L., FISCHER, N. D., JONES, R. D. and PILLSBURY, H. C. (1985) Comparisons of tracheostomy incisions in a pediatric model. *Annals of Otology, Rhinology and Laryngology*, **94**, 450–453

GERSON, C. R. and TUCKER, G. F. (1982) Infant tracheotomy. *Annals of Otology, Rhinology and Laryngology*, **91**, 413–416

GOODALL, E. W. (1934) The story of tracheostomy. *British Journal of Childhood Diseases*, **31**, 167–176

HOME, F. (1765) *An enquiry into the Natural Causes and Cure of Croup.* Edinburgh: Kincaid and Bell

LINE, W. S., HAWKINS, D. B., KAHLSTROM, E. J., MACLAUGHLIN, E. F. and ENSLEY, J. C. (1986) Tracheotomy in infants and young children: the changing perspective, 1970–1985. *The Laryngoscope,* **96,** 510–515

MALLORY, G. B., REILLY, J. S., MOTOYAMA, E. K., MUTICH, R., KENNA, M. A. and STOOL, S. E. (1985) Tidal flow measurement in the decision to decannulate the pediatric patient. *Annals of Otology, Rhinology and Laryngology,* **94,** 454–457

MUKHERJEE, D. K. (1979) The changing concepts of tracheostomy. *Journal of Laryngology and Otology,* **93,** 899–907

NELSON, T. G. (1958) *Tracheostomy: A Clinical and Experimental Study.* Baltimore: Williams and Wilkins

OKAFOR, B. C. (1983) Tracheostomy in the management of paediatric airway problems. *Ear, Nose and Throat Journal,* **62,** 50–55

PRACY, R. (1976) Tracheostomy tubes. In *Scientific Foundations of Otolaryngology,* edited by R. Hinchcliffe and D. Harrison, p. 766–772. London: William Heinemann Medical Books

PRACY, R. (1979) Intubation of the larynx, laryngotomy and tracheostomy. In *Scott-Brown's Diseases of the Ear, Nose and Throat,* 4th edn, edited by J. Ballantyne and J. Groves, pp. 567–586. London: Butterworths

QUINEY, R. E., SPENCER, M. G., BAILEY, C. M., EVANS, J. N. G. and GRAHAM, J. M. (1986) Management of sub-glottic stenosis: experience from two centres. *Archives of Disease in Childhood,* **61,** 686–690

REILLY, J. S. and MYER, C. M. (1985) Excision of suprastomal granulation tissue. *The Laryngoscope,* **95,** 1545–1546

RODGERS, B. M., BROOKS, J. J. and TALBERT, J. L. (1979) Pediatric tracheostomy: long term evaluation. *Journal of Pediatric Surgery,* **14,** 258–263

RODGERS, J. H. (1980) Decannulation by external exploration of the tracheostomy in children. *Journal of Laryngology and Otology,* **94,** 454–457

SALMON, L. F. W. (1957) Tracheostomy: the evolution of an operation. *Guy's Hospital Gazette,* **71,** 233–242

SASAKI, C. T., FUKUDA, H. and KIRCHNER, J. A. (1973) Laryngeal abductor activity in response to varying ventilatory resistance. *Transactions of the American Academy of Ophthalmology and Otolaryngology,* **77,** 403–410

SONI, N. K., CHATTERJI, P. and THIND, S. S. (1984) Tracheostomy in children. *Indian Journal of Paediatrics,* **51,** 45–47

SWIFT, A. C. and ROGERS, J. H. (1987) The changing indications for tracheostomy in children. *Journal of Laryngology and Otology* (in press)

TEPAS, J. J., HERDY, J. H., SHERMETA, D. W. and HALLER, J. A. (1981) Tracheostomy in neonates and small infants: problems and pitfalls. *Surgery,* **89,** 635–639

TUCKER, J. A. and TUCKER, G. F. (1979) A clinical perspective on the development and anatomical aspects of the infant larynx and trachea. In *Laryngo-Tracheal Problems in the Pediatric Patient,* edited by G. B. Healy and T. J. I. McGill, pp. 3–8. Springfield, Illinois: Charles C. Thomas

WETMORE, R. F., HANDLER, S. D. and POTSIC, W. P. (1982) Pediatric tracheostomy experience during the past decade. *Annals of Otology, Rhinology and Laryngology,* **91,** 628–632

YUNG, M. W. and SNOWDON (1984) Respiratory resistance of tracheostomy tubes. *Archives of Otolaryngology,* **110,** 591–595

33

Home tracheostomy care

Gillian M. Tym

Despite the advances in paediatric laryngeal surgery (Cotton and Evans, 1981), there are a number of children who need to have a tracheostomy for a prolonged period. Nursing these children in hospital is not only expensive and impractical, but separates them from the contact and security of family life which may be detrimental to their development. Ideally a child with a tracheostomy is best cared for at home. Occasionally, there will be patients for whom home care is not suitable and, in this case, hospital life must be made as normal as possible.

However, parents from all walks of life can be taught tracheostomy management and become confident, capable and responsible for their child at home. It is the responsibility of medical and nursing staff to prepare parents slowly and compassionately so that they gain confidence in all aspects of tracheostomy management.

Adjustment to tracheostomy

The idea of taking a newly tracheostomized child home may be daunting. It will quickly become evident that the child will put new pressures and constraints on normal daily routine. Parental reaction to a tracheostomy can vary from terror to over confidence, guilt or anger. Others are merely relieved to see their child free from stridor. Parents need repeated reassurance that these different feelings are normal reactions.

There are definite advantages in parents communicating with other happy tracheostomized children and their families; this leads to the realization they are not unique and so helps them to gain confidence. Friendships often form between parents and in time this can lead to mutual support. For example, at a practical level, those living in the same locality could exchange babysitting favours.

Training for home care

Training for home care begins at the earliest opportunity, preferably before surgery, with the teaching of basic anatomy. Simple line drawings may help to explain the functions of the larynx and trachea. Parents need to appreciate and understand:

(1) the reasons why their child has an artificial airway
(2) the extent to which normal laryngeal functions have been impaired by the formation of a tracheostomy.

They need to visualize the oesophagus and trachea as separate tubes for eating and breathing and appreciate that special precautions must be taken now that inspired air is no longer warmed, filtered or humidified.

Parents must learn the skills at their own pace. This takes time and patience on behalf of the ward team. It is essential they receive a unified teaching programme. There must be absolute uniformity of instruction from all members of staff.

In order for parents to learn tracheostomy management as quickly as possible, it is important they spend as much time as they can manage with the child in hospital.

At first they will simply observe the techniques. Gradually, with gentle encouragement, they will become increasingly competent to carry out these procedures under supervision and eventually have full confidence to undertake the task alone.

They will need education in the following:

(1) stoma and skin care
(2) irrigation and suction
(3) changing the tracheostomy tapes
(4) changing the tracheostomy tube
(5) chest physiotherapy
(6) detection and management of complications
(7) resuscitation
(8) supplies and equipment for home use and the care of plastic and silver tracheostomy tubes
(9) cleaning and sterilization of all equipment
(10) problems associated with the tracheostomized child at home
(11) available help in the community.

Nursing technique

Stoma and skin care

Once a tracheostomy is established the tract usually epithelializes quickly and minimal skin care is necessary. Gentle cleaning with normal saline or a mild antiseptic solution will help keep the skin dry, clean, and free from irritation and infection. Creams and ointments should be avoided.

If the skin should become sore, it must be cleaned more frequently, and a non-adherent dressing applied; this is changed when necessary. (Cotton wool based dressings should not be used; they disintegrate and fragments may be inhaled.)

Granulomata around the tube sometimes occur and are treated with topical applications of silver nitrate.

Irrigation and suction

Whenever possible the child should be encouraged to cough and clear accumulated mucus from the trachea. If, however, the secretions cannot be cleared in this manner, it is important they are made less tenacious by the instillation of 0.5–1 ml isotonic saline into the trachea prior to suction.

With washed hands a clean catheter is inserted, just beyond the end of the tracheostomy tube. Suction is applied as the catheter is withdrawn, with a rotating motion. If further suctioning is required a new clean catheter should be used each time. Each suction should not take more than 20–30 seconds. The frequency of applying suction varies from child to child. Secretions usually become less plentiful as the child becomes accustomed to his tube and a daily routine is established away from the hospital environment.

Hospital staff wear disposable gloves for suction to prevent cross-infection, but there is no need for parents to wear gloves. They should, however, pay special attention to handwashing and person-al hygiene before performing any of the procedures. Suction should be performed prior to feeds or mealtimes and be avoided immediately afterwards if possible.

Changing the tapes

Tapes should be changed daily or whenever they become dirty or wet. It is often desirable to perform tape changing as a routine after the child's bath in the evening. At this time they are often sleepy and will offer less resistance.

It is advisable to have two adults present. If necessary the child can be restrained by wrapping in a towel or blanket. The child is laid down and the neck extended over a pillow or rolled up nappy. One person holds the tube in place while the other cuts and removes the old tapes, and cleans the area around the stoma.

New tapes are attached by tying three knots on one side of the tube and a bow on the other. The first person should continue to hold the tube in place until the tension has been checked.

Checking the tension

The importance of obtaining the correct tension must be stressed repeatedly to the parents, as one of the causes of home tracheostomy fatality is a displaced tube.

With the child sitting up with his neck flexed forward, it should be possible to insert just one finger between the tapes and the neck (*Figure 33.1*). Adjust the bow until the correct tension is

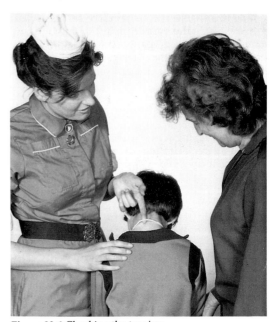

Figure 33.1 Checking the tension

obtained. Once satisfied that the tapes are correctly tensioned, the bow is secured by tying it with three knots.

Changing the tracheostomy tube

This must be the most traumatic aspect of tracheostomy management and it is very natural and right that parents should view tube changing with some anxiety. Parents should be reassured that changing of the tube is safe if the taught routine is followed. It is normal for the child to cough, cry or protest; they usually become more cooperative as they get older. It is usually sufficient to change the tube once a week and it is advisable to do so prior to feeds or meal times. However, if secretions are tenacious the tube is more likely to become crusted and will need to be changed more frequently.

Special precautions

(1) There must always be two adults present for a routine tube change.
(2) Good lighting is essential.
(3) Meticulous attention to handwashing and sterility of the tube is essential.
(4) Spare tube and suction apparatus must be available.
(5) Suction is applied and the stoma cleaned before changing the tube.

Procedure

While one person extends the neck and holds the chin, the second person cuts the tapes and removes the old tube with one hand, and gently but quickly inserts the new tube with the other. The tapes are tied and tension checked carefully.

Chest physiotherapy

Once a child has been discharged from hospital, secretions tend to diminish and the need for chest physiotherapy is eliminated.

However, if the child suffers from a respiratory infection, the secretions will become more plentiful and it is then advisable that the parents administer safe chest percussion. It is essential that a physiotherapist teaches the family how to do this prior to discharge.

Detection and management of complications
Respiratory tract infections

There is a significant decrease in the frequency of respiratory tract infections once the tracheosto-mized child is at home. Parents must be made aware of normal and abnormal conditions for their child. They should be taught to watch for fever, loss of appetite, and change in colour, consistency or amount of tracheal secretions.

They should appreciate that it may become necessary to increase the frequency of suctioning, to increase the fluid intake, and to give regular chest physiotherapy. Either the general practitioner or hospital physician should be informed and relevant antibiotics commenced if indicated. Clinical trials have shown that S-carboxymethyl-cysteine (Mucodyne) reduces the viscosity of sputum. It improves the ability to cough up bronchial secretions without adverse side-effects (Edwards *et al.*, 1976).

It is useful for the parents to have a few sputum traps at home so that specimens can be obtained for culture when necessary.

Resuscitation

There is a mortality associated with a tracheosto-mized child in hospital which is slightly increased when the child is nursed at home. To minimize this risk it is absolutely essential that the parents are taught cardiopulmonary resuscitation prior to discharge. It is a difficult issue to raise for the nurse, doctor and parent. It must be handled efficiently and with sensitivity. It is important that the family have quick access to a telephone in the event of an emergency.

Equipment and supplies for home use

It is advisable to keep all tracheostomy equipment on a clean, well lit surface next to the child's bed. All electrical appliances should be checked prior to discharge from hospital.

Electric suction machine *(Figure 33.2)*

Several different designs of machine are available. Essentially it should be reliable, light and easy to clean with a regulator switch to ensure optimal suction. Correct tubing and connectors should be supplied with the pump. Any filter in the unit should be changed weekly.

Portable suction unit *(Figure 33.3)*

It is essential that parents are provided with a small portable suction unit, operating independently of the electricity supply, such as a foot pump. This enables the child and family to have

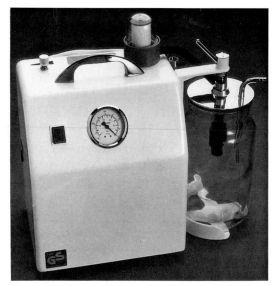

Figure 33.2 Electric suction pump

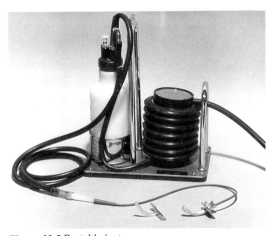

Figure 33.3 Portable foot pump

freedom from the confines of home, and should there be an electricity power cut, this form of suction will be reliable and sufficient until normal power is restored.

Catheters

There are many different designs of catheter available. Rubber catheters which cause less tissue damage, are soft but not disposable, whereas the plastic disposable catheters are slightly stiffer. However, since the catheters will be used by only one patient, it is usually possible to clean and re-use all of them.

Tracheostomy tubes

Disposable

There are several companies who manufacture disposable paediatric tracheostomy tubes (for example Warne/Franklin, England; Portex Ltd., England; Shiley Ltd., England) (*Figure 33.4*). Hospital preference usually determines the type to be used.

In all cases these tubes can be sterilized at home and re-used on several occasions before discarding. Extended tubes (*Figure 33.5*) can be used to prevent small infants with 'double chins' accidentally occluding their airways while sleeping.

The parents should be given four or five sterile tubes to take home and told to carry a spare with them at all times in case of emergency.

Advantages of plastic tubes (Stool, Campbell and Johnson, 1968)

(1) They are more pliable at body temperature and conform well to the trachea, reducing the danger of tracheal ulceration.

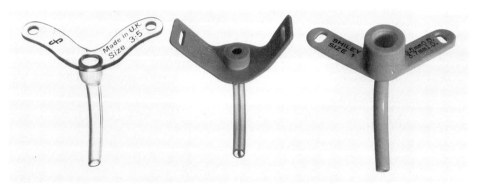

Figure 33.4 Warne Franklin, Portex and Shiley plastic tubes

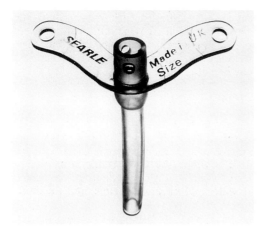

Figure 33.5 GOS extended tube

(2) The length of the tube can be easily shortened for neonates.
(3) The tube is relatively inexpensive.
(4) Plastic causes less inflammatory reaction and healing around the tube is rapid.

Di Santi valves

Di Santi valves (*Figure 33.6*) are designed to fit snugly into all sizes of the 'Great Ormond Street' (GOS) pattern plastic tracheostomy tube (Warne Franklin, England). The valve closes on expiration and vocalization can occur, either due to air leak around the tube or through a fenestration which can be carefully cut into the plastic.

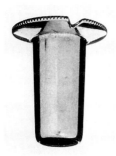

Figure 33.6 Di-Santi valve

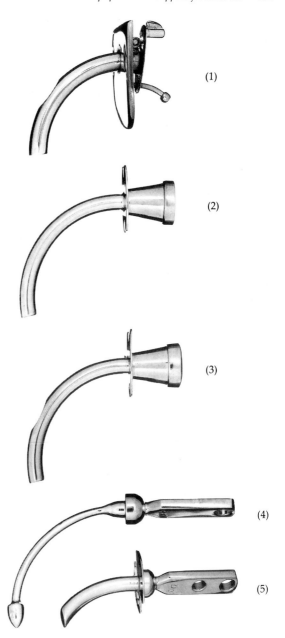

Figure 33.7 Five parts of silver Alder Hey tube

Silver tracheostomy tubes

There are advantages and disadvantages associated with silver tracheostomy tubes. The most commonly used 'Alder Hey' tube (Downs Surgical plc, England) consists of five parts (*Figure 33.7*):

(1) a fenestrated outer tube
(2) plain inner valve
(3) a fenestrated speaking valve

(4) introducer
(5) blocker.

These tubes are individually made and parts are not interchangeable.

Advantages

(1) They are reusable.
(2) They have an inner valve which is easily removed for cleaning.

(3) When the fenestration is correctly aligned within the airway, air passes up through the vocal cords and vocalization occurs (*Figure 33.8*). The position of the fenestra should be checked by lateral neck X-rays prior to discharge.

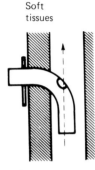

Figure 33.8 Silver tube in correct alignment

Disadvantages

(1) They are expensive.
(2) They are slightly more unsightly than plastic tubes.
(3) Occasionally it is difficult to align the fenestra within the airway and tissue damage can occur (*Figure 33.9*).

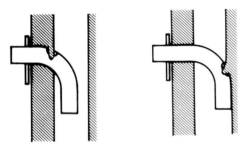

Figure 33.9 Two incorrect alignments of a silver tube

(4) It is sometimes difficult to clean under the flanges of the tube.
(5) Some children are allergic to the tubes.

Special precautions with silver tubes

(1) *Always* insert tube with introducer in position and *always* remove the tube with plain valve in position. In both cases the risk of soft tissue damage is minimized.
(2) *Always* remove the valved speaking tube and replace it with the plain tube when the child is put down to rest or sleep. There is a significant risk of the valve remaining closed due to accumulation of secretions.

(3) It is always safer to perform suction with the plain inner tube in position. *Never* perform suction through the valved speaking tube. The valve can be damaged or part of the catheter may be cut off and inhaled.

Syringes and saline

Syringes should be provided for insertion of saline into the trachea. If necessary saline can be prepared at home by mixing one teaspoon of non-iodized salt to 1.8 litres (one pint) of cooled boiled water, which should be stored in sterile containers.

Humidifiers

These are very expensive and there are only a few children who require humidification at home. It may be indicated for those with severe lower airway disease or those with extremely tenacious secretions.

Cleaning and sterilization of equipment

Parents should be encouraged to care for the equipment provided and to clean it regularly. All non-metallic items can be cleaned in hot soapy water and then immersed in a sterilizing fluid such as Milton (sodium hypochlorite) (Richardson, Vicks Ltd., England). Metal items should be either sterilized in spirit and then rinsed with cooled boiled water, autoclaved or boiled.

Day-to-day problems (Tym, 1986)

Once nursing techniques are mastered, the parents will start to ask specific questions pertaining to the child's daily routine. These issues create as many worries as the nursing care. Severe stress can be put on a family caring for a tracheostomized child 24 hours a day, 7 days a week. Single parent families will need even greater support. All family members and relatives should be encouraged to learn the care and help at home.

Sometimes the parents can gain confidence and independence by taking their child away from the ward environment for increasing periods of time prior to discharge.

Discipline

Parents should not blame the tracheostomy for any lack of discipline in the home. Initially parents often consider their child is weak and feel sorry for him. In the end the child becomes manipulative and the boss of the family, everything revolving around him. The family should treat the child as any other, taking into consideration three important points:

(1) suction equipment is available at all times
(2) the child is protected from water, sand and wind
(3) the child is never left alone with anyone who cannot manage the tracheostomy.

Speech and language development

A child with a tracheostomy may be considered at risk in the development of his speech and language skills. Fortunately, many children manage to vocalize, either by using the air leak around the tube or by use of a valved fenestrated tube. In all cases children should be referred to a speech therapist for assessment around one year of age, or earlier if parents so wish. Parents must be directed to encourage language development in their child at all times.

Clothing

Clothing which is excessively fluffy or with a high neckline should be avoided. A thin scarf over the tracheostomy may be of value, especially on windy days, to prevent particles from entering the trachea.

Sleeping

Small babies should sleep in the same room as their parents. Bells or cradle plays attached to the child's bed will usually warn of distress, since a child in respiratory distress will not lie quietly but will thrash around and create noise from the attached bells or cradle play. Toddlers and older children can sleep alone. An intercom should be used. These are fairly cheap and can be purchased from several large stores. The microphone may be placed in the child's room while the auxillary end may be placed anywhere in the house or even outdoors.

Parents can become extremely exhausted from deprivation of sleep and where possible they should alternate the night care.

Feeding

Feeding does not usually present a problem. Parents should not allow young siblings to feed the tracheostomized child without supervision. They should also avoid performing suction or routine tube changing immediately after a feed as this may cause vomiting.

Bathing and hairwashing

These children can bath normally in shallow water. They should not take a shower. Hair should be washed with the child laid on his back with a controlled spray of water directed backwards.

Schooling

Children with tracheostomies may attend either normal or special schools depending on the area in which they live. Arrangements must be made with teaching staff for them to be carefully observed and staff must be competent in all care.

Travelling

The parents must be encouraged to have a bag of equipment especially for travelling. When away from home they must always carry:

(1) portable suction with catheters
(2) spare tracheostomy tube and tapes
(3) a pair of scissors
(4) saline and syringe
(5) tissues.

Parental freedom

It is important that a third person be trained to take care of the child. One of the major difficulties for parents is the inability to leave home. In some cases it may be possible to exchange babysitting favours with parents of another tracheostomized child in the same area.

Play (Figure 33.10)

A child with a tracheostomy must not go swimming but may paddle under close supervision. Parents must be told to keep their child away from loose, fine, dry sand which is easily inhaled. Any article which could be inhaled should be kept well out of reach of the child.

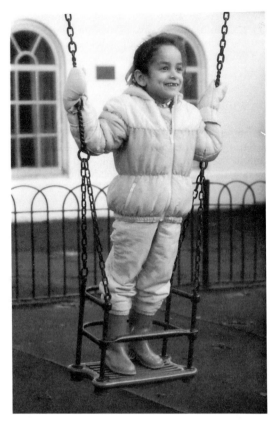

Figure 33.10 A tracheostomized child happily playing

Support from the community

Community care workers (general practitioners, health visitors, district nurses, etc.) must be informed about the child prior to discharge home, so that they can be prepared to give maximum support. Social workers may be able to offer financial help. As time goes by, a routine is established and community workers will have a smaller part to play in home care.

Parents must be reassured that they can contact either medical or nursing staff at the hospital day or night for advice. They must not feel isolated.

There is now a registered charity for these children at home – ACT (Aid for Children with Tracheostomies) which aims to give encouragement, support and practical advice.

Checklist for home care

Before discharge:

(1) parents must be capable in all nursing techniques
(2) they must be able to care for all the equipment provided
(3) community health workers and the general practitioner must be informed.

In conclusion, it must be stated that there is a slightly increased mortality risk in nursing these children at home. However, with proper teaching, instruction and back up from the community and local hospital, the risk is significantly minimized.

Thus children with a tracheostomy who are otherwise well, can, and should be cared for at home.

References

COTTON, R. and EVANS, J. N. G. (1981) Laryngotracheal reconstruction in children, five year follow-up. *Annals of Otology, Rhinology and Laryngology*, **90**, 516–520

EDWARDS, G. F., STEEL, A. E., SCOTT, J. K. and WARREN JORDAN, J. (1976) S-carboxymethylcysteine in the fluidification of sputum and treatment of chronic airway obstruction. *Chest*, **70**, 506–513

STOOL, S. E., CAMPBELL, J. R. and JOHNSON, D. G. (1968) Tracheostomy in children: the use of plastic tubes. *Journal of Paediatric Surgery*, **3**, 402–407

TYM, G. M. (1986) *Tracheostomy – A Guide for Parents*. A Hospital for Sick Children, London publication

34

Stenosis of the larynx

J. N. G. Evans

Stenosis of the larynx is more frequent than tracheal stenosis; in a review of 752 cases of stridor seen at The Hospital for Sick Children, Great Ormond Street, London, laryngeal pathology accounted for 88% of the cases (Evans, 1986). The major cause of airway obstruction was as a result of congenital anomalies of the larynx and trachea. Holinger (1980) noted in his review of 219 patients with stridor, that it was caused by a congenital anomaly of the larynx or trachea in 87.2% of the patients. Congenital laryngeal anomalies are discussed in Chapter 26.

The incidence of acquired subglottic stenosis is increasing, resulting from the increased survival rate of preterm infants ventilated for bronchopulmonary dysplasia and hyaline membrane disease. The precise incidence of subglottic stenosis following intubation is difficult to establish. It is certainly less than the high figure of up to 20% reported in the late 1960s and early 1970s, the true incidence probably lying between 1 and 8% (Parkin, Stevens and Jung, 1976; Strong and Passy, 1977; Papsidero and Pashley, 1980; Ratner and Whitfield, 1983). This figure almost certainly underestimates the true incidence since, sadly, many low-birth-weight infants do not survive, and minor degrees of subglottic stenosis may go undetected. Some are recognized only later as a result of persistent stridor following an upper respiratory tract infection, or as an incidental finding on intubation for general anaesthesia.

Aetiology and pathology

Many factors are involved in the creation of subglottic stenosis due to intubation; these include the material from which the tube is made, the shape and size of the tube (Marshak and Grundfast, 1981; Gould and Howard, 1985), its method of fixation and, above all, the skill and care which the intubated patient receives. Increased awareness of all these factors is extremely important if the incidence of subglottic stenosis is to be reduced further.

There are two varieties of acquired laryngeal stenosis related to intubation: *soft* and *hard* stenosis. In the soft stenosis, acute inflammatory oedema of the mucosa and submucosal connective tissue occurs (Rasche and Kuhns, 1972; Hawkins, 1978). Mucosal ulceration (*see Plate 3a*) will then supervene, because of mucosal abrasion resulting from poor fixation of the endotracheal tube, or because of pressure if the endotracheal tube is too large. The process of ulceration will be accelerated by infection; good aseptic technique and strict hygiene will, therefore, minimize the infective complications of intubation. Chemical irritation from rubber or plastisizers used to soften plastic tubes may further aggravate the process of mucosal ulceration, as will any residue of chemicals used in the sterilization of the tubes, for example ethylene oxide (Guess and Stetson, 1970). The process of ulceration eventually exposes the perichondrium of the cricoid cartilage causing perichondritis and chondritis. This is usually associated with the production of granulation tissue and fibrosis (*see Plate 3b*). The stenosis associated with infection of the cricoid cartilage is of the hard variety. Hard stenosis may be further subdivided into two categories: fibrous and cartilaginous (Holinger, 1982). The fibrous stenoses can be dilated but tend to re-stenose (*see Plate 3c*), whereas the cartilaginous stenoses cannot be dilated.

Subglottic stenoses may also occur as a result of acute infection of the larynx (*see* Chapter 30) and of blunt trauma to the neck in hanging injuries. The incidence of direct laryngeal trauma as a result of road traffic accidents has declined as a consequence of legislation prohibiting the transport of children under the age of 5 years in the front passenger seat of cars, and the compulsory wearing of seat belts by older children. Iatrogenic stenosis of the larynx may also occur as a result of prolonged treatment of juvenile laryngeal papillomata and the injudicious use of the CO_2 laser. Whatever the aetiological factor, the end result is a scarred contracted laryngeal opening. Although the number of cases of acquired subglottic stenosis is increasing due to increased survival rates of preterm infants of low birth weight, the actual incidence of subglottic stenosis is falling due to the improved care of preterm babies who are intubated endotracheally. The histological nature of the cricoid cartilage of preterm babies has been noted by Hawkins (1978) to be hypercellular with a scant gel-like matrix, and it may be that it is more distensible; this would account for the fact that these tiny babies may tolerate endotracheal intubation for several weeks without gross damage to the subglottic larynx.

There is certainly no point in laying down arbitrary time scales for endotracheal intubation before a tracheostomy becomes necessary. In general, it is essential to use an endotracheal tube that is as small as possible and which allows a leak of air during positive pressure ventilation. If the air leak disappears and a smaller endotracheal tube cannot be used, then a cricoid split procedure as advocated by Cotton and Seid (1980) and Frankel *et al.* (1984) may allow a further period of between 10 and 14 days intubation before tracheostomy is necessary due to developing perichondritis or chondritis of the cricoid. It has been suggested by Quiney *et al.* (1986) that, even if chondritis of the cricoid is present, epithelialization of the laryngeal mucosa may occur around the endotracheal tube – an argument for prolonged undisturbed intubation!

The investigation of the patient with acquired laryngeal stenosis is similar to that required for congenital laryngeal anomalies and is dealt with in Chapter 26.

Treatment of laryngeal stenosis

The treatment of laryngeal stenosis is one of the most controversial topics in paediatric otolaryngology. Therapeutic procedures range from repeated dilatation, prolonged laryngeal stenting with or without the use of steroids, the use of the CO_2 laser to create an airway with or without tracheos-

tomy, to early tracheostomy and open surgical operation on the child's larynx.

Congenital subglottic stenosis

Congenital subglottic stenosis is on the whole less severe than acquired stenosis and, in some cases, mild congenital subglottic stenosis can be treated without performing a tracheostomy (*see Plate 3d*). Holinger (1982) reported a series of 24 infants with severe subglottic stenosis, six of whom were treated with the CO_2 laser so avoiding tracheostomy.

Almost half of the patients with congenital subglottic stenosis will require a tracheostomy (Cotton and Myer, 1984). Most of these patients will be decannulated within 2–5 years without requiring any operative procedure on the larynx. The process of natural resolution makes the effect of treatment difficult to assess. This difficulty is compounded by the fact that there are two basic types of congenital subglottic stenosis, the first being the result of soft tissue abnormality, the second of abnormalities of the cricoid cartilage (*see Plate 3e*).

Soft tissue abnormalities

Submucosal fibrosis, hyperplasia of the submucous glandular tissue and frank granulation tissue usually occur as a result of intubation (Holinger, 1982). The hyperplasia of the submucous glandular tissue may be so exuberant as to present as submucous retention cysts (Mitchell *et al.*, 1987) (*see Plate 3f*) and these cysts respond well to deroofing with the CO_2 laser, cup forceps or diathermy.

Abnormalities of the cricoid

In the review by Morimitsu *et al.* (1981) of congenital cricoid stenosis, 12 cases had a large anterior lamina with a very small posteriorly sited airway having an average diameter of 1.9 mm. In one case, there was a thickened posterior lamina (*see Plate 3g*) and, in another, the cricoid cartilage itself was oval. Tucker *et al.* (1979) also described a trapped first tracheal ring as an abnormality associated with subglottic stenosis. Thickening of the cricoid with a small posterior lumen is certainly the author's experience. The clinical importance of identifying thickening of the cricoid is fundamental, since these cases do not respond to dilatation and treatment with the CO_2 laser is also likely to be unsuccessful. After a period of observation of approximately one year, in the case of neonates, or until the child's weight exceeds 10 kg, an open procedure on the larynx should be considered.

An open procedure on the larynx is also necessary in acquired stenosis were there is a hard cicatrix which has formed as a result of cricoid perichondritis.

Dilatation

The soft tissue stenoses may respond to simple dilatation whereas dilatation is contraindicated, and may indeed be harmful, in patients with abnormalities of the cricoid cartilage.

Steroids

The use of steroids as an adjunct to dilatation and simple excision of scar tissue either by CO_2 laser or cup forceps might be expected, on theoretical grounds, to aid decannulation. Baker and Whitaker (1950) demonstrated that the administration of corticosteroids during wound healing stopped fibroplasia and the growth of granulation tissue. Successful decannulation after the intralesional injection of steroids was reported by Waggoner, Belenky and Clark (1973). Peerless, Pillsbury and Peerless (1981) showed that the inhalation of beclomethasone dipropionate was an excellent adjunct therapy for the treatment of laryngeal stenosis. Birck (1970) reported seven patients with subglottic stenosis who were successfully decannulated within 2 months of treatment which involved dilatation and systemic administration of steroids. In spite of their occasional reports of successful treatment with steroids, most practitioners have not found them to be helpful in the management of subglottic stenosis because the delayed healing process increases the patient's susceptibility to infection and thereby delays epithelial healing. It is the practice of the author to use systemic steroids in a dose of 0.5 mg/kg to reduce oedema after bronchoscopy in a difficult case, for example after the removal of a foreign body from the trachea of a young child.

Endoscopic resection

Various endoscopic methods of resection have been employed and include infant urethral resectoscopes (Downing and Johnson, 1979) and cryogenic probes (Rodgers and Talbot, 1978). It is probably true to say that the majority of paediatric otolaryngologists who specialize in the management of laryngeal stenosis would favour the use of the CO_2 laser for endoscopic resection (Strong *et*

al. 1979; Friedman, Healy and McGill, 1983; Carruth *et al.*, 1986). The successful endoscopic management of laryngeal stenosis depends upon careful patient selection. Simpson *et al.* (1982) reviewed 60 cases of laryngeal stenosis, 31 of whom had subglottic stenosis, and he was able to identify factors which indicated where endoscopic treatment was likely to be unsuccessful. These included cases of combined laryngeal and tracheal stenosis, particularly if the stenotic areas were wide or circumferential or if they were accompanied by significant loss of cricoid or tracheal cartilage.

If abundant scar tissue was present involving at least 1 cm of larynx or trachea vertically, the scar tissue was circumferential or the posterior commissure was involved and the arytenoids were fixed, then an unsuccessful outcome was likely.

If bacterial infection of the trachea associated with perichondritis occurred prior to treatment, an unsuccessful outcome was noted in 87.5% of the cases.

If these adverse factors are noted, then an open operation upon the larynx is advised and if there has been evidence of perichondritis with significant cartilage loss, it is essential to wait for at least 6 months to one year before attempting an open operation. This interval allows the active inflammatory process to resolve and increases the chance of a successful outcome of a procedure which may involve free grafts of cartilage where infection is likely to prejudice the success of the operation.

Open operations

Many surgical procedures for the correction of subglottic stenosis have been described; in the main they involve the use of autogenous grafts, hyoid bone (Abedi and Frable, 1983), sternohyoid myo-osseous flaps (Close, Lozano and Schaeffer, 1983) and nasal septal cartilage (Toohill, Martinelli and Janowak, 1976). The techniques of laryngotracheoplasty (Evans and Todd, 1974) and laryngotracheal reconstruction using free costal cartilage grafts (Cotton, 1978) are the most popular and will be discussed in some detail (Cotton and Evans, 1981).

Laryngotracheoplasty

This technique is used in congenital subglottic stenosis where the cricoid cartilage is abnormally thick; it may also be used in cases of laryngeal webs where there is often an associated anomaly of the cricoid cartilage. In this procedure, a midline incision is made through the thyroid cartilage and cricothyroid membrane, a castellated

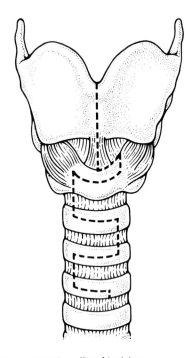

Figure 34.1 Castellated incision

incision (*Figure 34.1*) then being fashioned through the cricoid cartilage and involved tracheal rings. The larynx is opened from above and the vocal cords separated at the anterior commissure under direct vision. Once the larynx is opened, a submucosal dissection and removal of the scar tissue is made using scissors designed for microscopic surgery. As much laryngeal mucosa as possible is saved to line the stenotic segment. If the cricoid is abnormally thick, cartilage may be pared or cored from its internal surface to increase the lumen (*Figure 34.2*). An internal stent consisting of a 'swiss-roll' of Silastic sheeting (*Figure 34.3*) is inserted and the cartilaginous laryngeal and tracheal pegs are sutured in their displaced position. The Silastic roll is secured by a transfixion suture (*Figure 34.4*) which is brought out over the strap muscles and buried subcutaneously. The Silastic roll is removed endoscopically 6 weeks later.

Laryngotracheal reconstruction

This procedure is indicated where there has been loss of cartilage due to perichondritis and chondritis in acquired stenosis. If the stenosis is confined to the anterior part of the larynx and upper trachea, then it is only necessary to insert the cartilage graft anteriorly (*Figure 34.5*). A standard laryngofissure incision is made and a free graft of

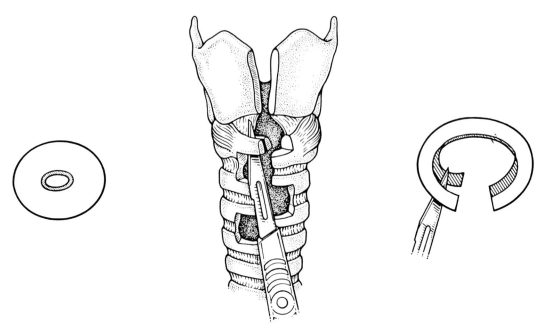

Figure 34.2 The coring out of the abnormally thick cricoid

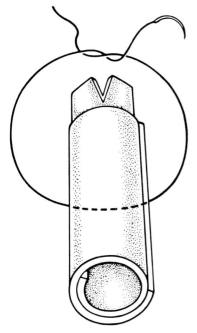

Figure 34.3 Internal stent of rolled Silastic (swiss roll)

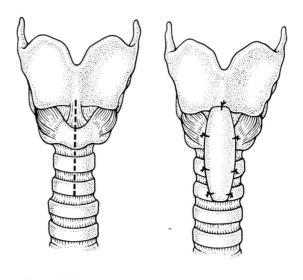

Figure 34.5 Laryngotracheal reconstruction showing the fixation of the anterior graft of costal cartilage

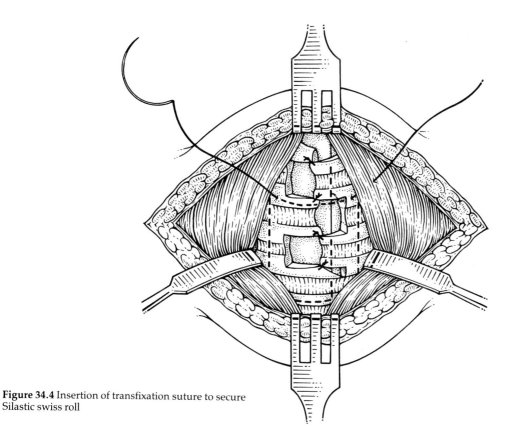

Figure 34.4 Insertion of transfixation suture to secure Silastic swiss roll

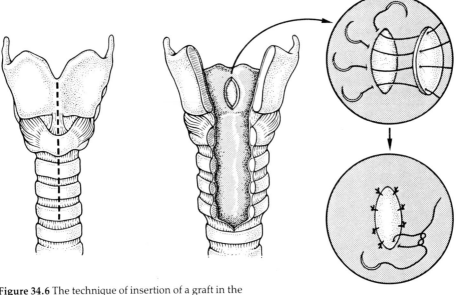

Figure 34.6 The technique of insertion of a graft in the posterior lamina of the cricoid

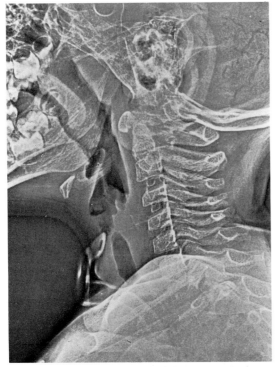

Figure 34.7 Xerogram showing subglottic stenosis after intubation following cardiac surgery

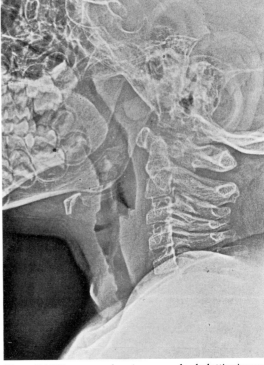

Figure 34.8 Xerogram showing normal subglottic airway after laryngotracheoplasty

costal cartilage is inserted. The cartilage graft is taken from the costal margin and trimmed until it exactly fits the defect, the perichondrial surface is placed internally and the graft is sutured in position using 5/0 polypropylene sutures.

If the scarring involves the posterior part of the glottis with interarytenoid fixation (*see Plate 3h*), the posterior lamina of the cricoid is divided and a smaller graft of costal cartilage inserted, as described by Rethi (1956) (*Figure 34.6*). If combined anterior and posterior stenoses are present or if the stenosis is complete, combined anterior and posterior grafts may be used.

Stenting

The author prefers to stent the larynx and upper trachea in most cases, the best material probably being a Silastic swiss-roll because it has the advantage of being self-adjusting. Rigid stents, such as the Montgomery Silastic laryngeal stent, the Montgomery T tube or the Aboulker Teflon stent (Aboulker *et al.*, 1966), do not have this advantage and, if the selected stent is too big, it may cause further damage to the laryngeal and tracheal mucosa. The Silastic stent is usually retained for 6 weeks, but in severe cases it may be retained for 6 months and in one of the author's cases the stent was retained for 2 years before successful decannulation (Evans, Batch and Leitch, 1986).

The management of laryngeal stenosis in infants and young children should be conservative, since in the majority of cases the stenosis will improve with laryngeal growth. The utmost gentleness must be employed in the inspection and endoscopic treatment of the infant larynx. Open surgical procedures are only to be recommended when it has been established by careful endoscopic assessment that the laryngeal lumen has not increased in size. The surgeon should be prepared to graft the larynx or to perform laryngotracheoplasty and often the appropriate procedure can only be determined when the cricoid cartilage is exposed at operation (*Figure 34.7* and *34.8*). Currently, the efficacy of operations on the larynx has been established and it has been shown that there is a reasonable prospect of achieving decannulation in the majority of cases. One can at least give the parents of these children a reasonably accurate prognosis, and the hope that their child can be restored to normality and to a state that is no longer dependent on tracheostomy.

References

ABEDI, E. and FRABLE, M. A. S. (1983) Conjoint hyoid bone segment for the repair of severe laryngeal stenosis. *Archives of Otolaryngology*, **109**, 482–484

ABOULKER, P., STERKERS, J. M., DEMALDENT, J. E., and

SAUTON, P. (1966) Modifications apportees a l'intervention de Rethi. *Annals of Otology and Laryngology*, **83**, 98–106

BAKER, B. L. and WHITAKER, W. L. (1950) Interference with wound healing by the local action of adrenocortical steroids. *Endocrinology*, **46**, 544–551

BIRCK, H. B. (1970) Endoscopic repair of laryngeal stenosis. *Transactions of the American Academy of Ophthalmology and Otolaryngology*, **74**, 140–143

CARRUTH, J. A. S., MORGAN, N. J., NIELSEN, M. S., PHILLIPPS, J. J. and WAINWRIGHT, A. C. (1986) The treatment of laryngeal stenosis using the CO_2 laser. *Clinical Otolaryngology*, **11**, 145–148

CLOSE, L. G., LOZANO, A. J. and SCHAEFFER, S. D. (1983) Sternohyoid myo-osseous flap for acquired subglottic stenosis in children. *The Laryngoscope*, **93**, 433–439

COTTON, R. T. (1978) Management of subglottic stenosis in infancy and childhood: review of a consecutive series of cases managed by surgical reconstruction. *Annals of Otology, Rhinology and Laryngology*, **87**, 649–657

COTTON, R. T. and EVANS, J. N. G. (1981) Laryngotracheal reconstruction in children. Five-year follow up. *Annals of Otology, Rhinology and Laryngology*, **90**, 516–520

COTTON, R. T. and MYER, C. M. (1984) Contemporary surgical management of laryngeal stenosis in children. *American Journal of Otolaryngology*, **5**, 360–368

COTTON, R. T. and SEID, A. B. (1980) Management of the extubation problem in the premature child: anterior cricoid split as an alternative to tracheostomy. *Annals of Otology, Rhinology and Laryngology*, **89**, 508–511

DOWNING, T. P. and JOHNSON, D. G. (1979) Excision of subglottic stenosis with the urethral resectoscope. *Journal of Pediatric Surgery*, **14**, 252–257

EVANS, J. N. G. (1986) Laryngeal and upper tracheal stenosis in children. *Proceedings of the Fourth International Congress of Paediatric Otorhinolaryngology*, edited by J. Hirschberg and Z. Labas. Kultura Budapest (in press)

EVANS, J. N. G., BATCH, A. J. G. and LEITCH, R. N. (1986) Tracheal problems in children. *Proceedings of the Fifth World Congress for Bronchology, 5th World Congress on Bronchoesophagology*, p. 147–150

EVANS, J. N. G. and TODD, G. B. (1974) Laryngotracheoplasty. *Journal of Laryngology and Otology*, **88**, 589–597

FRANKEL, L. R., ANAS, N. G., PERKIN, R. M., SEID, A. B., PETERSON, B. and PARK, S. M. (1984) Use of anterior cricoid split operation in infants with acquired subglottic stenosis. *Critical Care Medicine*, **12**, 395–398

FRIEDMAN, E. M., HEALY, G. B. and McGILL, T. J. I. (1983) Carbon dioxide laser management of subglottic and tracheal stenosis. *Otolaryngologic Clinics of North America*, **16**, 871–877

GOULD, S. J. and HOWARD, S. (1985) Histopathology of the larynx in the neonate following endotracheal intubation. *Journal of Pathology*, **146**, 301–311

GUESS, W. L. and STETSON, J. B. (1970) Tissue toxicity of rubber endotracheal tubes. *International Anaesthesiology Clinics*, **8**, 823–828

HAWKINS, D. B. (1978) Hyaline membrane disease of the neonate prolonged intubation in management: effect on the larynx. *The Laryngoscope*, **88**, 201–224

HOLINGER, L. D. (1980) Etiology of stridor in the neonate infant and child. *Annals of Otology, Rhinology and Laryngology*, **89**, 397–400

HOLINGER, L. D. (1982) Treatment of severe subglottic stenosis without tracheostomy: a preliminary report.

Annals of Otology, Rhinology and Laryngology, **91**, 407–412

MARSHAK, G. and GRUNDFAST, K. M. (1981) Subglottic stenosis. *Pediatric Clinics of North America*, **28**, 941–948

MITCHELL, D. B., IRWIN, B. C., BAILEY, C. M. and EVANS, J. N. G. (1987) Cysts of the infant larynx. *Journal of Laryngology and Otology* (in press)

MORMITSU, T., MATSUMOTO, I., OKADA, S., TAKAHASHI, M. and KOSUGI, T. (1981) Congenital cricoid stenosis. *The Laryngoscope*, **91**, 1356–1364

PAPSIDERO, M. J., PASHLEY, N. R. T. (1980) Acquired stenosis of the upper airway in neonates. *Annals of Otology, Rhinology and Laryngology*, **89**, 512–514

PARKIN, J. L., STEVENS, M. H. and JUNG, A. L. (1976) Acquired and congenital subglottic stenosis in the infant. *Annals of Otology, Rhinology and Laryngology*, **85**, 573–581

PEERLESS, S. A., PILLSBURY, H. R. and PEERLESS, A. G. (1981) Treatment of laryngeal stenosis a conservative new approach. *Annals of Otology, Rhinology and Laryngology*, **90**, 512–515

QUINEY, R. E., SPENCER, M. G., BAILEY, C. M., EVANS, J. N. G. and GRAHAM, J. M. (1986) Management of subglottic stenosis: experience from two centres. *Archives of Disease in Childhood*, **61**, 686–690

RASCHE, R. F. H. and KUHNS, L. R. (1972) Histopathologic changes in airway mucosa of infants after endotracheal intubation. *Paediatrics*, **50**, 632–637

RATNER, I. and WHITFIELD, J. (1983) Acquired subglottic stenosis in the very low birth weight infant. *American Journal of Diseases of Children*, **137**, 40–43

RETHI, A. (1956) An operation for cicatricial stenosis of the larynx. *Journal of Laryngology and Otology*, **70**, 283–293

RODGERS, B. M. and TALBERT, J. L. (1978) Clinical application of endotracheal cryotherapy. *Journal of Pediatric Surgery*, **13**, 662–668

SIMPSON, G. T., STRONG, M. S., HEALY, G. B., SHAPSHAY, S. M. and VAUGHAN, C. W. (1982) Predictive factors of success or failure in the endoscopic management of laryngeal and tracheal stenosis. *Annals of Otology, Rhinology and Laryngology*, **91**, 384–388

STRONG, R. M. and PASSY, V. (1977) Endotracheal intubation complications in neonates. *Archives of Otolaryngology*, **103**, 329–335

STRONG, M. S., HEALY, G. B., VAUGHAN, C. W., FRIED, M. P. and SHAPSHAY, S. (1979) Endoscopic management of laryngeal stenosis. *Otolaryngologic Clinics of North America*, **12**, 797–806

TOOHILL, R., MARTINELLI, D. and JANOWAK, M. (1976) Repair of laryngeal stenosis with nasal septal graft. *Annals of Otology, Rhinology and Laryngology*, **85**, 601–608

TUCKER, G. F., OSSOFF, R. H., NEWMAN, A. N. and HOLINGER, L. D. (1979) Histopathology of congenital subglottic stenosis. *The Laryngoscope*, **89**, 866–876

WAGGONER, L. G., BELENKY, W. M. and CLARK, C. E. (1973) Treatment of acquired subglottic stenosis. *Annals of Otology, Rhinology and Laryngology*, **82**, 822–826

35

Paediatric anaesthesia

E. F. Battersby

There is no difference between adult and paediatric practice in the basic concepts of anaesthesia. There are, however, very important differences in the anatomy and physiology which have a significant impact on the conduct and safety of the anaesthetic. These differences are at their extreme in the neonatal period – the first 28 days of life – but some remain of importance until 4–5 years of age (Table 35.1). Of equal importance is the infant's psychological development, particular problems being experienced at 2–3 years of age with the emergence of independence, but the continuing need for security. Those who practice otolaryngological anaesthesia and surgery must appreciate the nature of the cardiorespiratory changes if the perianaesthetic period is to be conducted without

morbidity, and the optimum conditions provided so that the correct diagnosis and treatment can be established. In no other branch of surgery is an understanding of each other's problems, cooperation and communication between surgeon and anaesthetist more important to the welfare of the patient.

Neonatal physiology

The respiratory system

Major changes occur in the respiratory system with the adaptation to extrauterine life and the gaseous expansion of the lung during the first few breaths. Lung growth continues albeit at a reducing rate until about 5 years of age.

Table 35.1 Normal values in full-term infants compared with adults

	Infant	Adult
Weight (kg)	3.0	70
Surface area (m^2)	0.19	1.8
Surface area/weight (m^2/kg)	0.06	0.03
Respiratory frequency (breaths/minute)	30–40	12–16
Tidal volume (V_T) (ml/kg)	6–8	7
Dead space (V_D) (ml/kg)	2–2.5	2.2
V_D/V_T	0.3	0.3
Vital capacity (VC) (ml/kg)	35–40	50–60
Thoracic gas volume (TGV) (ml/kg)	35–40	30
Functional residual capacity (FRC) (ml/kg)	27–30	30
Lung compliance (C_L) (ml/cmH$_2$O)	5–6	200
Specific compliance (C_L/FRC) (ml/cmH$_2$O per ml)	0.04–0.06	0.04–0.07
Airways resistance (R_{aw}) (cmH$_2$O/l per s)	25–30	1.6
Work of breathing (g/cm per l)	2000–4000	2000–7000
Resting alveolar ventilation (V_A) (ml/kg per minute)	100–150	60
Resting oxygen consumption (V_{O_2}) (ml/kg per minute)	6.8	3.3

Anatomy of the airway

The neonate has a relatively large head and a short neck. The larynx lies opposite the lower border of the vertebral body of C4 and does not reach the adult position of C5–6 until 4 years of age. The epiglottis is inclined to the posterior pharyngeal wall at an angle of 45° and the glottis is in a more anterior position than in the adult. The tongue is relatively large. This combination of a high forward-looking larynx and a large tongue makes endotracheal intubation difficult if using a curved laryngoscope with the blade placed in the vallecula. A straight blade of the Magill type with the tip posterior to the epiglottis at the anterior commissure gives optimum conditions for endotracheal intubation. By one year of age changes towards the adult position have occurred so that either method of intubation is satisfactory.

Both straight and curved laryngoscopes should be available when anaesthetizing the small infant. The narrowest part of the airway is the cricoid ring which is complete and may not accept an endotracheal tube which has passed through the glottis. The cricoid is slightly elliptical in shape and in a newborn infant weighing 2.5 kg should have a sagittal diameter of 0.5 cm, a coronal diameter of 0.55 cm and a surface area of 0.25 cm². The variations in size and rate of growth of the cricoid cartilage were discussed by Too-Chung and Green (1974). Minimal oedema at the cricoid ring may reduce the airway by up to 60% in the neonate. The trachea is about 4 cm in length. Unless measurement of endotracheal tube length and fixation are carried out meticulously accidental extubation or bronchus intubation readily occur. Air entry to both lungs should always be checked after intubation in an infant.

The lung

Oxygen consumption in the normal newborn infant at neutral environmental temperature is 7 ml/kg per minute which is twice that of the adult on a weight basis. This requires a minute alveolar ventilation of 150 ml/kg per minute, twice that of the adult, which is achieved largely by an increased respiratory rate because of a relatively small inspiratory reserve volume in the neonate. There is a higher dead space ventilation per minute because of the higher rate of breathing. Falls in inspired oxygen concentration will rapidly affect arterial oxygen concentration. Airway resistance is high due to the small bore of the airways but an intrathoracic pressure change of only 5 cmH₂O is needed for normal tidal breathing. However, airway resistance forms a larger fraction of total resistance than in the adult, and infants are particularly at risk from the development of small airway obstruction.

Chest wall compliance in the neonate is about five times as great as lung compliance, whereas these are about equal in the adult. This more flexible chest wall means that relatively little work is required to move the chest cage in quiet breathing, but provides a rather unstable chest cage if the work of breathing is markedly increased due to airway obstruction or non-compliant lungs. The clinical assessment of increased work of breathing may be very difficult in the neonate as chest cage retraction and paradoxical breathing can leave the impression of good chest expansion in the presence of minimal alveolar ventilation. Increasing respiratory rates above 60 breaths per minute indicate the need for continuing close observation. Serial blood gas analysis is more helpful in the assessment of the neonate than it is in the older child.

The relatively low outward recoil force of the chest wall is probably the cause of the tendency of the newborn lung to stabilize with a relatively low functional residual capacity (FRC). This is also likely to be the cause of the tendency to peripheral airway closure with increased intrapulmonary shunting, hypoxia and peripheral gas trapping. These problems can be helped by the use of a continuous distending pressure applied to the airway (*Figure 35.1*). This forms an important

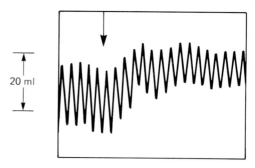

Figure 35.1 Change in functional residual capacity with continuous positive airway pressure (10 cmH₂O)

aspect of the management of both respiratory failure and general anaesthesia in the newborn.

The healthy newborn infant uses about 1% of his energy expenditure in breathing, and about 75% of this is to overcome elastic resistance and 25% flow resistance. A respiratory rate of 30–40 breaths per minute is the most efficient with regard to energy consumption. Increases in airway resistance or pulmonary stiffness will increase the work of breathing considerably so that it represents a very significant percentage of metabolic rate. Both these factors are likely to increase intrapulmonary shunting and consequently lower oxygen availability. Some reversal of this trend is achieved by the use of continuous positive airway pressure (CPAP) (Gregory *et al.*, 1971; Cogswell *et al.*, 1975).

The circulation

Major changes occur in the circulation at birth with the loss of the low resistance vascular bed of the placenta and the opening up of the high resistance pulmonary vascular bed. Pulmonary vascular resistance decreases dramatically after aeration of the lungs, but remains labile for some time until there is regression of the smooth muscle in the terminal arteriolar wall. A partial return to the circulation *in utero* may occur if the pulmonary vascular resistance rises and fetal anastomotic channels such as the ductus arteriosus and foramen ovale re-open. This is called a transitional circulation and up to 70–80% of the cardiac output may shunt right to left through these channels resulting in severe systemic desaturation. The pulmonary arteriolar smooth muscle constricts in response to hypoxaemia, hypercapnia and acidosis. This damaging triad may be present in the neonate with severe airway obstruction and aggressive treatment is required if cerebral damage from hypoxia or venous congestion is to be prevented.

The neonate has less myocardial contractile muscle mass than the adult, and severe hypoxaemia and acidosis may cause a 25% fall in cardiac output. Cardiac stroke volume remains relatively fixed in the neonatal period and cardiac output is closely related to cardiac rate, falling significantly at pulse rates below 100 per minute.

Several anaesthetic techniques which cause cardiac slowing will also cause a major fall in cardiac output.

The response to postural changes is less efficient so that hypovolaemia and head-up tilting are less well tolerated than in the older child. Normal pulse rates and blood pressure in childhood are shown in *Tables 35.2* and *35.3*.

Table 35.2 Normal heart rate
(beats per minute)

Age	Average rate
Preterm	150 ± 20
Term	135 ± 20
1 month	160 ± 20
6 months	140 ± 20
1 year	120 ± 20
2 years	110 ± 20
5 years	90 ± 20
10 years	80 ± 20

Table 35.3 Normal blood pressure (mmHg)

Age	Blood pressure	Average range Systolic	Average range Diastolic
Neonate	80–50	80 ± 15	50 ± 15
6 months	90–60	90 ± 20	60 ± 10
1 year	95–65	95 ± 30	65 ± 20
2 years	100–65	100 ± 25	65 ± 25
5 years	95–55	95 ± 15	55 ± 10
10 years	110–60	110 ± 15	60 ± 10

Temperature control

The neonate is adversely affected by exposure to an environmental temperature which is outside a very narrow range just below normal body temperature. The smaller the newborn the narrower is this neutral temperature range and the nearer it approaches normal body temperature. There are several reasons for this; the newborn has a surface area nearly three times that of the adult relative to body mass, and an insulating layer of subcutaneous tissue which at best is only half that of the adult and is frequently very much less. The normal mechanisms of cutaneous vasoconstriction and dilatation do take place, but they can only compensate for very modest changes in environmental temperature.

About 70% of heat loss takes place by convection, radiation and conduction, and this can be greatly reduced by keeping the baby covered and nursed in a microclimate. This applies equally during transportation, induction of anaesthesia, application of monitoring equipment, surgery and recovery. Some exposure is necessary for adequate observation and the effects of this can be reduced by a warm draught-free operating theatre and the use of heating appliances such as an air mattress.

The principal mechanism for temperature maintenance in the neonate is increased heat production from the oxidation of triglycerides present in the brown fat deposits. The reaction is mediated via the sympathetic nervous system. Metabolism can increase threefold with a large increase in oxygen consumption, but this does not compensate for the large heat losses which occur in an unfavourable thermal environment. This metabolic response to cold is inhibited by hypoxia, which it may help to create and by hypoglycaemia, prematurity and general anaesthesia.

Day admission surgery

Trends in patient care over the last decade have revived the popularity of day-stay surgery and there has been considerable interest and activity in this concept in the paediatric field. This has recently been reviewed by Keneally (1985). The benefits quoted are minimal separation and anxiety for the child, coupled with less disruption for the family and there is probably a reduced risk of hospital-acquired infection. Economic benefits are considerable, although in the short term, introduction of day case work may be more expensive for an individual hospital. More complex and expensive work may occupy the beds released and the day care area may require a higher level of staffing because of the compression of activity into a shorter period of time. If savings are to be achieved, day care must be organized in such a way that it does not require the employment of staff during unsocial hours such as night time, weekends and holiday periods.

The requirements for safe and successful day case work are organization, careful case selection and a high standard of surgery and anaesthesia. The concept of 'inpatient for a day' expressed by Atkinson (1982) is important and haematological investigations and X-rays that are deemed necessary must be undertaken and the results seen before surgery commences. Case selection is important and reflects factors associated with the patient and with the operation. Patients should have a reasonable journey, adequate living conditions and be free of intercurrent infections. However, patients with long-term illnesses or malformations that have been fully investigated and are stable may be suitable for day-stay admission if the surgery and anaesthesia are unlikely to cause destabilization.

The type of surgery should preferably be less than one hour's duration, not enter body cavities, be unlikely to suffer postoperative bleeding, and have only moderate pain that can be controlled by a local block or a mild oral analgesic. Operations suitable for day admission include minor nose operations such as diathermy to turbinates, antral washout, antrostomy, and polypectomy. Minor surgery to the pinna, excision of accessory auricles, myringotomy, ventilation tube insertion and some patients for adenoidectomy are suitable, but the author's own policy does not include tonsillectomy because of the need for analgesic agents and the risk of haemorrhage during the first 24 hours. Laryngoscopy for minor stridor and some patients receiving laser treatment may be suitable for day discharge, but if doubt exists it is wise to warn parents that overnight admission may be necessary in the event of a more lengthy or major procedure being performed.

Anaesthesia has no particular restrictions but older ambulant children should not need premedication. Infants can be given premedication if indicated and it should be remembered that it is often easier for a parent to take home a sleepy toddler than one who is wide awake and fractious. Premedication, intravenous and postoperative analgesics which are associated with nausea and vomiting should be avoided if at all possible, and if used, should be coupled with an antiemetic. Muscle relaxants are not contraindicated, but suxamethonium should be avoided in older children as its use is sometimes associated with postoperative muscle pains in ambulant patients. Endotracheal intubation should not be withheld if the operation suggests its need, but it must be atraumatic with a loose-fitting tube.

Patients should be maintained under supervision for 3–4 hours after regaining consciousness and must be checked by a competent medical person before discharge. Parents should be advised about feeding, analgesics and possible significant postoperative complications, before discharge.

Airway obstruction

Airway obstruction forms a major part of infant otolaryngology and ranges from the urgent diagnosis and relief of severe life-threatening obstruction to assessment of a variety of causes of stridor in the infant. The implication of some of the causes may mean a prolonged, difficult and disruptive period for both the parents and patient, often with a long-term tracheostomy and much surgery. Other diagnoses mean repeated inactivity and reassurance of the parents that significant and worrying stridor will eventually disappear. Nothing is more damaging to parental security and ability to manage than changing and conflicting diagnoses and management regimens. Anaesthetists must be able to provide the surgeon with the operating conditions that allow the correct diagnosis to be made.

The newborn infant rarely presents with airway obstruction in the first days of life, but when this occurs it requires urgent and expert management. The older infant may present for the diagnosis and appropriate treatment of stridor. Over recent years small infants are sometimes seen who have been difficult to extubate or who have stridor appearing after satisfactory and successful care in a preterm neonatal intensive care unit where respiratory support has been required. Finally, older infants and young children who have been leading normal healthy lives may suddenly appear with an acute infective upper airway obstruction which is life-threatening. These will usually appear in non-specialist units and require prompt and correct management if damaging side-effects or loss of life are to be avoided. Stridor in paediatric patients has been reviewed by Maze and Bloch (1979).

The neonate

Airway obstruction is responsible for nearly all the otolaryngology admissions in the first 2 weeks of life and is the result of some form of developmental malformation. Infants with a lesser degree of congenital airway obstruction, or acquired lesions, will present later in infancy. Newborns presenting in the first 2 weeks of life will have serious problems which are likely to require urgent diagnosis and treatment, and the medical and anaesthetic management differs slightly from that in the older infant. The causes are shown in *Table 35.4*.

Table 35.4 Causes of respiratory obstruction in the newborn

Nose
(1) Bilateral postchoanal atresia
(2) Absent nose

Pharynx
(1) Maxillofacial deformities associated with mandibular hypoplasia such as Treacher Collins syndrome and Pierre Robin syndrome
(2) Macroglossia – Beckwith syndrome
– haemangioma
(3) Lymphangioma – cystic hygroma
(4) Haemangioma

Supraglottis
(1) Isolated cysts – vallecular or epiglottic
(2) Multiple cysts – cystic hygroma

Glottis
(1) Bilateral vocal cord palsy – central nervous system and vagus nerve lesions
(2) Laryngomalacia and atresia

Subglottis
(1) Congenital stenosis or web
(2) Haemangioma

Trachea
(1) Tracheomalacia – unstable trachea
(2) Microtrachea – small closed cartilage rings
(3) Localized web or stenosis
(4) Extrinsic compression – vascular ring with localized tracheomalacia
– any intrathoracic tumour

Airway obstruction that is severe or prolonged or has bouts of near total obstruction may be fatal or result in permanent neurological damage from cerebral hypoxia or intraventricular haemorrhage. Feeding is difficult, glycogen stores may be rapidly utilized and blood glucose may fall to a level which causes cerebral neuronal damage – below 1.7 mmol/l (30 mg %). Feeding by nasogastric tube is necessary but may aggravate the airway obstruction as the newborn is an obligate nose breather. The neonatal trachea is soft and will collapse with respiratory effort in the presence of an obstructive lesion elsewhere in the airway, thus the differentiation from tracheomalacia may be difficult.

The classic signs of infant airway obstruction are stridor, intercostal indrawing, chest recession which is usually severe because of the compliant nature of the rib cage, and a respiratory rate increasing above 60 breaths per minute. The above may not be so obvious in the first days of life and the main signs may be non-specific, with an irregular breathing pattern, apnoeic attacks, intermittent cyanosis, bradycardia and peripheral circulatory failure. If doubt exists about the diagnosis because of atypical presentation, a rapid screen to distinguish from congenital heart disease, or primary pulmonary or intrathoracic pathology must take place, remembering that congenital malformations are often multiple.

Clinical examination must include a check for facial, mouth and neck malformations, and patency of the posterior choana and oesophagus using a nasogastric tube. Assessment of cardiac and liver size and the presence of femoral pulses is an essential preliminary cardiac screen. A plain X-ray of neck, chest and abdomen is necessary to rule out pneumothorax, diaphragmatic hernia and other intrathoracic and thoracic inlet pathology. If doubt about heart disease exists then an electrocardiograph (ECG) and two-dimensional echocardiogram should be performed, but X-ray contrast studies of the oesophagus to define a vascular ring may be omitted at this stage because of the danger of aspiration. Blood gas estimation is neither diagnostic of any one pathology nor the degree of obstruction, but an indication of the well-being of the neonate which is sometimes a difficult assessment. Normal values of blood gases at 24 hours of age are shown in *Table 35.5*. Serial blood gases are only marginally helpful in making a decision to proceed to a surgical assessment of the obstruction which should, if possible, be carried out before these values deteriorate.

Table 35.5 Normal blood gases at age 24 hours

pH	7.35	7.35
P_aCO_2	4.5 kPa	34 mmHg
P_aO_2	10.6 kPa	80 mmHg
Base excess	−4 mmol/l	−4 mmol/l

Diagnostic laryngoscopy should be undertaken in an operating theatre with full surgical and theatre teams present. Premedication with atropine 0.1 mg intramuscularly helps to dry secretions and to stabilize a more rapid pulse rate, which maintains cardiac output. A precordial stethoscope, ECG, intravenous cannula and warm draught-free theatre are essential. Preoxygenation using a tight-fitting mask, end expiratory pressure and assisted ventilation allows some further assessment of the degree of obstruction prior to attempted awake laryngoscopy and endotracheal intubation. Problems with visualization of the glottis due to facial or pharyngeal malformations will already have been noted, and unexpected solitary supraglottic cysts are always anterior to the glottic opening. The passage of a laryngoscope will improve the airway in supraglottic pathology.

A problem with insertion of an endotracheal tube through a normal-looking glottis is always due to a subglottic stenosis or web, which is not easily recognizable at first laryngoscopy. If an 8 FG rigid neonatal preformed Cole pattern endotracheal tube cannot be inserted, then a tracheostomy will almost certainly be necessary. This will require oxygen and halothane to be administered with assisted ventilation holding the tube impacted onto the stenosis, through the glottis, and local infiltration of the neck with 0.5 or 1% lignocaine.

Once intubated, anaesthesia should commence with oxygen and halothane 2%. The larynx should be sprayed with 10 mg of lignocaine and any additional monitoring applied. When settled, laryngoscopy and bronchoscopy can be carried out on a spontaneously breathing patient, so that a full assessment of the dynamic status of the trachea and larynx is possible. During any hypoventilation or breath holding, assisted or controlled ventilation is carried out via the ventilating Storz-Hopkins bronchoscope. The 2.5 mm bronchoscope is difficult to use as a ventilating bronchoscope as a consequence of the high gas flow resistance. Laryngoscopy is performed during emergence using 100% oxygen and spontaneous breathing. If continuing temporary airway assistance is required then a nasotracheal or nasopharyngeal tube can be inserted and the neonate allowed to breathe humidified air and oxygen via a circuit allowing controlled continuous positive airway pressure.

The infant

The older neonate, infant or young child may present with upper airway obstruction from congenital or acquired causes (*Table 35.6*). The diagnosis is based on the presence of stridor. Stridor that is positional and only inspiratory suggests a functional supraglottic cause, and unremitting inspiratory and expiratory stridor – often referred to as two-way stridor – indicates anatomical subglottic or tracheal obstruction. The degree of obstruction is largely a clinical assessment based on the work required to achieve adequate alveolar ventilation. The more effort

required and the more compliant the chest cage, the greater the use of accessory muscles and the more indrawing and chest cage retraction present. Blood gases are well maintained unless there is a concomitant pulmonary problem as is frequently seen in laryngotracheobronchitis. As obstruction increases more respiratory effort is required but eventually fatigue occurs. Serious hypoventilation with less stridor, less chest retraction and rapidly deteriorating blood gases supervenes. Urgent relief is required as hypoxia, apnoea, cerebral damage and cardiac arrest rapidly follow. Obstruction must never be allowed to progress to this state. Indicators of deterioration include reluctance to drink, a respiratory rate rising above 60 breaths per minute, a rising pulse rate, sweating, pallor and a poor peripheral circulation. Factors contributing to deterioration are dehydration and secretion retention.

Most infants presenting to the anaesthetist have mild to moderate airway obstruction and are referred for diagnosis by microlaryngoscopy and bronchoscopy, and treatment if appropriate. The surgical requirements are a still, oxygenated spontaneously breathing patient who can be maintained almost awake, and without laryngospasm, so that a careful assessment of cord and cricoarytenoid movement can be made. The basic technique requires good topical anaesthesia of the larynx and a light inhalational anaesthetic. Premedication consists of intramuscular atropine. Good drying of pharyngeal secretions is essential, so that topical anaesthesia is effective, thus making adequate preoperative starvation mandatory. Sedation should be avoided. Induction with

Table 35.6 Acquired airway obstruction in infants (congenital causes *see Table 35.4*)

Infective stridor
  croup
  epiglottitis
  diphtheria
  retropharyngeal and tonsillar abscess
  cellulitis floor of mouth and neck

Trauma
  foreign body
  external trauma
  chemical and thermal burns
  intubation and instrumentation – subglottic oedema
  long-term intubation
    granuloma
    web
    cricoarytenoid fixation
  recurrent laryngeal nerve damage – cord palsy

Neoplasia
  laryngeal papillomatosis
  tumours thoracic inlet or chest

halothane/oxygen is satisfactory and once consciousness is lost the use of a tight-fitting mask and semi-occlusion of the T-piece bag achieves considerable raised airway pressure. Functional stridor will reduce or disappear, but stridor caused by a fixed obstructive lesion such as a subglottic stenosis will only improve minimally.

While anaesthesia deepens using up to 4% halothane/oxygen, monitoring and an intravenous infusion are established and a decision made whether to intubate using deep anaesthesia or muscle relaxant. If mask ventilation is difficult a muscle relaxant must not be used and if any doubt exists a preliminary look at the larynx will indicate the safety of muscle paralysis. The larynx is sprayed using a metered dose 10% lignocaine spray with a maximum dose of 4–5 mg/kg. Pelton *et al.* (1970) reported on the safety of this preparation in a dose up to 3 mg/kg, but over many years the author has used the larger maximum dose with no clinically definable problems and excellent clinical conditions (Eyres *et al.*, 1978).

A modest-sized plastic nasotracheal tube is inserted through the glottis which allows a crude estimate of subglottic size and maintains anaesthesia during transport, the setting up of the suspension laryngoscope, and preliminary assessment. The tube is then removed to the nasopharynx and oxygen/halothane insufflated for any minor surgery, and the patient is allowed to wake up with the laryngoscope tip positioned in the vallecula, while vocal cord and cricoarytenoid movement is assessed. The use of an injector attachment to the laryngoscope is unsatisfactory under about 7–8 years of age, as the gas jet causes distortion to the glottis, ventilation is usually inadequate and a functional assessment is impossible. Bronchoscopy is carried out first if the primary lesion is likely to be tracheal and is only performed at the end if the laryngoscopy is negative. Bronchoscopy is contraindicated in the presence of a significant subglottic stenosis, as postoperative oedema may precipitate an acute respiratory obstructive episode. Prophylactic intravenous dexamethasone (0.5–1 mg/kg) is given and is helpful, although it has not proved helpful in chronic subglottic oedema. Nebulized racemic adrenaline has also been widely used and is effective (0.05 ml/kg of 2.25% solution).

Diagnostic bronchoscopy is performed with the Storz-Hopkins ventilating bronchoscope as its optical and lighting system provides excellent clarity of view. The system can be readily sealed and used as a ventilating bronchoscope, but in the sizes below 5 mm the antifog sheath must not be used as the gas flow resistance for both spontaneous breathing and intermittent positive pressure ventilation is too high. The sheath is replaced by a spacing block which prevents the telescope from projecting beyond the end of the bronchoscope. The 2.5 mm bronchoscope has a high gas flow resistance with the telescope in position and its use in this mode is accompanied by considerable airway obstruction.

An alternative is to use the telescope on its own, with spontaneous breathing, which is necessary anyway to establish a diagnosis of generalized or localized tracheomalacia. Much of the visual quality is lost if this bronchoscope is used without the telescope, with proximal lighting and a magnification lens, but it is sealed and can be used in a ventilating mode. *Table 35.7* demonstrates the airway resistance measured in the smaller bronchoscopes. The tip of the larger size paediatric bronchoscopes is slightly elliptical, but as it must pass the cricoid ring which is almost circular and the narrowest structure in the normal airway, the larger diameter is the most relevant. *Table 35.8* shows bronchoscope tip sizes and the appropriate size instrument for normal patients in the lower age group.

The alternative Negus bronchoscope is not possible to seal and is therefore used with

Table 35.7 Storz-Hopkins bronchoscopes

| | Gas flow resistance (cmH$_2$O/l per s) | | | |
| | Measured at 5 l flow | | Measured at 10 l flow | |
Bronchoscope size (mm)	Bronchoscope only	Bronchoscope and telescope	Bronchoscope only	Bronchoscope and telescope
2.5	42	1512	80	2700
3.0	21	40	30	65
3.5 (short)	12	16	15	26
3.5 (long)	12	34	19	39
4.0	8	20	15	25
5.0	6	12	12	18

Battersby and Ridley (unpublished data)

Table 35.8 Storz-Hopkins bronchoscopes

Bronchoscope size (nominal) (mm)	Internal diameter (mm)	Maximum external diameter (mm)	Age normal airway
2.5	3.0	4.0	Neonate
3.0	4.0	5.0	Neonate– 6 months
3.5	4.6	5.6	6–18 months
4.0	6.0	7.0	18 months – 3 years
5.0	6.8	8.0	3–8 years

spontaneous breathing or in a paralysed or deeply anaesthetized patient with the Venturi injector (Sanders, 1967). Magnification can be provided by the use of a small telescope which is mounted on a moveable arm. Although the view for diagnostic assessment is inferior to that provided by the Storz-Hopkins bronchoscope, the Negus instrument is often easier to use with grasping and holding forceps as they can be manipulated directly. The Negus bronchoscope is tapered with a wide bore proximal opening, thus allowing the use of a high pressure injector jet and gas entrainment to ventilate the lungs.

There is a need to restrict either driving pressure or jet size in smaller patients to prevent barotrauma to the lungs; in addition, over-ventilation with CO_2 washout and removal of inhalational anaesthetic agent can occur very rapidly. In practical terms, it is easier to leave the driving pressure at standard anaesthetic machine pipeline pressure (60 psi, 413 kPa) and to reduce jet size. Bethune *et al.* (1972) recommended appropriate jet sizes for different bronchoscopes using a standard pipeline driving pressure (*Table 35.9*). Miyasaka, Sloan and Froese (1980) reported on the use of jet injectors in both tapered and tubular bronchoscopes, and confirmed the safety of a 19 gauge jet in the smaller size Negus bronchoscopes.

Anaesthesia can be maintained in a stabilized patient by running oxygen and inhalational agent

Table 35.9 Negus bronchoscope injectors

Negus bronchoscope	Injector size	Maximum pressure (cmH$_2$O)	Peak flow (l/minute)
Suckling	19	15	27
Infant	19	18	45
Child	19	18	75
Adolescent	18	24	110
Adult (small)	16	28	180

down the bronchoscope side arm, thus enriching entrained gas with some inhalational agent, or by the use of intermittent injection or infusion of an appropriate short-acting intravenous anaesthetic agent. Total muscle relaxation is not essential all the time in smaller patients as apnoea frequently occurs from CO_2 washout, but better conditions are usually provided if muscle paralysis is used. The newer agents, atracurium and vecuronium, given by injection or infusion are very satisfactory. Bronchoscopic assessment or operation on the lower airway through a tracheostome is easy and either spontaneous breathing or intermittent positive pressure ventilation presents no problems provided that the proximal bronchoscope side holes are first occluded, otherwise gas leakage makes ventilation impossible.

The ability to change from spontaneous breathing to intermittent positive pressure ventilation and back again during microlaryngoscopy and bronchoscopy allows a full assessment of organic and functional pathology to be carried out quickly and safely. Neither anaesthetic technique is always entirely adequate on its own, but muscle paralysis prevents functional assessment and should never be induced until there is certainty that ventilation will be achieved.

Monitoring is all important and requires close continuous clinical observation, a precordial stethoscope, ECG and pulse oximetry to ensure safety at all times. This is a field where pulse oximetry would seem to have an essential role as a monitor, as the earliest significant subclinical sign encountered is a fall in arterial oxygen saturation.

Acute infective obstruction

Acute epiglottitis and croup are the principal acute infective causes of airway obstruction in childhood. They are of especial importance because of their widespread occurrence and potential danger to life. The clinical course and management of both conditions is very different and is dealt with fully in Chapter 30, but there are important implications for anaesthesia.

Acute epiglottitis

Acute epiglottitis is less common and is caused by infection with *Haemophilus influenzae*. The time course is acute and death from airway obstruction as a result of the hugely swollen and inflamed epiglottis may occur within a few hours of the onset of symptoms. Breathing is easier in the sitting position, but swallowing is difficult so that the characteristic picture is of a child with rapid onset mild stridor, sitting forward and dribbling. Attempted diagnosis by awake pharyngoscopy is dangerous as it may precipitate a respiratory arrest. Lateral X-ray of the neck is likely to be diagnostic, but is frequently unnecessary. If it is required then it must be undertaken in the intensive care unit or operating theatre where full facilities and personnel for airway rescue are present. The clinical picture is so characteristic and may change so rapidly that urgent anaesthesia and endotracheal intubation are indicated in all patients once the clinical diagnosis is made. Any preliminary disturbing episode that may precipitate acute airway obstruction should be avoided.

Anaesthesia is induced in the sitting position with oxygen (100%) and halothane, as recommended by Hannallah and Rosales (1978). As consciousness is lost the patient is placed flat and positive end expiratory pressure and ventilatory assistance are applied via a tight-fitting mask while an assistant applies monitoring equipment and sets up an intravenous infusion. Muscle relaxants must not be given. Endotracheal intubation is carried out orally with a smaller than usual size of tube of adequate length and rigid enough to manipulate through the oedematous supraglottis. The essentials are reliable and duplicate equipment, a range of endotracheal tube sizes already checked, and competent assistance. Otolaryngological surgical and nursing staff and functioning bronchoscopes must be available as, although it is usually feasible to insert an endotracheal tube, it is sometimes extremely difficult.

Oedema begins to resolve rapidly and within 10 minutes is frequently lessening or has been displaced so that the change from an oral to a long-term nasotracheal tube is always easier. The nasotracheal tube should be small enough to insert easily and for the tip to lie at mid-trachea. Fixation must be satisfactory and over many years the method described by Reid and Tunstall (1966) has proved reliable. Sedation will be required initially and the most satisfactory drugs to use are diazepam, morphine or nasogastric chloral hydrate. The dose ranges are shown in *Table 35.10*.

All patients with long-term nasotracheal tubes who breathe spontaneously are attached to a continuous flow, humidified, oxygen enriched circuit where a continuous positive end expiratory pressure of a few centimetres of water can be maintained, otherwise significant pulmonary atelectasis will occur. Because of the rapid response to antibiotics and airway relief, oedema resolves rapidly and extubation is frequently possible within 24 hours, so that there is no place for tracheostomy in the management of this condition.

Acute laryngotracheobronchitis

Acute laryngotracheobronchitis or croup is a viral infection of the entire airway, but its initial clinical presentation is stridor, with slowly increasing upper airway obstruction. The condition has a prolonged course and only a small proportion of patients come to need airway relief. Large airway secretions may be extremely difficult to remove by coughing because of their viscosity, dyspnoea and subglottic oedema. The increased viscosity reflects dehydration which occurs because of the rapid respiratory rate and unwillingness to drink. Early and adequate intravenous fluid replacement is an integral part of the treatment of this condition. If lower airway infection and secretions are significant then hypoxaemia may occur.

Indications for airway relief are clinical and are based on continuous close observation of the patient, assessing the respiratory work used to achieve alveolar ventilation and the degree of chest cage instability. A rising respiratory rate, increasing chest retraction, inability to cough, agitation, restlessness and fatigue, are indicators that relief is required. Serial blood gases are usually of little help, although a falling arterial Po_2 due to peripheral lung secretions may indicate the need for earlier relief.

Oral tracheal intubation under general anaesthesia relieves the obstruction caused by subglottic oedema and allows aspiration of retained airway secretions. A small dose of intravenous diazepam 0.1–0.2 mg/kg may be given at the commencement of anaesthesia if the infant is very agitated. Oxygen/halothane is a suitable induction agent and assisted ventilation quickly allows a level of anaesthesia where laryngoscopy is well tolerated. Visualization of the larynx is easy as supraglottic oedema is insignificant, but the subglottis may cause considerable resistance to the passage of even a very small bore tube. It is essential that a variety of tube sizes of adequate length is available and that they can be made stiffer by the use of a semirigid tube introducer.

The use of a short-acting muscle relaxant is contraindicated. The principle of not giving short-acting muscle relaxants to patients with airway obstruction, until it is known with absolute certainty that the airway can be secured, must be followed at all times. There is no exception. After initial clearance of airway secretions the oral tube

Table 35.10 Sedating agents in intensive care units

Chloral hydrate	20–30 mg/kg	Oral nasogastric tube
Morphine		
infusion	0.5 mg/kg in 50 ml at 2 ml/hour	5% dextrose
bolus	0.1–0.2 mg/kg	intravenously
Diazepam	0.1–0.2 mg/kg	intravenously

is changed to a nasotracheal tube of correct size and length which is fixed in position. The nasotracheal tube must be several sizes smaller than would be used for routine anaesthesia and preferably should allow a small air leak.

Resolution of laryngotracheobronchitis is slow so that intubation is likely to be necessary for several days. Sedation, physiotherapy and good hydration are essential. There is still some controversy about the type of airway management of those few patients who need relief and both nasotracheal intubation and tracheostomy have their advocates. There are, however, large series of patients who have been managed successfully by nasotracheal intubation. Tracheostomy is not without problems such as tube blockage, displacement to the anterior mediastinum and inability to decannulate due to tracheal wall damage at the tracheostome site. There seems no adequate reason for not using nasotracheal intubation for this self-limiting condition, but the management of the intubated patient must be of a high standard.

Microlaryngeal surgery

The suspension laryngoscope allows a number of surgical procedures to be carried out on the larynx and, in many instances, there has been no need for a preliminary tracheostomy. Anaesthesia must take place with the patient's airway shared and the anaesthetic airway not obtrusive in the glottis. This is difficult in the small child where the glottic diameter may only be 5–8 mm. A number of techniques have proved satisfactory although none are devoid of problems.

Endotracheal anaesthesia and insufflation

Spontaneous breathing with deep inhalational anaesthesia, using halothane and sometimes additional methoxyflurane, is combined with topical anaesthesia of the larynx. A small-sized tracheal tube is positioned either anteriorly or posteriorly in the glottis while the major part of the surgical procedure is carried out, and is then withdrawn to the pharynx for the final part of the operation. The disadvantages are some obstruction to the surgical field initially and no control of ventilation latterly, but in practice, the technique is very satisfactory for relatively short procedures on the glottis. No special equipment is required.

Jet ventilation

This is a derivative of the Sanders bronchoscopic jet ventilation, but as there is no tapered tube there is no Venturi effect and so little gas entrainment. The jet is pressurized at 30–60 psi (207–413 kPa) and a near normal ventilatory rate is used. The injector jet system has been shown to maintain satisfactory blood gases (Spoerel and Greenway, 1973) and can be used for a relatively long period of time. Deep anaesthesia is necessary initially with topical anaesthesia to the larynx and complete muscle paralysis throughout the procedure. Anaesthesia may need to be maintained by intravenous supplementation with methohexitone or propofol. The jet can be sited on the laryngoscope blade but this is unsatisfactory in the lower age groups. It is difficult to maintain alignment with the trachea as glottic distortion occurs, surgery may interfere with ventilation or blood and debris may be blown into the trachea.

The jet may also be sited in the mid-trachea as described by Benjamin and Gronow (1979). The 'Ben-jet' has four small soft side flanges near the tip so that the jet is maintained in the mid-tracheal diameter thus avoiding damage to the tracheal mucosa and recoil as the jet is pressurized. The paediatric tube is 16 G and measured at 5 cm and has been found satisfactory in infants over 3 years of age. This size of jet requires a driving pressure well below standard compressed gas pipeline pressure and this has been achieved by use of the Komesaroff bronchoflator (Komesaroff and McKie 1972) which allows adjustment of the driving pressure. It is essential that the peak jet pressure is not too high and that the expiratory phase, which takes place through the glottis, is not obstructed at any time.

Muscle relaxation must be fully maintained during the procedure without the danger of sudden unexpected glottic closure, and the operative procedure must not occlude the glottis at any time. Failure to observe these provisos has resulted in serious barotrauma to the lungs with bilateral pneumothoraces. This technique should only be used by an experienced team because of the potential for serious complications.

High frequency positive pressure ventilation

The use of high frequency positive pressure ventilation has been reviewed by Sjöstrand (1980). The technique has been used for laryngoscopy and bronchoscopy (Eriksson and Sjöstrand 1977) and has been administered by a transglottic insufflation catheter (Borg, Eriksson and Sjöstrand, 1980) and via a percutaneous transtracheal catheter

(Klain and Smith, 1977), thus avoiding any glottic tube. The use of a percutaneous transtracheal catheter is not without risk and it does not seem an acceptable method of catheter placement in infants requiring repeated endoscopy.

The advantages of high frequency positive pressure ventilation are the reduced risk of barotrauma as the peak inspiratory pressure is usually below that required for conventional positive pressure ventilation. There is improved intrapulmonary gas distribution and, as there is no entrainment, the delivered gas mixture can be precisely controlled. However as expiration is continuous and takes place around the catheter or endoscope an open glottis is essential and full muscle paralysis must be maintained at all times. Borg, Eriksson and Sjöstrand (1980) recommend a frequency of 60 breaths per minute with a fixed inspiratory time of 22%. Much higher frequencies have been used, although there seems little advantage in their use during laryngeal surgery. Carbon dioxide elimination may become inadequate at frequencies over 100–150 breaths per minute, although experimental evidence using percutaneous transtracheal jet ventilation suggests that it may be possible to use much higher frequencies safely (Smith, Klain and Babinski, 1980). This technique requires the use of a specially designed high frequency jet ventilator. As chest movement, the traditional method of assessment of ventilation is not present, careful and close monitoring of the patient is mandatory and should involve the use of pulse oximetry (Yelderman and New, 1983).

Specific conditions
Choanal atresia

Bilateral choanal atresia may be membranous or bony, but in either case, nasal breathing is completely obstructed. The neonate alternates between normal crying and rest which results in cyanosis and apnoea as breathing becomes obstructed. Temporary relief is obtained by insertion of a small plastic airway which can be strapped in position until surgical relief is obtained. During this period orogastric tube feeding is necessary as the baby cannot feed and breathe.

Anaesthesia consists of awake intubation in the neonate with a tube that is kink proof under a tongue blade as the approach is similar to that for a tonsillectomy. Maintenance with nitrous oxide and oxygen and a muscle relaxant such as atracurium or vecuronium with intermittent positive pressure ventilation by hand using a T-piece and bag is satisfactory. Monitoring and temperature maintenance are necessary. The approach is usually to drill from the nose through the posterior choanae using a shielded dental drill, until an adequate-sized dilator can be passed into the pharynx. More rarely a transpalatal approach is used and this may involve blood loss of a magnitude that requires replacement. Splints made from a plastic nasal endotracheal tube are inserted into each nostril and fixed in position with a heavy nylon tie around the nasal septum. These provide a patent nasal airway so that termination of anaesthesia is trouble-free, and they are left in position for about 6 weeks. Dilatation of the posterior choanae may be required after the splints have been removed.

Supraglottic cysts

These are rare and are usually single but may be multiple in association with cystic hygroma. Single cysts are always anterior and may present with episodes of airway obstruction in between periods of apparent normality, but they can nearly always be seen on a good quality lateral X-ray of the neck. The surgical treatment is to deroof the cyst and marsupialize the base which is frequently wide and usually in the vallecula. This is undertaken using the suspension laryngoscope and endotracheal anaesthesia. Inhalational anaesthesia with oxygen 100% and halothane should be used and orotracheal intubation performed as soon as possible. This may be difficult with large cysts but the glottic opening is always found posteriorly. In extreme difficulty the cyst may be partially aspirated with a needle attached to a suction unit. Once the larynx is intubated the area should be sprayed with topical lignocaine and, if practical, the tube changed to a nasotracheal tube as this sits in a better position when using the suspension laryngoscope. Anaesthesia may be continued with nitrous oxide, oxygen and halothane, but preferably with the use of a muscle relaxant and intermittent positive pressure ventilation as rapid complete awakening is required. Awake extubation is usually trouble-free and as tissue damage is minimal, postoperative oedema is unlikely.

Multiple cysts associated with cystic hygroma are unpredictable and range from small pedunculated cysts on the epiglottis and aryepiglottic folds to cystic tissue in the pyriform fossa, pharyngeal wall and tongue. Anaesthesia is managed as for a solitary cyst, but the surgical interference should be minimal and only to relieve obstructive symptoms. The more severe forms of cystic hygroma cannot be excised totally and some postoperative obstruction may persist so that rapid and complete awakening is required. Occasionally adequate relief is impossible and tracheostomy is required but this will usually be associated with a major resection of cystic hygroma from the neck.

Laryngeal cleft

Patients with posterior laryngeal cleft are unable to achieve competent glottic closure during swallowing and so have frequent episodes of aspiration. The more extreme forms extending to the upper trachea and oesophagus develop severe aspiration pneumonias from very early in life. They are initially managed with a low tracheostomy and gastrostomy feeding and later have a direct repair via an anterior laryngofissure approach or a lateral pharyngotomy. The minor forms are usually not diagnosed until later because the recurrent bouts of chestiness are not initially attributed to aspiration. Direct laryngoscopy can easily overlook the defect as the superficial appearance of the glottis may be normal but a probe will readily reveal the deficiency of interarytenoid tissue. The minor forms that are associated with aspiration are closed by direct suture using the suspension laryngoscope.

Laryngeal papillomatosis

Laryngeal papillomatosis is caused by a viral infection, probably with a DNA virus of the papova group. Management depends on the extent of the infection and the degree of airway obstruction, and is based on the destruction of individual papillomata by burning. In the upper airway this is most easily and atraumatically accomplished by the use of the carbon dioxide laser and in the lower airway by bronchoscopic diathermy. A few of the more severe and intractable clinical states require a long-term tracheostomy for safe and adequate management.

The carbon dioxide laser is used with an operating microscope and the invisible CO_2 laser beam is marked by a visible helium neon laser. The beam can be directed very accurately and the depth of tissue destruction controlled by a combination of power and exposure time. There is minimal damage to the surrounding areas so that there is little pain and oedema with good healing and minimal scarring (McGill, Freidmann and Healy, 1983). The use of the laser poses some anaesthetic problems, the principal difficulty being the ignition of rubber and plastic endotracheal tubes, combustion being supported by the anaesthetic gas mixture. The laser beam passes through gas mixtures which will only ignite, explode or decompose if a non-metallic solid object first absorbs the beam and produces heat. The beam is deflected and the energy scattered by metallic objects. The essential protective requirements are that all endotracheal and tracheostomy tubes and injectors should be metal or metal foil wrapped. Reflecting impregnated plastic wrap is

unsatisfactory. All theatre personnel must wear protective glasses to avoid accidental corneal burns. The patient's eyes, mouth and exposed areas which could be accidentally burned must be protected by moist gauze swabs.

Anaesthesia can be maintained with one of several techniques but all require good topical anaesthesia of the glottis. The author's preference at present is spontaneous breathing with nitrous oxide, oxygen and halothane via a foil wrapped endotracheal tube which is withdrawn to the pharynx for the final part of the laser procedure. This is a safe and simple technique which works well in the smaller patients. Alternatively, a muscle relaxant technique with ventilation using either an intratracheal jet or a supraglottic laryngoscopic jet has been recommended (Simpson and Strong, 1983; Norton, 1983), although the latter becomes increasingly unsatisfactory with smaller patients. Lower tracheal diathermy is easily managed using a muscle relaxant technique and a ventilating bronchoscope.

Laryngotracheoplasty

Laryngotracheoplasty is the operative correction of a subglottic or upper tracheal stenosis and the same approach may be used for direct closure of a posterior laryngotracheal cleft or surgical excision of a subglottic haemangioma. The patient will already have a low tracheostomy which should not have been allowed to stenose and the chest must be as clear of secretions as can be achieved immediately prior to operation. The surgical approach is through a small collar incision immediately above the tracheostome. The cricoid ring is enlarged by a stepped incision (Evans and Todd, 1974) or, if too abnormal or if the upper tracheal ring is stenosed, a costal cartilage graft is inserted. The trachea and cricoid may be closed over a rolled silastic splint which is left in place for 6 weeks.

Anaesthesia consists of any technique using muscle paralysis and intermittent positive pressure ventilation. The glottis is sprayed with lignocaine and the chest cleared of any viscid secretions by the use of normal saline and suction. The most stable airway conditions are achieved by the use of a cuffed armoured tube inserted into the trachea via the tracheostome and taken through 180° to connect with the anaesthetic circuit over the thorax. It is essential that the cuff is entirely in the trachea, otherwise it is likely to extrude during the operation, and the tube tip must be clear of the carina so that both lungs are ventilated. If the baby is too small to allow the use of a flexible cuffed tube a shortened preformed plastic tube provides a stable airway, but allows an air leak into the operation site and may allow tracheal aspiration of blood. The shoulders are placed over a sandbag and the neck extended. Extensive monitoring is required and must include a precordial stethoscope, an airway pressure gauge and disconnection alarm. Close continuous monitoring of the ventilatory state is essential. Electrocardigraph, blood pressure and pulse oximetry monitoring should be routine.

Intravenous fluids must be continued postoperatively as the silastic splint, if too long, may sometimes result in aspiration. Chest physiotherapy is important as there is nearly always a short-term deterioration in the chest status with an increase in secretions. If a rib graft has been taken, a postoperative chest X-ray to exclude a pneumothorax must be carried out.

Tracheostomy

The principal indication for tracheostomy in the infant is for the long-term bypass of congenital or acquired upper airway obstructive lesions while growth and corrective surgery takes place. Most airway maintenance for respiratory support is managed by long-term nasotracheal intubation, but this may be changed to a tracheostomy in some patients with intractable cardiorespiratory or neurological disease where the duration of intermittent positive pressure ventilation is many months. Tracheostomy should be performed under endotracheal general anaesthesia on a still, non-congested and oxygenated patient. Oxygen/halothane is a suitable induction agent but a short-acting muscle relaxant such as suxamethonium should be avoided in difficult obstructive lesions, or if there is recent demyelination from neurological disease. If the subglottis is narrow, intubation in smaller patients may be possible using the rather stiff 8 FG Cole pattern neonatal resuscitation tube (internal diameter 1.5 mm, external diameter 2.5 mm). Maintenance can be managed by any method, but muscle paralysis and intermittent positive pressure ventilation ensures oxygenation and prevents venous congestion due to coughing. An intravenous cannula and full monitoring are essential.

The neck is fully extended over a sandbag in the small infant, but only moderately extended in the child as there is the risk of making the tracheostomy in the thoracic trachea. The tracheal incision should be vertical through the third and fourth rings without excision of cartilage. The tracheal incision can be opened by the use of plastic surgical skin hooks, so that insertion of the tracheostomy tube under direct vision is easy once the endotracheal tube is withdrawn to just above the opening. The tracheostomy tube is tied firmly in place before the endotracheal tube is finally removed. Nylon stay sutures on the tracheal wall either side of the incision help to open the trachea in the event of early accidental decannulation, although the risk of making a false passage into the anterior mediastinum is still considerable. Conventional tracheostomy dilators are no help in this emergency situation. The operation must be followed by a chest X-ray to check the position of the tube, but more importantly to exclude a pneumothorax. The tracheostomy is initially most easily managed using a plastic tube, but after one week the tube may be changed to another type if more appropriate.

Foreign body

Inhaled foreign body is commonest in the 1–3-year-old age group and, although a wide range of small objects has been incriminated, the most universal is a peanut fragment. There is frequently a history suggestive of inhalation and X-ray signs of obstructive emphysema. Bronchoscopic removal under general anaesthesia is performed in nearly all instances and involves identifying the nature and location of the foreign body, its removal with the appropriate type of forceps, and a check bronchoscopy to ensure that removal is complete. Adequate preoperative starvation and an intramuscular atropine premedication are essential prerequisites, induction of anaesthesia being by inhalational oxygen/halothane or a small dose of intravenous thiopentone. A short-acting muscle relaxant such as suxamethonium allows the application of good topical anaesthesia to the trachea and glottis prior to orotracheal intubation. Anaesthesia is deepend with oxygen/halothane up to 4% during spontaneous breathing, while an intravenous infusion and full monitoring are applied. The addition of 0.5% methoxyflurane helps to prevent rapid emergence from anaesthesia.

In theatre, the endotracheal tube is exchanged for a bronchoscope and the foreign body is located. It is preferable at this stage to allow spontaneous breathing to continue with 100% oxygen and the appropriate amount of halothane to maintain a deep level of anaesthesia, but if necessary, ventilatory assistance can be carried out by ventilation through the Storz-Hopkins bronchoscope or use of the Venturi injector on the Negus bronchoscope. It is not unusual for several attempts to be necessary to grasp the foreign body and remove it up the trachea and it is usually essential to remove the bronchoscope and foreign body together through the glottis. The bronchoscope must be reinserted to check that removal is complete. The combination of a stable base of deep inhalational anaesthesia and the ability to carry out intermittent positive pressure ventilation via the bronchoscope provides the anaesthetist with good control and allows the surgeon considerable flexibility in approach.

The exercise may be prolonged due to inexperience of the operator or difficulty in manipulating the available forceps to grasp the object. If the foreign body has not been removed within 45 minutes the procedure should be abandoned and rescheduled with a more experienced operator or different equipment.

Peanut fragments that have been inhaled for more than 24 hours cause a severe localized bronchitis due to release of irritant products. Some foods fragment and need to be removed by suction. In either case, bronchoscopy must be followed by efficient physiotherapy and a short course of a prophylactic antibiotic. As several insertions of the bronchoscope may be necessary a possible sequel is the development of subglottic oedema and a single prophylactic dose of dexamethasone should be given and repeated if stridor becomes apparent. The intravenous infusion line should be kept for 10 hours to maintain hydration until a complete and uneventful recovery has occurred.

Vascular ring

Malformations of the aortic arch may cause compression of the trachea and oesophagus, although the malformation may not always be a complete ring. The most common type of defect is some form of double aortic arch. The degree of compression is determined partly by the type of vascular malformation present and by its severity. Symptoms are stridor, feeding difficulty and aspiration, and these are present at birth in 50% of patients, but nearly all have presented by 6 months of age (Roesler *et al.*, 1983). Diagnosis is by history, chest X-ray and contrast oesophagogram, which should be performed in all patients. Great care is needed in the severely obstructed neonate in the first days of life where there is the danger of serious aspiration. Bronchoscopy is unlikely to alter the surgical management and, as it may increase oedema at the obstruction site, it is best avoided just before surgery.

The operation involves division and sometimes reimplantation of the aberrant vessel or abnormal arch, and complete dissection of the oesophagus and trachea from surrounding fibrous tissue is necessary to achieve satisfactory relief. The more severe forms are associated with a localized tracheal malformation or tracheomalacia at the site of the compression and this results in some residual stridor which occurs in under 10% of patients. If significant stridor persists, bronchoscopy is essential to determine the extent of any tracheomalacia. Anaesthesia is managed with topical anaesthesia, oxygen/halothane and spontaneous breathing, so that segmental tracheal collapse can be readily identified, but as chest aspiration may have been severe, coughing and breath holding may require intermittent positive pressure ventilation to maintain satisfactory oxygenation. Occasionally undiagnosed vascular ring may present to the otolaryngology department for assessment of stridor in infancy.

Otitis media and adenotonsillectomy

The last decade has seen several changes in the surgical management of otitis media and pharyngeal lymphoid tissue hypertrophy. The increased incidence of otitis media with effusion has led to surgical middle ear drainage by myringotomy, ventilation tube insertion and adenoidectomy at the earlier age of 2–3 years. The effective treatment with antibiotics of acute bacterial tonsillitis has resulted in a more conservative approach to tonsillectomy and a reduction in the number of older children requiring tonsillectomy for recurrent tonsillitis.

The 2–3-year-old child is at one of the most difficult ages in terms of the psychological impact of hospitalization and operation. Children at this age are often truculently independent and persistently test the environment in their exploration of developing independence – at the same time they are totally dependent on their own family for support and security. The most satisfactory means of coping with this situation is a good rapport between medical and nursing staff and the parents, with as much ward involvement for the parents as is possible.

This requires effort, understanding, tact and patience in informing the more aggressive and insecure parents and encouraging the timid or apparently disinterested parent. Education should commence at the first outpatient consultation with information about hospitalization and operations in children. A number of books are available to help parents discuss this with their children and many hospitals produce their own advisory pamphlets. These should be available at the first outpatient visit, and an opportunity made for parents to ask questions relating to the operation and hospitalization at a later visit. From the child's point of view the essentials are kindness, honesty and an attitude of calmness and security from all the strangers in whose care he is placed.

Hospital admission should be for the shortest time practical, with unrestricted visiting if a parent is unable to be resident in hospital with the child. A parent should be with the child soon after consciousness has returned after the operation, and there are certainly no medical grounds for restricting parental access post-tonsillectomy. In contrast, the family needs to keep a sense of proportion and to realize that tonsillectomy is a major operation, the patient will not feel well afterwards and is not helped by a large family gathering at the bedside on operation day. With a sympathetic and informative attitude on the part of all hospital staff there are few problems.

The anaesthetic management for adenotonsillectomy is frequently difficult and requires an experienced anaesthetist if disasters are to be avoided. The requirements are:

(1) a reasonable but safe level of sedation and analgesia
(2) quiet non-depressed breathing with complete absence of airway obstruction during the surgery, so that bleeding due to a raised venous pressure is avoided
(3) the prevention of aspiration of blood both during surgery and afterwards by rapid awakening and the return of an active cough reflex
(4) an adequate fluid intake must be maintained during the day without stimulating vomiting.

Myringotomy and ventilation tube insertion

These procedures are well suited to day admission. Premedication should be given if the child would benefit or the anaesthetic technique requires it, but as there is little postoperative discomfort it may well be better avoided, particularly if the child faces a significant journey home. A mild non-emetic analgesic such as codeine phosphate or DF 118 may be given intramuscularly during the anaesthetic. Induction by inhalational nitrous oxide, oxygen, halothane or intravenous thiopentone, is entirely satisfactory with maintenance by nitrous oxide, oxygen and halothane administered using a T-piece circuit, face mask and oropharyngeal airway. Endotracheal intubation using a loose-fitting tube may be preferable in patients where the airway is difficult to maintain and repeated minor movement of the head makes the use of a microscope difficult. A similar situation occurs in patients with a very narrow external auditory meatus so that positioning under the microscope is critical for both vision and ventilation tube insertion. This is usually not the best position for airway maintenance.

Adenotonsillectomy

Adenoids are removed because they cause obstruction to the eustachian tubes and the nasopharyngeal airway. Tonsils are removed because of recurrent bouts of acute tonsillitis, peritonsillar abscess, or more rarely, oropharyngeal airway obstruction. Serious degrees of upper airway obstruction are not uncommon. This may be aggravated by the presence of congenital maxillofacial and mandibular malformations such as occur in Treacher Collins and Pierre Robin syndromes. Disproportion may be present in other congenital disorders such as Down's syndrome and the mucopolysaccharidoses. In some of these patients the upper airway obstruction may be associated with considerable anaesthetic difficulties in airway maintenance and endotracheal intubation. Postoperative improvement may be minimal.

Chronic upper airway obstruction may cause the development of the sleep apnoea syndrome with disordered central control of respiration and incoordination of the oropharyngeal musculature which may take some time to correct after removal of the obstruction (Guilleminault, Tilkian and Dement, 1976; Brouillette, Fernbach and Hunt, 1982; Bradley and Phillipson, 1985; Thach, 1985).

Episodes of hypoxaemia may continue in the immediate postoperative period. Hypoxaemia and hypercapnia may cause pulmonary vasoconstriction with right heart hypertrophy and more rarely right heart failure (Macartney, Panday and Scott, 1969). Klein and Reynolds (1986) reported the use of continuous insufflation of the pharynx as a means of helping to improve the preoperative status of children suffering from the sleep apnoea syndrome. Catley *et al.* (1985) have shown that, in adults, postoperative disturbances of respiration and sleep are associated with the use of opiate analgesia and result in episodes of hypoxaemia. Oxygen therapy corrects the hypoxaemia, but not the respiratory disturbances (Jones *et al.*, 1985). There is every reason to believe that a similar state of affairs is present post-adenotonsillectomy in children who have exhibited obstructive sleep apnoea. It may be that failure to appreciate this has been the cause of some of the perioperative tragedies associated with adenotonsillectomy.

Preoperative assessment of the patient must include a history relating to airway obstruction and disturbed sleep patterns, bleeding tendencies in the patient or near relative, and recent ingestion of acetylsalicylic acid (aspirin) as this may cause a prolongation of the bleeding time due to platelet dysfunction. A minor degree of increased bleeding time which has little effect on an operation may be disastrous in an adenotonsillectomy and the operation should be postponed until the haematological status is fully assessed. Many patients requiring adenoidectomy have a chronic purulent nasal discharge and this is not an indication to postpone operation. A story of pyrexia, vomiting, loss of appetite, and listlessness in the preceding 48 hours is an indication to postpone the operation as the likely cause will be a virus infection, which may be insignificant, but could be the prodroma of one of the childhood infectious diseases. Personal experience indicates that relatively few patients require postponement.

Premedication

In no other operation is it so important to adjust the type and dose of premedication to suit both the preoperative status of the patient and the intended anaesthetic technique. Premedication forms an integral part of the overall anaesthetic management. Patients who have severe upper airway obstruction from adenoidal hypertrophy and a history of a disturbed sleep pattern should receive intramuscular atropine only. The same applies to patients with less severe obstruction but coexisting maxillofacial deformities as these will not be relieved by surgery.

Children under the age 6–7 years are better premedicated with trimeprazine and atropine, which provide reasonable sedation, are given orally and have a significant antiemetic effect. A mild analgesic such as codeine phosphate is given intramuscularly just prior to extubation as trimeprazine is devoid of any analgesic action. Children over 6–7 years of age, where the indications for surgery are more likely to be recurrent tonsillitis rather than adenoidal obstruction, benefit from more analgesia, and papaveretum and hyoscine in reduced dose is satisfactory. Disadvantages are the less adequate cardiac vagal block from the hyoscine, so that adenoidal currettage may cause bradycardia unless additional intravenous atropine is given at induction, and there is an increased incidence of vomiting, so that an antiemetic is necessary.

Induction

Patients premedicated with trimeprazine are given an inhalational induction with halothane or cyclopropane, the newer inhalational agents, enflurane and isoflurane, being less satisfactory for induction. Endotracheal intubation is carried out using suxamethonium. Patients premedicated with an opiate are given intravenous thiopentone and a muscle relaxant to facilitate endotracheal intubation.

Maintenance

Anaesthesia for adenotonsillectomy was traditionally carried out using ether insufflation and a Boyle Davis gag; the newer inhalational agents are unsatisfactory and have an inadequate safety margin for this technique. The introduction of the Doughty (1957) split tongue blade and compression proof endotracheal tube connectors has allowed orotracheal intubation to provide safe access for both surgeon and anaesthetist. Modern preformed plastic tubes may compress under the tongue blade if the gag requires excessive opening or traction in a patient with difficult oral access. Maintenance with nitrous oxide, oxygen and halothane with spontaneous breathing is satisfactory in those premedicated with trimeprazine, but it is a difficult technique if opiates are used, as irregular breathing and hypoventilation occur. Deep anaesthesia with palatal relaxation is difficult to achieve and is then followed by delayed awakening. This can be avoided by the use of a medium-duration muscle relaxant, such as atracurium or vecuronium, and positive pressure ventilation. Both spontaneous breathing and controlled ventilation have their advocates, both are satisfactory provided that the other aspects of the anaesthetic are adjusted appropriately.

Awakening

Termination of the anaesthetic is the most critical time and one is faced with a choice of awake extubation usually preceded by coughing, straining and increased bleeding, or deep extubation with the possibility of aspiration, laryngospasm and hypoxia during emergence. In practice, children given only trimeprazine and halothane can be extubated deeply, regain consciousness very quickly and almost never exhibit laryngospasm. Patients given opiates, thiopentone and halothane have a high incidence of serious laryngospasm if extubated deeply and may take a considerable time to wake up. They should always be extubated awake and this is more easily achieved with the use of muscle relaxants and minimal or no halothane. If there has been pre-existing serious airway obstruction or anatomical difficulty in intubation, extubation must only take place when fully awake.

Bleeding must be controlled, and the mouth, pharynx and postnasal space cleared of blood clot prior to extubation. This should be in the 'tonsil position' on the side and head down, so that any residual blood can drain out through the mouth and nose. Close competent supervision of the patient must be maintained in the theatre until emergence from anaesthesia is complete, with no bleeding, a good cough reflex and a purposeful response to spoken commands. Restlessness during emergence from anaesthesia is not uncommon after tonsillectomy and is caused by pain which should be treated. Codeine phosphate intramuscularly is satisfactory, followed by paracetamol when swallowing is manageable. However, continuing restlessness later in the day is much more likely to be the result of a combination of bleeding, airway obstruction or aspiration and should not be treated with analgesics. A careful clinical examination of the operation site and the patient's cardiorespiratory status is required. Blood volume should be restored if indicated and consideration given to reoperation for bleeding.

Monitoring

Basic in-theatre monitoring requires an ECG, blood pressure measurement, and a precordial stethoscope. As surgery often takes place in conditions of reduced lighting and there is the ever present danger of endotracheal tube obstruction, a pulse oximeter (Yelderman and New, 1983) should become a high priority monitor.

The in-theatre blood loss associated with adenotonsillectomy has been variously reported as ranging from 5 to 10% of the circulating blood volume (75–80 ml/kg) with an occasional patient losing up to 20%. This means that although few patients require blood, many come close to a volume loss which needs replacement. Continuing postoperative loss can be extremely difficult to estimate as much of the blood is swallowed. An intravenous cannula is an integral part of this operation and should remain *in situ* until recovery is clearly satisfactory. Crystalloid fluid should always be given to patients under 13 kg body weight. Older children manage very well without intravenous fluids, but the fluid balance status should be noted until there is no doubt about the adequacy of oral intake. Fluid should be given if minor bleeding continues, there is vomiting, excessive insensible loss in hot weather, or there are additional medical problems where fluid and calorie restriction is contraindicated.

The bleeding tonsil

The bleeding tonsil or adenoid bed presents one of the more high risk situations in anaesthesia. Most patients who require reoperation have never really stopped bleeding and a little more patience at the original operation would have averted the situation. The common error is to underestimate the blood loss which is difficult to assess as much of it is swallowed. The danger signs are restlessness, pallor, tachycardia, poor peripheral circulation

and swallowing. Vomiting blood clot usually means that a significant loss has occurred. Bleeding that has continued for 2 hours does not usually stop until clot has been cleared from the bleeding site and a decision to reoperate should be made before the patient's condition deteriorates. Blood should be cross-matched early and blood volume restored before reoperation.

The most important factors in theatre are usually technical as most mortality and morbidity occur through loss of control of the airway with aspiration, obstruction and hypoxaemia. Induction of anaesthesia should take place with the patient on the side with the head down, so that clot vomited in early induction is not aspirated. Because of residual sedation and anaesthesia, loss of consciousness is readily achieved with halothane and oxygen. Intubation, which may require a smaller size tube than that used during the initial procedure, can be carried out using suxamethonium and cricoid pressure, after first visualizing the pharynx so that any obstructive clot can be cleared. Rapid sequence thiopentone and suxamethonium has been advocated, but thiopentone is contraindicated if hypovolaemia exists and there is little time to remove obstructive clot from the pharynx before hypoxaemia occurs. Ventilation via a face mask may precipitate massive regurgitation of clot from the stomach.

Important factors are the use of a technique which is familiar, to have adequate competent assistance and correctly functioning equipment with duplicate endotracheal tube, laryngoscope and high level wide bore suction. Once the airway is secured and the lungs ventilated with oxygen the endotracheal tube should be aspirated to remove any blood and a wide bore stomach tube used to clear the stomach. However, it is virtually impossible to empty the stomach of clot completely and vomiting always occurs during emergence, so that extubation must be delayed until consciousness has returned. Postoperatively little analgesia is required and is contraindicated in the presence of a postnasal pack. Maintenance intravenous fluid should always be given until the following day. Continuing oozing demands that a full coagulation screen and bleeding studies are performed without delay if this has not been undertaken already, and fresh frozen plasma or platelets given as indicated.

The ear

Major ear surgery in the very young is confined to exploration of congenital middle ear atresia with reconstruction of an external auditory meatus so that a hearing aid may be used. Older children may require a myringoplasty if infection has badly damaged the tympanic membrane, sometimes exploration of the ossicles, and more rarely exploration of the mastoid air cells to remove chronic infection and cholesteatoma and allow adequate drainage.

The anaesthetic requirements are a stationary bloodless field so that an operating microscope can be used, preservation of the facial nerve if necessary by monitoring its function, prevention of tympanic membrane graft displacement by nitrous oxide-induced pressure changes in the middle ear, and prevention of postoperative vomiting.

Congenital defects of the ear

Defects in development of the first and second branchial arches give rise to a condition known as hemifacial microsomia. Asymmetric hypoplasia of the malar, maxilla and mandible occurs and there is deformity or absence of the pinna, external auditory meatus and middle ear. A further progression of this deformity known as Goldenhar's syndrome involves the cervical spine and the heart, the usual defects being a ventriculoseptal defect or tetralogy of Fallot. Treacher Collins syndrome is an autosomal dominant mandibulofacial dysostosis which includes mandibular hypoplasia, often severe, and malformation of the pinna and external auditory meatus. Conductive deafness occurs in 40% of patients.

Exploration of the middle ear, followed by the formation of an epithelial lined external auditory meatus allows a hearing aid to be used to maximize residual hearing. Some cosmetic reconstruction of the pinna is usually necessary and the surgery is likely to be staged. Although the anaesthetic requirements are simple, considerable difficulty may be experienced in airway maintenance on induction and awakening, and in endotracheal intubation. This is because the oropharyngeal airway is narrow as a result of micrognathia and relative macroglossia due to posterior displacement of the tongue. Maxillary and palatal abnormalities may narrow the nasopharyngeal airway. The larynx is high as a consequence of the mandibular hypoplasia and mouth opening may be restricted.

Anaesthetic management requires careful assessment of any upper airway obstruction and avoidance of longer-acting sedating agents if any obstruction is present. An inhalational induction technique with halothane is satisfactory and spontaneous breathing with a face mask is usually trouble free once an appropriate-sized oropharyngeal airway can be used. The use of continuous distending pressure will relieve minor degrees of airway obstruction. Intravenous access can be set up while anaesthesia is deepened to a level at which laryngoscopy can be performed and a visual assessment made of the pharynx and larynx.

Intubation requires a precise and careful technique with a range of tube sizes and laryngoscopes available. Visualization of the larynx is aided by a firm posterior push on the larynx provided this does not cause distortion, lateral displacement or glottis closure. The use of a semirigid gum elastic bougie is helpful in directing a tube into an anteriorly placed larynx. Elevation of the shoulders converts a difficult intubation into one which is impossible. The use of a short-acting muscle relaxant makes laryngoscopy neither easier nor more difficult – it does, however, place a finite time limit on the procedure before hypoxia ensues. Careful documentation of the technique used and degree of difficulty encountered must be kept as this may allow the use of a different technique on a subsequent occasion.

In practice, it is nearly always possible to intubate orotracheally these patients in the younger age group, although a small percentage may present difficulties. Rarely, older children with these syndromes may be impossible to intubate by conventional means, but they can usually be identified by careful preoperative assessment, so that a decision can be made to use a different technique such as a fibreoptic scope or a technique using awake intubation under local anaesthesia (Edens and Sia, 1981).

Assessment includes the measurement of mouth opening which should be greater than 2 cm, and the prominence of the upper dentition and its occlusal relationship to the lower teeth. Plain X-rays of the head and neck may show cervical vertebral abnormalities such as fusion or hemivertebrae. Nichol and Zuck (1983) have shown that if the distance between the posterior arch of the atlas vertebra and the occiput is narrow, extension of the head will cause anterior bowing of the cervical spine, which may lift the larynx out of view. Delegue *et al.* (1980) have stressed the importance of the maxillopharyngeal angle which is created by the intersection of a line along the upper teeth and one along the posterior pharyngeal wall. Angles below 90° are associated with inability to visualize the glottis by direct laryngoscopy, while angles greater than 100° are associated with easy visualization provided that the mouth opens.

Once intubation is accomplished in the more difficult patients, anaesthesia should be maintained with a muscle relaxant, intermittent positive pressure ventilation and minimal supplement, so that extubation can be carried out with the return of full consciousness at the end of the operation and thus avoid postoperative airway obstructive problems.

Myringoplasty and mastoidectomy

Graft procedures on the tympanic membrane or operations on the ossicular chain are always carried out using the microscope and the requirements are a stationary and bloodless field.

Bleeding may be arterial or venous in origin and the poorest fields are most likely to be associated with venous bleeding. This will occur if the pressure in the internal jugular vein or superior vena cava is raised (*Figures 35.2* and *35.3*), and the causes usually relate to poor anaesthetic technique such as partial airway obstruction in a spontaneously breathing patient, a high mean airway pressure in a ventilated patient, or abdominal compression. Careful positioning on the theatre

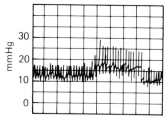

Figure 35.2 Venous pressure in the superior vena cava. Effect of operator's arm resting across the upper abdomen of a 15-month-old infant

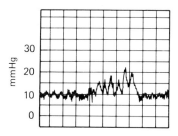

Figure 35.3 Venous pressure in the superior vena cava. Effect of moderate bag inflation of lungs in a 5-year-old child

table is essential to prevent venous obstruction from causes such as tight clothing, drapes or cables lying across the neck. There should be enough head-up tilt – 15°–20° – to lower the venous filling level in the external jugular vein well below the angle of the jaw.

Arterial bleeding has only a loose relationship with peak systolic pressure, although bleeding will increase with high arterial pressure and be less at pressures below 85 mmHg. Cardiac output increases with cardiac rate in children, until severe tachycardia occurs, and bleeding is always more

significant if the rate is elevated. The damaging effects of a stormy induction with crying, coughing and straining, last up to half an hour or more due to increased catecholamine secretion, with a higher cardiac rate and arterial pressure and venous congestion. Heavy sedating premedication may be indicated if the patient is unwilling and apprehensive.

Anaesthetic techniques which provide an impeccable airway, no increase in mean airway pressure, a modest reduction in P_aCO_2, some peripheral vascular dilatation and a normal or reduced cardiac rate, will always provide satisfactory operating conditions if the patient is positioned correctly on the operating table. For the majority of patients there is little difference between a technique employing spontaneous breathing with any of the currently used inhalational agents, or muscle paralysis with *d*-tubocurarine and modest hyperventilation. Hypoventilation and obesity are better managed using a mechanical ventilation technique, as are operations expected to take much longer than one hour.

Any well-managed anaesthetic will probably produce a peak arterial pressure of about 85 mmHg measured in the arm at the level of the heart. This represents a lower cerebral arterial pressure depending on the degree of head-up tilt. The mean arterial pressure in the brain should not be maintained below 50 mmHg.

Local vasoconstriction by the use of topically applied adrenaline 1:1000 is effective and there is no evidence of systemic absorption – this may be all that is required to produce good conditions.

Reduction of peak arterial pressure below 80 mmHg will usually require the use of a specific hypotensive agent, and the choice currently rests between three agents.

Trimetaphan camsylate (Arfonad)

This is the most widely used of the older group of drugs causing hypotension by autonomic ganglion blockade. Anderson (1955) showed that children are relatively resistant to its use, so that it must be given as a 0.2% solution in 5% glucose from a microdrop burette giving set. Dosage should be reduced if halothane is used. Its disadvantage is the development of a compensatory tachycardia which, in the fit older child, may be severe and cause poorer operating conditions even though the arterial pressure is lower. This can be prevented by the use of a small dose of a beta blocker such as practolol or propranolol. The histamine releasing effect of Arfonad may cause severe bronchospasm in susceptible patients and asthma is an absolute contraindication to its use. Newer agents are probably easier to manage.

Sodium nitroprusside (Nipride)

This is a powerful direct acting peripheral vascular dilator which produces a profound hypotension rapidly, but fairly transiently, as there is rapid conversion to cyanide and later thiocyanate which are inactive. Its administration requires precision as it is a very potent drug and it should be given by a slow infusion syringe pump in a solution of 1.5 mg/kg in 5% glucose in a 50 ml syringe, starting at a rate of 0.2–0.4 ml/hour which gives a dose of 0.1–0.2 μg/kg per minute. Satisfactory control of the blood pressure should be achieved with a dose of 1–3 μg/kg per minute, and if this is arrived at by a very slow increase in dose, tachycardia and tachyphylaxis may be avoided. Doses above 8 μg/kg per minute lead to excessive levels of cyanide in the blood which inhibit cellular oxidative metabolism and lead to a profound metabolic acidosis. Cyanide and thiocyanate interfere with the metabolism of vitamin B_{12} (cyanocobalamin) so that Nipride is contraindicated in vitamin B_{12} deficiency, poor liver function and Leber's optic atrophy. Blood pressure measurement must be carried out accurately and frequently – at least at minute intervals – using an automated machine such as a Dinamap or Arteriosonde. Dose increase must be so slow that serious overshoot with profound hypotension does not occur between blood pressure readings, and this is a difficult technique. If rapid production of a low arterial pressure is required then an indwelling arterial monitor line is mandatory. Ear surgery does not warrant the use of Nipride in this way.

Labetalol (Trandate)

This is the most satisfactory agent from the practical point of view. It induces hypotension by blocking α-adrenoreceptors in the peripheral arterioles and there is some concurrent β-blockade so that compensatory tachycardia is avoided. Modest reductions in both pulse rate and systemic pressure occur readily and there is a synergistic action with halothane. Administration is by incremental intravenous boluses commencing with a dose about 0.2 mg/kg and repeated at 5-minute intervals until the desired effect is achieved. This will always be at a dose below the maximum of 1 mg/kg. As the mean duration of effect is about one hour there is no sudden rebound hypertension which may occur with both trimetaphan and nitroprusside, however, postoperative postural hypotension may occur for some hours. Labetalol should be avoided in asthmatics as bronchospasm may be induced and excessive bradycardia is responsive to atropine in increased dosage.

Nitroglycerine is a direct acting peripheral vascular dilator which probably affects the venous system more than the arterial system. Its use in adults suggests that it is a safe, easy to use agent causing modest and controllable hypotension with few side-effects. Its use as an in-theatre hypotensive agent in children has not yet been clearly defined.

The indications for specific hypotensive drugs in ear surgery are minimal and their use must be carefully equated with the small but definite increased risk to the patient. They should never be used in an attempt to compensate for a poorly given general anaesthetic. When they are required labetalol is currently the most satisfactory agent to use, although further assessment may shift in favour of nitroglycerine.

Graft displacement

Tympanic membrane graft displacement is a theoretical and at times a practical problem if nitrous oxide is used for the anaesthetic. There is a 34-fold difference in the blood:gas partition coefficients between nitrous oxide (0.46) and nitrogen (0.013). After commencement of anaesthesia there is rapid diffusion of nitrous oxide into air-containing body cavities, reaching a peak in about 30 minutes. The body cavity either undergoes distension, or if non-distensible is subject to a significant increase in pressure. The middle ear will intermittently lower this pressure a little by discharge through the eustachian tube if it is patent. When nitrous oxide is withdrawn middle ear pressure will become negative once the cavity is closed and this may cause displacement of an underlay graft. To avoid this, nitrous oxide should be withdrawn 20 minutes before the middle ear is closed, and anaesthesia continued with oxygen or oxygen/air, and an increased dose of an inhalational agent, so that consciousness does not return. There should be a firm agreement between surgeon and anaesthetist about the use of nitrous oxide before the operation commences, so that the anaesthetic can be planned in a rational manner.

Fluid and electrolyte balance

Infants and small children have a high metabolic rate and therefore a high calorie and water turnover so that prolonged periods of fluid deprivation are not well tolerated. There is evidence that the postoperative well-being of patients is better if fluid depletion is avoided. All patients coming to theatre suffer some withholding of food and fluid because of the danger of vomiting or regurgitating and aspirating gastric contents during general anaesthesia. This is particularly important in otolaryngological surgery because of the site of the operation and the frequent application of topical anaesthesia to the larynx. No food is given for at least 6 hours before anaesthesia, but 5% glucose solution may be given up to 4 hours before the operation. Minimal gastric effects are seen from the osmotic pressure of oral 5% glucose. These times will sometimes be longer because of variations in the operating schedule, but should never be shorter.

After tonsillectomy, fluid intake may be delayed because of pain on swallowing, and after ear surgery there is a high incidence of vestibular disturbance resulting in nausea or vomiting. Antiemetic drugs induce drowsiness and this may cause delay in adequate oral intake. Infants with serious airway obstruction are always likely to have a significant fluid deficit particularly if nasogastric tube feeding has not been commenced. Many infants and young children are likely to suffer significant fluid depletion during the first 12 hours postoperatively and benefit from intravenous fluid replacement. Serious electrolyte disturbances are unlikely so that the principal concern is a satisfactory fluid maintenance regimen.

Normal daily requirements of fluid and electrolytes

Many methods have been used for calculating daily water requirements based on either body weight or surface area. For practical purposes the information must be simple and prescribed in terms such that nursing staff can readily relate it to the moment-to-moment management of an intravenous burette infusion. For this reason prescriptions should be in millilitres per hour derived from basic data in millilitres per kilogram per hour, although calculations dealing with major fluid and electrolyte imbalances should be based on 24-hour estimations. Basic water requirements for healthy non-surgical infants are shown in *Table 35.11*.

Carbohydrate

The infant metabolic rate is nearly twice that of the adult and the glucose requirement is about 5 g/kg per day. This can be supplied if all the daily maintenance fluid contains 5% glucose. Underweight neonates with little carbohydrate reserves tend to become hypoglycaemic with glucose levels below 1.7 mmol/l (30 mg%). If levels below this are maintained for several hours in full-term neonates, severe cortical neuronal damage is likely

and non-specific symptoms such as fits, twitching and apnoea may occur. If oral or nasogastric feeding cannot be instituted, glucose 10% should be given until blood glucose levels are satisfactory, although excessive amounts may cause an osmotic diuresis especially in the preterm baby. Routine 6-hourly blood glucose estimations are required in the at-risk group.

Ware and Osborne (1976) reported postoperative hypoglycaemia in infants when preoperative starvation was prolonged, but other reports have failed to substantiate this. It seems that infants will not become hypoglycaemic provided preoperative starvation is not excessive and oral intake commences within 4 hours of surgery. Prolonged withholding of food due to swallowing difficulties, vomiting, increased demand as a result of pyrexia, glycogen storage disorders or diabetes, require that intravenous glucose is given.

Sodium

The daily requirement of sodium in the neonate is about 1–2 mmol/kg per day, and this requirement will be met if daily maintenance fluid contains one-fifth normal saline. Surgery in the adult increases aldosterone secretion and thus some sodium retention. Studies in children show no increase in aldosterone secretion for moderate surgery which will include most otolaryngological surgery, although increased aldosterone secretion is seen after major abdominal surgery. Gastric secretion in infancy has a higher sodium content than in the adult and gastrointestinal fluid loss must be replaced with normal saline. Insensible fluid loss from the skin has a sodium content equivalent to one-third normal saline, but fluid lost through the respiratory tract is only water.

Table 35.11 Normal daily water requirements

Neonate		
Days of age	*ml/kg per hour*	*ml/kg per day*
1	2	50
5	4	100
10	6	150
15	6–7.5	150–180
Infants and children		
Body weight (kg)		
2	7.5	180
5	6	150
10	5	120
15	4	100
20	3	75
25	2.5	60
40	2	50

Potassium

The daily requirement of potassium is about 0.5–1 mmol/kg per day. Ninety eight per cent of total body potassium is intracellular and serum potassium more often reflects pH than total body potassium content. There is an obligatory daily renal loss of potassium and additional loss in gastric aspirate or diarrhoea. Respiratory alkalosis will depress serum potassium and this may be important for cardiac rhythm if operative or postoperative hyperventilation occurs in a dehydrated infant. Routine postoperative fluid comprising one-fifth normal Hartman's solution and 5% glucose contains 1 mmol/l of potassium, but if intravenous fluid is required beyond 24 hours this will need to be increased by the addition of 0.5 g KCl to 500 ml of intravenous fluid (13.4 mmol/l). Quantities greatly in excess of this will be needed if there is a large potassium loss, which is unlikely to occur in otolaryngological practice. If serum potassium remains persistently below 3 mmol/l, additional KCl, at the rate of 0.5–1 mmol per hourly fluid volume, may be safely given until the serum level reaches 3.5 mmol/l, provided that there is ECG monitoring, adequate urine output and careful control of the intravenous infusion rate.

Calcium

Hypocalcaemia may occur in the first days of life probably as a result of immaturity of the parathyroid glands. Slightly later hypocalcaemia may occur in babies fed on cow's milk which has a high phosphate content and so precipitates insoluble calcium phosphates in the gut. Hypocalcaemia may present with non-specific neurological irritability and fits such as are seen in hypoglycaemia. Treatment with calcium gluconate (1 ml/kg of 20% calcium gluconate as bolus) is required if there are symptoms or a serum ionized calcium level below 0.7 mmol/l. A serum ionized calcium level above 0.3 mmol/l is adequate for blood clotting and above 0.5 mmol/l for efficient myocardial contractility. Problems with calcium are unlikely to occur in otolaryngological practice outside the neonatal age group.

Calcium chloride 10% remains the drug of choice as a first line myocardial stimulant in acute resuscitation, particularly where the acute low cardiac output or arrest is associated with anaesthesia or hypoxia. The only contraindication is extreme hypokalaemia or digitalis intoxication, neither of which is likely in otolaryngological surgery. The dose is 0.25 ml/kg of calcium chloride 10%.

Intraoperative fluids

Intraoperative fluid may be given as intravascular volume replacement in the form of blood, plasma or other colloid, or as extracellular fluid replacement in the form of water-containing electrolytes, both may be necessary.

Intravascular replacement

Intraoperative blood loss of 10% or less of the calculated circulating blood volume (*Table 35.12*) does not require replacement unless the haemoglobin is below 1.55 mmol/l (10 g/dl) or considerable postoperative loss is anticipated. Losses of

Table 35.12 Average blood volume

Age	Blood volume (ml/kg)
Newborn	80–85
6 weeks–2 years	75–80
2 years–15 years	70–75

20% or over should be replaced with whole blood with an additional allowance of 5 ml/kg. Further volume will be required if postoperative loss continues. Between 10–20% loss replacement will be indicated if the haemoglobin is below 1.7 mmol/l (11 g/dl), significant postoperative loss is anticipated, or further staged surgery is to follow shortly.

Crystalloid replacement

The fluid maintenance requirement under anaesthesia has been estimated at 3–4 ml/kg per hour. Additional factors which add to this amount are the use of dry gas which requires humidification in the patient's upper airway. An additional water content of about 2.5 ml/l of minute ventilation per hour is required to saturate gas in a non-rebreathing system.

Translocation of extracellular fluid into areas where it is removed from effective circulation occurs in the first few hours of surgery. The quantities are extremely variable depending on the site of surgery and the degree of manipulation and trauma involved, but range from 1 ml/kg per hour in minor surgery which will include most otolaryngological procedures, to 10 ml/kg per hour in upper abdominal surgery.

Incompletely corrected preoperative loss is likely to be minimal in otolaryngology except in the case of emergency relief of airway obstruction where pre-existing fluid deficits may be considerable.

Usually in otolaryngology, if maintenance fluid is given, then little more than basic requirements are necessary and a one-fifth normal salt solution in 5% glucose is satisfactory.

Postoperative fluid

The minimum fluid requirements for the first 24–48 hours postoperatively are a similar volume to the intraoperative requirements, namely 3–4 ml/kg per hour. This quantity requires to be increased depending on environmental factors such as temperature, humidity, pyrexia, airway obstruction and the use of infra-red heaters, which all affect the insensible loss, sometimes considerably. Additional volumes of the appropriate electrolyte content are required to make up gastrointestinal loss. Maintenance fluid should be given as 5% glucose in one-fifth Ringer's lactate solution. In the presence of continuing pyrexia, sweating and acidosis, two-fifths of the volume should be Ringer's lactate solution. If hydration is satisfactorily maintained, then an average urine output of 0.3–0.5 ml/kg per hour in the neonate and 0.5–1 ml/kg per hour in the infant, should be achieved readily without recourse to diuretics. Early return to oral feeding should be possible after most otolaryngological surgery.

References

ANDERSON, S. M. (1955) Controlled hypotension with Arfonad in paediatric surgery. *British Medical Journal*, **2**, 103–104

ATKINSON, R. S. (1982) Anaesthesia for day-case surgery. *Recent Advances in Anaesthesia and Analgesia*, **14**, 81–88

BENJAMIN, B. and GRONOW, D. (1979) A new tube for microlaryngeal surgery. *Anaesthesia and Intensive Care*, **7**, 258–263

BETHUNE, D. W., COLLIS, J. M., BURBRIDGE, N. J. and FORSTER, D. M. (1972) Bronchoscope injectors. A design for use with pipeline oxygen supplies. *Anaesthesia*, **27**, 81–83

BORG, U., ERIKSSON, I. and SJÖSTRAND, U. (1980) High-frequency positive-pressure ventilation (HFPPV). A review based upon its use during bronchoscopy and for laryngoscopy and microlaryngeal surgery under general anaesthesia. *Anesthesia and Analgesia*, **59**, 594–603

BRADLEY, T. D. and PHILLIPSON, E. A. (1985) Pathogenesis and pathophysiology of the obstructive sleep apnoea syndrome. *Medical Clinics of North America*, **69**, 1169–1185

BROUILLETTE, R. T., FERNBACH, S. K. and HUNT, C. E. (1982) Obstructive sleep apnoea in infants and children. *Journal of Paediatrics*, **100**, 31–40

CATLEY, D. M., THORNTON, C., JORDAN, C., LEHANE, J. R., ROYSTON, D. and JONES, J. G. (1985) Pronounced episodic oxygen desaturation in the postoperative period. Its association with ventilatory pattern and analgesic regimen. *Anesthesiology*, **63**, 20–28

COGSWELL, J. J., HATCH, D. J., KERR, A. R. and TAYLOR, B. (1975) Effects of continuous positive airway pressure on lung mechanics of babies after operation for congenital heart disease. *Archives of Disease in Childhood*, **50**, 799–804

DELEGUE, L., ROSENBERG-REINER, S., GHNASSIA, M. D., MANLOT, G. and GUILBERT, M. (1980) L'intubation trachéale chez les enfants atteints de dysmorphie cranio-faciales congénitales. *Anesthesia Analgesia Reanimation*, **37**, 133–138

DOUGHTY, A. G. (1957) A modification of the tongue blade of a Boyle Davis Gag. *The Lancet*, **1**, 1074

EDENS, E. T. and SIA, R. L. (1981) Flexible fibreoptic endoscopy in difficult intubations. *Annals of Otology, Rhinology and Laryngology*, **90**, 307–309

ERIKSSON, I. and SJÖSTRAND, U. (1977) A clinical evaluation of high frequency positive pressure ventilation (HFPPV) in laryngoscopy under general anaesthesia. *Acta Anaesthesiologica Scandinavica Supplementum*, **64**, 101–110

EVANS, J. N. G. and TODD, G. B. (1974) Laryngotracheoplasty. *Journal of Laryngology and Otology*, **88**, 589–597

EYRES, R. L., KIDD, J., OPPENHEIM, R. and BROWN, T. C. K. (1978) Local anaesthetic plasma levels in children. *Anaesthesia and Intensive Care*, **6**, 243–247

GREGORY, G. A., KITTERMAN, J. A., PHIBBS, R. H., TOOLEY, W. H. and HAMILTON, W. K. (1971) Treatment of idiopathic respiratory distress syndrome with continuous positive airway pressure. *New England Journal of Medicine*, **284**, 1333–1340

GUILLEMINAULT, C., TILKIAN, A. and DEMENT, W. C. (1976) The sleep apnoea syndromes. *Annual Review Medicine*, **27**, 465–484

HANNALLAH, R. and ROSALES, J. K. (1978) Acute epiglottitis: current management and review. *Canadian Anaesthetist's Society Journal*, **25**, 84–91

JONES, J. G., JORDAN, C., SCUDDER, C., ROCI, E. D. A. and BARROWCLIFFE, M. (1985) Episodic postoperative oxygen desaturation: the value of added oxygen. *Journal of the Royal Society of Medicine*, **78**, 1019–1022

KENEALLY, J. P. (1985) Day-stay surgery in paediatrics. *Clinics in Anaesthesiology – Paediatric Anaesthesia*, **3**, 679–696

KLAIN, M. and SMITH, R. B. (1977) High-frequency percutaneous transtracheal jet ventilation. *Critical Care Medicine*, **5**, 280–287

KLEIN, M. and REYNOLDS, L. G. (1986) Relief of sleep-related oropharyngeal airway obstruction by continuous insufflation of the pharynx. *The Lancet*, **1**, 935–939

KOMESAROFF, D. and McKIE, B. (1972) The bronchoflator. A new technique for bronchoscopy under general anaesthesia. *British Journal of Anaesthesia*, **44**, 1057–1068

MACARTNEY, F. J., PANDAY, J. and SCOTT, O. (1969) Cor pulmonale as a result of chronic nasopharyngeal obstruction due to hypertrophied tonsils and adenoids. *Archives of Disease in Childhood*, **44**, 585–592

McGILL, T., FREIDMANN, E. M. and HEALY, G. B. (1983) Laser surgery in the paediatric airway. *Otolaryngologic Clinics of North America*, **16**, 865–870

MAZE, A. and BLOCH, E. (1979) Stridor in pediatric patients. *Anesthesiology*, **50**, 132–145

MIYASAKA, K., SLOAN, I. A. and FROESE, A. B. (1980) An evaluation of the jet injector (Sanders) technique for bronchoscopy in paediatric patients. *Canadian Anaesthetists' Society Journal*, **27**, 117–124

NICHOL, H. C. and ZUCK, D. (1983) Difficult laryngoscopy – the 'anterior' larynx and the atlanto-occipital gap. *British Journal of Anaesthesia*, **55**, 141–144

NORTON, M. L. (1983) Anaesthesia for laser surgery in laryngobronchoesophagoscopy. *Otolaryngologic Clinics of North America*, **16**, 785–791

PELTON, D. A., DALY, M., COOPER, P. D. and CONN, A. W. (1970) Plasma lidocaine concentrations following topical aerosol application to the trachea and bronchi. *Canadian Anaesthetists' Society Journal*, **17**, 250–255

REID, D. H. and TUNSTALL, M. E. (1966) The respiratory distress syndrome of the newborn. A method of treatment using prolonged nasotracheal intubation and intermittent positive pressure respiration. *Anaesthesia*, **21**, 72–80

ROESLER, M., DE LEVAL, M., CHRISPIN, A. and STARK, J. (1983) Surgical management of vascular ring. *Annals of Surgery*, **197**, 139–146

SANDERS, R. D. (1967) Two ventilating attachments for bronchoscopes. *Delaware Medical Journal*, **39**, 170–175

SIMPSON, G. T. and STRONG, M. S. (1983) Recurrent respiratory papillomatosis. The role of the carbon dioxide laser. *Otolaryngologic Clinics of North America*, **16**, 887–894

SJÖSTRAND, U. (1980) High-frequency positive pressure ventilation (HFPPV): a review. *Critical Care Medicine*, **8**, 345–364

SMITH, B. R., KLAIN, M. and BABINSKI, M. (1980) Limits of high frequency percutaneous transtracheal jet ventilation using a fluidic logic controlled ventilator. *Canadian Anaesthetists' Society Journal*, **27**, 351–356

SPOEREL, W. E. and GREENWAY, R. E. (1973) Technique of ventilation during endolaryngeal surgery under general anaesthesia. *Canadian Anaesthetists' Society Journal*, **20**, 369–377

THACH, B. T. (1985) Sleep apnoea in infancy and childhood. *Medical Clinics of North America*, **69**, 1289–1315

TOO-CHUNG, M. A. and GREEN, J. R. (1974) The rate of growth of the cricoid cartilage. *Journal Laryngology and Otology*, **88**, 65–70

WARE, J. and OSBORNE, J. P. (1976) Postoperative hypoglycaemia in small children. *British Medical Journal*, **2**, 499–501

YELDERMAN, M. and NEW, W. (1983) Evaluation of pulse oximetry. *Anesthesiology*, **59**, 349–352

Further reading

BENNETT, E. J. and BOWYER, D. E. (1985) Fluid balance. *Clinics in Anaesthesiology – Paediatric Anaesthesia*, **3**, 569–595

HATCH, D. J. and SUMNER, E. (1986) *Neonatal Anaesthesia and Perioperative Care*, 2nd edn, Current Topics in Anaesthesia Series. London: Edward Arnold

36

Cystic fibrosis

R. Dinwiddie

Cystic fibrosis is an autosomal recessive disease which affects approximately one in 2000 children born in the UK (Kuzemko, 1986). It is thought to be due to a primary gene defect which, although not yet precisely identified, appears to lie on the long arm of chromosome number 7 (Wainwright *et al.*, 1985). The disease is commonest in people of European caucasoid origin and its incidence is highest in countries populated by peoples of this genetic background. The disease is seen less frequently in Asians and in Negroes and is extremely rare in Chinese peoples.

The basic defect is not yet known precisely, but the clinical and diagnostic features stem almost entirely from the abnormalities of exocrine glandular secretions which occur throughout the body. The systems most affected clinically are the respiratory system and the digestive tract. There is also a high level of sodium in the sweat which can be used for specific diagnostic purposes (Gibson and Cooke, 1959). The disease is life-long and results in progressive deterioration of pulmonary function with age. It may also be associated with major problems in other systems such as the liver leading to cirrhosis, and the reproductive system causing infertility in males. These aspects are discussed in more detail later.

Antenatal diagnosis and screening

Antenatal diagnosis is presently available in two forms, either as an amniocentesis at 18–20 weeks' gestation or by chorionic villus sampling at 8–10 weeks. At amniocentesis, phenylalanine inhibitable intestinal alkaline phosphatase activity is measured; its activity is less inhibited than in normal individuals. This test, if positive, carries a reliability approaching 92% (Brock *et al.*, 1985). If negative there is a 3% chance of the infant being affected. More recently, chorionic villus sampling has become possible using new DNA genetic probes which can be used at 8–10 weeks of gestation (Farrall *et al.*, 1986). This, however, requires familial gene mapping of both parents and affected children before pregnancy begins. If the test proves positive it is highly reliable with an overall false negative rate of less than 5% and a false positive rate of less than 0.04%.

Neonatal screening for cystic fibrosis is also available utilizing the presence of an elevated plasma immunoreactive trypsin which can be measured on dried blood spot (Guthrie) test cards in the neonatal period (Kuzemko and Heeley, 1983). This substance remains elevated for approximately the first 3 months of life, after which it drops to normal or low values. This test is therefore useful for screening in the neonatal period and early infancy but is not of help subsequently. Screening with this technique in the UK has shown an incidence of approximately one in 2100 live births. The false positive rate is less than 0.05% on initial testing and drops to less than 0.001% on repeat testing. The false negative rate is also extremely low (Kuzemko, 1986).

The sweat test remains at present the only definitive diagnostic test. This is performed with the use of pilocarpine iontophoresis and the collection of sweat thereafter for sodium or chloride analysis (Gibson and Cooke, 1959). Classically, a value of these substances in excess of 70 mmol/l on a sample weighing in excess of 100 mg is diagnostic in the presence of appropriate clinical symptoms. However, the concentration of sodium in sweat tends to rise naturally with age and may also be elevated to the higher end of the normal range in patients with asthma. In some of these cases it may be extremely difficult to make the diagnosis (Hodson *et al.*, 1983) and pancreatic function tests may have to be performed to aid in the diagnosis. The virtual absence of pancreatic bicarbonate and low levels of the enzymes trypsin, lipase and amylase are typical of the patient with cystic fibrosis (Hadborn *et al.*, 1968).

Presentation

Neonatal

Cystic fibrosis may present in many different forms. The early presentations in the neonatal period are shown in *Table 36.1*.

Table 36.1 Neonatal presentation

Prenatal diagnosis
Meconium ileus
Meconium perforation and peritonitis
Obstructive jaundice
Neonatal screening – raised immunoreactive trypsin
Positive sweat test (sibling with cystic fibrosis)

Meconium ileus is the commonest presenting feature in this period. This will be the mode of presentation in 10–15% of all cases of cystic fibrosis (Donnison, Schwachman and Gross, 1966). Babies with this condition fail to pass stools after birth and rapidly develop abdominal distension secondary to intestinal obstruction which is caused by the sticky inspissated faecal material. These changes have been noted as early as 20 weeks by ultrasound *in utero*, some babies even develop intrauterine perforation. Treatment is usually surgical and may involve resection of the small bowel followed by end-to-end anastomosis (Dinwiddie, 1983). Some cases may respond to simple gastrografin enema. Particular attention should be paid to the baby's general condition in the perioperative period since they are prone to lower respiratory tract infection following ventilation. They may also develop infections either in the chest or due to septicaemia and may have particular nutritional difficulties until bowel function is restored. Those who present with meconium ileus now have almost as good a prognosis as those who present in later life (Wilmott *et al.*, 1983).

Infancy

The common modes of presentation in infancy are shown in *Table 36.2*. The most frequent presentation is with a combination of failure to thrive,

recurrent loose stools despite a large appetite, and frequent respiratory tract infections (Goodchild and Dodge, 1985a). Many infants are misdiagnosed as having food allergy or intolerance or possibly coeliac disease. The stools are typically pale, fatty and frequent. They tend to float and have an offensive pungent penetrating odour which can be virtually diagnostic.

Table 36.2 Presentation in infancy

Failure to thrive
Recurrent loose stools
Recurrent lower respiratory tract infection
Anaemia and oedema
Rectal prolapse
Heat exhaustion

A less common presentation is with anaemia and hypoproteinaemia secondary to the nutritional deficiencies (Neilson and Larsen, 1982). The baby frequently tastes salty when kissed and this too may be an important diagnostic clue. Rectal prolapse may result from the frequent loose stools and cystic fibrosis should always be considered in the infant who presents with this problem. Treatment is usually successful when the appropriate diagnosis is made and dietary management is commenced. In hot countries excessive salt loss through the sweat may result in major electrolyte imbalance or heat exhaustion with associated hyponatraemia and hypokalaemia (Kessler and Anderson, 1951).

A number of infants will present with recurrent respiratory infections or persistent respiratory symptoms after common viral infections such as bronchiolitis. If there is a productive cough, evidence of persistent hyperinflation or indrawing of respiratory muscles which continues after the acute phase is passed, this diagnosis should certainly be considered and a chest X-ray should be performed. A small number of patients will present with staphylococcal pneumonia and empyema and again cystic fibrosis should be considered in this group. The prognosis for children who present with these forms of pulmonary infection in infancy is not always as poor as might be thought since the lung is rapidly growing and developing at this stage and, if it can be protected from further major insult, there is considerable room for recovery for a period of time.

Childhood and adolescence

A number of patients will present in later childhood, adolescence or even in adult life with symptoms due to cystic fibrosis. These patients tend to have a milder form of the illness as seen clinically, at least initially. The different presentations seen at this stage are shown in *Table 36.3*.

Table 36.3 Presentation in childhood and adolescence

Recurrent wheeze, cough and purulent sputum production
Nasal polyps and sinusitis
Biliary cirrhosis
Meconium ileus equivalent
Diabetes mellitus
Heat exhaustion
Male infertility

Cystic fibrosis should certainly be considered in this group of patients particularly when symptoms are persistent or recurrent. Some of these cases are detected when a sibling is diagnosed as having cystic fibrosis and the rest of the family is reviewed. Some will have atopic features and may be thought to have asthma which can be particularly difficult to control, or have frequent respiratory infections. Suspicion should also be raised when there is evidence of chronic bronchial line shadowing on the chest X-ray or if there is any suggestion of finger clubbing when there is no other obvious reason for this. Allergic disorders, including rhinitis and asthma, are common in patients with cystic fibrosis (Wilmott, 1985) and this may obscure the diagnosis in some cases. A small number of patients with cystic fibrosis appear virtually asymptomatic, these are usually the siblings of known cases who, on screening with a sweat test, have high sweat sodium values. They represent one end of the spectrum of the illness and there must undoubtedly be a number of people who have the illness but who have virtually no symptoms and are never diagnosed.

Management

Management of the patient with cystic fibrosis is complex because it is a multisystem disease which therefore needs the involvement of a number of disciplines. Attention should not only be paid to the purely medical aspects, but also to the psychological, social, genetic, educational and occupational implications of the illness. While the diagnosis and management of the complications are best dealt with in a specialized cystic fibrosis clinic, much of the patient's care can now be undertaken by other sympathetic and involved hospital practitioners and family doctors. As more and more patients enter adult life in reasonable health, the value of combined care between hospital and general practitioner is greater than ever before.

Pulmonary disease
Pathology

The major changes in the lungs occur as a consequence of bacterial colonization resulting in persistent infection. This also leads to the production of increasingly viscid pulmonary secretions which are difficult to clear and result in marked airway obstruction with further infection and subsequently bronchiectasis (Tomashefski, Vawter and Reid, 1983). Initially there is a low grade chronic bronchitis and bronchiolitis, but as the disease progresses the airways become more permanently distorted, thickened and damaged by the infective process. This leads to areas of collapse with microabscess formation and other areas of overinflation and air trapping. The bronchial walls typically become thickened and this produces the classical signs seen on the chest X-ray (Chrispin and Norman, 1974). As a consequence of this chronic state, airway obstruction, which can result in wheezing, also occurs and this may have, in addition, an underlying allergic or asthmatic basis. It is important to test the patient for bronchodilator responsiveness if he is wheezing since not all bronchodilators work effectively in patients with cystic fibrosis (Mitchell *et al.*, 1978). As the disease progresses the more common pathogens, particularly *Staphylococcus aureus* and *Pseudomonas aeruginosa*, may become permanent residents of the lower respiratory tract (Wilmott *et al.*, 1983). These assume varying degrees of pathogenicity, but often result in the need for frequent or continuous antibiotic treatment to suppress their activity.

Upper respiratory tract problems are also common in cystic fibrosis and include chronic sinusitis, allergic rhinitis and frequently nasal polyposis (Drake-Lee and Pitcher-Wilmott, 1982). These are due to a combination of chronic infection and sometimes underlying allergy. The nasal polyps tend to grow slowly but ultimately result in significant nasal obstruction with breathing difficulties and recurrent headaches. When removed they tend to return again and many patients require repeated surgery for this problem.

Management of the lung

Management of the pulmonary complications is aimed at minimizing the effect of chronic infection, clearing the lung of the viscid secretions and treating any underlying asthma which may be present. The major modes of pulmonary management are shown in *Table 36.4*.

Physiotherapy is the most important part of treatment for the lung and is required on a daily basis in virtually all cases (Hodson and Gaskell

Table 36.4 Pulmonary management of cystic fibrosis

Chest physiotherapy
Forced expiratory technique (FET)
Physical exercise
Antibiotics – intermittent or continuous
Antifungal agents
Bronchodilators
Sodium cromoglycate (Intal)
Steroids – oral or inhaled
Inhaled mucolytics

1983). The frequency and timing will depend on each patient. It is important to continue this on a regular basis because it prevents the accumulation of secretions and allows the patient to be physically trained in receiving this treatment. This is particularly important when an infection supervenes and the frequency and intensity must be increased. When the patient regularly produces sputum, physiotherapy should be carried out three times daily for 10–15 minutes. Older children and adults can successfully perform their own physiotherapy using the forced expiratory technique (FET) (Pryor *et al.*, 1979). This is a special method of chest percussion, postural drainage and coughing which is successful in clearing sputum once it has been properly demonstrated by an appropriately trained physiotherapist. Physical exercise is helpful in the management of the lung, but does not replace physiotherapy as a means of clearing the lung secretions (Geddes, 1984). Any underlying exercise-induced wheezing should also be treated with β-agonists or with sodium cromoglycate.

Antibiotics

Antibiotic therapy is frequently required for lung infection in patients with cystic fibrosis. The antibiotics may be administered by different regimens including continuous therapy throughout life with antistaphylococcal agents, antibiotic therapy in the early years to reduce colonization with *Staphylococcus* or other pathogens, or intermittent therapy during exacerbations of respiratory infection (*Table 36.5*) (Goodchild and Dodge, 1985b). The most common present practice is to administer antibiotics as required in relation to symptoms and the presence of significant pathogens. Recent studies have demonstrated an increase in bacterial induced symptoms, even during intercurrent viral infections (Stroobant, 1986), so it is important to cover these with antibiotics as well.

The two major pulmonary pathogens in cystic fibrosis are *Staphylococcus aureus* and *Pseudomonas aeruginosa* (Pitt, 1986). These often become perma-

nent residents of the lower respiratory tract and when they are persistently cultured from the sputum it is virtually impossible to eradicate them. Treatment is therefore aimed at suppressing their activity and reducing their effect on the production of chronic bronchiectasis.

Staphylococci may be treated with intensive oral therapy but in severe cases hospital admission is required for intravenous treatment. *Pseudomonas* requires parenteral therapy, either in hospital or at home, and this is usually given in the form of two antibiotics, an aminoglycoside in combination with either a ureidopenicillin, such as azlocillin or a third generation cephalosporin such as ceftazidime. The usual treatment period is for 2 weeks and this is combined with intensive physiotherapy and nutritional support. Recently, aerosol antibiotics have been used more frequently for the treatment of Pseudomonas infections with some success and selected patients with chronic symptoms may well benefit from this form of treatment on a daily basis at home, either for short periods or even continuously for a period of many months (Hodson, Penketh and Batten, 1981). Ciprofloxacin is a new oral antipseudomomas agent which has been used in this situation but resistant organisms have already emerged.

Inhaled mucolytic agents may be helpful in those with particularly thick or viscid sputum and there is some evidence that these may be particularly useful when combined with inhaled antibiotic therapy (Heaf, Webb and Matthew, 1983). Whenever possible, the response to this treatment should be measured by the use of lung function tests as, in some cases, the lung function deteriorates when these agents are given.

Wheezing is a common feature in the lung disease of cystic fibrosis and may be due to airway

Table 36.5 Antibiotics in cystic fibrosis

Antistaphylococcal
  flucloxacillin
  erythromycin
  trimethoprim
  fusidic acid
  chloramphenicol
Other antibiotics
  amoxycillin
  cephalosporins
  doxycycline
Antipseudomonas agents
  gentamicin
  tobramycin
  amikacin
  carbenicillin
  cefotaxime
  ceftazidime
  ciprofloxacin

obstruction secondary to infection. Many cases, however, have associated asthmatic symptoms and these should be treated vigorously with the usual agents, including β-agonists, theophylline, sodium cromoglycate and steroids if necessary (Wilmott, 1985). Again, the response to the treatment should be assessed by lung function tests whenever possible.

Other pulmonary complications which may be encountered include haemoptysis, seen more commonly in the adolescent or adult patient with more advanced lung disease (Batten and Matthew, 1983). Most cases will stop bleeding spontaneously but occasionally bronchoscopy followed by angiography and embolization of the vessel may be necessary.

Pneumothorax is not uncommon in adults and requires treatment with the usual measures including high oxygen concentration if tolerated, intercostal chest drainage and pleurodesis or pleurectomy after a period of 7–10 days if the lesion has not resolved (Penketh *et al.*, 1982).

Advanced cases show evidence of cor pulmonale and this will require treatment with diuretics and more intensive treatment of the underlying lung infection. Its onset is usually associated with worsening of the prognosis.

Alimentary problems

Abnormalities of bowel function are one of the major features of cystic fibrosis. Eighty-five per cent of patients have clinically abnormal pancreatic function and require pancreatic enzymes in varying quantities. The features of the disordered bowel function may present in a number of different ways including the following: meconium ileus (10–15%), steatorrhoea with pale, offensive, fatty stools in the presence of large appetite, and third, anaemia and hypoproteinaemia secondary to nutritional deficiency. Abnormalities of the bowel have been seen *in utero* as early as 18 weeks and also form the basis of the microvillar enzyme tests based on the intestinal alkaline phosphatase which may be measured in amniotic fluid obtained by amniocentesis (Brock *et al.*, 1985).

Meconium ileus

Babies with meconium ileus usually present with intestinal obstruction in the first 24–48 hours of life. They often require surgery to remove areas of necrotic bowel and to aid in the release of the sticky, viscid meconium which has caused the intestinal obstruction. A number of babies respond to treatment with gastrografin enema, but the remainder require operative surgery. It is

important to maintain the baby's nutrition at this time until bowel function is restored and this may be undertaken with intravenous feeding or enteral feeds including breast milk where possible, low fat high carbohydrate formula or Pregestemil if necessary (Dinwiddie, 1983). Most of these children will require pancreatic supplements from an early age and the dose of these should be modified to result in normal weight gain and growth and in the passage of normal stools which do not contain an excess of fat. All infants will require vitamin supplementation including A, B, C, D and usually E.

Later problems

Later abdominal complications may occur in infancy and childhood including intussusception, adhesion obstruction, stricture formation at a previous anastomotic site and low grade appendicitis. A few infants with cystic fibrosis present with rectal prolapse secondary to the malabsorption and this diagnosis should always be considered in young children with this condition.

Once weaned, the child should be given a diet with a normal fat content and the dosage of pancreatic supplements adjusted accordingly. The new enteric coated, acid resistant preparations, such as Creon and Pancrease, allow a higher lipase delivery to the duodenum and thus enable the fat content of the diet to be normal.

Another complication of cystic fibrosis in the older patient is meconium ileus equivalent, also termed distal intestinal obstruction syndrome. This presents with abdominal pain, distension and failure to pass stools. This results from inspissated stool obstructing the caecum in particular, although there is usually also significant generalized faecal loading present. Treatment is medical and consists of oral gastrografin or oral acetylcysteine. Recently a specialized non-absorbed electrolyte mix has proved successful in relieving symptoms (Cleghorn *et al.*, 1986). If the patient fails to respond to these measures, then a gastrografin enema is usually successful. Enzyme therapy may need to be increased or decreased during the acute phase and readjusted again when the nutritional intake is restored. Those with chronic or recurrent symptoms may benefit from the use of cimetidine to diminish gastric acidity.

Other abdominal complications of cystic fibrosis include oesophageal varices in the presence of advanced liver disease and hypersplenism. These may result in recurrent haematemesis and, at present, treatment involves endoscopic sclerosis in order to prevent further bleeding episodes (Stamatakis *et al.*, 1982). About 15% of patients have liver disease of significance resulting in the longer term in biliary cirrhosis, ascites due to hypoproteinaemia and anaemia, neutropenia and thrombocytopenia because of hypersplenism. Those with significant liver disease will require additional vitamin K as part of their daily supplementation.

Other problems in cystic fibrosis

Diabetes mellitus

As many as 5% of older patients with cystic fibrosis may develop diabetes mellitus. A higher number will have abnormal glucose tolerance tests, although not clinical symptoms. This probably results from pancreatic fibrosis. It is more commonly seen in the adolescent or adult. Control of the diabetes is in the usual form with dietary measures and insulin if necessary. This clearly requires expert dietary advice.

Arthropathy

A small number of patients with cystic fibrosis complain of recurrent joint pains mainly affecting the larger joints and associated with low grade or minimal X-ray change. This may be secondary to their chronic inflammatory lung disease but the aetiology of this condition is not clear (Phillips and David, 1986). Treatment is usually conservative and symptomatic with drugs such as paracetamol, although the patient's liver function should be checked before these are used on a chronic basis.

Fertility

Almost all cystic fibrosis males are infertile due to fibrosis of the vas deferens, reduced sperm count and motility. Male sexual activity is otherwise normal.

Many adult females with cystic fibrosis have produced normal, healthy children (Cohen, di Sant'Agnese and Friedlanders, 1980). They have significant reduction of overall fertility secondary to their chronic lung disease, and abnormalities of the mucus in the reproductive tract. The risk of a female with cystic fibrosis producing a child with this condition is one in 50. The breast milk of females with cystic fibrosis may be excessively salty and, if this is the case, breast feeding should be avoided.

Psychological problems

The psychological support of the family with cystic fibrosis is one of the most important parts of treatment. Because the patient has a chronic and life-limiting disease, much support has to be given by a number of health care professionals. There are marked effects on family life, both in terms of the patient's chronic ill health and also because of their need for frequent hospital visits and admissions and the time and expense that this involves. The psychological stress of the dying patient and the trauma of one or more family members being lost with the illness provides a great stress over an extended period. Sympathetic and supportive help and understanding is vital for these families on a long-term basis (Bywater, 1984).

Prognosis

The overall prognosis for patients with cystic fibrosis has greatly improved over the last 20 years. It is estimated that 60–70% of newborn infants with the illness may now expect to reach adult life (Wilmott *et al.*, 1983) and 50% of those alive at 17 are still alive at the age of 30. Increasing numbers of older adults in their third and fourth decades are now being recorded. Many adults with cystic fibrosis have undertaken useful jobs and entered a wide variety of professions (Norman and Hodson, 1983).

The recent genetic advances in the location of the cystic fibrosis gene bring with them great promise for major changes in the understanding of the disease and the possibility of greatly improved treatments in the near future.

References

BATTEN, J. C. and MATTHEW, D. J. (1983) The respiratory system. In *Cystic Fibrosis,* edited by M. E. Hodson, A. P. Norman and J. C. Batten, ch. 6, p. 123. London: Baillière-Tindall

BROCK, D. H. J., BARRON, L., BEDGOOD, D. and HAYWARD, C. (1985) Prospective prenatal diagnosis of cystic fibrosis. *The Lancet,* **1,** 1175–1178

BYWATER, E. M. (1984) Coping with a life-threatening illness: an experiment in parent's groups. *British Journal of Social Work,* **14,** 117–127

CHRISPIN, A. R. and NORMAN, A. P. (1974) The systematic evaluation of the chest radiograph in cystic fibrosis. *Pediatric Radiology,* **2,** 101–106

CLEGHORN, G. J., STRINGER, D. A., FORSTNER, G. G. and DURIE, P. R. (1986) Treatment of distal intestinal obstruction syndrome in cystic fibrosis with a balanced intestinal lavage solution. *The Lancet,* **1,** 8–11

COHEN, L. F., DI SANT'AGNESE, P. A. and FRIEDLANDERS, J. (1980) Cystic fibrosis and pregnancy. A national survey. *The Lancet,* **2,** 842–844

DINWIDDIE, R. (1983) Meconium ileus. In *Cystic Fibrosis,* edited by M. E. Hodson, A. P. Norman and J. C. Batten, ch. 11, pp. 202–204. London: Baillière-Tindall

DONNISON, A. B., SHWACHMAN, H. and GROSS, R. E. (1966) A review of 164 children with meconium ileus seen at the Children's Medical Center, Boston. *Pediatrics,* **37,** 833–837

DRAKE-LEE, A. B. and PITCHER-WILMOTT, R. W. (1982) The clinical and laboratory correlates of nasal polyps in cystic fibrosis. *International Journal of Pediatric Otorhinolaryngology,* **4,** 209–214

FARRALL, M., HAI-YANG, L., RODECK, C. H., WARREN, R., STANIER, R., SUPER, M. *et al.* (1986) First trimester prenatal diagnosis of cystic fibrosis with linked DNA probes. *The Lancet,* **1,** 1402–1404

GEDDES, D. M. (1984) Physical exercise and cystic fibrosis. In *Cystic Fibrosis: Horizons,* edited by D. Lawson, pp. 114–133. Chichester: Wiley

GIBSON, L. E. and COOKE, R. E. (1959) A test for concentration of electrolytes in sweat in cystic fibrosis of the pancreas utilising pilocarpine by iontophoresis. *Pediatrics,* **23,** 545–549

GOODCHILD, M. and DODGE, J. A. (1985a) Editors. Clinical and diagnostic features. In *Cystic Fibrosis, Manual of Diagnosis and Management,* 2nd edn, ch. 3, pp. 27–46. London: Baillière-Tindall

GOODCHILD, M. and DODGE, J. A. (1985b) Editors. Management of respiratory disease. In *Cystic Fibrosis, Manual of Diagnosis and Management,* 2nd edn, ch. 5, pp. 53–56. London: Baillière-Tindall

HADORN, B., ZOPPI, G., SHMERLING, D., PRADER, A., McINTYRE, I. and ANDERSON, C. M. (1968) Quantitative assessment of exocrine pancreatic function in infants and children. *Journal of Pediatrics,* **73,** 39–50

HEAF, D. P., WEBB, G. J. and MATTHEW, D. J. (1983) *In vitro* assessment of combined antibiotic and mucolytic treatment of *Pseudomonas aeruginosa* infections in cystic fibrosis. *Archives of Disease in Childhood,* **58,** 824–826

HODSON, M. E. and GASKELL, D. V. (1983) Physiotherapy. In *Cystic Fibrosis,* edited by M. E. Hodson, A. P. Norman and J. C. Batten, ch. 13, pp. 219–241. London: Baillière-Tindall

HODSON, M. E., PENKETH, A. R. L. and BATTEN, J. C. (1981) Aerosol carbenicillin and gentamicin treatment of *Pseudomonas aeruginosa* infections in patients with cystic fibrosis. *The Lancet,* **2,** 1137–1139

HODSON, M. E., BELDON, I., POWER, R., DUNCAN, F. R., BAMBER, M. and BATTEN, J. C. (1983) Sweat tests to diagnose cystic fibrosis in adults. *British Medical Journal,* **286,** 1381–1383

KESSLER, W. R. and ANDERSON, D. H. (1951) Heat prostration in fibrocystic disease of the pancreas and other conditions. *Pediatrics,* **8,** 648–656

KUZEMKO, J. A. (1986) Screening, early neonatal diagnosis and prenatal diagnosis. *Journal of the Royal Society of Medicine,* **79,** (suppl. 12), 2–5

KUZEMKO, J. A. and HEELEY, A. F. (1983) Diagnostic methods and screening. In *Cystic Fibrosis,* edited by M. E. Hodson, A. P. Norman and J. C. Batten, ch. 2, pp. 21–30. London: Baillière-Tindall

MITCHELL, I., COREY, M., WOENNE, R., KRASTINS, I. R. B. and LEVISON, H. (1978) Bronchial hyperreactivity in cystic fibrosis and asthma. *Journal of Pediatrics,* **93,** 744–748

NEILSON, O. H. and LARSEN, B. F. (1982) The incidence of anaemia, hypoproteinaemia and oedema in infants as presenting symptoms of cystic fibrosis. *Journal of Pediatric Gastroenterology and Nutrition,* **1,** 355–359

NORMAN, A. P. and HODSON, M. E. (1983) Emotional and social aspects of treatment. In *Cystic Fibrosis,* edited by M. E. Hodson, A. P. Norman and J. C. Batten, ch. 14, pp. 242–259. London: Baillière-Tindall

PENKETH, A. R. L., KNIGHT, R. K., HODSON, M. E. and BATTEN, J. C. (1982) Management of pneumothorax in adults with cystic fibrosis. *Thorax,* **32,** 850–853

PHILLIPS, B. M. and DAVID, T. J. (1986) Pathogenesis and management of arthropathy in cystic fibrosis. *Journal of the Royal Society of Medicine,* **79,** (suppl. 12), 44–50

PITT, T. L. (1986) Biology of *Pseudomonas aeruginosa* in relation to pulmonary infection in cystic fibrosis. *Journal of the Royal Society of Medicine,* **9,** (suppl. 12), 13–18

PRYOR, J. A., WEBBER, B. A., HODSON, M. E. and BATTEN, J. C. (1979) Evaluation of the forced expiratory technique as an adjunct to postural drainage in treatment of cystic fibrosis. *British Medical Journal,* **2,** 417–418

STAMATAKIS, J. D., HOWARD, E. R., PSACHAROPOULOS, H. T. and MOWATT, A. P. (1982) Injection sclerotherapy for oesophageal varices in children. *British Journal of Surgery,* **69,** 74–75

STROOBANT, J. (1986) Viral infection in cystic fibrosis. *Journal of the Royal Society of Medicine,* **79,** (suppl. 12), 19–22

TOMASHEFSKI, J. F., VAWTER, G. F. and REID, L. (1983) Pulmonary pathology. In *Cystic Fibrosis,* edited by M. E. Hodson, A. P. Norman and J. C. Batten, ch. 3, pp. 31–35. London: Baillière-Tindall

WAINWRIGHT, B. J., SCAMBLER, P. J., SCHMIDTKE, J., WATSON, E. A., HA-YANG, L., FARRALL, M. *et al.* (1985) Localisation of cystic fibrosis locus to human chromosome 7 cen-q 22. *Nature,* **318,** 384–385

WILMOTT, R. W. (1985) Allergy and infection in cystic fibrosis. In *Neonatal and Pediatric Respiratory Medicine,* edited by A. S. Milner and R. J. Martin, ch. 10, pp. 190–210. London: Butterworths

WILMOTT, R. W., TYSON, S. L., DINWIDDIE, R. and MATTHEW, D. J. (1983) Survival rates in cystic fibrosis. *Archives of Disease in Childhood,* **58,** 835–838

37

Diseases of the oesophagus

Lewis Spitz

Embryology

The oesophagus and trachea first become identifiable as separate structures when the embryo is 22–23 days old, as a median ventral diverticulum in the developing foregut. Shortly thereafter, the primitive stomach appears as a fusiform enlargement immediately caudal to the diverticulum. The oesophagus develops from the short area between the tracheal diverticulum and the stomach. As the trachea and oesophagus elongate, ridges appear in the lateral walls. Fusion in the midline of these ridges separates the trachea from the oesophagus. The separation process commences caudally, proceeds cranially and is complete between days 34 and 36 of gestation. Elongation of the oesophagus also begins in the distal portion and is complete at 7 weeks (that is relative to the rest of the developing fetus).

The circular musculature of the oesophagus appears in the sixth week and by the end of that week innervation by the vagus nerve has commenced. During the seventh and eighth weeks, the epithelium of the oesophagus proliferates to such an extent that the lumen is virtually, but not completely, occluded. Initially, the epithelium is ciliated, but it is gradually replaced by stratified squamous epithelium.

Oesophageal atresia

This was a uniformly fatal congenital abnormality until 1939 when the first two survivors were reported independently by Ladd and Levin (Levin, 1941; Ladd, 1944). Both infants required multiple procedures – cervical oesophagostomy,

feeding gastrostomy, and subsequent reconstruction. The first success with primary repair of the defect, which paved the way to future developments, was described by Haight in 1941 (Haight and Towsley, 1943). It is now rare for an infant with oesophageal atresia to succumb from the anomaly, unless it is associated with additional complex life-threatening anomalies or extreme prematurity (Rickham, Stauffer and Cheng, 1977; O'Neill, Holcomb and Neblett, 1982; Louhimo and Lindahl, 1983).

Incidence

The incidence of abnormalities in oesophageal development is one in 3000–4000 live births (Myers, 1974). There does not appear to be any standard genetic pattern of inheritance, although the condition has been documented in siblings, in one and very occasionally in both twins and in two generations.

Embryology

The anomaly is thought to arise between the third and sixth weeks of intrauterine development. The precise cause and mechanism are unknown. Failure of complete separation of the foregut from the respiratory tract would appear to be the final common pathway for the development of the various types of defects. Oesophageal atresia may occur as an isolated anomaly but at least 40% of cases have additional malformations.

Types of anomaly

The variety and incidence of the different types of tracheo-oesophageal abnormalities are shown in *Figure 37.1*. These are as follows:

(1) oesophageal atresia with distal tracheo-oesophageal fistula – 87%
(2) oesophageal atresia without tracheo-oesophageal fistula – 6–7%
(3) oesophageal atresia with proximal tracheo-oesophageal fistula – 2%
(4) oesophageal atresia with proximal and distal tracheo-oesophageal fistula – <1%
(5) tracheo-oesophageal fistula without oesophageal atresia – 3–4%.

Associated anomalies

Additional congenital malformations are found in about one-half of infants with tracheo-oesophageal anomalies. The various systems affected are as follows (multiple defects occur in many patients) (Holder *et al.*, 1964; German, Mahour and Woolley, 1976):

(1) cardiovascular defects – 34%
(2) gastrointestinal (excluding anorectal) anomalies – 14%
(3) genitourinary anomalies – 12%
(4) anorectal malformations – 11%
(5) skeletal defects – 11%
(6) respiratory anomalies – 6%
(7) genetic/chromosomal defects – 2%
(8) miscellaneous anomalies – 10%.

The VATER complex of associated anomalies was described by Quan and Smith (1973). (The acronym stands for V = vertebral, A = anorectal, T-E = tracheo-oesophageal fistula and (o)oesophageal atresia, R = radial and renal dysplasia.)
Ventricular septal defects are the single most common cardiac malformation (Greenwood and Rosenthal, 1976). Of the gastrointestinal anomalies, malrotation of the midgut occurs most frequently, followed by Meckel's diverticulum and duodenal atresia or stenosis. A variety of genitourinary anomalies occurs in association with oesophageal atresia, the most serious being renal agenesis (Potter's syndrome) which is incompatible with survival. The anorectal anomalies are

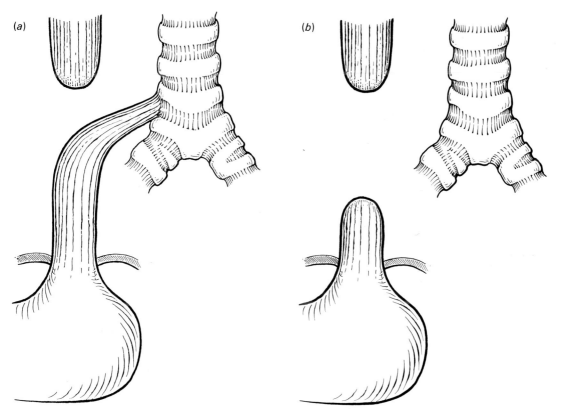

(a)

(b)

Figure 37.1 Types of oesophageal atresia. (*a*) Oesophageal atresia with distal tracheo-oesophageal fistula, 87%; (*b*) oesophageal atresia without tracheo-oesophageal fistula, 6–7%;

(c)

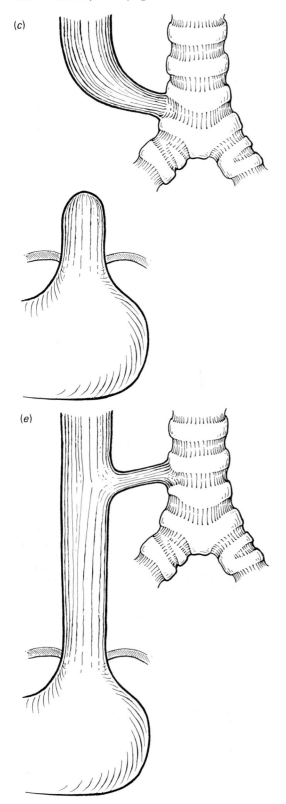

(d)

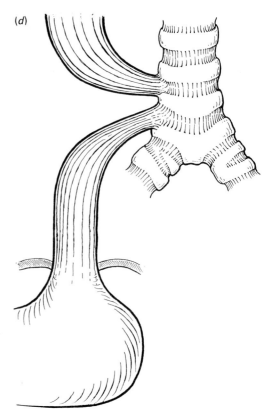

Figure 37.1 (c) oesophageal atresia with proximal tracheo-oesophageal fistula, 2%; (d) oesophageal atresia with proximal and distal tracheo-oesophageal fistula, <1%; (e) tracheo-oesophageal fistula without oesophageal atresia, 3–4%

equally divided between the supralevator (high) and translevator (low) defects.

Diagnosis

Polyhydramnios occurs in approximately 30% of mothers of infants with oesophageal atresia. Antenatal ultrasound scan may be diagnostic of oesophageal atresia without fistula as a result of failure to demonstrate the presence of intragastric fluid. The infant, at birth, is 'excessively mucusy' and requires repeated suction as it is unable to swallow saliva. Failure to recognize the anomaly at this stage will expose the infant to choking episodes and aspiration pneumonitis with the first feed. The diagnosis is confirmed by passing a large calibre (no. 10 French) firm catheter through the mouth and into the stomach. The position of arrest of the tube is confirmed on a chest X-ray (*Figure 37.2*). If the tube enters the stomach, there is no

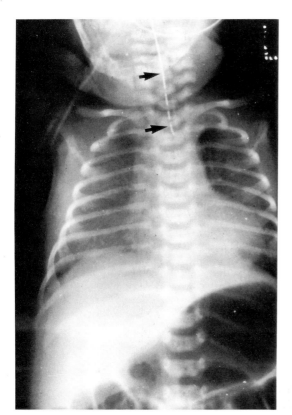

Figure 37.2 Plain X-ray of the chest and upper abdomen in an infant with oesophageal atresia. The radiopaque tube can be seen in the upper oesophagus. Gas in the intestines indicates the presence of a distal tracheo-oesophageal fistula

oesophageal atresia. In the majority of cases with this condition, the tube cannot be advanced more than 10 cm beyond the lower gum margin. It is important to include the abdomen on the original X-ray in order to assess the presence of intestinal gas shadows (*Figure 37.3*). Gas within the gastrointestinal tract implies the presence of a distal tracheo-oesophageal fistula while the distribution of the gas may indicate an additional intestinal anomaly, for example duodenal atresia or malrotation. The chest radiograph should be assessed for pulmonary pathology and the configuration of the heart shadow may be indicative of cardiac defects, for example, Fallot's tetralogy.

Management

Treatment of infants with oesophageal atresia should be concentrated in large centres where the surgical expertise, supportive services (anaesthesia, radiology, pathology) and specialized nursing care are available. Transfer to such centres should be effected promptly without exposing the infant to the risks of aspiration pneumonitis. The infant is transported in a portable incubator either in the 45° upright or in the prone position in order to discourage reflux of gastric juice in the distal tracheo-oesophageal fistula, while continuous suction of the upper pouch prevents aspiration of saliva (Spitz, Wallis and Graves, 1984). Definitive repair may have to be postponed in the presence of aspiration pneumonitis which generally responds very rapidly to broad-spectrum antibiotics and vigorous chest physiotherapy (Koop, Schnaufer and Broennie, 1974; Randolph, Altman and Anderson, 1977; Grosfeld and Ballantine, 1978; Ito, Sugito and Nagaya, 1984). In the infant with severe respiratory distress requiring mechanical ventilatory support, consideration should be given to emergency ligation of the distal tracheo-oesophageal fistula to facilitate respiratory support and to prevent overdistension of the stomach and intestine (Jones *et al.*, 1980; Filston *et al.*, 1982).

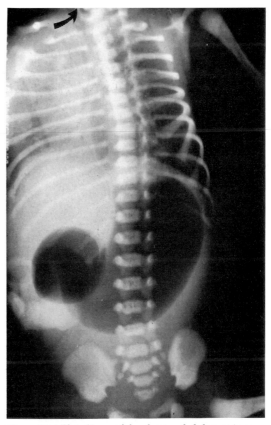

Figure 37.3 Plain X-ray of the chest and abdomen in an infant with oesophageal atresia – the tip of the catheter can be seen at the thoracic inlet. The gas pattern in the abdomen indicates the presence of a duodenal atresia ('double bubble')

(a)

(b)

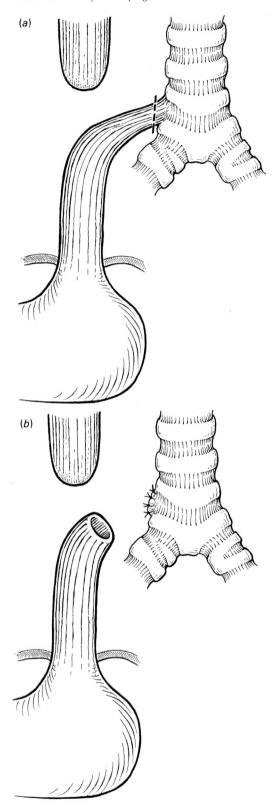

The operative procedure is carried out under general endotracheal anaesthesia. Access is ideally via a right posterolateral extrapleural approach through the fourth or fifth intercostal space (deLorimier and Harrison, 1985). After dividing the azygos vein, the distal oesophagus is identified and traced proximally to the fistulous entrance into the trachea. Mobilization of the distal oesophagus should be kept to a minimum as the blood supply to it is segmentally derived directly from small aortic branches and excessive devascularization would expose the anastomosis to impaired healing. The fistula is divided and the tracheal defect closed with fine interrupted non-absorbable sutures (5.0 Prolene). The proximal blind end of the oesophagus is identified and mobilized in the apex of the chest as extensively as required to effect an anastomosis with as little tension as possible. The end-to-end anastomosis is performed using a single layer of full thickness 5.0 or 6.0 polyglycolic acid or Prolene sutures (*Figure 37.4*). A Livaditis (1973) oesophagomyotomy and/

(c)

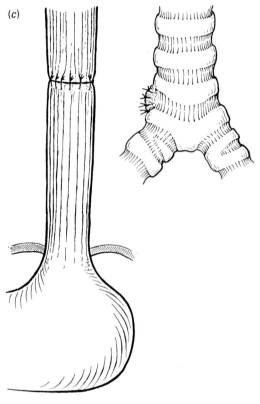

Figure 37.4 The technique of operative repair of oesophageal atresia with distal tracheo-oesophageal fistula. (*a*) Division of distal tracheo-oesophageal fistula. (*b*) Closure of tracheal defect with interrupted sutures. (*c*) End-to-end oesophago–oesophageal anastomosis with single layer of interrupted sutures

or the use of mechanical ventilation for a few days postoperatively may be effective in reducing the incidence of anastomotic complications.

The passage through the nose of a fine silastic transanastomotic tube into the stomach or the fashioning of a gastrostomy will allow early enteral feeding postoperatively.

A contrast oesophagogram performed between 7 and 10 days postoperatively will determine the anastomotic integrity following which oral feeds may be introduced.

Patients with a long-gap between the proximal and distal segment (particularly those with an isolated oesophageal atresia) require special attention. The alternative approaches available are to delay repair pending differential growth of the oesophageal segments towards each other (3–6 months), or to perform a cervical oesophagostomy and carry out an oesophageal substitution (deLorimier and Harrison, 1986) at a later stage – colonic interposition (Waterston, 1969), gastric tube (Anderson and Randolph, 1978), or gastric transposition (Spitz, 1984).

Results and prognosis

A total of 148 infants with tracheo-oesophageal anomalies were treated at The Hospital for Sick Children, London in the period 1980–1985. The infants were allocated into risk groups according to the definitions of Waterston, Bonham-Carter and Aberdeen (1962, 1963) (*Table 37.1*). Group C infants were subdivided into those with associated anomalies compatible or incompatible with survival. The survival rates in this series are shown in *Table 37.2*.

Table 37.1 Risk groups for children with tracheo-oesophageal anomalies

Group	Birthweight (g)	Associated anomaly	Pneumonia
A	>2500	None	None
B	1800–2500	None or moderate	±
C	<1800	Severe and/or multiple	±

Table 37.2 Survival rates of 148 children with tracheo-oesophageal anomalies

Group	Number	Percentage	Survivors	Percentage Survival	
A	66	45	66	100	
B	35	24	30	86	88.7%
C1	41	28	30	73	
C2	6	4	0	–	

Anastomotic complications were most frequent when silk was used for the repair. Anastomotic leaks occurred in 21% of cases (24 patients) of which all but four healed on conservative treatment. Anastomotic strictures developed in 17% but the vast majority responded to one or two dilatations. Recurrent tracheo-oesophageal fistulae were identified (Ein *et al.*, 1983) in 12% of infants and all required surgical closure.

Other complications included severe gastro-oesophageal reflux (20%) and tracheomalacia (Wailoo and Emery, 1979) (16%). These were responsible for life-threatening apnoeic attacks or recurrent pneumonia. Nissen fundoplication (Ashcraft *et al.*, 1977; Jolley *et al.*, 1980) and aortopexy (Filler, Rosillo and Lebowitz, 1976; Benjamin, Cohen and Glasson, 1976) respectively were dramatically successful in alleviating the symptoms.

Swallowing difficulties may persist for many years as a result of the inherent oesophageal dysmotility, affecting the distal segment in particular (Laks, Wilkinson and Schuster, 1972). The infant gradually learns to cope with this problem unless there is an associated anatomical defect (anastomotic stricture, gastro-oesophageal reflux, distal oesophageal stenosis). These infants are also prone to recurrent respiratory infections during the first few years of life (Martin and Alexander, 1985).

Mortality in oesophageal atresia is directly related to the severity of associated congenital anomalies particularly cardiac defects (Koop, Schnaufer and Broennie, 1974; Rickham, Stuaffer and Cheng, 1977; Myers, 1979; Holder, 1986).

Achalasia

Achalasia is a motility disorder of the oesophagus characterized by an absence of peristalsis and a failure of relaxation of the lower oesophageal sphincter (Henderson, 1966; Payne and King, 1983).

Incidence

Achalasia is rare in children (Azizkhan, Tapper and Eraklis, 1980). The incidence is one per 100 000 and approximately 5% of all patients are symptomatic before the age of 15 years (Herman and Moersch, 1929; Olsen *et al.*, 1951). There are few reports of achalasia occurring in siblings (London *et al.*, 1977; Stoddard and Johnson, 1982) and it has been reported in association with a number of syndromes, for example Riley-Day. Evidence for a familial incidence of the disease is lacking. Both sexes are equally affected.

Aetiology and pathogenesis

The aetiology of achalasia is unknown. Oesophageal dysmotility also occurs in Chaga's disease, scleroderma, oesophageal atresia, diabetes and secondary to gastro-oesophageal reflux, but the unique feature of achalasia is the constantly non-relaxing lower oesophageal sphincter.

Numerous theories exist regarding the pathogenesis of the condition, the primary defect being described variously as neurogenic, myogenic and hormonal. There is evidence suggesting that it is the result of an abnormality of parasympathetic innervation. Absence of ganglion cells in the myenteric plexus in the dilated portion of the oesophagus with normal ganglion cells in the distal non-dilated segment have been described (Gallone, Peri and Galliera, 1982). This, however, is not a constant feature and is reflected in the variable reports of the histopathology of some of the specimens of oesophageal muscle. These range from the total absence of ganglia, to the presence of normally ganglionated muscle or abnormal ganglion cell morphology. Histochemical staining for acetylcholinesterase may reveal the presence of ganglion cells and nerve trunks in the myenteric plexus, although their numbers are slightly reduced. Recent reports using electron microscopy (Friesen, Henderson and Hanna, 1983) and intestinal polypeptide hormonal assay

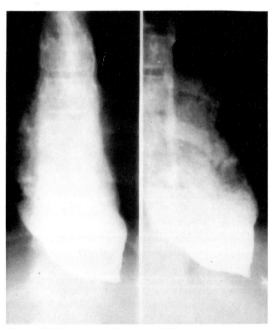

Figure 37.5 Barium swallow in a child with achalasia of the oesophagus with the classical 'rat-tail' deformity of the distal end

support the theory that this is a neurogenic disorder (Aggestrup *et al.*, 1983).

Diagnosis

Symptomatology

The principal symptoms of achalasia in childhood consist of vomiting, dysphagia, chest pain and weight loss. Dysphagia with the sensation of food sticking in the lower oesophagus and postprandial vomiting are the most frequent presenting symptoms. Retrosternal or epigastric pain occurs in one-third of the patients and in a few cases it is the primary presenting symptom. Weight loss of varying extent occurs in one-half of the patients. Nocturnal regurgitation may give rise to respiratory symptoms and recurrent respiratory infections may be experienced. A constant feature is the prolonged delay in establishing the precise diagnosis. The average duration of symptoms prior to diagnosis is 24 months and many children are treated for long periods for 'cyclic vomiting' or for 'anorexia nervosa' before achalasia is diagnosed.

Radiological features

The plain chest radiograph may show a dilated food-filled oesophagus with an air-fluid level in the distal third. In addition, there may be radiological signs of repeated aspiration pneumonitis. The chief characteristics on barium oesophagogram are a dilated oesophagus, the absence of a stripping wave, uncoordinated oesophageal contractions and obstruction at the oesophagogastric junction with prolonged retention of barium in the oesophagus. Failure of relaxation of the lower oesophageal sphincter leads to classical rat-tail deformity of funnelling and narrowing of the distal oesophagus (*Figure 37.5*).

Endoscopy

Oesophagoscopy contributes little to the diagnosis, but retained food may be found within the dilated oesophagus. The main value of endoscopy is to exclude organic causes of obstruction in the oesophagus.

Oesophageal manometry

The diagnosis of achalasia is best confirmed by oesophageal motility studies using a constantly perfused catheter technique. The criteria for the diagnosis are:

(1) a high pressure (>30 mmHg) lower oesophageal sphincter zone

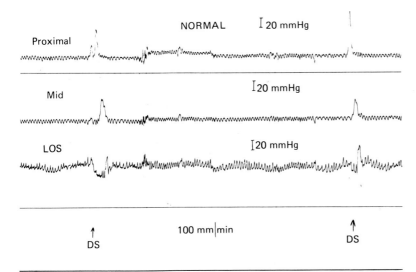

Figure 37.6 Oesophageal motility study in a normal child showing a progression of the peristaltic waves through the oesophagus (DS = dry swallow)

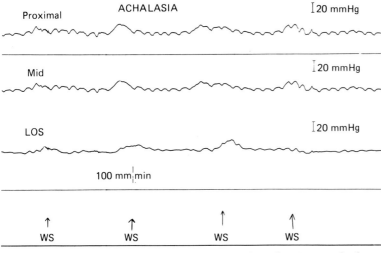

Figure 37.7 Oesophageal motility in a child with achalasia showing completely incoordinate oesophageal contractions (WS = wet swallow)

(2) failure of the lower oesophageal sphincter to relax in response to swallowing
(3) absence of propulsive peristalsis
(4) uncoordinated tertiary contractions in the body of the oesophagus (*Figures 37.6* and *37.7*).

Treatment

Three treatment options are available for the management of achalasia – pharmacological manipulation, forceful dilatation and oesophageal myotomy with or without the addition of an antireflex procedure.

Pharmacological treatment

The manipulation of oesophageal motility disorders using pharmacological and dietary measures has been disappointing. Recent reports of the use of isosorbide dinitrate and nifedipine have been more encouraging (Blackwell, Holt and Heading, 1981; Gelfond, Rosen and Gilat, 1982). Nifedipine is a calcium entry blocker and since calcium ions are directly responsible for the activity of myofibrils and consequently the tension generated, their use in reducing the pressure in the lower oesophageal sphincter in achalasia, or for the vigorous oesophageal contractions which occur in diffuse oesophageal spasms, seems logical. Prostaglandin E_2 has also been employed with some success. Its value in the long-term treatment of achalasia remains to be proven.

Forceful dilatation

Good palliation may be obtained by forceful dilatation. The most commonly used dilator consists of a single bag of fixed diameter which is inflated with water (Plummer) or air (Browne-McHardy, Rider-Moeller).

Forceful dilatation has been advocated as the treatment of choice in adults. Fellows, Ogilvie and Atkinson (1983) showed that following pneumatic dilatation in adults only 10% of patients subsequently required cardiomyotomy. In general, the results of pneumatic dilatation in children have been variable. Success rates, ranging from 40 to 60% have been reported in children (Payne, Ellis and Olsen, 1961; Berquist *et al.*, 1983). The aim of forceful dilatation is to disrupt the muscle fibres of the lower oesophageal sphincter. There is, however, no evidence that the muscle fibres tear rather than stretch. Vantrappen and Janssens (1983) were unable to distinguish histologically between sphincter segments in dogs and monkeys subjected to forceful dilatations and those from normal control patients. In general, older children respond better to pneumatic dilatation (Azizkhan, Tapper and Eraklis, 1980). A report of 899 adult patients treated at the Mayo Clinic (Payne and King, 1983) concluded that myotomy was more successful and safer than dilatation, poor results being obtained twice as frequently following dilatation as after myotomy. The incidence of perforation following pneumatic dilatation varies from 1 to 5% (Bennett and Hendrix, 1970; Vantrappen *et al.*, 1971; Fellows, Ogilvie and Atkinson, 1983).

Surgical procedure

Cardiomyotomy as originally described by Heller in 1914 is the basis of all surgical procedures. The controversies concern the length of the oesophageal myotomy, the distance which the myotomy extends onto the stomach and the necessity for including an additional antireflux procedure (Jara *et al.*, 1979; Ballantine, Fitzgerald and Grosfeld, 1980; Buick and Spitz, 1985).

Myotomy may be performed either via an abdominal approach or by a left thoracotomy through the bed of the seventh or eighth rib.

Taking care to protect the vagus nerves, a 5–7 cm incision is made through the muscle of the distal oesophagus. The incision is deepened down through the muscle to the mucosa. Particular care must be taken to avoid opening the mucosa. The muscle wall is dissected laterally off the mucosa so that at least half the circumference of the oesophagus is exposed and the mucosa pouts freely through the incision. Ellis, Gibb and Crozier (1980) insist that to avoid reflux the incision should not extend for more than a few millimetres onto the stomach. If a longer incision is made onto the stomach wall, an antireflux procedure in the form of a short lax (floppy) Nissen fundoplication should be added to the procedure (*Figure 37.8*).

Oesophageal foreign bodies

Over 90% of ingested foreign bodies pass uneventfully through the gastrointestinal tract. Of those that are held up, this mostly occurs in the oesophagus (Spitz, 1971).

Anatomy

There are four sites of anatomical narrowing in the oesophagus where foreign bodies are likely to impact. These are at the postcricoid region, the level of the aortic arch, the level of the left main bronchus, and the level of the diaphragmatic hiatus (Slovis, Tyler-Werman and Solightly, 1982). Eighty per cent of impacted foreign bodies are held up at the level of the cricopharyngeus. Impaction may also occur at sites of pathological narrowing, for example strictures secondary to peptic oesophagitis, corrosive strictures, anastomotic strictures or congenital stenosis.

Clinical presentation

In the majority of cases there will be a clear history of ingestion of a foreign object. The child will present with acute symptoms of coughing, choking, excessive salivation, dysphagia or vomiting (Nandi and Ong, 1978; O'Neill, Holcomb and Neblett, 1983). If the foreign body remains impacted, adaptation may occur and the child will select foods which can be managed without producing symptoms (Giordano *et al.*, 1981; O'Neill, Holcomb and Neblett, 1983). In other cases, there is no definite history or acute symptomatology and presentation occurs in an obscure fashion, for example chronic respiratory symptoms (stridor, wheezing, recurrent pneumonia) (Goldsher, Eliachar and Joachims, 1978) anorexia, haematemesis or pyrexia of unknown origin.

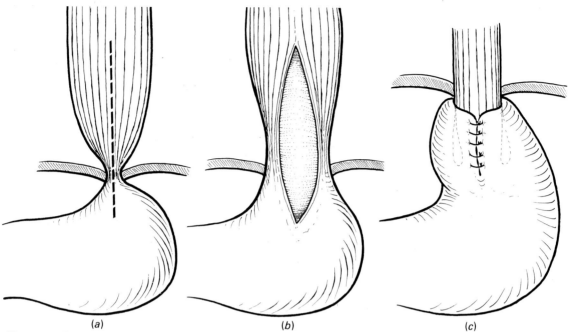

Figure 37.8 Operative procedure for achalasia – myotomy combined with a loose fundoplication. (*a*) Line of incision of myotomy from distal oesophagus through gastro-oesophageal junction onto body of the stomach. (*b*) Myotomy completed. Mucosa bulging through defect in the muscle. The muscularis should be separated from the mucosa for half the circumference of the oesophagus. (*c*) Loose (floppy) fundoplication around distal 1.5–2.5 cm of oesophagus

Diagnosis

The diagnosis will be confirmed on straight posteroanterior (PA) and lateral X-ray of the chest in those cases with a radiopaque foreign body ingestion. Further investigations are essential in patients in whom a foreign body is suspected but not evident on the plain X-ray. In these cases, a barium oesophagogram (Sharp, 1986), computerized tomography (Crenshaw, 1977) or endoscopy should be undertaken. In particular, it is the radiolucent foreign object which causes diagnostic difficulties. An aluminium can top can easily escape detection on plain X-ray (*Figures 37.9* and *37.10*) (Spitz and Hirsig, 1982).

Treatment

All foreign bodies lodged in the upper third of the oesophagus as well as sharp objects in the lower oesophagus should be removed using direct endoscopy. Rounded objects may be dislodged by means of a Foley balloon catheter. Rounded objects in the lower half of the oesophagus may be observed for 24–48 hours in anticipation of their spontaneous passage into the stomach following which passage through the rest of the gastrointestinal tract can be confidently predicted (Spitz, 1971). Associated strictures of the oesophagus should be dilated and subsequently subjected to further investigation and definitive treatment.

Complications

Problems usually arise in proportion to the duration of impaction (Clerf, 1975). Possible complications include ulceration, stricture formation, tracheo-oesophageal fistula, erosion through the wall of the oesophagus with mediastinal abscess or penetration into major blood vessels (Sharp, 1986). Perforation may also occur during attempts at endoscopic removal of a sharp object.

Corrosive injury to the oesophagus

Accidental ingestion of caustic substances has become relatively uncommon as a result of government legislation regulating their use in commercially available drain cleaners (Leape, 1986).

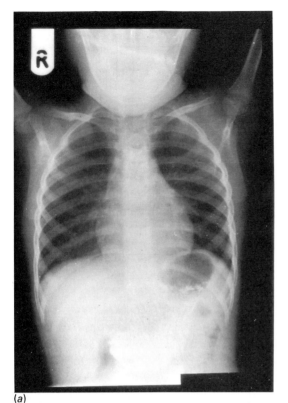

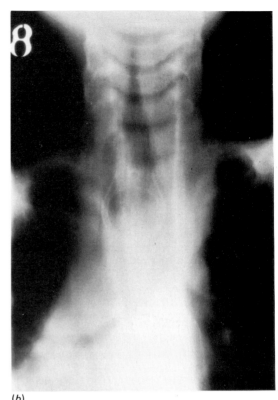

(a)   (b)

Figure 37.9 Radiolucent foreign body. (*a*) Plain X-ray of the chest in a child presenting with dysphagia. (*b*) Tomograph of same patient showing ring top lodged in upper oesophagus

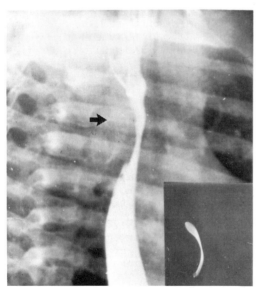

Figure 37.10 Barium swallow in an infant with dysphagia and respiratory symptoms. There is an indentation in the posterior wall of the upper oesophagus. This was caused by an abscess resulting from migration of a can tab (inset) through the oesophagus into the superior mediastinum

Pathophysiology

Caustic soda (sodium hydroxide) ingestion can cause severe injury to the oropharynx, oesophagus or stomach. The strong alkali rapidly penetrates the body tissues producing an intense acute inflammatory reaction and oedema. If the concentration of the solution is high, transmural penetration occurs with resulting destruction of the musculature of the oesophagus, penetration into the perioesophageal tissues with mediastinitis or frank perforation of the oesophagus. The acute phase is followed by sloughing of the necrotic tissue and replacement by granulation tissue. The final outcome varies from complete resolution in the mild case to extensive fibrosis of the entire oesophagus in the severely damaged cases. The extent and severity of the injury are directly related to the concentration of the lye injested (liquid lye is more damaging than the granular form), the quantity ingested and the duration of contact (Ashcraft and Padula, 1974).

Clinical presentation

There is extensive oedema and swelling of the mouth and lips and the child is unable to swallow.

Chest pain is indicative of mediastinitis while abdominal pain will occur if large quantities of lye reach the stomach. There may be haematemesis, dyspnoea, stridor and the other respiratory symptoms develop as a consequence of the resulting oedema or from direct laryngeal injury. Fibrosis of the lips and temporomandibular joint may develop as a result of severe oropharyngeal burns (*Figure 37.11*).

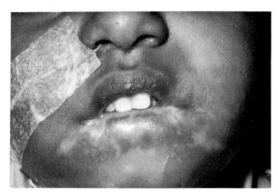

Figure 37.11 Fibrosis of the lips following severe oropharyngeal burns secondary to caustic soda ingestion

Diagnosis

It is important to ascertain whether the lye was actually ingested or whether it entered the oral cavity only. Early endoscopic examination, within 12–24 hours of the injury, should be undertaken to determine whether or not the oesophagus is affected. Assessment of the extent of oesophageal burn is not possible at this early stage and if the endoscopic examination is terminated once evidence of oesophageal injury is encountered, the risk of perforation is minimal (Leape, 1986).

An early contrast oesophagogram will reveal the extent of the injury, determine the presence of a perforation and act as a baseline for evaluating future stricture formation (*Figure 37.12*).

Treatment

Emergency

Vomiting should not be induced. The lye should be neutralized by ingestion of milk or, if this is not available, by water. Admission to hospital of all suspected cases is imperative.

Continued management

Initial treatment should consist of broad-spectrum antibiotics, intravenous fluids and prednisone 2 mg/kg per day (Haller and Bachman, 1963). If on endoscopy no oesophageal injury is found, treatment is stopped and the patient is discharged. If a burn is found, antibiotics are continued for 10 days and steroids for 3 weeks. Oral feeds are commenced as soon as the child is able to tolerate fluids. A gastrostomy for feeding purposes may be necessary in cases with severe burns. In these patients the opportunity should be taken to pass a string through the oesophagus to act as a guide for future dilatations.

A repeat oesophagogram is carried out 3 weeks after ingestion of the lye and oesophageal dilatations are commenced if a stricture is found. The dilatations are repeated at regular intervals until the stricture is eliminated. Ninety per cent of oesophageal strictures will respond to dilatation, the remaining cases will require oesophageal replacement.

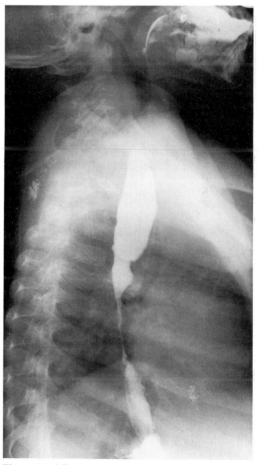

Figure 37.12 Barium oesophagogram in a child following ingestion of caustic soda. There is extensive stricture formation of the distal half of the oesophagus

Gastro-oesophageal reflux

Incompetence of the lower oesophageal sphincter is a common occurrence in newborn infants. In the vast majority of these infants maturation of the sphincter mechanism develops during the first year of life as the infant assumes the sitting and then the upright position (Carre, 1959).

Pathophysiology

Gastro-oesophageal reflux may or may not be associated with an anatomical hiatus hernia. A sliding hiatus hernia is generally associated with reflux while a rolling hernia (paraoesophageal) causes symptoms by virtue of its intrathoracic volume or secondary to complications such as haemorrhage or perforation as a consequence of peptic ulceration or volvulus of the stomach. A paraoesophageal hernia always requires surgical correction (Ellis, Crozier and Shea, 1986) (*Figure 37.13*).

Acid-pepsin reflux into the lower oesophagus results in a chemical inflammation of the squamous mucosa which is ill equipped to resist the digestive enzymes. In the early stages there is an inflammatory cell infiltration with erythema of the mucosa. With continuing reflux the mucosa becomes friable and bleeds on contact. Later, ulceration develops which may proceed to stricture formation as fibrous tissue is laid down as a consequence of transmural damage.

Acid-pepsin reflux
↓
Erythema
↓
Friability of the mucosa
↓
Ulcerative oesophagitis
↓
Stricture formation

Clinical presentation (Ramenofsky, 1986)

Early infancy

The infant presents with recurrent vomiting which may be projectile and may even mimic pyloric stenosis. The vomitus generally contains ingested milk only, but haematemesis in the form of fresh blood or of 'coffee-grounds' may occur as a result of ulcerative oesophagitis. With repeated vomiting, the infant fails to gain weight at the expected rate and develops severe constipation. Presentation with recurrent respiratory infections or apnoeic attacks will be discussed under aspiration syndromes.

Later childhood

Persistent vomiting is still the major symptom in older children, but the problem may only occur in the form of night vomiting of mucus which is noted on the pillow in the morning. Heartburn caused by oesophagitis and dysphagia from

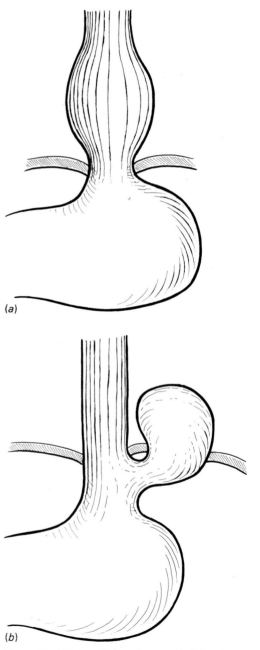

Figure 37.13 Types of hiatus hernia. (*a*) sliding hiatus hernia; (*b*) paraoesophageal ('rolling') hiatus hernia

ulcerative oesophagitis or stricture formation assume more prominence at this age. Hypochromic microcytic anaemia may develop as a consequence of constant slow blood loss into the oesophagus from ulcerative oesophagitis. Asthma or recurrent respiratory infections may develop from recurrent aspiration of gastric content.

Associated anatomical defects

Gastro-oesophageal reflux is more common in patients with corrected oesophageal atresia, diaphragmatic hernia or defects of the anterior abdominal wall, for example exomphalos. Precipitating causes are malrotation of the midgut and other causes of gastric outlet obstruction, for example pyloric stenosis or antral dysmotility.

Neurological abnormalities

The association between gastro-oesophageal reflux and severe mental retardation and other neurological abnormalities has only recently been appreciated. An estimated 10% of retarded children in institutional care manifest vomiting as a major problem. The tendency is to ascribe the vomiting to psychological causes and this had led to prolonged delay in diagnosis exposing the child to the development of complications from the reflux. Severe failure to thrive, iron deficiency anaemia, recurrent bouts of pneumonia and strictures frequently occur in these children (Abrahams and Burkitt, 1970; Sondheimer and Morris, 1979; Spitz, 1982).

Aspiration syndromes

Recurrent episodes of pneumonia (Ashcraft, Holder and Amoury, 1981; Jolley *et al.*, 1981), attacks of asthma and apnoeic episodes resulting in near-miss sudden infant death syndrome have been ascribed to aspiration of gastric contents (Beckwith, 1973; Leape *et al.*, 1977; Herbst, Books and Bray, 1978; Fontan *et al.*, 1984). Near-miss sudden infant death syndrome results from either laryngospasm (Downing and Lee, 1975) or reflex bradycardia (Kenigsberg *et al.*, 1983).

Unusual presentation

Abnormal head and neck contortions in association with ulcerative oesophagitis were first described by Sandifer in 1964 (Kinsbourne, 1964). The range of symptoms has been extended to torticollis, tics, dystonia and irritability. Protein-losing enteropathy may occur as a result of ulcerative oesophagitis.

Diagnosis

A range of investigations has been applied to establish the presence and severity of gastro-oesophageal reflux (Darling, 1975; McCauley, Darling and Leonidas, 1979).

Barium oesophagogram

The patient should be kept warm and comfortable during the examination. No attempt should be made to induce reflux by means of abdominal compression or other provocative manoeuvres. The patient is screened in the lateral, supine and prone positions. Particular attention is paid to the following details:

(1) anatomy of the oesophagus and the presence of strictures (*Figure 37.14*), ulcerative oesophagitis (*Figure 37.15*), abnormal narrowing or displacement should be noted
(2) peristaltic activity: primary contractions of the oesophagus occur during deglutition, secon-

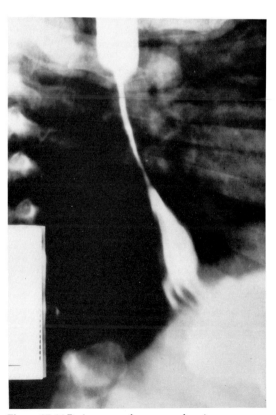

Figure 37.14 Barium oesophagogram showing an extensive stricture in the distal oesophagus and an associated sliding hiatus hernia

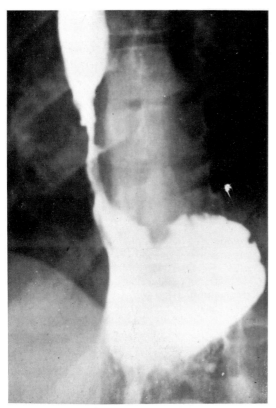

Figure 37.15 Barium oesophagogram showing extensive narrowing and ulcerative oesophagitis in the distal oesophagus with an associated sliding hiatus hernia

dary waves clear any residual content and may be normal, while tertiary waves are feeble attempts at contraction which are generally incoordinated and are always abnormal
(3) hiatus hernia: the presence of a sliding or paraoesophageal hernia will become evident during the examination
(4) the degree of gastro-oesophageal reflux is graded according to the highest level of the refluxed barium content:
grade 1 – distal oesophagus
grade 2 – proximal/thoracic oesophagus
grade 3 – cervical oesophagus
grade 4 – continuous gastro-oesophageal re-flux
grade 5 – aspiration of barium into the tracheobronchial tree
grade 6 – delayed reflux on the 30 minute X-ray film
The rate of clearance of refluxed barium should also be noted
(5) evidence of gastric outlet obstruction or duodenal malrotation.

Oesophageal pH monitoring

Measurement of the pH in the distal oesophagus by means of an intraluminal pH probe is currently the most accurate method of documenting reflux (Jolley *et al.*, 1978, 1979; Boix-Ochoa, Lafuente and Gil-Vernet, 1980; Sondheimer, 1980; Ramenofsky and Leape, 1981). The recordings are monitored continuously over a 24-hour period. pH levels below 4 are regarded as significant and during the 24-hour recording the following parameters are examined:

(1) number of episodes when pH falls below 4
(2) duration of each reflux episode
(3) number of reflux episodes lasting more than 5 minutes
(4) total duration of reflux expressed as a percentage of recording time.

Oesophageal manometry

This is best measured by continuous infusion open-tipped catheters. A high pressure zone is normally present at the lower oesophageal sphincter. There is good correlation between reflux and decreased lower oesophageal pressure in adults, but measurements of the sphincter pressure in children is much more variable. Euler and Ament (1977) suggested that lower oesophageal pressure values may be useful in predicting those cases which would eventually require surgical treatment.

Endoscopy and oesophageal biopsy

Endoscopic examination of the oesophageal mucosa is required to document the degree of oesophagitis and should be supplemented by endoscopic biopsy to provide histopathological grading of inflammatory cell infiltration. Four grades of oesophagitis may be found at endoscopy:

grade I   – erythema of the mucosa
grade II – friability of the mucosa
grade III – ulcerative oesophagitis
grade IV – stricture formation.

Scintiscanning

Technetium (^{99}Tc) sulphur colloid scans have been used in an attempt to define the presence of gastro-oesophageal reflux over a longer period than during the barium examination (Christie and Rudd, 1978; Jona, Sty and Glickich, 1981). They also provide evidence of pulmonary aspiration in delayed scans taken 24 hours later. Aspiration may also be confirmed by the presence of lipid-laden macrophages in tracheal aspirates.

Management

Medical treatment

Feeds

Small frequent feeds thickened with cornflour or Nestargel should be given to infants with reflux (Herbst, 1986).

Position

The 60° upright position used to be recommended but it was found that the infant slumps forward in this position, thus increasing the intra-abdominal pressure. The position most frequently adopted now is the 30° head elevated prone position (Orenstein and Whittington, 1983).

Antacids

Simple antacids such as magnesium or aluminium hydroxide are more effective in the liquid form. Antacids combined with alginic acid (Gaviscon) form a foam level in the fundus of the stomach which discourages reflux (Cucchiara *et al.*, 1984).

Hydrogen receptor antagonists (cimetidine, ranitidine)

These agents are particularly useful in the presence of severe oesophagitis in promoting healing and in achieving symptomatic relief of heartburn (Cucchiara *et al.*, 1984).

Other drugs

Drugs which increase the lower oesophageal pressure, for example metaclopramide, bethanechol, domperidone etc., also stimulate gastric emptying (McCallum *et al.*, 1983).

Surgical treatment

The indications for a surgical approach are (Spitz and Kirtane, 1985):

(1) established oesophageal stricture
(2) failure of conservative medical measures
   (a) in the presence of an anatomic anomaly, for example oesophageal atresia, malrotation, exomphalos, etc.
   (b) in the presence of associated neurological damage. The response to medical treatment is notoriously poor and the additional nursing burden imposed by repeated vomiting adds significantly to the social stress of the family
   (c) apnoeic episodes and repeated respiratory infections which do not respond promptly
   (d) failure to thrive in spite of adequate treatment.

With the exception of near-miss sudden infant death syndrome, failure of medical treatment should not be considered until the treatment has been attempted for at least 3 weeks in hospital or 6–12 weeks at home.

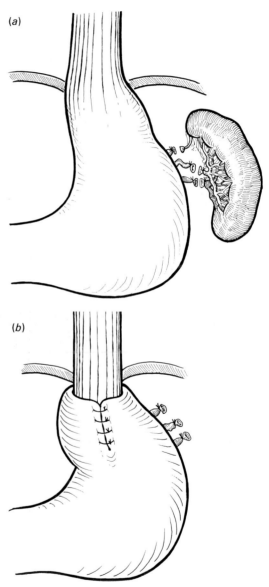

Figure 37.16 The operative technique for Nissen fundoplication. (*a*) The oesophagus is exposed at the hiatus and mobilized for a short distance into the posterior mediastinum. The short gastric vessels are ligated and divided. The hiatus is narrowed to prevent recurrences of the hernia. (*b*) The fundus of the stomach is wrapped around the distal 2–3 cm of oesophagus and sutured in position with interrupted non-absorbable sutures including the suture in the anterior (extramucosal) wall of the oesophagus

The most widely adopted surgical procedure for the correction of reflux is Nissen fundoplication. This involves wrapping the fundus of the stomach around the distal 2–4 cm of oesophagus. The wrap should be lax and short to allow free passage of food through the oesophagus and to permit the patient to eructate, while at the same time preventing reflux (*Figure 37.16*). Postoperative complications are more frequent in patients with established strictures and in debilitated children with severe retardation. Referral for surgery is invariably delayed in those children and earlier surgery may avoid many of the postoperative problems (Spitz, 1982).

Congenital oesophageal stenosis

Stenosis of the oesophagus most commonly arises from acquired lesions, for example reflux oesophagitis, corrosive ingestion, foreign body impaction or secondary to surgical resection and anastomosis. Congenital stenosis is a rare anomaly which may be either caused by a membranous web or diaphragm, or may arise as a result of intramural deposits of tracheobronchial cartilagenous tissue. The latter pathology has been most frequently reported in association with oesophageal atresia and/or tracheo-oesophageal fistula (Nishina, Tsuchida and Saito, 1981).

Clinical features

In the presence of a complete web, presentation is similar to that of oesophageal atresia with symptoms occurring on the first day of life. In other cases, symptoms may develop at any stage of life through to adulthood but generally arise in early infancy. The symptoms include dysphagia, vomiting with food ingestion, failure to thrive, recurrent respiratory infections and foreign body impaction.

Diagnosis

Gastro-oesophageal reflux as a cause of the stenosis should always be excluded. The barium oesophagogram will identify the site of the lesion. Congenital webs are most commonly located in the middle third of the oesophagus and appear as shelf-like projections within the oesophageal lumen. Tracheobronchial remnants are generally located in the lower third of the oesophagus or at the gastro-oesophageal junction and they cause sharp narrowing at this point. The precise nature and anatomical location of the lesion should be confirmed on endoscopic examination.

Treatment

Dilatation alone may be sufficient for many cases of oesophageal webs. Surgical resection of tracheobronchial cartilagenous tissue is generally recommended (Scherer and Grosfeld, 1986).

References

ABRAHAMS, P. and BURKITT, B. F. E. (1970) Hiatus hernia and gastro-oesophageal reflux in children and adolescents with cerebral palsy. *Australian Paediatric Journal*, **6**, 41–46

AGGESTRUP, S., UDDMAN, R., SUNDLER, F. *et al.* (1983) Lack of vasoactive intestinal polypeptide nerves in esophageal achalasia. *Gastroenterology*, **84**, 924–927

ANDERSON, K. D. and RANDOLPH, J. G. (1978) Gastric tube interposition. A satisfactory alternative to the colon for esophageal replacement in children. *Annals of Thoracic Surgery*, **25**, 521–525

ASHCRAFT, K. W., GOODWIN, C. D., AMOURY, R. A. and HOLDER, T. M. (1977) Early recognition and aggressive treatment of gastroesophageal reflux following repair of esophageal atresia. *Journal of Pediatric Surgery*, **12**, 317–321

ASHCRAFT, K. W., HOLDER, T. M. and AMOURY, R. A. (1981) Treatment of gastroesophageal reflux in children by Thal fundoplication. *Journal of Thoracic Cardiovascular Surgery*, **82**, 706–712

ASHCRAFT, K. W. and PADULA, R. T. (1974) The effect of dilute corrosives on the esophagus. *Pediatrics*, **53**, 226–232

AZIZKHAN, R. G., TAPPER, D. and ERAKLIS, A. (1980) Achalasia in childhood: a 20-year experience. *Journal of Pediatric Surgery*, **15**, 457–461

BALLANTINE, T. V. N., FITZGERALD, J. F. and GROSFELD, J. L. (1980) Transabdominal esophagomyotomy for achalasia in children. *Journal of Pediatric Surgery*, **15**, 457–461

BECKWITH, J. B. (1973) The sudden infant death syndrome. *Current Problems in Pediatrics*, **3**, 3–37

BENJAMIN, R., COHEN, D. and GLASSON, M. (1976) Tracheomalacia in association with congenital tracheoesophageal fistula. *Surgery*, **79**, 504–508

BENNETT, J. R. and HENDRIX, T. R. (1970) Treatment of achalasia with pneumatic dilatation. *Modern Treatment*, **7**, 1217–1228

BERQUIST, W. E., BYRNE, W. J., AMENT, M. E., FONKALSRUD, E. W. and EULER, A. R. (1983) Achalasia: diagnosis, management and clinical course in 16 children. *Pediatrics*, **71**, 798–805

BLACKWELL, J. N., HOLT, S. and HEADING, R. C. (1981) Effect of nifedipine on oesophageal motility and gastric emptying. *Digestion*, **21**, 50–56

BOIX-OCHOA, J., LAFUENTE, J. M. and GIL-VERNET, J. M. (1980) Twenty-four hour pH monitoring in gastroesophageal reflux. *Journal of Pediatric Surgery*, **15**, 74–78

BUICK, R. G. and SPITZ, L. (1985) Achalasia of the cardia in children. *British Journal of Surgery*, **72**, 341–343

CARRE, I. (1959) The natural history of the partial thoracic stomach (hiatus hernia) in children. *Archives of Disease in Childhood*, **34**, 344–353

CHRISTIE, D. and RUDD, T. G. (1978) Radionuclide test for gastroesophageal reflux in children. *Pediatric Research*, **12**, 432

CLERF, L. H. (1975) Historical aspects of foreign bodies in the air and food passages. *Southern Medical Journal*, **68**, 1449–1454

CRENSHAW, R. T. (1977) 'Pop Top' ingestion: a technique for localization. *Journal of the American Medical Association*, **237**, 1928–1929

CUCCHIARA, S., STAIANO, A., ROMANIELLO, G. *et al.* (1984) Antacids and cimetidine treatment for gastro-oesophageal reflux and peptic oesophagitis. *Archives of Disease in Childhood*, **59**, 842–847

DARLING, D. B. (1975) Hiatal hernia and gastroesophageal reflux in infancy and childhood: analysis of the radiologic findings. *American Journal of Roentgenology, Radium and Therapeutic Nuclear Medicine*, **123**, 724–736

deLORIMIER, A. A. and HARRISON, M. R. (1985) Esophageal atresia: embryogenetics and management. *World Journal of Surgery*, **9**, 250–257

deLORIMIER, A. A. and HARRISON, M. R. (1986) Esophageal replacement. In *Pediatric Esophageal Surgery*, edited by K. W. Ashcraft and T. M. Holder, pp. 89–136. Orlando: Grune and Stratton

DOWNING, S. E. and LEE, J. C. (1975) Laryngeal chemosensitivity: a possible mechanism for sudden infant death. *Pediatrics*, **55**, 640–649

EIN, S. H., STRINGER, D. A., STEPHENS, C. A. *et al.* (1983) Recurrent tracheoesophageal fistula: seventeen year review. *Journal of Pediatric Surgery*, **18**, 436–441

ELLIS, F. H., CROZIER, R. E. and SHEA, J. A. (1986) Paraesophageal hiatus hernia. *Archives of Surgery*, **121**, 416–420

ELLIS, F. H., GIBB, S. P. and CROZIER, R. E. (1980) Esophagomyotomy for achalasia of the esophagus. *Annals of Surgery*, **192**, 157–161

EULER, A. R. and AMENT, M. E. (1977) Value of esophageal manometric studies in the gastroesophageal reflux in infancy. *Pediatrics*, **59**, 58–61

FELLOWS, I. W., OGILVIE, A. L. and ATKINSON, M. P. (1983) Pneumatic dilatation in achalasia. *Gut*, **24**, 1020–1023

FILLER, R. M., ROSILLO, P. J. and LEBOWITZ, R. L. (1976) Life threatening anoxic spells caused by tracheal compression after repair of oesophageal atresia: correction by surgery. *Journal of Pediatric Surgery*, **11**, 739–748

FILSTON, H. C., CHITWOOD, W. R., SCHKOLNE, B. and BLACKMAN, L. R. (1982) The Fogarty balloon catheter as an aid to management of the infant with esophageal atresia and tracheoesophageal fistula complicated by severe RDS or pneumonia. *Journal of Pediatric Surgery*, **17**, 149–151

FONTAN, J. P., HELDT, G. P., HEYMAN, M. B. *et al.* (1984) Esophageal spasm associated with apnea and bradycardia in an infant. *Pediatrics*, **73**, 52–55

FRIESEN, D. L., HENDERSON, R. D. and HANNA, W. (1983) Ultrastructure of the esophageal muscle in achalasia and diffuse esophageal spasm. *American Journal of Clinical Pathology*, **79**, 319–325

GALLONE, L., PERI, G. and GALLIERA, M. (1982) Proximal gastric vagotomy and anterior fundoplication as complementary procedures to Heller's operation for achalasia. *Surgery, Gynecology and Obstetrics*, **155**, 337–341

GELFOND, M., ROSEN, P. and GILAT, T. (1982) Isosorbide dinitrate and nifedipine treatment of achalasia: a clinical, manometric and radionuclide evaluation. *Gastroenterology*, **83**, 963–969

GERMAN, J. C., MAHOUR, G. H. and WOOLLEY, M. M. (1976) Esophageal atresia and associated anomalies. *Journal of Pediatric Surgery*, **11**, 299–306

GIORDANO, A., ADAMS, G., BORIES, L. *et al.* (1981) Current management of esophageal foreign bodies. *Archives of Otolaryngology*, **107**, 249–251

GOLDSHER, M., ELIACHAR, I. and JOACHIMS, H. Z. (1978) Paradoxical presentation in children of foreign bodies in trachea and oesophagus. *The Practitioner*, **220**, 631–632

GREENWOOD, R. D. and ROSENTHAL, A. (1976) Cardiovascular malformations associated with tracheoesophageal fistula and esophageal atresia. *Pediatrics*, **57**, 87–91

GROSFELD, J. L. and BALLANTINE, T. V. (1978) Esophageal atresia and tracheoesophageal fistula: effect of delayed thoracotomy on survival. *Surgery*, **84**, 394–402

HAIGHT, C. and TOWSLEY, H. A. (1943) Congenital atresia of the esophagus with tracheoesophageal fistula and end-to-end anastomosis of esophageal segments. *Surgery, Gynecology and Obstetrics*, **76**, 672–688

HALLER, J. A. and BACHMAN, K. (1963) The comparative effect of current therapy of experimental caustic burns of the esophagus. *Journal of the American Medical Association*, **186**, 262

HELLER, E. (1914) Extramukose Cardiaplastik beim chronische Cardiospasm mit Dilatation des Oesophagus. *Mitteilungen Grenzgebiete Medizinische Chirurgie*, **27**, 141

HENDERSON, R. D. (1966) *The Esophagus: Reflux and Primary Motor Disorders*, pp. 149–179. Baltimore/London: Williams & Wilkins

HERBST, J. J. (1986) Medical treatment of gastroesophageal reflux. In *Pediatric Surgery*, edited by K. W. Ashcraft and T. M. Holder, pp. 181–191. Orlando: Grune and Stratton

HERBST, J. J., BOOKS, L. S. and BRAY, P. F. (1978) Gastroesophageal reflux in the 'near miss' sudden infant death syndrome. *Journal of Pediatrics*, **92**, 73–75

HERMAN, J. and MOERSCH, M. D. (1929) Cardiospasm in infancy and in childhood. *American Journal of Diseases of Children*, **38**, 294–298

HOLDER, T. M. (1986) Esophageal atresia and tracheoesophageal fistula. In *Pediatric Esophageal Surgery*, edited by K. W. Ashcraft and T. M. Holder, pp. 29–52. Orlando: Grune and Stratton

HOLDER, T. M., CLOUD, D. T., LEWIS, J. E. and PILLING, G. P. (1964) Esophageal atresia and tracheoesophageal fistula. A survey of its members by the surgical section of the American Academy of Pediatrics. *Pediatrics*, **34**, 542–549

ITO, T., SUGITO, T. and NAGAYA, M. (1984) Delayed primary anastomosis in poor-risk patients with esophageal atresia associated with tracheoesophageal fistula. *Journal of Pediatric Surgery*, **19**, 243–247

JARA, F. M., TOLEDO-PEREYRA, L. H., LEWIS, J. W. and MAGILLIGAN, D. J., JR (1979) Long-term results of esophagomyotomy for achalasia of the esophagus. *Archives of Surgery*, **114**, 935–936

JOLLEY, S. G., HERBST, J. J., JOHNSON, D. G., BOOK, L. S., MATLAK, M. E. and CANDON, V. R. (1979) Patterns of postcibal gastroesophageal reflux in symptomatic infants. *American Journal of Surgery*, **138**, 946–950

JOLLEY, S. G., JOHNSON, D. G., HERBST, J. J., PENA, A. R. and GARNIER, R. C. (1978) An assessment of gastroesophageal reflux in children by extended pH monitoring of the distal esophagus. *Surgery*, **84**, 16–24

JOLLEY, S. G., JOHNSON, D. G., HERBST, J. J. and MATLAK, M. E.

(1981) The significance of gastroesophageal reflux patterns in children. *Journal of Pediatric Surgery*, **16**, 859–865

JOLLEY, S. G., JOHNSON, D. G., ROBERTS, C. C. *et al.* (1980) Patterns of gastroesophageal reflux in children following repair of esophageal atresia and distal tracheoesophageal fistula. *Journal of Pediatric Surgery*, **15**, 857–862

JONA, J. Z., STY, J. R. and GLICKICH, M. (1981) Simplified radioisotope technique for assessing gastroesophageal reflux in children. *Journal of Pediatric Surgery*, **16**, 114–117

JONES, T. B., KIRCHNER, S. G., LEE, F. A. and HELLER, R. M. (1980) Stomach rupture associated with esophageal atresia, tracheoesophageal fistula and ventilatory assistance. *American Journal of Roentology*, **134**, 675–677

KENIGSBERG, K., GRISWOLD, P. G., BUCKLEY, B. J., GOOTMAN, N. and GOOTMAN, P. M. (1983) Cardiac effects of esophageal stimulation: possible relationship between gastroesophageal reflux (GER) and sudden infant death syndrome (SIDS). *Journal of Pediatric Surgery*, **18**, 542–545

KINSBOURNE, M. (1964) Hiatus hernia with contortions of the neck. *The Lancet*, **1**, 1058–1061

KOOP, C. E., SCHNAUFER, L. and BROENNIE, A. M. (1974) Esophageal atresia and tracheoesophageal fistula: supportive measures that affect survival. *Pediatrics*, **54**, 558–564

LADD, W. E. (1944) The surgical treatment of esophageal atresia and tracheoesophageal fistula. *New England Journal of Medicine*, **230**, 625–637

LAKS, B. H., WILKINSON, R. H. and SCHUSTER, S. R. (1972) Long-term results following correction of esophageal atresia and tracheoesophageal fistula. A clinical and cinefluorographic study. *Journal of Pediatric Surgery*, **7**, 591–597

LEAPE, L. L. (1986) Chemical injury of the esophagus. In *Pediatric Esophageal Surgery*, edited by K. W. Ashcraft and T. M. Holder, pp. 73–88. Orlando: Grune and Stratton

LEAPE, L. L., HOLDER, T. M., FRANKLIN, J. D., AMOURY, R. A. and ASHCRAFT, K. W. (1977) Respiratory arrest in infants secondary to gastroesophageal reflux. *Pediatrics*, **60**, 924–928

LEVIN, N. L. (1941) Congenital atresia of the esophagus with tracheoesophageal fistula: report of successful extrapleural ligation of fistulous communication and cervical esophagostomy. *Journal of Thoracic Surgery*, **10**, 648–657

LIVADITIS, A. (1973) Esophageal atresia: a method of overbridging large segmental gaps. *Zeit Kinderchirugie*, **13**, 298–306

LONDON, F. A., RAAB, D. E., FULLER, J. and OLSEN, A. M. (1977) Achalasia in three siblings: a rare occurrence. *Mayo Clinical Proceedings*, **52**, 97–100

LOUHIMO, I. and LINDAHL, H. (1983) Esophageal atresia: primary result of 500 consecutively treated patients. *Journal of Pediatric Surgery*, **18**, 217–229

McCALLUM, R. W., FINK, S. M., LERNER, E. and BARKOWITZ, D. M. (1983) Effects of metroclopramide and bethanecol on delayed gastric emptying present in gastroesophageal reflux patients. *Gastroenterology*, **84**, 1573–1577

McCAULEY, R. G., DARLING, D. B. and LEONIDAS, J. C. (1979) Gastroesophageal reflux in infants and children: a

useful classification and reliable physiologic technique for its demonstration. *American Journal of Roentology*, **130**, 47–50

MARTIN, L. W. and ALEXANDER, F. (1985) Esophageal atresia. *Surgical Clinics of North America*, **65**, 1099–1113

MYERS, N. A. (1974) Oesophageal atresia: the epitome of modern surgery. *Annals of the Royal College of Surgeons, England*, **54**, 277–287

MYERS, N. A. (1979) Oesophageal atresia and/or tracheo-oesophageal fistula. A study of mortality. *Progress in Paediatric Surgery*, **13**, 141–165

NANDI, P. and ONG, G. B. (1978) Foreign body in the oesophagus: review of 2394 cases. *British Journal of Surgery*, **65**, 5–9

NISHINA, T., TSUCHIDA, Y. and SAITO, S. (1981) Congenital esophageal stenosis due to tracheobronchial remnants and its associated anomalies. *Journal of Pediatric Surgery*, **16**, 190–193

OLSEN, A. M., HARRINGTON, S. W., MOERSCH, H. J. and ANDERSEN, H. A. (1951) The treatment of cardiospasm: analysis of a twelve year experience. *Journal of Thoracic Surgery*, **22**, 164–187

O'NEILL, J. A., HOLCOMB, G. W. and NEBLETT, W. W. (1982) Recent experience with esophageal atresia. *Annals of Surgery*, **195**, 739–745

O'NEILL, J. A., HOLCOMB, G. W. and NEBLETT, W. W. (1983) Management of tracheobronchial and esophageal foreign bodies in childhood. *Journal of Pediatric Surgery*, **18**, 475–479

ORENSTEIN, S. R. and WHITTINGTON, P. E. (1983) Positioning for prevention of infant gastroesophageal reflux. *Journal of Pediatrics*, **103**, 534–537

PAYNE, W. S., ELLIS, F. H., JR and OLSEN, A. M. (1961) Treatment of cardiospasm (achalasia of the esophagus) in children. *Surgery*, **50**, 731–735

PAYNE, W. S. and KING, R. M. (1983) Treatment of achalasia of the esophagus. *Surgical Clinics of North America*, **63**, 963–970

QUAN, L. and SMITH, D. W. (1973) The VATER association. *Journal of Pediatrics*, **82**, 104–107

RAMENOFSKY, M. L. (1986) Gastroesophageal reflux. Clinical manifestations and diagnosis. In *Pediatric Esophageal Surgery*, edited by K. W. Ashcraft and T. M. Holder, pp. 151–179. Orlando: Grune and Stratton

RAMENOFSKY, M. L. and LEAPE, L. L. (1981) Continuous upper esophageal pH monitoring in infants and children with gastroesophageal reflux, pneumonia, and apnoeic spells. *Journal of Pediatric Surgery*, **16**, 374–378

RANDOLPH, J. G., ALTMAN, R. P. and ANDERSON, K. D. (1977) Selective surgical management based upon clinical status in infants with esophageal atresia. *Journal of Thoracic and Cardiovascular Surgery*, **74**, 335–342

RICKHAM, P. P., STAUFFER, U. G. and CHENG, S. K. (1977) Oesophageal atresia: triumph or tragedy. *Australian and New Zealand Journal of Surgery*, **47**, 138–143

SCHERER, L. R. and GROSFELD, J. L. (1986) Congenital esophageal stenosis, esophageal duplication, mesenteric cyst and esophageal diverticulum. In *Pediatric Esophageal Surgery*, edited by K. W. Ashcraft and T. M. Holder, pp. 53–71. Orlando: Grune and Stratton

SHARP, R. J. (1986) Esophageal foreign bodies. In *Pediatric Esophageal Surgery*, edited by K. W. Ashcraft and T. M. Holder, pp. 137–149. Orlando: Grune and Stratton

SLOVIS, C. M., TYLER-WERMAN, R. and SOLIGHTLY, D. P.

(1982) Massive foreign object ingestion. *Annals of Emergency Medicine*, **11**, 433–435

SONDHEIMER, J. M. (1980) Continuous monitoring of distal esophageal pH: a diagnostic test for gastroesophageal reflux in infants. *Journal of Pediatrics*, **96**, 804–807

SONDHEIMER, J. M. and MORRIS, B. A. (1979) Gastroesophageal reflux among severely retarded children. *Journal of Pediatrics*, **94**, 710–714

SPITZ, L. (1971) Management of ingested foreign bodies in childhood. *British Medical Journal*, **4**, 469–472

SPITZ, L. (1982) Surgical treatment of gastroesophageal reflux in severely mentally retarded children. *Journal of the Royal Society of Medicine*, **75**, 525–529

SPITZ, L. (1984) Gastric transposition via the mediastinal route for infants with long-gap esophageal atresia. *Journal of Pediatric Surgery*, **19**, 149–154

SPITZ, L. and HIRSIG, J. (1982) Prolonged foreign body impaction in the oesophagus. *Archives of Disease in Childhood*, **57**, 551–553

SPITZ, L. and KIRTANE, J. (1985) Results and complications of surgery for gastro-oesophageal reflux. *Archives of Disease in Childhood*, **60**, 743–747

SPITZ, L., WALLIS, M. and GRAVES, H. F. (1984) Transport of the surgical neonate. *Archives of Disease in Childhood*, **59**, 284–288

STODDARD, C. J., JOHNSON, A. G. (1982) Achalasia in siblings. *British Journal of Surgery*, **69**, 84–85

VANTRAPPEN, G., HELLEMANS, J., DILOOF, W., VALEMBOIS, P. and VANDENBROUCKE, J. (1971) Treatment of achalasia with pneumatic dilatations. *Gut*, **12**, 268–275

VANTRAPPEN, G. and JANSSENS, J. (1983) To dilate or operate? That is the question. *Gut*, **24**, 1013–1019

WAILOO, M. P. and EMERY, J. L. (1979) The trachea in children with tracheoesophageal fistula. *Histopathology*, **3**, 329–338

WATERSTON, D. J. (1969) Reconstruction of the esophagus. In *Pediatric Surgery*, edited by W. T. Mustard, M. M. Ravitch and W. H. Snyder, pp. 400. Chicago: Year Book Medical

WATERSTON, D. J., BONHAM-CARTER, R. E. and ABERDEEN, E. (1962) Oesophageal atresia: tracheo-oesophageal fistula. A study of survival in 218 infants. *The Lancet*, **1**, 819–822

WATERSTON, D. J., BONHAM-CARTER, R. E. and ABERDEEN, E. (1963) Congenital tracheo-oesophageal fistula in association with oesophageal atresia. *The Lancet*, **2**, 55–57

Volume index

Cumulative index

This index is intended as a general guide only of the main heading entries covered in the six volumes of *Scott-Brown's Otolaryngology*, and is not comprehensive. For more detailed treatment of a subject refer to the individual volume indexes.

Entries are indexed by volume and page number, volume numbers are indicated by **bold** type.